LIPID METABOLISM

Edited by **Rodrigo Valenzuela Baez**

Lipid Metabolism
http://dx.doi.org/10.5772/2928
Edited by Rodrigo Valenzuela Baez

Contributors

Rodrigo Valenzuela B., Alfonso Valenzuela B., Claudia Borza, Danina Muntean, Cristina Dehelean, Germaine Săvoiu, Corina Şerban, Georgeta Simu, Mihaiela Andoni, Marius Butur, Simona Drăgan, Jason L. Burkhead, Svetlana Lutsenko, Line M. Grønning-Wang, Christian Bindesbøll, Hilde I. Nebb, Jasmina Dimitrova-Shumkovska, Leo Veenman, Inbar Roim, Moshe Gavish, Paul K. Crellin, Chu-Yuan Luo, Yasu S. Morita, Yasuo Uchiyama, Eiki Kominami, Alicia Huazano-García, Mercedes G. López, Fang Hu, Yingtong Zhang, Yuanda Song, Heather M. White, Brian T. Richert, Mickey A. Latour, Heli Putaala, Bożena Waszkiewicz-Robak, Miguel A. Martín-Acebes, Ángela Vázquez-Calvo, Flavia Caridi, Juan-Carlos Saiz, Francisco Sobrino, Luca Siracusano, Viviana Girasole, Christine Tayeh, Béatrice Randoux, Frédéric Laruelle, Natacha Bourdon, Delphine Renard-Merlier, Philippe Reignault, Yuanxin Yan, Eli Borrego, Michael V. Kolomiets, Yong Zhang, Heping Zhang

Published by InTech
Janeza Trdine 9, 51000 Rijeka, Croatia

Publishing Process Manager Sandra Bakic
Technical Editor InTech Prepress, Novi Sad
Cover InTech Design team

Additional hard copies can be obtained from orders@intechopen.com

Lipid Metabolism, Edited by Rodrigo Valenzuela Baez
p. cm.
ISBN 978-953-51-0944-0

For EU product safety concerns:
IN TECH d.o.o., Prolaz Marije Krucifikse Kozulić 3, 51000 Rijeka, Croatia,
info@intechopen.com or visit our website at intechopen.com.

Meet the editor

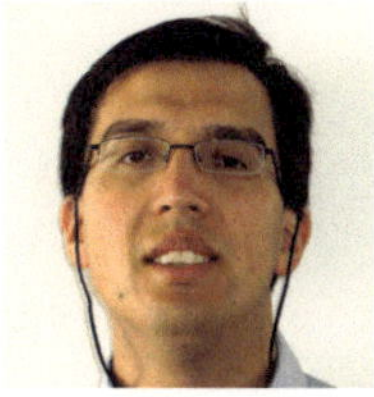

Rodrigo Valenzuela Baez completed Pre-graduate studies (Nutritionist) at University of Chile (2003), Magister in Nutrition and Food Technology, University of Chile (2007), Doctoral degree in Nutrition and Foods, University of Chile (2012). Currently he is a Research Scientist in Food Sciences and Assistant Professor, Fats and Oils Section, Food and Nutrition Research Laboratory, School of Nutrition and Dietetics, Faculty of Medicine, University of Chile, Santiago, Chile. Dr. Baez's teaching areas are: Food Science and Nutrition, Fats and Oils in Human Nutrition. His current research areas are in: Lipid in Health and Disease, Metabolism and cytoprotection by long-chain polyunsaturated fatty acids from marine origin, bioconversion of n-3 and n-6 fatty acids from vegetable and marine oils, physiological effects of n-3 fatty acid as functional food.

Contents

Preface

Fats and oils are a large group of chemical structures different in shape, size and physicochemical characteristics, collectively identified as lipids. Ancestrally, lipids were fundamental components in the early human diet, providing an important and valuable amount of energy (9 kcal / g 37.7 kJ / g) and other components, such as essential fatty acids, fat soluble vitamins and sterols (such as cholesterol and/or phytosterols). The different structural characteristics of lipids give them multiple biochemical, physiological and nutritional functions, being transcendental to our body and allowing, among other functions, the development and growth of highly specialized tissues, such as the brain.

Lipids have been important in the evolution of many species and especially for the human being. At present a significant number of studies have demonstrated the role of lipids in the development, prevention and / or treatment of various acute and chronic diseases. The present book, "Lipid Metabolism", discuss in its various chapters the importance of lipid metabolism in humans and other species.

The first section of the book is dedicated to the structure and general metabolism of lipids, with emphasis on the structural and metabolic differences of each lipid. Regarding lipid metabolism, the main features from their absorption and digestion are also discussed, highlighting in particular the complexity of lipoprotein metabolism.

At molecular level lipid metabolism is even more complex. Some chapters revise and discuss the close relationship between some lipids and i) the cell membrane structure ii) the regulation of intracellular signaling pathways, iii) the direct interaction with gene transcription factors iv) the regulation of gene expression, and v) the effect of lipid peroxidation in cellular metabolism. All these interactions involving lipid metabolic products show the relevance of these molecules in the maintenance of normal structural, organic and systemic cellular activity.

Currently, a central element in the study of lipid metabolism is the participation of these molecules in the development and the prevention of certain diseases, especially those of chronic non communicable nature such as, obesity, insulin resistance, diabetes mellitus, atherosclerosis, cardiovascular disease and cancer. It is well known the association of some saturated fatty acids, such as palmitic acid (C16: 0) or of cholesterol, with the increased risk of cardiovascular diseases, or the effect of the imbalance of omega-6 and omega-3 fatty acids in the course of inflammatory process and its posterior resolution.

An interesting aspect of lipid metabolism refers to its importance in plants where, such as in animals, lipids represent more than an energy reservoir, highlighting as regulatory elements in the metabolism and in the functional properties of many vegetables, and having a direct impact on the health and nutrition of the human and animal population.

Collectively, the book intent to be a systematic and comprehensive review of lipid structure and metabolism. Special emphasis is made to the functional characteristics of some lipids, such as membrane phospholipids. Some chapters discuss the molecular aspects of lipid metabolism, its interaction with oxidative stress, and particularly the close relationship of some lipids with health and disease.

Rodrigo Valenzuela Baez, Nutricionist. Msc. PhD.
Assistant Professor
Fats and Oils in Food and Nutrition Research
Nutrition and Dietetics School
Faculty of Medicine
University of Chile
Santiago,
Chile

Section 1

Introduction to Lipid Metabolism

Chapter 1

Overview About Lipid Structure

Rodrigo Valenzuela B. and Alfonso Valenzuela B.

Additional information is available at the end of the chapter

http://dx.doi.org/10.5772/52306

1. Introduction

The term lipid is used to classify a large number of substances having very different physical - chemical characteristics, being its solubility in organic non-polar solvents the common property for their classification. Lipids are composed of carbon, hydrogen and oxygen atoms, and in some cases contain phosphorus, nitrogen, sulfur and other elements. In this context, fats and oils are the main exponents of lipids present in foods and in nutritional processes [1,2], being diverse fatty acids and cholesterol the most representative molecules due their important metabolic and nutritional functions [3,4]. The structural, metabolic and nutritional importance of lipids in the body is supported by numerous investigations in different biological models (cellular, animals and humans). Lipids have been instrumental in the evolution of species, having important role in the growth, development and maintenance of tissues [5,6]. A clear example of this importance is the elevated fatty acid concentration present in nerve tissue, especially very long-chain polyunsaturated fatty acids [7,8].

Fatty acids are, among lipids, of crucial relevance in the structure and physiology of the body because: i) forms an integral part of phospholipids in cell membranes; ii) are the primary source of energy (9 kcal /g or 37.62 kjoules/g); iii) in infants, provide more than 50% of the daily energy requirements; iv) some fatty acids are of essential character and are required for the synthesis of eicosanoids and docosanoids (of 20 and 22 carbon atoms, respectively), such as leukotrienes, prostaglandins, thromboxanes, prostacyclins, protectins and resolvins), and; v) some of them may act as second messengers and regulators of gene expression [9,10]. Besides fatty acids, cholesterol is another lipid that has important functions in the body, among which are: i) together with phospholipids is important in the formation of cell membranes; ii) constitutes the skeleton for the synthesis of steroid hormones (androgens and estrogens); iii) from its structure is derived the structure of vitamin D, and; iv) participates in the synthesis of the bile salts and the composition of bile secretion [11].

Lipids play a key role in the growth and development of the organism, where the requirements of these molecules (mainly fatty acids) will change depending on the age and physiological state of individuals [12]. Furthermore, lipids have crucial participation both, in the prevention and/or in the development of many diseases, especially chronic non-communicable diseases [13], affecting the lipid requirements in humans [14]. As food components, lipids are also important because: i) are significant in providing organoleptic characteristics (palatability, flavor, aroma and texture); ii) are vehicle for fat soluble vitamins, pigments or dyes and antioxidants, and; iii) may act as emulsifying agents and/or promote the stability of suspensions and emulsions [15].

Fats and oils, the most common lipids in food, are triacylglyceride mixtures, i.e. structures formed by the linking of three different or similar fatty acids to the tri-alcohol glycerol [16]. A fat is defined as a mixture of triacylglycerides which is solid or pasty at room temperature (usually 20 °C). Conversely, the term oil corresponds to a mixture of triglycerides which is liquid at room temperature. In addition to triacylglycerides, which are the main components of fats and oils (over 90%), these substances frequently contain, to a lesser extent, diacylglycerides, monoacylglycerides, phospholipids, sterols, terpenes, fatty alcohols, carotenoids, fat soluble vitamins, and many other minor chemical structures [17,18]. This chapter deals with the general aspects of lipids, especially those related to the chemical structure and function of these molecules.

2. Fatty acids

Fatty acids are hydrocarbon structures (containing carbon and hydrogen atoms) formed by four or more carbons attached to an acidic functional group called carboxyl group. The chemical and physical properties of the different fatty acids, such as their solubility in non-polar solvents and the melting point, will depend on the number of carbon atoms of the molecule. [19]. The higher the number of carbon atoms of the chain the higher will be melting point of the fatty acid. According to the chain length fatty acids are referred as short-chain fatty acids, those having four (C4) to ten (C10) carbons; as medium-chain fatty acids those having twelve (C12) to fourteen (C14) carbons; long-chain fatty acids to those of sixteen (C16) to eighteen carbons (C18); and very long-chain fatty acids those having twenty (C20) or more carbon atoms. Molecules having less than four carbon atoms (C2; acetic acid and C3; propionic acid) are not considered fatty acids due their high water solubility. On the other side, fatty acids of high number of carbon atoms are not frequent, however are present in significant amount in the brain of vertebrates, including mammals and human. In the human brain have been identified fatty acids as long as 36 carbon atoms [20].

The link between carbons in fatty acids, correspond to a covalent bond which may be single (saturated bond) or double (unsaturated bond). The number of unsaturated bonds in the same molecules can range from one to six double bonds. Thus, the more simple classification of the fatty acids, divided them in those that have not double bonds, named saturated fatty acids (SAFA), and fatty acids that have one or more double bonds, collectively named unsaturated fatty acids. In turn, when the molecule has one unsaturation it is classified as monounsaturated fatty acid (MUFA) and when has two to six unsaturations are classified as polyunsaturated fatty acids (PUFAs) [21]. The presence of unsaturation or double bonds in fatty acids is represented by denoting the number of carbons of the molecule followed by an indication of the number of double bonds, thus: C18:1 corresponds to a fatty acid of 18 carbons and one unsaturation, it will be a MUFA. C20: 4 correspond to a molecule having 20 carbons and four double bonds, being a PUFA. Now, it is necessary to identify the location of the unsaturations in the hydrocarbon chain both in MUFAs and PUFAs [22].

3. Nomenclature of fatty acids

According to the official chemical nomenclature established by IUPAC (International Union of Practical and Applied Chemistry) carbons of fatty acids should be numbered sequentially from the carboxylic carbon (C1) to the most extreme methylene carbon (Cn), and the position of a double bond should be indicated by the symbol delta (Δ), together to the number of the carbon where double bonds begins. According to this nomenclature: C18: 1, Δ9, indicates that the double bond is between carbon 9 and 10 [23]. However, in the cell the metabolic utilization of fatty acids occurs by the successive scission of two carbon atoms from the C1 to the Cn (mitochondrial or peroxisomal beta oxidation). This means that as the fatty acid is being metabolized (oxidized in beta position), the number of each carbon atom will change, creating a problem for the identification of the metabolic products formed as the oxidation progress. For this reason R. Holman, in 1958, proposed a new type of notation that is now widely used for the biochemical and nutritional identification of fatty acids [24]. This nomenclature lists the carbon enumeration from the other extreme of the fatty acid molecule. According to this notation, the C1 is the carbon farthest from the carboxyl group (called as terminal or end methylene carbon) which is designed as "n", "ω" or "omega". The latter notation is the most often used in nutrition and refers to the last letter of the Greek alphabet [25]. Thus, C18: 1 Δ9 coincidentally is C18: 1 ω-9 in the "ω" notation, but C18: 2 Δ9, Δ12, according to this nomenclature ω would be C18: 2 ω-6. What happens with fatty acids having more than a double bond? Double bonds are not randomly arranged in the fatty acid structure. Nature has been "ordained" as largely incorporate them in well-defined positions. Most frequently double bonds in PUFAs are separated by a methyl group (or most correctly methylene group) forming a **-C=C-C-C=C-** structure which is known as "unconjugated structure", which is the layout of double bonds in most naturally occurring PUFAs [26]. However, although much less frequently, there are also present "conjugated structures" where double bonds are not separated by a methylene group, forming a **-C=C-C=C-** structure. This particular structural disposition of double bonds, i.e conjugated structures, is now gaining much interest because some fatty acids having these structures show special nutritional properties, they are called "conjugated fatty acids". Most of them are derived from the unconjugated structure of linoleic acid (C18:2 ω-6) [27,28].

For the application of the "ω" nomenclature and considering the "order" of double bonds in unsaturated fatty acids having unconjugated stucture, it can be observed that by pointing the location of the first double bond, it will automatically determined the location of the subsequent double bonds [29]. Thus, C18: 1 ω-9, which has a single double bond at C9 counted from the methyl end, correspond to oleic acid (OA), which is the main exponent of the ω-9 family. Oleic acid is highly abundant both in vegetable and animal tissues. C18: 2 ω-6 corresponds to a fatty acid having double bonds at the C6 and C9 (for unconjugated fatty acids it is not necessary to indicate the position of the second or successive double bonds). This is linoleic acid (LA), the main exponent of the ω-6 family and which is very abundant in vegetable oils and to a lesser extent in animal fats [30]. C18: 3, ω-3 corresponds to a fatty acid having double bonds at C3, C6 and C9. It is alpha-linolenic acid (ALA), the leading exponent of the ω-3 family. ALA is a less abundant fatty acid, almost exclusively present in the vegetable kingdom and specifically in land-based plants [31]. Within (LCPUFAs), C20: 4, ω-6 or arachidonic acid (AA); C20: 5, ω-3 or eicosapentaenoic acid (EPA) and; C22 : 6, ω-3 or docosahexaenoic acid (DHA), are of great nutritional importance and are only found in ground animal tissues (AA) and in aquatic animal tissues (AA, EPA and DHA) and in plants of marine origin (EPA and DHA) [32].

The increase of double bonds in fatty acids significantly reduces its melting point. Thus, for a structure of the same number of carbon atoms, if it is saturated may give rise to a solid or semisolid product at room temperature, but if the same structure is unsaturated, may originate a liquid or less solid product at room temperature. Figure 1 shows the classification of fatty acids according to their degree of saturation and unsaturation and considering the notation "ω", and table 1 shows different fatty acids, showing the C nomenclature, their systematic name, their common name and the respective melting point.

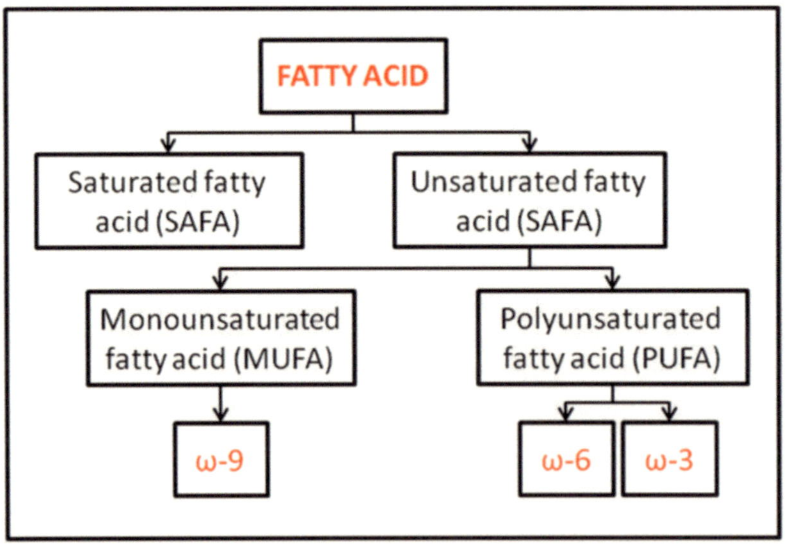

Figure 1. Classification of fatty acids according to their degree of saturation and unsaturation and considering the notation " ω".

Nomenclature	Systematic name	Common name	Melting point °C
	Saturated Fatty Acid		
C 4:0	Butanoic	Butiric	-5.3
C 6:0	Hexaenoic	Caproic	-3.2
C 8:0	Octanoic	Caprilic	16.5
C10:0	Decanoic	Capric	31.6
C12:0	Dodecanoic	Lauric	44.8
C14:0	Tetradecanoic	Miristic	54.4
C16:0	Hexadecanoic	Palmitic	62.9
C18:0	Octadecanoic	Estearic	70.1
C20:0	Eicosanoic	Arachidic	76.1
C22:0	Docosanoic	Behenic	80.0
C24:0	Tetracosanoic	Lignocenic	84.2
	Unsaturated Fatty Acid		
C16:1	9-Hexadececoic	Palmitoleic	0.0
C18:1	9-Octadecenoic	Oleic	16.3
C18:1	11-Octodecenoic	Vaccenic	39.5
C18:2	9,12-Octadecadienoic	Linoleic	-5.0
C18:3	9,12,15-Octadecatrienoic	Linolenic	-1.0
C20:4	5,8,11,14-Eicosatetraenoic	Arachidonic	49.5

Table 1. Different fatty acids, showing the C nomenclature, their systematic name, their common name and the respective melting point.

4. Mono-, di- and triacylglycerides

The structural organization of fatty acids in food and in the body is mainly determined by the binding to glycerol by ester linkages. The reaction of a hydroxyl group of glycerol, at any of its three groups, with a fatty acid gives rise to a monoacylglyceride. The linking of a second fatty acid, which may be similar or different from the existing fatty acid, gives rise to a diacylglyceride. If all three hydroxyl groups of glycerol are linked by fatty acids, then this will be a triacylglyceride [33]. Monoacylglycerides, by having free hydroxyl groups (two) are relatively polar and therefore partially soluble in water. Different monoacylglycerides linked to fatty acids of different lengths are used as emulsifiers in the food and pharmaceutical industry [34]. The less polar diacylglycerides which have only one free hydroxyl group are less polar than monoacylglycerides and less soluble in water. Finally, triacylglycerides, which lack of free hydroxyl groups are completely non-polar, but highly soluble in non-polar solvents, which are frequently used for their extraction from vegetable or animal tissues, because constitutes the energy reserve in these tissues [35]. Diacylglycerides and monoacylglycerides are important intermediates in the digestive and absorption process of fats and oils in animals. In turn, some of these molecules also perform other metabolic functions, such as diacylglycerides which may act as "second messengers" at the intracellular level and are also part of the composition of a new generation of oils nutritionally designed as "low calorie oils" [36]. When glycerol forms mono-, di-, or triacylglycerides, its carbon atoms are not chemically and structurally equivalent. Thus, carbon 1 of the glycerol is referred as carbon (α), or sn-1 (from "stereochemical number"); carbon 2 is referred as carbon (β), or sn-2, and carbon 3 as (γ), or sn-3. It is important to note that the notation "sn" is currently the most frequently used [37]. This spatial structure (or conformation) of mono-, di- and triacygglycerides is relevant in the digestive process of fats and oils (ref). Figure 2 shows the structure of a monoacylglceride, a diacylglyceride and a triacylglyceride, specifying the "sn-" notation.

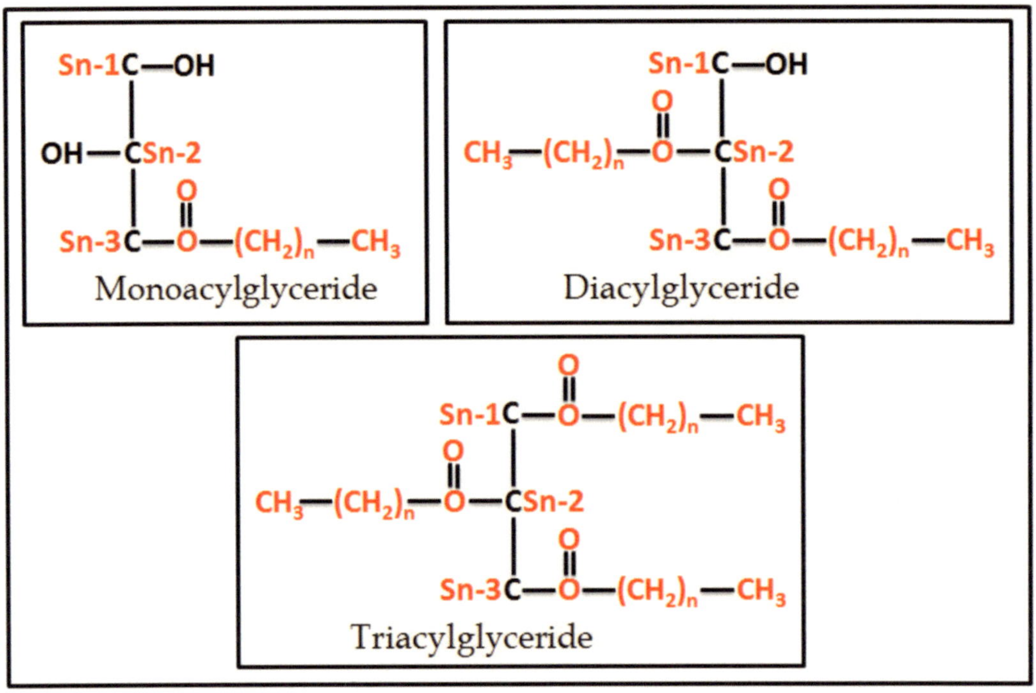

Figure 2. Structure of a monoacylglyceride, a diacylglyceride and a triacylglyceride, specifying the "sn-" notation

5. Essential fatty acids

The capability of an organism to metabolically introduce double bonds in certain positions of a fatty acid or the inability to do this, determines the existence of the so-called non-essential or essential fatty acids (EFAs). According to this capability, mammals, including primates and humans, can introduce a double bond only at the C9 position of a saturated fatty acid (according to "ω" nomenclature) and to other carbons nearest to the carboxyl group, but not at carbons nearest the C1 position [38]. This is the reason why OA is not an EFA. In contrast, mammals can not introduce double bonds at C6 and C3 positions, being the reason why AL and ALA are EFAs. By derivation, the AA is formed by the elongation and desaturation of LA, and EPA and DHA, which are formed by elongation and desaturation of ALA, become also essential for mammals when their respective precursors (LA and ALA, respectively) are nutritionally deficient [39]. Figure 3 shows the chemical structure of a SAFA, such as the stearic acid (C18:0), AO, LA and ALA, exemplifying the "ω" notation of each and indicating the essential condition in relation to the position of their unsaturated bonds.

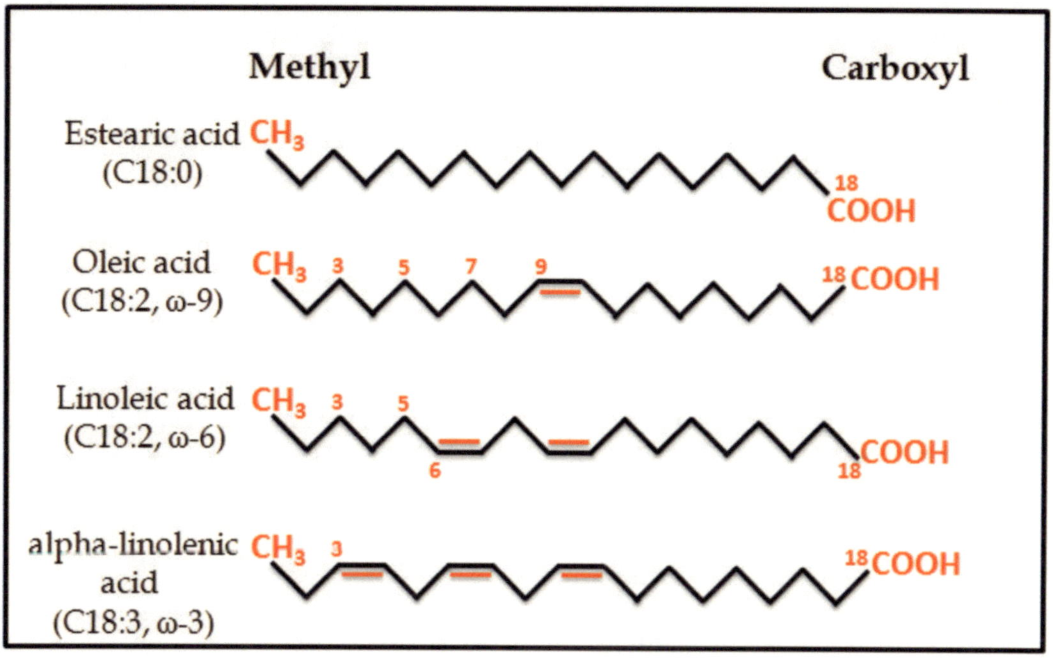

Figure 3. The chemical structure of a SAFA, such as the stearic acid (C18:0), AO, LA and ALA, exemplifying the "ω" notation of each and indicating the essential condition in relation to the position of their unsaturated bonds

6. Isomerism of fatty acids

According to the distribution of double bonds in a fatty acid and to its spatial structure, unsaturated fatty acids may have two types of isomerism: geometrical isomerism and positional isomerism. By isomerism it is referred to the existence two or more molecules having the same structural elements (atoms), the same chemical formula and combined in equal proportions, but having a different position or spatial distribution of some atoms in the molecule [40].

6.1. Geometrical isomers of fatty acids

Carbon atoms forming the structure of the fatty acids possess a three-dimensional spatial structure which forms a perfect tetrahedron. However, when two carbons having tetrahedral structure are joined together through a double bond, the spatial conformation of the double bond is modified adopting a flat or plane structure [41]. Rotation around single bonds (C-C) is entirely free, but when they are forming a double bond (C=C), this rotation is impeded and the hydrogen atoms that are linked to each carbon involved in the bond may be at the same side or opposed in the plane forming the double bond. If hydrogen atoms remain at the same side, the structure formed is referred as *cis* isomer (denoted as "*c*"). When hydrogen atoms remain at opposite sides the structure formed is referred as *trans* isomer (denoted as "*t*", *trans*: means crossed) [42]. Figure 4 shows the *cis – trans* geometric isomerism of fatty acids. The *cis* or *trans* isomerism of fatty acids confers them very different physical properties, being the melting point one of the most relevant [43]. Table 2 shows the melting point of various *cis – trans* geometric isomers of different fatty acids. It can be observed substantial differences in the melting point of *cis-* or *trans* isomers for the same fatty acid. Melting point differences bring to the geometrical isomers of a fatty acid very different biochemical and nutritional behavior. Fatty acids having *trans* isomerism, especially those of technological origin (such as generated during the partial hydrogenation of oils), have adverse effect on humans, particularly referred to the risk of cardiovascular diseases [44]. It is noteworthy that the majority of naturally occurring fatty acids have *cis* isomerism, although thermodynamically is more stable the *trans* than the *cis* isomerism, whereby under certain technological manipulations, such as the application of high temperature (frying process) or during the hydrogenation process applied for the manufacture of shortenings, *cis* isomers are easily transformed into *trans* isomers [45].

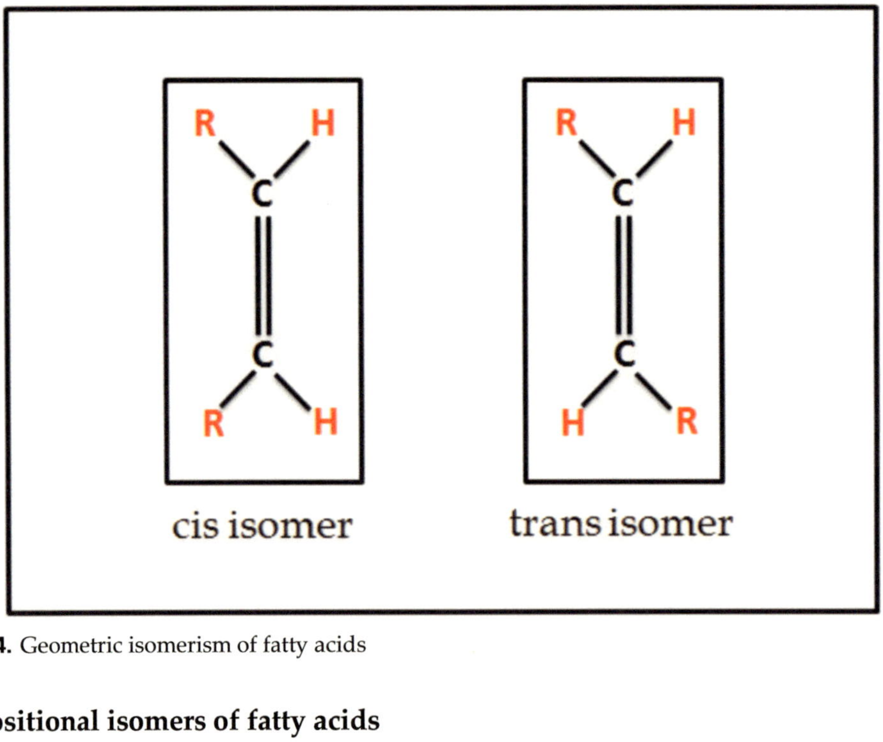

Figure 4. Geometric isomerism of fatty acids

6.2. Positional isomers of fatty acids

Positional isomerism refers to the different positions that can occupy one or more double bonds in the structure of a fatty acid. For example, oleic acid (C18:1 Δ9c), is a common fatty acid in vegetable oils, particularly in olive oil, but vaccenic acid (C18:1 Δ11t) is more common in animal fats. This is a double example, since both fatty acids are geometric isomers (oleic acid *cis* and vaccenic acid *trans*) and at the same time positional isomers, since oleic acid has a double bond at the Δ9 position and vaccenic acid at the Δ11 position [46].

Fatty acid	Isomerism	Melting point (°C)
C12:0	------	44.2
C16:0	------	62.7
C18:0	------	69.6
C18:1	Cis	13.2
C18:1	Trans	44.0
C18:2	cis, cis	-5.0
C18:2	trans, trans	18.5
C18:3	cis, cis, cis	11.0
C20:3	trans, trans, trans	29.5

Table 2. Changes in the melting point of various *cis – trans* geometrical isomers of different fatty acids

In general, all fatty acids naturally present positional isomerism of their more frequent molecular structure. However, these isomers occur in very low concentrations. Unlike the known biochemical and nutritional effects of *trans* geometric isomers, there is little information about the biological effects of positional isomers and for the majority of them these effects are considered as not relevant, except for some conjugated structures, such as conjugated linoleic acid (C18:2, Δ9, Δ11, CLA), a geometric and positional isomer of the most common linoleic acid, for which it has been attributed various health properties, especially those related to anti-inflammatory and lipolytic actions, but up to date the scientific evidence for these properties are considered insufficient [47]. Such as geometrical isomerism, the technological manipulation of fatty acids (i.e. temperature and/or hydrogenation) increases the number and complexity of the positional isomers [48]. Figure 5 summarizes the positional and geometric isomers of unsaturated fatty acids.

7. Phospholipids

Phospholipids are minor components in our diet because less than 4-5% of our fat intake corresponds to phospholipids. However, this does not detract nutritionally important to these lipids, since they are important constituents of the cellular structure having also relevant metabolic functions [49]. Life, in its origin, would not have been possible without the appearance of phospholipids, as these structures are the fundamental components of all cellular membranes. Phospholipids have structural and functional properties that distinguish them from their counterparts, triacylglycerides. In phospholipids positions sn-1 and sn-2 of the glycerol moiety are occupied by fatty acids, more frequently polyunsaturated fatty acids, linked to glycerol by ester bonds. The sn-3 position of glycerol is linked to orthophosphoric acid [50]. The structure which is formed, independent of the type of fatty acid that binds at sn-1 and sn-2, is called phosphatidic acid. The presence of phosphate substituent at the sn-3 position of the glycerol gives a great polarity to this part of the molecule, being non-polar the rest of the structure, such as in triacylglycerides. This double feature, a polar extreme and a non-polar domain due the presence of the two fatty acids characterizes phospholipids as amphipathic molecules (*amphi*: both; *pathos*: sensation) [51].

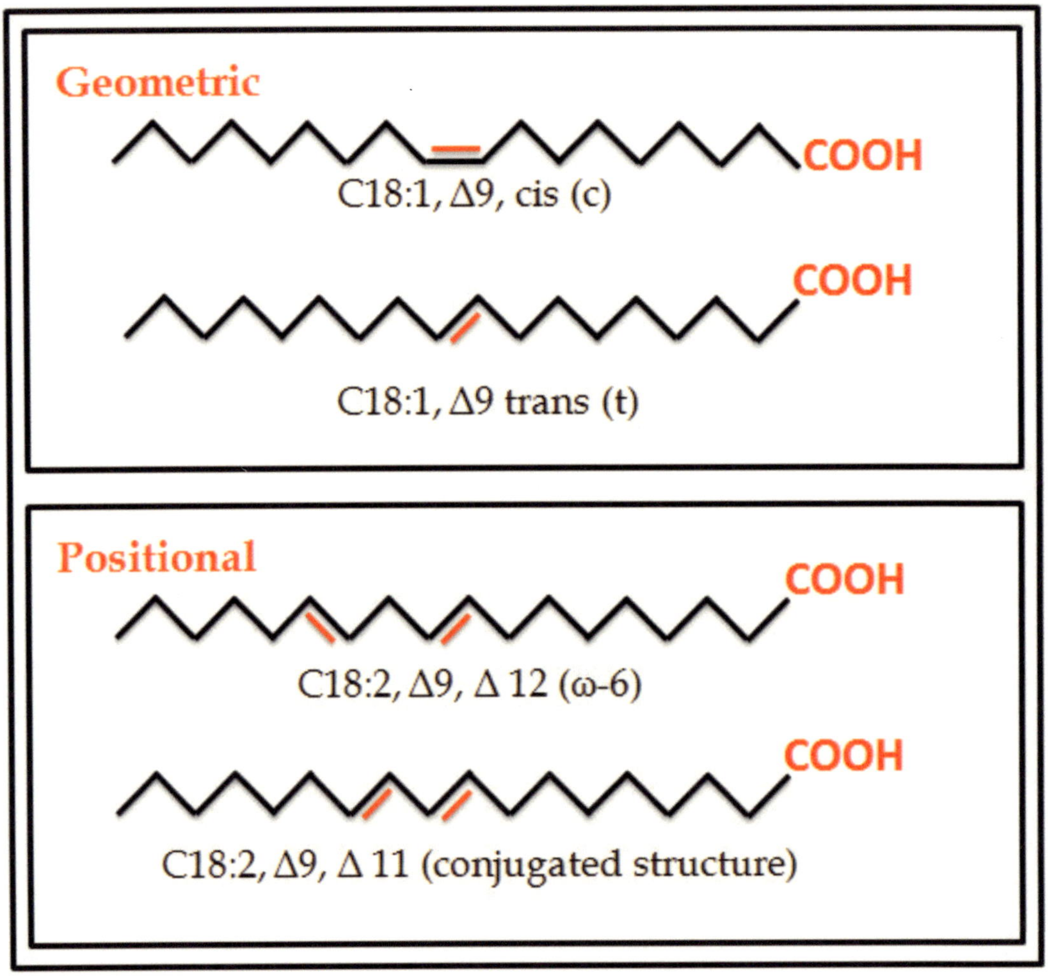

Figure 5. Positional and geometric isomers of unsaturated fatty acids

The structure of phospholipids is usually simplified representing the polar end as a sphere and the fatty acids as two parallel rods. Figure 6 shows the chemical structure of phosphatidic acid in its simplified representation. The amphipathic character of phosphatidic acid can be increased by joining to the phosphate different basic and polar molecules that increases the polarity to the extreme of the sn-3 position. When the substituent of the phosphate group is the aminoacid serine it is formed phosphatidylserine; when it is etanolamine it is formed phosphatidylethanolamine (frequently known as cephalin); when choline is the substituent it is formed phosphatidylcholine (well known as lecithin); and when the substituent is the polyalcohol inositol it is formed phosphatidylinositol, a very important molecule involved in cell signaling. [52].

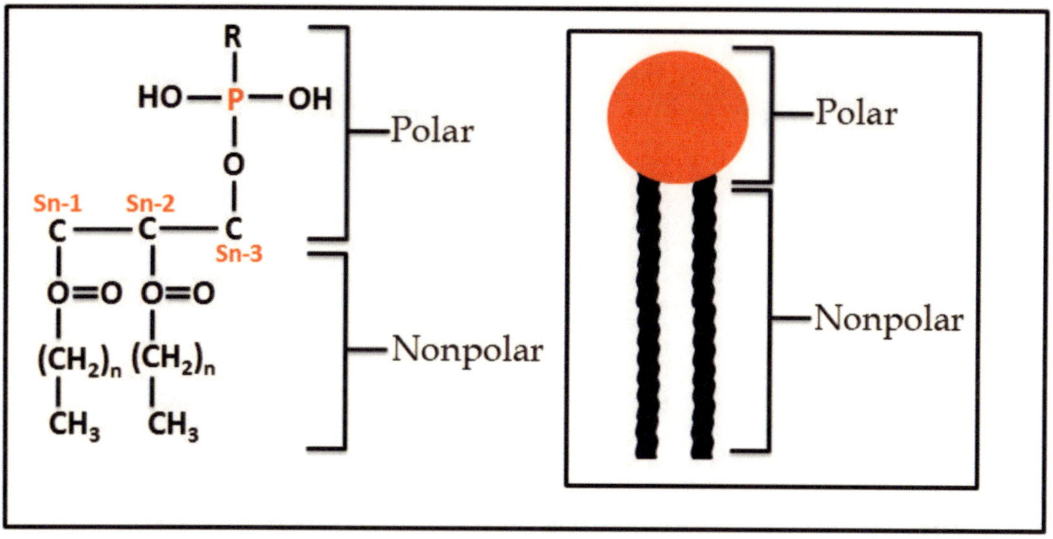

Figure 6. Chemical structure of phosphatidic acid and its simplified representation

These more complex phospholipids are much more common than phosphatidic acid, since this is only the structural precursor of the above molecules. Figure 7 shows the structure of various phospholipids. A number of other molecules are also classified as phospholipids, but are structurally different. Cardiolipin is a "double" phospholipid in which two phosphatidic acid molecules are attached through their phosphates by a molecule of glycerol. Cardiolipin is a very important in the structure of the inner membrane of mitochondria and due their molecular volume it is the only immunogenic phospholipid (which stimulates the formation of antibodies) [53]. Plasmalogens are other lipid molecules related to phospholipids. In these molecules the substituent at sn-1 position of the glycerol is not a fatty acid, but a fatty alcohol which is linked to glycerol by an ether linkage. Phosphatidalethanolamine (different than phosphatidylethanolamine) is an abundant plasmalogen in the nervous tissue [54]. Phosphatidalcholine, the plasmalogen related to phosphatidylcholine, is abundant in the heart muscle. Another structures related to phospholipids are sphingolipids. In these structures glycerol is replaced by the amino alcohol; sphingosine. When the hydroxyl group (alcoholic group) of sphingosine is substituted by phosphocholine, it is formed sphingomyelin, which is the only sphingolipid that is present in significant amount in human tissues as a constituent of myelin that forms nerve fibers [ref]. Platelet activating factor (PAF) is an unusual glycerophospholipid structure. In this molecule position sn-1 of glycerol is linked to a saturated alcohol through an ether bond (such as in plasmalogens) and at the sn-2 binds an acetyl group instead of a fatty acid. PAF is released by a variety of cells and by binding to membrane receptors produces aggregation and degranulation of platelets, has potent thrombotic and inflammatory effects, and is a mediator of anaphylactic reactions [55].

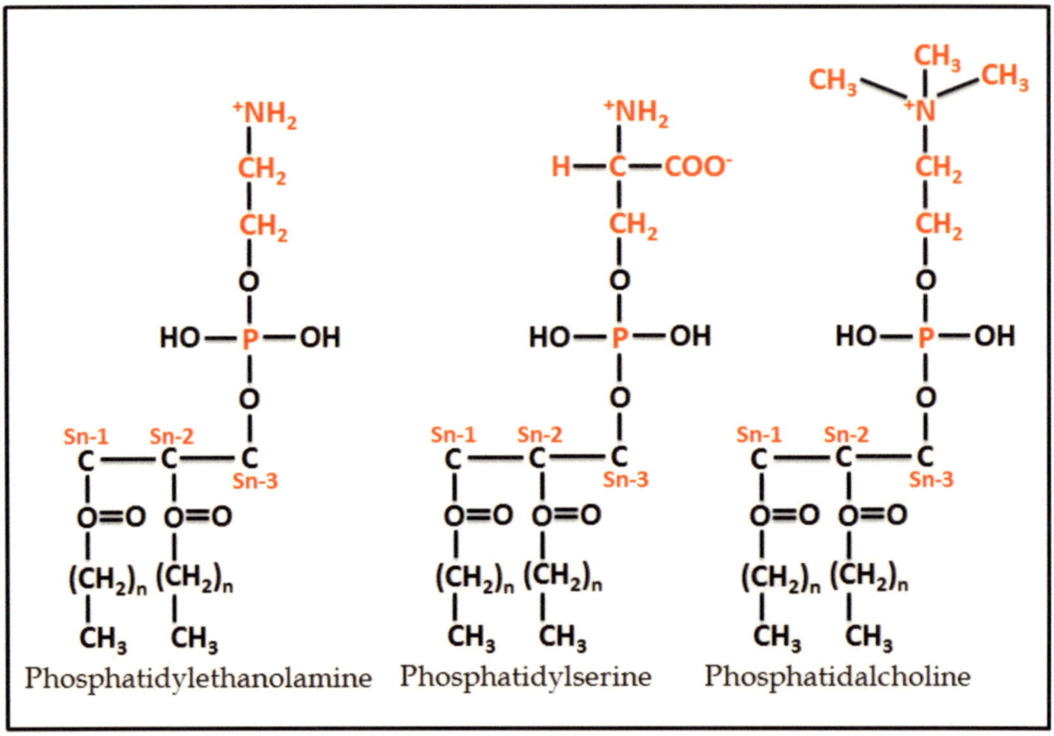

Figure 7. Structure of various phospholipids

A fundamental aspect of phospholipids is their participation in the structure of biological membranes, and the structural characteristics of the fatty acids are relevant to determine the behavior and the biological properties of the membrane. As an example, a diet rich in saturated fatty acids result in an increase in the levels of these fatty acids into cell membrane phospholipids, causing a significant decrease in both, membrane fluidity and in the ability of these structure to incorporate ion channels, receptors, enzymes, structural proteins, etc., effect which is associated to an increased cardiovascular risk [56]. By contrast, a diet rich in monounsaturated and/or polyunsaturated fatty acids produce an inverse effect. At the nutritional and metabolic level this effect is highly relevant because as the fatty acid composition of the diet is directly reflected into the fatty acid composition of phospholipids, changes in the composition of the diet, i.e. increasing the content of polyunsaturated fatty acids, will prevent the development of several diseases [57]. Figure 8 shows a simulation how the structural differences of the fatty acids which comprise phospholipids may affect the physical and chemical behavior of a membrane.

8. Sterols

Sterols are derived from a common structural precursor, the sterane or cyclopentanoperhydrophenanthrene, consisting in a main structure formed by four aromatic rings identified as A, B, C and D rings. All sterols have at carbon 3 of A ring a polar hydroxyl group being the rest of the structure non-polar, which gives them certain amphipathic character, such as phospholipids. Sterols have also a double bound at carbons 5 and 6 of ring B [58]. This double bond can be saturated (reduced) which leads to the formation of stanols, which together with plant sterols derivatives are currently used as hypocholesterolemic agents when incorporated into some functional foods. At carbon 17 (ring D) both sterols as stanols have attached an aliphatic group, consisting in a linear structure of 8, 9 or 10 carbon atoms, depending on whether the sterol is from animal origin (8 carbon atoms) or from vegetable origin (9 or 10 carbon atoms) [59]. Figure 9 shows the structure of cyclopentanoperhydrophenanthrene and cholesterol. Often sterols, and less frequent stanols, have esterified the hydroxyl group of carbon 3 (ring A) with a saturated fatty acid (usually palmitic; C16:0) or unsaturated fatty acid (most frequent oleic; C18:1 and less frequent linoleic acid; C18:2. The esterification of the hydroxyl group eliminates the anphipaticity of the molecule and converts it into a structure completely non-polar. Undoubtedly among sterols cholesterol is the most important because it is the precursor of important animal metabolic molecules, such as steroid hormones, bile salts, vitamin D, and oxysterols, which are oxidized derivatives of cholesterol formed by the thermal manipulation of cholesterol and that have been identified as regulators of the metabolism and homeostasis of cholesterol and sterols in general [60].

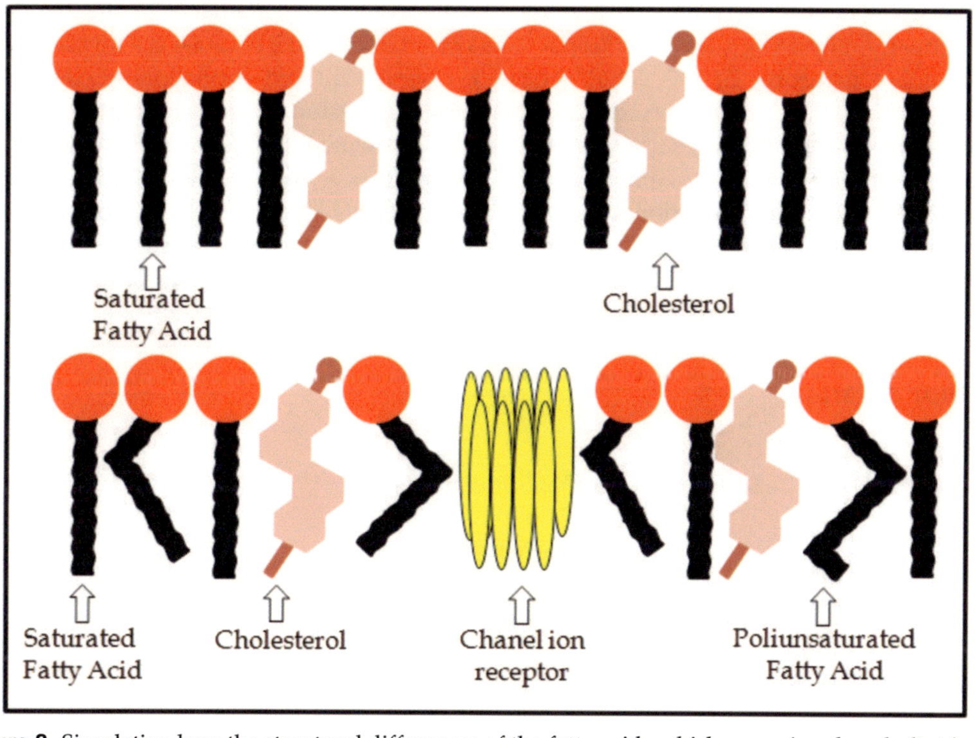

Figure 8. Simulation how the structural differences of the fatty acids which comprise phospholipids may affect the physical and chemical behavior of a membrane

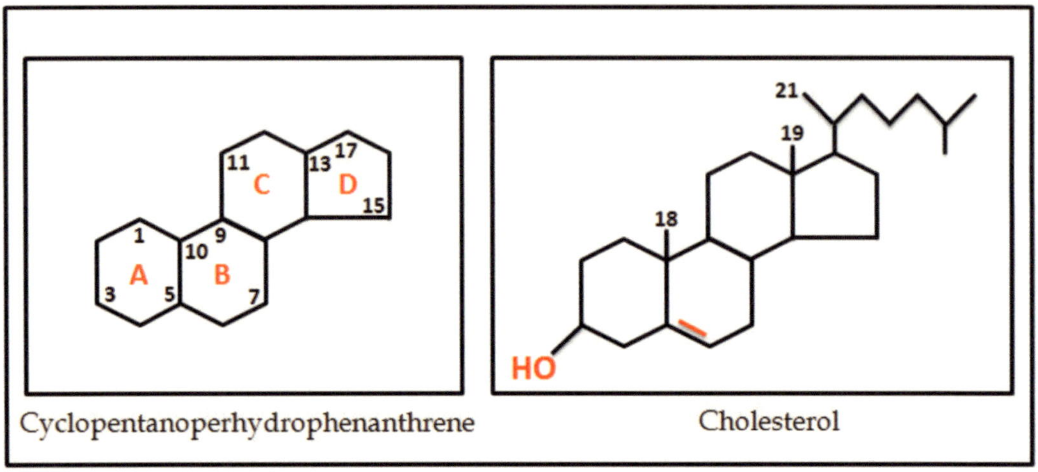

Figure 9. Structure of cyclopentanoperhydrophenanthrene and cholesterol

9. Conclusions

Lipids are a large and wide group of molecules that are present in all living organism and also in foods and characterized by particular physicochemical properties, such as their non polarity and their solubility in organic solvents. Some lipids, in particular fatty acids and sterols, are essential for animal and plant life. Lipids are key elements in the structure, biochemistry, physiology, and nutritional status of an individual, because are involved in: i) the cellular structure; ii) the cellular energy reserve, iii) the formation of regulatory metabolites, and; iv) in the regulation and gene expression, which directly affects the functioning of the body. Another important aspect related to lipids is their important involvement, either in the treatment and/or the origin of many diseases which can affect humans. Structural and functional characteristics of lipids, discussed in this chapter, will allow you to integrate those metabolic aspects of these important and essential molecules in close relationship of how foods containing these molecules can have a relevant influence in the health or illness of an individual.

Author details

Rodrigo Valenzuela B.
Nutrition and Dietetics School, Faculty of Medicine, University of Chile, Santiago Chile

Alfonso Valenzuela B.
Lipid Center, Nutrition and Food Technology Institute, University of Chile, Faculty of Medicine, University of Los Andes, Santiago Chile

Acknowledgement

The authors are grateful from FONDECYT, FONDEF and INNOVA-Chile the support of their research.

10. References

[1] Carpenter K. (1998). Early ideas on the nutritional significance of lipids, *J. Nutr.* 128, 423S-426S.

[2] Orešič M. (2009). Metabolomics, a novel tool for studies of nutrition, metabolism and lipid dysfunction. *Nutrition, Metabolism and Cardiovascular Diseases*, Vol 19, pp. 816-24.

[3] Burlingame B, Nishida C, Uauy R. et al. (2009). Fats and fatty acids in human nutrition; joint FAO/WHO Expert Consultation. *Ann. Nutr. Metab.*, Vol 55, pp. 1-3.

[4] Food and Agriculture Organization of the United Nations (FAO). (2010). Fats and fatty acids in human nutrition Report of an expert consultation. *Food and Nutrition.* Paper 91, pp. 9-19.

[5] Valenzuela A. (2009). Docosahexaenoic acid (DHA), an essential fatty acid for the proper functioning of neuronal cells: Their role in mood disorders. *Grasas & Aceites*, Vol 60, pp. 203-12.

[6] Simopoulos A. (2011), Evolutionary aspects of diet: the omega-6/omega-3 ratio and the brain. *Mol Neurobiol*, Vol 44, pp. 203-15.

[7] Valenzuela R, Bascuñán K, Valenzuela A, et al. (2009). Omega-3 fatty acids, neurodegenerative and psychiatric diseases: A new preventive and therapeutic approach. *Rev Chil Nutr*, Vol 36, pp. 1120-28.

[8] Campoy C, Escolano-Margarit M, Anjos T, et al. (2012). Omega 3 fatty acids on child growth, visual acuity and neurodevelopment. *Br J Nutr*. 2012, Vol 107, Suppl 2:S85-106.

[9] Weylandt K, Chiu C, Gomolka B, et al. (2012). Omega-3 fatty acids and their lipid mediators: towards an understanding of resolvin and protectinformation. *Prostaglandins Other Lipid Mediat.* Vol 97, pp. 73-82.

[10] Zúñiga J, Cancino M, Medina F, et al. (2011). N-3 PUFA supplementation triggers PPAR-α activation and PPAR-α/NF-κB interaction: anti-inflammatory implications in liver ischemia-reperfusion injury. *PLoS One.* Vol 6, pp. e28502.

[11] Dawson P, Lan T, and Rao A. (2009). Bile acid transporters *J. Lipid Res.* Vol 50, pp. 2340-57.

[12] Dietary fats and coronary heart disease. (2012). Willett WC. *J Intern Med*. Vol 272, pp. 13-24.

[13] Valenzuela R, and Videla L. (2011). The importance of the long-chain polyunsaturated fatty acid_n-6/n-3 ratio_in development of non-alcoholic fatty liver associated with obesity. *Food Funct*. Vol 2, pp. 644-8.

[14] Katan M, Zock P, and Mensink R. (1994). Effects of fats and fatty acids on blood lipids in humans: an overview. *Am. J. Clin. Nutr.*, Vol 60, pp. 1017S-22S.

[15] Valenzuela A, Delplanque B, and Tavella M. (2011). Stearic acid: a possible substitute for trans fatty acids from industrial origin. *Grasas & Aceites*. Vol 62, pp. 131-38.

[16] Lee Y, Tang T, and Lai O. (2012). Health Benefits, Enzymatic Production, and Application of Medium and Long-Chain Triacylglycerol(MLCT) in Food Industries: A Review. *J Food Sci.* doi: 10.1111/j.1750-3841.2012.02793.x

[17] Asensio C, Nepote V, and Grosso N. (2011) Chemical stability of extra-virgin_olive oil added with oregano essential oil. *J Food Sci.* Vol 76, pp. S445-50.

[18] Saggini A, Anogeianaki A, Angelucci D, et al. (2011). Cholesterol and vitamins: revisited study. *J Biol Regul Homeost Agents.* Vol 25, pp. 505-15.

[19] Fahy E, Subramanium S, Brown A, et al. (2005). A comprehensive classification system for lipids. *J. Lipid Res.* Vol 46, pp. 839-61.

[20] Kuipers R, Luxwolda M, Offringa P, et al. (2012). Fetal intrauterine whole body linoleic, arachidonic and docosahexaenoic acid contents and accretion rates. *Prostaglandins Leukot Essent Fatty Acids.* Vol 86, pp 13-20.

[21] Rodríguez E, Giri M, Rottiers R et al. Fatty acid composition of erythrocyte phospholipids is related to insulin levels, secretion and resistance in obese type 2 diabetics on Metformin. *Clinica Chimica Acta,* Vol 346. pp. 145-52.

[22] Gurr MI. (1992). Dietary lipids and coronary heart desease: Old evidence, new persspective *Prog in Lip Res.* Vol 31, pp 195-243.

[23] Martin D, Muriel E, Antequera T, et al. Quantitative changes in the fatty acid profile of lipid fractions of fresh loin from pigs as affected by dietary conjugated linoleic acid and monounsaturated fatty acids during refrigerated storage. *J. Food Composition and Analysis.* Vol 22, pp. 102-11.

[24] Arnauld S, Fidaleo M, Clémencet MC, et al. (2009). Modulation of the hepatic fatty acid pool in peroxisomal 3-ketoacyl-CoA thiolase B-null mice exposed to the selective PPARalpha agonist Wy14,643. *Biochimie.* Vol 91, pp. 1376-86.

[25] Harris W, Miller M, Tighe A, et al. (2008). Omega-3 fatty acids and coronary heart disease risk: Clinical and mechanistic perspectives *Atherosclerosis,* Vol 197, pp. 12-24.

[26] Osorio N, Ribeiro M, da Fonseca M, et al. (2008). Interesterification of fat blends rich in ω-3 polyunsaturated fatty acids catalysed by immobilized *Thermomyces lanuginosa* lipase under high pressure *J Mol Catalysis B: Enzymatic,* Vol 52. pp. 58-66.

[27] Skerratt J, Nichols P, Bowman J, et al. (1992). Occurrence and significance of long-chain (ω-1)-hydroxy fatty acids in methane-utilizing bacteria. *Organic Geochemistry.* Vol 18, pp. 189-94.

[28] Ansari G, Bhupendra S, Kaphalia M, et al. (1995). Fatty acid conjugates of xenobiotics *Toxicology Letters.* Vol 75, pp. 1-17.

[29] Michl J, and West R. Conformations of linear chains. (2000). Systematics and suggestions for nomenclature. Acc Chem Res. Vol 33, pp. 821-3.

[30] Din J, Newby D, and Flapan A, (2004). Omega 3 fatty acids and cardiovascular disease—fishing for a natural treatment. *BMJ.* Vol 3, pp. 30-35.

[31] Kris-Etherton P, Taylor D, Yu-Poth S, et al. (2000). Polyunsaturated fatty acids in the food chain in the United States. *Am J Clin Nutr. Vol 71. pp.* S179-88.

[32] Kris-Etherton P, Harris W, Appel LJ for the Nutrition Committee. (2002). AHA scientific statement. Fish consumption, fish oil, omega-3 fatty acids, and cardiovascular disease. *Circulation.* Vol 106. pp. 2747-57.

[33] Kishi T, Carvajal O, Tomoyori H, et al.(2002). Structured triglycerides containing medium-chain fatty acids and linoleic acid differently influence clearance rate in serum of triglycerides in rats *Nutrition Research,* Vol 22, pp. 1343-51.

[34] Carpentier Y, Simoens C, Siderova V, et al. (1997). Recent developments in lipid emulsions: relevance to intensive care. *Nutrition,* Vol 13, pp. 73-78.

[35] Irene Cetin, Gioia Alvino, Manuela Cardellicchio. (2009). Long chain fatty acids and dietary fats in fetal nutrition. *J Physiol*. Vol 15, pp. 3441–51.

[36] Rekha S, Singhal A, Gupta P, et al. Low-calorie fat substitutes. *Trends in Food Science & Technology*. Vol 2, pp. 241-44.

[37] Morita O, Knapp J, Tamaki Y, et al. (2008). Safety assessment of dietary diacylglycerol oil: A two-generation reproductive toxicity study in rats. *Food and Chemical Toxicology*, Vol 46, pp. 3059-68.

[38] Blasbalg T, Hibbeln J, Ramsden C, et al. (2011). Changes in consumption of omega-3 and omega-6 fatty acids in the United States during the 20th century. *Am J Clin Nutr*. Vol 93, pp. 950-62.

[39] Le H, Meisel J, de Meijer V, et al. (2012). The essentiality of arachidonic acid and docosahexaenoic acid. *Prostaglandins Leukot Essent Fatty Acids*. Vol 81, pp. 165-170.

[40] Valenzuela A, and Morgado N. (1999). Trans fatty acid isomers in human health and in the food industry. *Biol Res*. Vol 32, pp. 273-87.

[41] Micha R, King I, Lemaitre R, et al. (2010). Food sources of individual plasma phospholipid trans fatty acid isomers: the Cardiovascular Health Study. *Am J Clin Nutr*. Vol 91, pp. 883-93.

[42] Minville-Walz M, Gresti J, Pichon L, et al. (2012). Distinct regulation of stearoyl-CoA desaturase 1 gene expression by cis and trans C18:1 fatty acids in human aortic smooth muscle cells. *Genes Nutr*. Vol 7, pp. 209–16.

[43] Valenzuela A. (2008). Trans fatty acids I. Origin and effects in human health. *Rev Chil Nutr*. Vol 35, pp. 162-71.

[44] Micha R, and Mozaffarian D. (2008). Trans Fatty Acids: Effects on Cardiometabolic Health and Implications for Policy. Prostaglandins Leukot Essent Fatty Acids. Vol 79, pp. 147-52.

[45] Kuhnt K, Baehr M, Rohrer C, et al. (2011). Trans fatty acid isomers and the trans-9/trans-11 index in fat containing foods. Eur J Lipid Sci Technol. Vol 113, pp. 1281–92.

[46] Seppänen-Laakso T, Laakso I, Backlund P, et al. (1996). Elaidic and trans-vaccenic acids in plasma phospholipids as indicators of dietary intake of 18:1 trans-fatty acids. *Journal of Chromatography B: Biomedical Sciences and Applications*. Vol 687, pp. 996, Pages 371-78.

[47] Dilzer A, and Park Y. (2012). Implication of conjugated linoleic acid (CLA) in human health. Crit Rev Food Sci Nutr. Vol 52, pp. 488-513.

[48] Izadifar M. (2005). Neural network modeling of trans isomer formation and unsaturated fatty acid changes during vegetable oil hydrogenation. *Journal of Food Engineering*. Vol 66, pp. 227-32.

[49] Green J, Liu Z, and Bazinet P. (2010). Brain phospholipid arachidonic acid half-lives are not altered following 15 weeks of N-3 polyunsaturated fatty acid_adequate or deprived diet. *J Lipid Res*. Vol 51, pp. 535–43.

[50] Koga Y, and Goldfine H. (1984). Biosynthesis of_phospholipids_in Clostridium butyricum: kinetics of synthesis of plasmalogens and the glycerol acetal of ethanolamine plasmalogen. J Bacteriol. Vol 159, pp 597–604.

[51] García-Sáinz J, and Fain J. (1980). Effect of insulin, catecholamines and calcium ions on phospholipidmetabolism in isolated white fat-cells. *Biochem J*. Vol 15, pp. 781–89.

[52] Castro-Perez J, Roddy T, Nibbering N, et al. (2011). Localization of Fatty Acyl and Double Bond Positions in_Phosphatidylcholines_Using a Dual Stage CID Fragmentation Coupled with Ion Mobility Mass Spectrometry. *J Am Soc Mass Spectrom*. Vol 22, pp. 1552-67.

[53] Huang Z, Jiang J, Tyurin V, et al. (2009). Cardiolipin_deficiency leads to decreased cardiolipin peroxidation and increased resistance of cells to apoptosis. *Free Radic Biol Med*. Vol 44, pp. 1935-44.

[54] Oleic- and Docosahexaenoic Acid-Containing_Phosphatidylethanolamines_Differentially Phase Separate from Sphingomyelin. Shaikh S, LoCascio D, Soni S, et al. (2010). *Biochim Biophys Acta*. Vol 1788, pp 2421-26.

[55] Esquenazi S, and Bazan H. (2010). Role of_Platelet-Activating Factor_in Cell Death Signaling in the Cornea: A Review. *Mol Neurobiol*. Vol 42, pp. 32-38.

[56] Gimenez M, Oliveros L, and Gomez N. (2011). Nutritional Deficiencies and Phospholipid Metabolism. *Int J Mol Sci*. Vol 12, pp 2408-33.

[57] Levantesi G, Silletta M, and Marchioli R. (2010). Uses and benefits of omega-3 ethyl esters in patients with cardiovascular disease. *J Multidiscip Healthc*. Vol 3, pp. 79-96.

[58] Gulati S, Liu Y, Munkacsi A, et al. (2011). Sterols and sphingolipids: Dynamic duo or partners in crime?. *Prog Lipid Res*. Vol 49, pp. 353-65.

[59] Izar M, Teganiv D, Kasmas S, et al. (2010). Phytosterols and phytosterolemia: gene–diet interactions *Genes Nutr*. Vol 6, pp. 17-26.

[60] Björkhem I. (2009). Are side-chain oxidized oxysterols regulators also in vivo?. *J Lipid Res*. Vol 50, pp. S213–18.

Section 2

Molecular Aspects of Lipid Metabolism

Chapter 2

Oxidative Stress and Lipid Peroxidation – A Lipid Metabolism Dysfunction

Claudia Borza, Danina Muntean, Cristina Dehelean, Germaine Săvoiu,
Corina Şerban, Georgeta Simu, Mihaiela Andoni,
Marius Butur and Simona Drăgan

Additional information is available at the end of the chapter

http://dx.doi.org/10.5772/51627

1. Introduction

Free radicals are chemical compounds with unpaired electron(s), therefore being considered very active molecules. The cells had developed their own antioxidant defence systems in order to prevent the free radicals synthesis and to limit their toxic effects. These systems consist of enzymes which breakdown the peroxides, enzymes which bind transitional metals or compounds which are considered scavengers of the free radicals. Reactive species oxidize the biomolecules that will further elicit tissue injury and cell death. Evaluation of free radicals involvement in pathology is rather difficult due to their short life time.

2. Biochemistry of reactive oxygen species (ROS)

Free radicals can be formed by three mechanisms.

- Homolytic cleavage of a covalent bond of a molecule, each fragment retaining one electron

$$X{:}\,Y \rightarrow X^{\cdot} + Y^{\cdot}$$

- Loss by a molecule of a single electron

$$A \rightarrow A^{\cdot} + e^{-}$$

- Addition by a molecule of a single electron

$$A\,e^{-} \rightarrow A^{-\cdot}$$

- Heterolytic cleavage – covalent bond electrons are held up by only one of the molecule's fragments. Basically, charged ions occur.

$$XY \rightarrow X:^{-} + Y$$

Oxygen activation is the main factor that induces enhanced formation of ROS. Due to its presence in the atmosphere, but also in the body, free radicals reaction with oxygen is inevitable. A second characteristic of oxygen refers to its electronic structure. Thus, O_2 has on the outer layer two unpaired electrons, each located on one orbital. Therefore, oxygen can be considered a free di-radical, but with a lower reactivity. Oxidation of this electron donor is achieved by spin inversion from the O_2 reaction with transition metals or by univalent reduction in two phases of one electron [5]. These two mechanisms underlie oxidation reactions that occur in nature. Although this process represents only 5%, following the univalent reduction of O_2, ROS occurs, with greater reactivity and toxicity, as is the hydroxyl radical OH.

In biological systems, the most important free radicals are oxygen derivate radicals formed by the following mechanisms:

O_2 reduction by the transfer of an electron will result in the synthesis of the superoxide anion ($O_2^{\cdot -}$). The formation of the superoxide anion is the first step of O_2 activation and occurs in the body during normal metabolic processes. In some cells, its production is continuous, which implies the existence of intracellular antioxidants [3].

$$O_2 + e^{-} \rightarrow O_{2-}$$

Tissue alteration by traumatic, chemical or infectious means causes cell lysis along with the release of iron from deposits or by the action of hydrolases on metalloproteinase.

Reduced transition metal autooxidation generates the superoxide anion. The reaction of transition metal ions with O_2 can be considered a reversible redox reaction, important in promoting ROS formation.

$$Fe^{2} + O_2 \rightarrow Fe^{3} + O_{2-}$$

$$Cu + O_2 \rightarrow Cu^{2} + O_{2-}$$

Degradation of H_2O_2 in the presence of transition metal ions leads to the formation of the most reactive and toxic ROS: the hydroxyl radical (OH.) (Fenton and Haber-Weiss reaction). To this radical, the body does not present antioxidant defense systems such as for the superoxide anion or hydrogen peroxide (H_2O_2). Although metallothioneins (natural antioxidants) are proteins that bind to metal ions, including Fe^{2+}, thus inhibiting the Haber-Weiss reaction, however they are found in too low concentrations in the body to be effective in the decomposition of the hydroxyl radical. But these reactions can be inhibited by specific scavengers for OH, such as mannitol and chelating agents: desferroxamine. However, chelators as EDTA stimulate this reaction.

The reduction of O_2 by two electrons leads to the formation of hydrogen peroxide, H_2O_2.

$$O_2 + 2e^- + 2H \rightarrow H_2O_2$$

H_2O_2 is often formed in biological systems via peroxide anion production.

$$2O_{2-} + 2H \rightarrow H_2O_2 + O_2$$

H_2O_2 is not a free radical, but falls within the category of reactive oxygen species that include not only free radicals but also its non-radical derivatives involved in producing these ROS. Of all free radicals, H_2O_2 is the most stable and the easiest to quantify. Intracellular formation of hydrogen peroxide, depending on the content of catalase, is the way by which the bactericidal mechanism is achieved in phagocytosis.

The formation of singlet oxygen ($^1O_2$). It represents an excited form of molecular oxygen, resulting from the absorption of an energy quantum. It is equated to a ROS due to its strong reactivity. Singlet oxygen has an electrophilic character, reacting with many organic compounds: polyunsaturated fatty acids, cholesterol, hydroperoxides or organic compounds containing S or N atoms, producing oxides. In plasma it is neutralized by the presence of antioxidants, especially albumin.

Singlet oxygen is formed in the following reactions:

- Reaction of hydrogen peroxide or hydroxyl radical with the superoxide anion
- Different enzymatic catalyzed reactions
- Decomposition of endoperoxides
- Degradation of hydroperoxides in liver microsomes

2.1. Free radicals resulting in lipid peroxidation propagation phase

Lipid peroxidation is a complex process consisting of three major phases: initiation, propagation and end of the reaction. The initiation phase is slow due to the need of accumulation of a sufficient quantity of ROS, followed by the activation process of oxygen which is the amplifier factor. The process' latency period is that which determines the continuation of reactions by altering the oxidative balance in favor of pro-oxidant factors. The evolution of these reactions is unpredictable due to the formation of own catalysts determining the complexity of the process [1].

Free radicals are very unstable, their lifetime being very short. Their reactivity results from their coupling at the end of the reaction, only for an unpaired electron to reappear, thus stimulate the propagation of the reaction by forming a new radical.

The end of the reaction occurs by:

- Free radical recombination among them or,
- Intervention of antioxidant systems with membrane or intracellular action: superoxide dismutase (SOD), catalase.

Peroxides and their decomposition products (aldehydes, lipofuscin) are the most stable and represent the final link of O_2 activation. They are produced directly by the hydroxyl or singlet oxygen radical. During these reactions, own catalysts are formed, represented by free radicals or degradation products that diversify and increase the oxidation reactions; the structures involved are diverse, and are represented by polyunsaturated fatty acids, hemoproteins, nucleic acids, carbohydrates or steroids [4].

3. The production of reactive oxygen species

3.1. Endogenous production

The electron transfer in the respiratory chain involves an incomplete reduction of molecular O_2 at a rate of 1-2% with the formation of superoxide anion and of singlet oxygen.

If the anion is released in a low in protons environment, it will initiate peroxidation, the substrate being formed by polyunsaturated fatty acids from cell membranes.

If the anion will reach a proton rich environment, dismutation will take place; this following auditioning an electron from another anion and by proton reaction will form hydrogen peroxide. Dismutation can occur spontaneously, but in this case it takes place very slowly or catalyzed by SOD, which increases 10^{10} the reaction rate to the body's pH. There is an inversely proportional relationship between reaction rate and pH value. The efficiency of this enzyme is proven by its presence in all aerobic cells, and cells exposed to oxygen action, as hepatocytes and erythrocytes, contain large amounts of SOD [6].

$$O_{2-} + e^{-} \rightarrow O_2^{-} + 2H \rightarrow H_2O_2$$

Superoxide anion production during mitochondrial respiration has a self-regulation mechanism. Superoxide anion formed in part by autoxidation of NADH dehydrogenase, can then induce this enzyme's inactivation, so the presence of SOD in the membrane matrix to achieve dismutation is absolutely necessary. It results that the two enzymes SOD and NADPH dehydrogenase are a metabolic control and energy preservation couple in the presence of oxygen [7].

The release of hydrogen peroxide is proportional to the partial pressure of O_2. In case of a cerebral or cardiac ischemia, extramitochondrial concentration decreases, disrupting oxidative phosphorylation and ATP levels. An inversely proportional relationship between mitochondrial H_2O_2 formation rate and lifetime exists. Thus, it was observed experimentally that old animals present an increase in lipid peroxide formation in the mitochondria as a result of increased production of superoxide anion compared with young animals.

Antimicrobial defense. Phagocytosis of bacterial germs is accompanied by a massive production of superoxide anions and other derivatives (OH^-, HOCl, H_2O_2, $1O_2$) from the leukocyte metabolism. A NADPH-dependent oxidase, activated by protein kinase C and arachidonic acid released under the action of phospholipase A allow anion synthesis with an increased consumption of O_2.

The sequence of reactions initiated in the membrane continues into the cytoplasm where a substantial amount of superoxide anion is formed which then is diffuses also extracellularly. Increased use of glucose occurs for energetic purposes and for restoring NADPH and oxygen consumption necessary for the production of ROS [8].

Hydrogen peroxide is toxic on the neutrophil, which is inhibited by the presence at this level of the three enzymes that degrade the excess of peroxide: GSH-peroxidase, catalase and myeloperoxidase.

The enzyme present in phagosome, myeloperoxidase, will catalyze in the presence of H_2O_2 and chloride ions, forming toxic halogenated derivatives.

$$H_2O_2 + Cl^- \rightarrow ClO^- + H_2O$$

In turn, hypochlorous acid can react with aminic groups or with the ammonium ion (NH_4) forming chloramines. In the presence of hydrogen peroxide, HOCl forms singlet oxygen. These products of activated leukocytes have bactericidal properties.

Based on the properties of leukocytes to emit chemiluminescence during phagocytosis, this method has a clinic utility. Chemiluminescence emission is due to formation of free radicals, lipid peroxides and prostaglandin synthesis, a process associated with phagocytosis. This property is suppressed by anesthesia, cytostatic agents and anti-inflammatory preparations. Drugs with anti-inflammatory effect inhibit the activity of cyclooxygenase, the enzyme involved in prostaglandin synthesis.

A deficiency in the leukocyte production of free radicals (septic granulomatosis) or decrease of myeloperoxidase activity (following corticotherapy) is characterized by particularly sensitivity to infections.

During phagocytosis, three cytotoxic and antimicrobial effect mechanisms take place:

- oxygen dependent mechanism involves activation of myeloperoxidase and other peroxidases
- Nitrogen compounds dependent mechanism involving participation of NO, NO_2, other nitrogen oxides and nitrites. In this mechanism both types of cytotoxic inorganic oxidants interact: oxygen and nitrogen reactive radicals.
- The third mechanism is independent of oxygen and nitrogen by changing phagolysosome pH that favors the action of antimicrobial substances present in the lysosomal or nuclear level.

The constitutive form of NO synthase is found in endothelial cells, neutrophils, neurons. The existence of the inducible form has been shown in macrophages, hepatocytes, endothelial cells, neutrophils and platelets. Glucocorticoids inhibit the expression of inducible NO synthase but not of the constitutive enzyme.

Nitrogen reactive radicals have a cytotoxic effect by inhibiting mitochondrial respiration, DNA synthesis, and mediate oxidation of protein and non-protein sulfhydryl groups.

Although NO has a protective role at the vascular level by a relaxing effect (EDRF), under certain conditions it may exert a cytotoxic effect, causing pathological vasodilatation, tissue destructions, inhibits platelet aggregation, modulates lymphocyte and immune response function.

Synthesis of prostaglandins. Phospholipase A_2 catalyzes the degradation of membrane phospholipids with arachidonic acid formation. Stimuli such as phagocytosis, antibody production, and immune complex formation, the action of bacterial endotoxins or cytokines stimulate the activation of this enzyme. There are two enzymatic forms: type I PLA_2, membrane bound, which is stimulated by Ca^{2+} at physiological pH, and the type II one, cytoplasmic, which is inhibited by Ca^{2+} and is active at acidic pH. Two enzymes, lipoxygenase and cyclooxygenase, bound to plasmic and microsomal membranes, convert arachidonic acid in derivatives such as: thromboxane, prostaglandins, leukotrienes [18].

Under the action of lipoxygenase, arachidonic acid is converted into a hydroperoxide: hydroperoxyeicosatetraenoic acid (HPETE) which will release the hydroxyl radical during its transformation into hydroxyeicosatetraenoic acid (HETE). Hill et al. have emphasized the role of glutathione peroxidase (GSH-Px) and of glutathione in this reaction: blocking the activity of this enzyme, they have noticed a significant decrease (of 66%) of HPETE conversion in HETE [14, 16].

Under the action of cyclooxygenase, arachidonic acid incorporates two oxygen molecules to form an endoperoxide, PGG; it loses the OH group to form PGH. This transformation, which is accompanied by the release of hydroxyl radical, exerts a negative retro-control to prostaglandin synthesis, inactivating the cyclooxygenase. Some of the products developed have a complex effect on the inflammatory process: thus, in the first phase, PGE_2 acts on cells from the vascular wall with a procoagulant effect, and in the late phase it has an inflammatory effect by inhibiting leukocyte activation and oxidative metabolism of these cells during phagocytosis. The byproducts resulting from this process will be the ones to modulate the intensity of the next phase [15, 22].

The two endoperoxides formed, PGG_2 and PGH_2, have an inducible role on the production of PCI_2 or TxA, being involved in the mechanism that ensures homeostasis of the vascular and platelet phase of hemostasis.

The other enzyme has a dual effect, and promotes the initiation of lipid peroxidation and the decomposition of resulting products of these reactions.

3.2. Exogenous production

The human body is subjected to aggression from various agents capable of producing free radicals. Thus, UVs induce the synthesis of ROS and free radicals generating molecules via photosensitizing agents.

Ingestion of alcohol causes ROS synthesis by different mechanisms: xanthine oxidase and aldehyde oxidase can oxidase the main metabolite of ethanol (acetaldehyde) resulting in superoxide anion.

Ethanol also stimulates the production of superoxide anion and, by inducing NADPH-oxidase synthesis, NADPH cytochrome reductase and P450 cytochrome.

The alcohol ingestion decreases the activity of protective enzymes (SOD, glutathione peroxidase). Also low serum concentrations of selenium and vitamin E have been found in alcoholics.

Toxic substances as nitrogen oxide and nitrogen dioxide in the environment are responsible for autoxidation of polyunsaturated fatty acids in lung alveoli. The reaction may be reversible or irreversible. $NO^{\cdot}$ and NO_2 may react with H_2O_2 produced by alveolar macrophages and can generate the hydroxyl radical.

The reduction of carbon tetrachloride (CCl_4) in $CCl_3^{\cdot}$ performed under the action of cytochrome P_{450} or in the presence of Fe_2 is another factor that induces autoxidation of polyunsaturated fatty acids, increasing lipid hydroperoxides concentration.

Anticancer drugs are able to synthesize free radicals, this process depending on the mode of action and their toxicity.

These drugs under the action of cytochrome P450-dependent enzymes produce the activation of O_2 with the formation of ROS which will attack GSH and other thiols (hemoglobin), causing the formation of lipid peroxides and activation of Ca^{2+}-dependent endonucleases.

These mechanisms can induce disturbances of the coagulation system (increased hemolysis), severe forms of cardiomyopathies, because of the low level of cardiac antioxidants (AO) [25].

4. Reactive oxygen species and oxidative stress

In physiological conditions a delicate balance exists between ROS production and the antioxidant capacity. A higher ROS production and/or a decreased antioxidant capacity is responsible for the harmful effects of free radicals or the oxidative stress (OS). Oxidative stress represents an important pathogenic mechanism involved in inflammation, cancerogenesis or aging [24].

End products of free radicals action, aldehydes, inhibit the activity of membrane enzymes (glucose-6-phosphate, adenylate cyclase). These aldehydes react selectively with proteins or enzymes containing SH groups and cause tissue destructions.

The emergence of OS is one of the most important pathogenic mechanisms involved in inflammation, carcinogenesis, radiation disease and aging.

The objective of various experimental models was to study erythrocyte response to oxidant substances action. Erythrocyte characteristics and test substance dosing allowed the evaluation of OS; these experiments can be extrapolated to explain various physiological or pathological processes in the body.

Oxidative stress is an ongoing process in the body, and under physiologic conditions there are effective mechanisms that negate its effects, thus high concentration of erythrocyte GSH and related enzyme equipment provide a defense against ROS.

Erythrocyte congenital enzyme deficiencies confer erythrocytes an increased sensitivity to OS.

A section of the body intensely studied to assess OS is the liver due to its role in the metabolism of a wide range of endogenous and exogenous products. Thus, by the metabolism of aromatic compounds, drugs or carcinogenic hydrocarbons in the live, a large amount of FR occurs, which will initiate in the next phase OS from this level.

Liver antioxidant systems are represented by SOD, GSH and dependent enzymes (transferase and peroxidase). Using ESR and spin trapping, FR resulting from chemical pollutants metabolism were identified, and a strong correlation between the functional impairment of the hepatic parenchyma, free radicals formation and decrease in GSH was noted. Under these conditions, free radicals of that substance occur which can cause tissue destructions also without O_2 activation.

The experimental poisoning of rats with alcohol (1.5 mmol/kg) showed significant decrease at one hour of ingestion of GSH, vitamin E and C along with hepatic necrosis and formation of lipid peroxides [2, 11].

GSH is an important protective factor against OS. Its level is interrelated with other antioxidants (vitamin C and E) that stimulate its preservation in reduced form.

Stress proteins. Structurally altered intracellular protein group, whose synthesis is induced by oxidative stress has been named stress proteins group. Of particular interest is the 32 kDa protein whose synthesis is induced by the action of ionizing radiation, hydrogen peroxide. This protein is a marker of generalized response to oxidative stress. Free radicals affect cytokines (endogenous pyrogens: IL-1, IL-2, TNF-a, IFN) that play a role in regulating signal transmission in response to stress which will cause the synthesis of these proteins. It is considered that SOD itself is a stress protein.

The tissue repair process is enzymatically catalyzed (repair enzymes) that break down damaged cellular particles, take intact aminoacids to synthesize new defense proteins.

5. The effects of reactive oxygen species

5.1. Oxygen free radicals – Intracellular messengers

Before discussing the negative effect of oxygen activation on the body, we should also take into consideration their involvement in certain physiological processes, when these ROS are produced in quantities which do not exceed the antioxidant capacity. Thus, the superoxide anion is produced by leukocytes during phagocytosis and in smooth muscle cells, epithelial cells, skin fibroblasts and endothelial cells [27].

The anion produced by macrophages and endothelial cells induces conformational changes of receptors on the LDL lipoprotein surface, allowing their recognition and involvement in atherogenesis [10, 12].

It is also involved in cascade-type metabolic reactions of arachidonic acid and in achieving platelet adhesion and aggregation function.

5.2. Lipid peroxidation

Formation of peroxides, especially lipid ones, is a consequence of the activation of O_2, the interconversion of reactive species and natural systems protection overcoming. In biological environments, the most favorable substrate for peroxidation is represented by polyunsaturated fatty acids (PUFA), components of cell and subcellular membranes.

Peroxidation is a complex process that includes three phases: initiation, propagation, end-decomposition, which interpose, so that only end products can be determined chemically: aldehydes (malondialdehyde), polymerized carbonyl compounds (lipofuscin) [9].

A radical character initiator (which may have different structures and origins, including peroxy ROO· radicals) removes a hydrogen atom from polyunsaturated fatty acid diallyl carbon, forming a favorable reactive center for oxygen action. The peroxy ROO· radicals which become hydroperoxides result. In fact, due to side reactions, other locations of the peroxide group per PUFA molecule occur [28].

5.3. Cell structural alterations

Since the formation of peroxides and their decomposition products, the sequence of reactions passes from a molecular level to a cellular one due to structural changes that occur in membranes: structural disorganization of the membrane and deterioration of pores crossing the double phospholipid layers. Peroxidation leads to changes in fatty acid qualitative composition of phospholipids composition with changing the ratio between PUFA and other acids. The first two effects induce the third, which consists in a decrease in membrane fluidity and altered active ion transport; these effects finally lead to changes in ion and other intracellular compounds concentration [26].

Numerous experimental studies have shown that tissue injury caused by free radicals determined at one point an imbalance of Ca^{2+} (i.e., increases in intracellular Ca^{2+} concentration). Under physiological conditions, there are effective homeostatic mechanisms (enzyme systems, protein transporters) to keep an optimum ratio between intracellular (0.1-0.4 microM) and extracellular of the mM order concentration. Overcoming these mechanisms (in this case by producing free radicals) determines the accumulation of calcium in the cell which will lead to structural membrane alterations, production of unsaturated lipids, efflux of GSH, its transition to an oxidized form and the creation of an intracellular oxidative potential [21, 23].

Experimental studies on isolated hepatocytes have shown the correlation between the cellular toxicity of calcium and the decrease of tocopherols levels, substances with strong antioxidant character.

Maintaining the cell functional state ultimately depends on the level of proteins containing SH groups. Thus, the role of GSH in protection against oxidative stress is precisely regeneration of protein SH groups which in turn will ensure intracellular calcium homeostasis. Vitamin E stabilizes ATPase activity dependent of calcium in the endoplasmic reticulum by maintaining SH groups in the structure of the enzyme in reduced state. Also, vitamin E is protective against the compounds resulting from lipid peroxidation: a molecule of alpha-tocopherol protects against 500 molecules of polyunsaturated fatty acids.

5.4. DNA destruction

The results of chromatographic technique used to determine the urinary excretion products resulting from scission of DNA in humans showed a normal excretion in average of 100 nmol products. This total represents 10^3 thymine molecules oxidized per day for each of the $6X10^{13}$ cells in the body.

Between eliminating these products and the specific metabolic rate (SMR) there is a linear correlation.

The specific metabolic rate of an organism is dependent on the O_2 use rate by its tissues and it is proportional to the free radicals production rate. In this case, the ratio between the total concentration of antioxidants (enzymatic and non-enzymatic systems) and the metabolic rate represents the protection degree of a tissue or body to free radicals. It seems that there is a genetic programming of the metabolic rate for each species and individual.

Looking at the hypothesis on free radicals involvement in aging, it has been shown that there is an inversely proportional relationship between the metabolic rate, free radicals production, respectively, and he maximum lifespan potential (MLP). Thus, on the evolutionary scale, metabolic rate decreased and lifespan increased, in mammals their product being constant.

One can calculate the lifespan energy potential (LEP), expressed in kcal-kg as follows: LEP 2.70 X MLP X SMR. This potential is directly proportional to the total concentration of antioxidants.

During aging, the formation of free radicals amplifies by exposure to prooxidant factors from the environment, and by the decreased antioxidant defense capacity.

At an intracellular level (especially in muscles and neurons), deposits of lipofuscin pigments, lipid peroxides and their breakdown products are formed.

These deposits are mainly localized in the myocardium, brain, and, by the age of 80, they represent 70% of cytoplasmic volume of neurons and 6% of that of myocardiocytes.

Experimental studies demonstrated that in 50 years a person accumulates 13.4 mg/lipofuscin/gram of myocardium, pigment formation taking place once with exceeding the absorption of 0.6 free radicals micromoles/gram of tissue.

There is an inversely proportional relationship between the formation of these products and the concentration of vitamin E in the body.

To control the effects of aging, ones requires a moderate diet, which reduces metabolic rate and O_2 consumption with an optimal concentration of lipids and a quantitatively and qualitatively balanced intake of antioxidants and other factors that enhance assimilation and their metabolism. It is also necessary to achieve a balanced interaction of endogenous antioxidants.

The antioxidants level varies greatly depending on the age of the body, that organ and subcellular components; thus an increase of GSH-Px activity was noted in mitochondria of cardiac cells and erythrocytes in the elderly, and a decrease of activity in liver and kidneys. The decrease of SOD activity in the liver of the elderly was highlighted and no significant changes in the concentration of intramitochondrial SOD in the heart were noted.

Also, there is a correlation between the intensity of DNA destructions caused by FR and xanthine oxidase concentration. This enzyme, present in low concentrations, in tissue or plasma, increases under tissue injury.

5.5. Effects on molecules

Free radicals are responsible for the inactivation of enzymes especially of serine proteases, the fragmentation of macromolecules (collagen, proteoglycans, hyaluronic acid), the formation of dimers, the protein aggregates in the cytoplasmic membranes. The most susceptible amino acids to their action are tryptophan, tyrosine, phenylalanine, methionine and cysteine.

Transition metal ions (Fe, Cu, Ni, Co, Cd) have a pro-oxidant action by intensifying reactions in which FR are formed and those in which the decomposition of lipid peroxides takes place. At the molecular level, Fe^{2+} ion contributes to the induction of oxidative stress by increasing non-enzymatic oxidation of catecholamines and GSH, promoting lipid peroxide decomposition and the formation of the most toxic free radicals, the hydroxyl radical. Fe^{2+}, under complexed form as transferrin, is inactive against peroxides. Fe^{2+} release from transferrin takes place under pH decrease as it does in hypoxia, leukocyte activation or in muscle tissue during strenuous physical exercise. Another source of free Fe^{2+} is represented by hemoglobin, which at low concentrations acts as a pro-oxidant favoring PUFA peroxidation. Proteins that bind Fe^{2+} have a different action: thus, ferritin has a pro-oxidant capacity, while hemosiderin and lactoferrin are antioxidants.

Bilirubin, resulting from the metabolism of hemoglobin, as transition metal ions, causes alterations in the membrane structure by initiating PUFA peroxidation. Bilirubin crosses the blood-brain barrier, inhibits oxidative phosphorylation and decreases AMPc and GSH concentration. Thus, the encephalopathy caused by intense hemolytic jaundice in neonates is correlated with elevated levels of bilirubin, blood lipid peroxides and GSH decrease.

The same changes were observed in hepatitis of various etiologies (viral, ethanolic) and were correlated with graded morphological changes of the steatosis type, up to the irreversible ones, cirrhosis, caused by exceeding the protective antioxidant systems.

The bilirubin has an antioxidant effect, enhanced by binding to albumin, its plasma transport form. This different behavior of bilirubin depends on the concentration and the environment, like ascorbic acid, which features a pro- and antioxidant character, widely accepted today.

6. Reactive oxygen species – Implications in cardiovascular pathology

Atherosclerosis (ATS) and its notable complication, coronary heart disease, still represent the major cause of premature death worldwide. Several lines of evidence suggest that the major risk factors (hypertension, diabetes mellitus, hyperlipemia, smoking) elicit oxidative stress at the luminal surface of vascular wall that will be further responsible for the oxidative damage of lipoproteins, formation of lipid peroxides, platelet aggregation and activation of macrophages [10]. LDL lipoproteins are the easiest to be oxidized because of their high PUFA content; at variance from native LDL, oxidatively modified LDLs are more avidly taken up by macrophages via the scavenger receptor thus generating the well-known "foam cells" of the atherosclerotic plaques. Experimental studies demonstrated that LDL can be oxidized by all of the major cells of the arterial wall (macrophages, endothelial cells, smooth muscle cells). Besides its rapid uptake by macrophages, oxidized LDL elicit a chemoatractive effect facilitating monocyte adhesion to the endothelium and a toxic affect at the level of endothelial cells by inhibiting the release of nitric oxide. *In vivo* identification of oxidized LDL in atherosclerotic plaques clearly established in the late 80s the oxidative-modification theory of ATS. Much effort was further directed towards identification of factors that influence the susceptibility of LDL particles to oxidation. Among these, the presence of small dense LDS particles, of preformed lipid peroxides, as well as glycation or binding of LDLs to proteoglycans were proven to facilitate oxidation [12].

Highly reactive aldehydes are one of the major causative factors in oxidative related cardiovascular pathology and ageing. Specific aldehydes (e.g., 4-hydroxynonenal acetaldehyde, acrolein) were reported to be transiently increased in the settings of heart failure and ischemia-reperfusion injury [13] and to interfere with transcriptional regulation of endogenous anti-oxidant networks in mitochondria [1]. Recently, accumulation of reactive aldehydes was studied from the point of view of the subsequent protein carbonylation and its implication in cardiovascular pathophysiology [4].

On the other hand, decreased antioxidant defense further contributes to the oxidative damage. Low concentration of GSH-peroxidase in the vascular wall creates conditions favorable to the actions of hydrogen peroxide and other FR on lipids and lipoproteins [28]. In physiological conditions, nitric oxide acts as an antioxidant, inhibiting LDL peroxidation and their destructive effect on interstitial proteoglycans. With the increased production of FR, NO may become a prooxidant factor, stimulating LDL peroxidation by a mechanism involving myoglobin. Deficiency of other protective factors will favor oxidative injury. Lipid-soluble antioxidants such as tocopherols and ubiquinol are present in the hydrophobic environment of the lipoproteins in order to protect PUFA from FR attack. *In vitro* experimental data showed that: i) exposure of LDL to oxidative stress will trigger lipid peroxidation only after the loss of its above mentioned antioxidants and ii) enrichment of LDL with vitamin E will make LDL oxidation more difficult [6].

Accordingly, the beneficial role of antioxidant supplementation has been extensively investigated in the past decades in a variety of animal models. Most investigators reported beneficial effects, i.e., prevention of atherosclerotic lesions with vitamin E supplementation, yet an early study by Keaney et al. mentioned a deleterious effect of high doses of tocopherol on endothelial-dependent relaxation in cholesterol fed rabbits [11]. Unfortunately, despite the promising observational experimental data, several prospective, double-blind, placebo-controlled trials did not support a causal relationship between vitamin C and E supplementation and a lower risk of coronary heart disease [21]. Similarly, lack of beneficial effect with long term vitamin E supplementation was recently reported in large clinical trial (the Women's Health Study) that addressed the role of antioxidant therapy in the primary prevention of heart failure [2].

These negative results may be related to the fact that antioxidant supplements could abolish the physiological role of ROS as signaling molecules [18], especially when considering that most cardiovascular patients are treated with "pleiotropic" drugs such as statins, angiotensin-converting enzyme inhibitors, angiotensin receptor blockers, that besides their major effects are reported to reduce ROS formation [23]. Indeed, a large body of evidence demonstrated unequivocally that reduced amounts of reactive oxgen species, most probably of mitochondrial origin [17] but not exclusively, are essential in regulating cardiovascular homeostasis [19] as well as the powerful mechanisms of endogenous cardioprotection at postischemic reperfusion, namely pre- and postconditioning [20].

In conclusion, increasing the level of endogenous antioxidants, as recently suggested via the supplimentation of weak "pro-oxidants" [8], and not chronic supplementation with large dose of exogenous antioxidants could become in the future a more appropriate approach to treat diseases that share oxidative stress as a common denominator.

Author details

Claudia Borza, Danina Muntean, Cristina Dehelean,
Germaine Săvoiu, Corina Şerban, Georgeta Simu, Mihaiela Andoni,
Marius Butur and Simona Drăgan
University of Medicine and Pharmacy "Victor Babeş" Timişoara, Romania

7. References

[1] Anderson EJ, Katunga LA, Willis MS. Mitochondria as a source and target of lipid peroxidation products in healthy and diseased heart. *Clin Exp Pharmacol Physiol* 2012, 39(2): 179-93.

[2] Chae CU, Albert CM, Moorthy MV, Lee IM, Buring JE – Vitamin E supplementation and the risk of heart failure in women *Circ Heart Fail* 2012, 5(2): 176-82.

[3] Cheesman KH, Slater TF - An introduction to free radical biochemistry, in *Free radicals Medicine: British Medical Bulletin*, 1993, vol 49, 3, 481-494.

[4] Fritz KS, Petersen DR. Exploring the biology of lipid peroxidation-derived protein carbonylation. *Chem Res Toxicol* 2011, 24(9): 1411-1419.

[5] Fulbert J C, Cals M-J - Les radicaux libres en biologie clinique: origine, role pathogene et moyens de defense, in *Pathologie Biology*, 1992, vol 40, 1, 66-77.

[6] Gutteridge JM, Halliwell B. Antioxidants: Molecules, medicines, and myths. *Biochem Biophys Res Commun* 2010, 393(4): 561-564.

[7] Halliwel B, Gutteridge C, Cross C - Free radicals, antioxidants and human disease. Where are you now?, *J Lab Clin Med*, 1993, 119 (6), 606-610.

[8] Halliwell B. Free radicals and antioxidants: updating a personal view. *Nutr Rev* 2012, 70(5): 257-265.

[9] Holley A, Cheesman K H - Measuring free radical reactions in vivo, in *Free radicals in Medicine: British Medical Bulletin*, 1993, vol 49, 3, 494-506.

[10] 10.Kawada T - Oxidative stress markers and cardiovascular disease: advantage of using these factors in combination with lifestyle factors for cardiovascular risk assessment. *Int J Cardiol* 2012, 157(1): 119-120.

[11] Keaney JF Jr, Gaziano JM, Xu A, Frei B, Curran-Celentano J, Shwaery GT, Loscalzo J, Vita JA – Low dose alpha-tocopherol improves and high-dose alpha tocopherol worsens endothelial dependent vasodilator function in cholesterol-fed rabbits. *Journal of Clinical Investigation*, 1994, 93(2):844-851.

[12] Lee R, Margaritis M, Channon KM, Antoniades C - Evaluating oxidative stress in human cardiovascular disease: methodological aspects and considerations. *Curr Med Chem* 2012, 19(16): 2504-20.

[13] Marczin N, El-Habashi N, Hoare GS, Bundy RE, Yacoub M - Antioxidants in myocardial ischemia-reperfusion injury: therapeutic potential and basic mechanisms. *Arch Biochem Biophys* 2003, 420 (2), 222-236.

[14] Mederle C, Raica M, Schneider F, Tănăsie G - The constrictor effect of acethylcoline by enhanced hydrogen peroxide in ovalbumin - sensitised rat tracheal muscle. *The Romanian - Hungarian Physiology Joint - Meeting, 1996, Szeged - Timişoara, Physiology*, 6, 2 (10).

[15] Mederle C, Schneider F, Mătieş R - Oxidative stress evaluation in experimental and clinical asthma. *Inter Rew Allerg Clinic Immunol*, III, 1997,1: 30-31.

[16] Mederle C, Schneider F, Raica M - Free radicals and mast cell reaction in tracheal muscle of rats sensitised with ovalbumin. *Allergy* (suppl), 1996, 31, 51: 188-189.

[17] Muntean DM, Mirica SN, Ordodi V, Răducan AM, Duicu OM, Gheorghiu G, Henţia C, Fira-Mlădinescu O, Săndesc D – Mitocondria: novel therapeutic target in cardioprotection. *Rev Rom Med Vet* 2008, 1(4): 406-412.

[18] Murphy MP, Holmgren A, Larsson NG, Halliwell B, Chang CJ, et al. Unraveling the biological roles of reactive oxygen species. *Cell Metab* 2011, 13(4): 361-6

[19] Otani H. Reactive oxygen species as mediators of signal transduction in ischemic preconditioning. *Antiox Redox Signal* 2004, 6(2): 449-469.

[20] Penna C, Mancardi D, Rastaldo R, Pagliaro P - Cardioprotection: a radical view. Free radicals in pre- and postconditioning. *Biochim Biophys Acta*, 2009, 1787(7): 781-93.

[21] Riccioni G, Frigiola A, Pasquale S, Massimo deG, D'Orazio N - Vitamin C and E consumption and coronary heart disease in men. *Front Biosci* 2012, 1(4): 373-380.

[22] Schneider F, Mederle C, Mătieş R, Săvoiu G, Goţia S, Mihalaş G I, Buftea A - Drug influence of morphological and functional response in contention stress by rats. *Fiziologia - Physiology*, 1992, 2, 2:27.

[23] Selvaraju V, Joshi M, Suresh S, Sanchez JA, Maulik N, Maulik G Diabetes, oxidative stress, molecular mechanism, and cardiovascular disease - an overview. *Toxicology Mech Met* 2012, 22(5): 330-5.

[24] Sies H - Oxidative stress: From Basic Research to Clinical Application: *The American Journal of Medicine: Proceedings of a Symposium: Oxidants and Antioxidants: Pathophysiological Determinants and Therapeutic Agents*: vol 91 (3C), 1991, (3C-31S).

[25] Tinkel J, Hassanain H, Khouri SJ - Cardiovascular antioxidant therapy: a review of supplements, pharmacotherapies, and mechanisms. *Cardiol Rev* 2012, 20(2): 77-83.

[26] Valko M, Leibfritz D, Moncol J, Cronin M, Mazur M, Telser J. Free radicals and antioxidants in normal physiological functions and human disease. *Int J Biochem & Cell Biol* 2007, 39, 44-84.

[27] Verceloti M G, Severson P S, Duane P, Moldow F - Hydrogen peroxide alters signal transduction in human endothelial cells. *J Lab Clin Med*, 1991, 117,1: 15-23.

[28] Yung LM, Leung FP, Yao X, Chen ZY, Huang Y. Reactive oxygen species in vascular wall. *Cardiovasc Hematol Disord Drug Tagets*. 2006, 6(1): 1-19.

Chapter 3

The Role of Copper as a Modifier of Lipid Metabolism

Jason L. Burkhead and Svetlana Lutsenko

Additional information is available at the end of the chapter

http://dx.doi.org/10.5772/51819

1. Introduction

1.1. Copper homeostasis in mammals

Dietary copper enters the body largely through the small intestine. Two membrane transporters are essential for this process. The high affinity copper uptake protein Ctr1 is responsible for making copper that enters via the apical membrane available in the cytosol for further utilization (1), whereas the copper-transporting ATPase ATP7A facilitates copper exit from the enterocytes into circulation (2) (Figure 1). Complete genetic inactivation of either transporter in experimental animals is embryonically lethal (3-5). However, partial inactivation or tissue specific inactivation of ATP7A or Ctr1, respectively, in either case is associated with copper accumulation in the intestine, impaired copper entry into the bloodstream, and severe copper deficiency in many organs and tissues (1). Copper deficiency, in turn, produces distinct metabolic changes that are discussed in detail in the following sections.

The majority of absorbed dietary copper is initially delivered to the liver. Hepatocytes utilize copper for their metabolic needs (such as respiration and radical defense); they also synthesize and secrete the major copper containing protein in serum, ceruloplasmin, and prevent copper overload in the body by exporting excess copper via the canalicular membrane into the bile (Figure 1). These two important functions of hepatocytes (the production of ceruloplasmin and the removal of excess copper) are performed by another transporter, the copper transporting ATPase ATP7B, which is homologous to ATP7A (6, 7). Inactivation of ATP7B in patients with Wilson's disease and in animal models is associated with marked copper overload in the liver and pathologic changes including marked lipid dysregulation in the liver and the serum (discussed in the later sections).

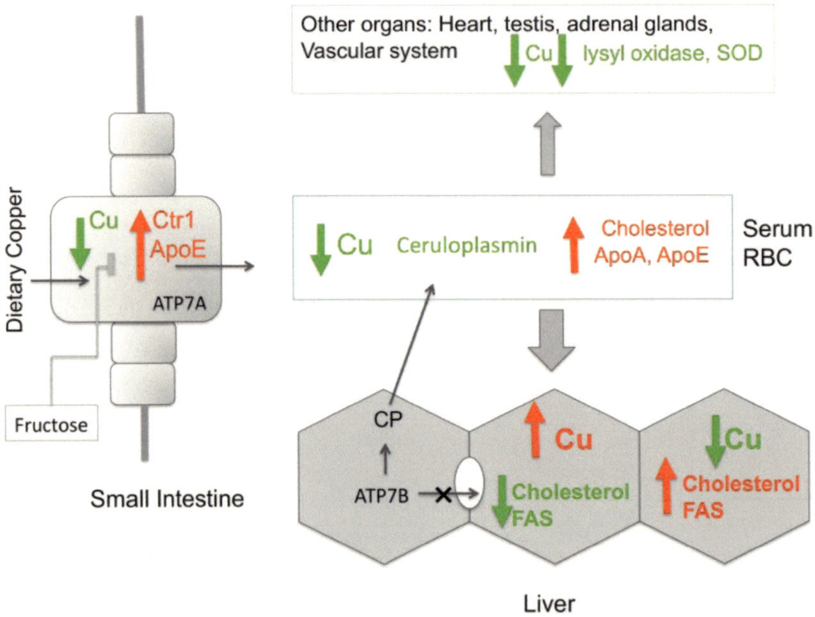

Figure 1. Copper homeostasis and lipid metabolism display functional interactions. Copper enters circulation via small intestine where copper transporters Ctr1 and ATP7A play the major role in the dietary copper absorption. Dietary copper deficiency is associated with a lower level of ceruloplasmin in the serum and increase in cholesterol and lipoproteins. Copper deficiency also upregulates the copper uptake protein Ctr1 in intestine; this compensatory effects is diminished by high fructose. In the liver, copper deficiency is associated with increased synthesis of cholesterol and higher expression of fatty acid synthase (FAS). Also, in the liver, the copper-transporting ATPase ATP7B mediates copper delivery to ceruloplasmin and copper export into the bile. Genetic inactivation of ATP7B in Wilson's disease is associated with copper overload and marked changes in lipid metabolism. Cholesterol biosynthesis is downregulated and both the serum and hepatic lipid profiles are altered.

The level of expression of copper transporters and their regulation varies between various organs (8). For example, ATP7B is the main transporter in hepatocytes, but it is absent from the adrenal gland, whereas opposite is true for ATP7A (9). Most of the tissues such as heart, brain, lung, placenta and kidneys express both copper-transporting ATPases along with the two copper uptake systems Ctr1 and Ctr2. As a result, the consequences of copper deficiency and copper overload are tissue specific, and certain organs such as heart or liver are more profoundly affected (see below). Recent studies also revealed an important homeostatic cross-talk between different organs in either copper deficiency or copper overload. For example, copper overload in the liver is accompanied by functional copper deficiency in the adrenal gland (9), whereas severe copper deficiency in the heart stimulates copper efflux from the liver (10), presumably to compensate for the deleterious effects of copper depletion.

The analysis of available literature also illustrates that variations in copper levels, either through the diet or as a result of genetic copper misbalance, have a profound effect on lipid metabolism. Significance of these observations is becoming more and more apparent given recent data that dietary influences (such as amount of fat in the diet) could be important modifiers of the course and severity of the disorders associated with copper misbalance (11). Reciprocally, copper deficiency has emerged as a factor in the development of Non-alcoholic Fatty-Liver Disease (NAFLD)(12, 13), although current reports paint complex picture (14) and further studies are needed. Despite ample phenotypic evidence in support of copper-lipid interactions, little mechanistic work has been done so far, and current understanding of this metabolic interaction at the molecular level is very limited. The goal of this review is to illustrate and emphasize the need for such detailed mechanistic investigations.

2. Copper deficiency

2.1. Copper in western diet

Copper deficiency has long been known to alter lipid metabolism; consequently, it has been proposed as a significant factor in human diseases associated with dyslipidemia (15). Copper deficiency is rarely diagnosed in humans, with a notable exception of a growing number of reports pointing to copper and other mineral insufficiencies as unintended consequences of bariatric surgeries (16-18). The under-detection of copper deficiency could be due to limitations of screening using serum or urine samples. Although liver is the main homeostatic organ for copper and has a high copper content, copper levels in serum and urine do not correlate well with a hepatic copper concentration (19), possibly masking deficiency in the liver.

Recent work using a categorical regression analysis of copper deficiency and excess shows a U-shaped dose-response curve. Compilation of data on toxicity due to copper excess and deficiency yielded a generalized linear model that was used to estimate adverse responses depending on copper dose or severity of copper limitation, as well as duration of copper misbalance (20). This model indicates that for humans the optimal intake level for Cu is 2.6 mg/day. The current United States Recommended Daily Intake is only 0.9 mg (US Food and Nutrition Board), whereas dietary study indicated that even 1.03 mg of Cu/day may be insufficient for adult men (21). The results of the third National Health and Nutrition Examination Survey (NHANES III, 2003) in the US showed that the mean daily intake of copper, depending on age, was 1.54–1.7 mg/day (±0.05 standard deviation (SD)) for men and 1.13-1.18 mg/d (±0.05 SD) for women. These results imply that a large portion of the population may have insufficient dietary copper intake and mild copper deficiency.

2.2. Low copper and human disease

Current data suggest that copper deficiency may be a common contributing factor in cardiovascular disease (CVD) and non-alcoholic fatty-liver disease (NAFLD) (22-24). As described above, surgical obesity treatment has also been strongly implicated in copper deficiency, likely by causing a diminished absorption of copper after a gastric bypass surgery (16-18). In addition, low copper levels were detected in organs, plasma and tissue of patients with several chronic diseases including cardiovascular disease, central nervous system, and musculoskeletal disorders (25). In fact, it was suggested that an ischemic heart disease could be largely attributed to copper deficiency (26), and that Cu deficiency and the high sugar consumption characteristic in the Western diet may interact in CVD (27). In a rat model, copper deficiency that reduces plasma levels of copper and ceruloplasmin also reduces copper content of the heart, liver, and testes. Coincidentally, heart zinc is also reduced, whereas hepatic iron levels rise (28), demonstrating the multifaceted effects of copper depletion on the overall body metal homeostasis.

Numerous studies in the rodent and other animal models (discussed below) provide strong indication of a significant link between copper deficiency and dyslipidemia. Specific studies linking human lipid response to copper deficiency are very limited. The available reports clearly illustrate the need for a better mechanistic insight. For example, studies using healthy male volunteers showed severe copper depletion with a diet containing 0.83 mg Cu/day, which is similar to levels in some contemporary diets. In these individuals, along with the diminished copper, the levels of serum copper-depended enzyme ceruloplasmin were reduced, as was copper-zinc superoxide dismutase activity in erythrocytes. In parallel, changes in lipid metabolism were evident. Cholesterol was elevated in the serum, and changes in the cholesterol levels were found to be more sensitive to copper levels than changes in hematology (29). These observations suggest that the dietary copper levels may be significant modifying factors in the disorders associated with lipid misbalance. Indeed, a role for copper deficiency is emerging in NAFLD (discussed below).

2.3. Low copper levels and hypercholesterolemia

Current data indicate that copper deficiency is associated with specific effects on systemic lipid metabolism. Although copper deficiency affects multiple organs (liver, heart, intestine, brain, adipose tissue), the liver and cardiovascular system appear more profoundly affected compared to other tissues. The effects of copper deficiency are partially reversible. In a middle-aged adult population with cardiovascular disease (CVD), copper supplementation was shown to raise the serum copper enzyme activities, but improvement of CVD measures was inconsistent (30). The same report also showed that copper supplementation reduced levels of oxidized serum LDL with statistical significance, but the results were inconsistent necessitating further research.

As described above, plasma cholesterol levels rise in human volunteers consuming a marginally low copper diet (29). In humans, the molecular mechanism behind this phenomenon has not yet been investigated in detail. However, much effort has been made characterizing the influence of copper deficiency on serum cholesterol as well as lipid profiles using animal models. These studies yielded wealth of useful information. Early work feeding rats a copper deficient diet revealed hypercholesterolemia, cardiac hypertrophy, hemorrhage, inflammation, and focal necrosis (31). This work also indicated that some of the cardiac pathology caused by copper deficiency could be linked to the lysyl oxidase deficiency. Lysyl oxidase (LOX) is a copper-dependent enzyme involved in the cross-linking of collagen and elastin. Aortas of copper-deficient rats showed deformation and loss of elasticity, though myocardial arteries were normal. Since lysyl oxidase is only one of the copper dependent enzymes required for proper heart functions (others include cytochrome C oxidase, cytosolic superoxide dismutase, dopamine beta-mono-oxygenase) the role of low copper in CVD may be realized through multiple mechanisms in addition to the altered lipid metabolism.

The development of cholesterolemia in response to copper deficiency has been explored in some detail in rats. Copper deficiency was found to be associated with the increased HDL and LDL levels (30% increase in HDL in one study). In addition, the plasma volume also increases, thus raising the available pool of cholesterol even more (22, 32). In effect, a 60% increase in total cholesterol may be observed (22). Overall, copper deficiency increases the absolute levels of cholesterol, but there is an argument whether the size of plasma cholesterol pool size may be a more powerful measure of cholesterol elevation. For example, the time course study of serum cholesterol in rats kept for 3-7 weeks on a copper deficient diet found that with time the plasma cholesterol concentration leveled off, but the pool size of cholesterol increased due to increases in the plasma volume (33). Curiously, the rates of HDL catabolism also increased, though the liver and the adrenal gland did not take up additional HDL in copper deficiency, suggesting one possible mechanism for dyslipidemia with respect to the HDL pool (34).

2.4. Serum lipoproteins: changes in structure, composition, and degradation

Rat models have proven to be especially consistent and valuable in studies of the dyslipidemia resulting from copper deficiency. Despite variations in the age, diet composition, and time on a copper deficient diet, an increase in the cholesterol concentration and/or pool was consistently reported in these animals. The lipids and lipoprotein components were analyzed in detail by al-Othman and co-workers and provided valuable data on changes in plasma pool size along with the composition and concentration of lipoproteins (33). These studies demonstrated no change in plasma phospholipid composition in copper deficient rats when compared to controls. In contrast, triglycerides, phospholipids, and cholesterol in LDL and HDL increased 2-fold or more. The VLDL composition of copper deficient animals changed most significantly with a 6-fold increase in triglycerides, 36% reduction in cholesterol and no change in phospholipid. An increase was observed in the VLDL particle size, but not the number of particles. In contrast, an increase in both size and number was seen for the LDL particles, whereas for the HDL particles an increase in the number of particles was observed, but no size change.

The composition of serum lipoproteins in copper deficient animals may also be influenced by shifts in the expression and distribution of apolipoproteins, linking physiological response in the liver to the observed changes in plasma cholesterol. The plasma levels of apolipoproteins A, B, and E increase in rats fed a copper deficient diet, consistent with the increased particle numbers and sizes (35-39). Remarkably, hepatic apoA1, ApoE and ApoB mRNA levels remain unchanged, suggesting that the alteration of the apolipoprotein levels is not due to an increase in transcription. Indeed, it was found that hepatic synthesis and secretion rates of apoA1 are upregulated (35), whereas the rates of synthesis of ApoB-48 and ApoB-100 are unchanged, despite an increase in secretion (37). Intestinal secretion of apoA-1 was also observed, providing yet another source for increased circulating apolipoproteins and cholesterol (40).

In copper deficiency, plasma HDL rich in apolipoprotein E (ApoE) accumulates and total ApoE binding to liver plasma membranes increases (also reported as a reduction in ApoE-free HDL binding). Interestingly, the cholesterol levels in the liver decrease with copper deficiency, despite an overall increase in hepatic cholesterol synthesis (41, 42). These changes in synthesis, binding properties, and redistribution of lipoproteins suggest some mechanisms through which copper deficiency affects serum cholesterol levels. Thus far, molecular investigations of copper deficiency have identified increased hepatic expression of SREBP1-responsive fatty-acid synthase, along with the increased nuclear localization of the mature SREBP1 transcriptional activator (24). Changes in the expression of other genes involved in the fatty acid synthesis have not been explored in any significant detail, although the mRNA levels for cholesterol 7-alpha hydroxylase were found decreased by 80%.

Changes in the plasma lipoprotein composition and structure are expected to influence the lipid content of red blood cells (RBC) through lipid exchange. Consequently, in copper deficiency changes in the RBC lipid composition are likely (43-45). Studies of the lipid profile of plasma and membranes of RBCs in copper deficiency support this view. Both cholesterol and phospholipid levels increase in the RBCs plasma membranes in Cu deficient rats, whereas the molar ratios of cholesterol:phospholipids and cholesterol:membrane protein are reduced (46). The phospholipid profiles change as well, with the increased stearic and docosadienoic acid content, and the lower levels of oleic and linolenic acid (47). A study assessing structural characteristics of the RBC membranes demonstrated a decrease in membrane fluidity and speculated that this could be the cause of hemolysis and anemia (48). Intriguingly, another study reported an increase in the RBC plasma membrane fluidity in copper deficient rats (49). This discrepancy may be due to experimental conditions. Motta and colleagues found that in copper deficiency, increased fluidity in RBCs plasma membrane can be seen alongside with higher rigidity due to enhanced susceptibility of triacylglycerol-rich lipoproteins to lipid peroxidation (50).

2.5. Copper-dependent lipid alteration in tissues

Given significant changes induced by copper deficiency in the serum and the liver, it is not surprising that the lipid and fatty-acid composition of other organs is also affected. Severe copper deficiency can be induced in C57BL mice by feeding dams a copper deficient diet and subsequently weaning pups to the same diet. These animals had lower levels of phospholipids in the liver and kidney, as well as lower triacylglycerols in kidneys (51). Lower proportion and total amount of di-homo-γ-linoleic acid was observed in all tissues of these mice, though levels of other lipids varied. Severe copper deficiency also induced hepatomegaly, reduced the brain weight, and reduced serum ceruloplasmin to 0.5% of control, indicating profound systemic effects.

The liver is an organ that experiences significant changes in lipid composition and membrane structure in response to copper deficiency. The loss of membrane fluidity in hepatic tissue has been reported and suggested to be caused by changes in the composition of unsaturated fatty acids and triacylglycerols of fatty acids (48). Other observed changes in membrane lipids associated with copper deficiency include a decreased ratio of monounsaturated:saturated C16 and C18 fatty acids in adipose tissue and a decreased fatty acid desaturase activity in liver microsomes (52). Phosphatidylcholine biosynthesis may also be affected, as choline phosphotransferase activity levels are lower both in the heart and liver tissue in copper deficient rats (53).

Concurrent with changes in lipid profiles and synthesis, copper deficiency decreases the total amounts of body fat and shifts metabolic fuel use from carbohydrate to fat. Respiratory quotient is reduced, but total energy intake is the same for animals kept on copper deficient and copper adequate diets (54). Young, weanling rats fed on a copper deficient diet for six weeks are leaner than controls, though they have increased serum cholesterol and triglycerides. Metabolically, whole body respiratory quotient decreases, reflected in a reduction of cardiac and adipose lipoprotein lipase, but not the skeletal muscle lipoprotein lipase (55). The change in fuel use may be related to upregulation of fatty acid synthesis. Copper deficiency does, however, decrease levels of hepatic cytochrome C oxidase (56).

The molecular mechanisms for these changes in lipid metabolism due to copper deficiency are understudied; as a result, current knowledge is limited. Increases in expression of specific apolipoproteins and increased transcription of gene for fatty acid synthase in the liver have been reported (see above), providing first insights into molecular players that are involved in response to low copper. Some key information has also been gained in one gene expression study. A transriptome analysis in the small intestine of copper deficient rats revealed upregulation of mRNA for proteins involved in cholesterol transport including apolipoprotein E and the lecithin:cholesterol acyltransferase providing mechanism for enhanced intestinal cholesterol secretion (57). The study also reported down-regulation of genes in the pathway for fatty acid beta-oxidation (both mitochondrial and peroxisomal). The results suggested a change in cell metabolism that reduced fatty acid oxidation, perhaps as a feedback to the decreased cytochrome C oxidase activity. The specific effects of copper deficiency may differ in tissues and serum. For example, in contrast to intestine, the activity of plasma lecithin:cholesterol acyltransferase (a risk factor for ischemic heart disease) is decreased in rats fed a copper deficient diet (58).

3. Functional interactions between copper, lipid, and other nutrients

3.1. Copper and dietary fat/lipid

Considering that copper deficiency influences systemic lipid metabolism, it would be interesting to know whether interactions between copper and lipid levels are reciprocal. In other words, it is important to determine whether dietary fat consumption, or changes in the type of fat consumed influences the activity or levels of copper-dependent enzymes. Changes in the ratios of saturated and unsaturated fatty acids have been noted in copper deficiency, and a cardioprotective effect of increasing proportion of polyunsaturated fatty acids was proposed (59). Curiously, feeding saturated fat in a copper deficient rat model increased hepatic copper as well as iron levels to a significant degree. Saturated fat consumption, however, did not change copper deficiency-induced lipid peroxidation, despite recovery of some hepatic copper. Copper-zinc superoxide dismutase (Cu/Zn-SOD) in the liver is less active in copper-deficient rats, whereas other hepatic antioxidant enzymes are unaffected by copper deficiency (56). This observation suggests that proper incorporation of copper in Cu/Zn-SOD may be key to preventing lipid peroxidation.

The effect of fatty acids on copper may also be mediated at the level of intestinal absorption. Experiments with the long chain fatty acids palmitate and stearate showed reduced levels of copper absorption from the jejunum (60) in response to treatment. In another study, direct cholesterol feeding of rabbits was used to model hypercholesterolemia and atherosclerosis. Adding cholesterol to 0.5% of diet triggered the redistribution of copper from the liver to plasma, with a 50% increase in plasma Cu and a 74% reduction in liver copper (61). Interestingly, copper supplementation in cholesterol-fed rabbits reduced atherosclerotic lesions (62). Further support for the importance of copper-lipid interactions in cardiac function is indicated by the observation that cardiomyopathy might be exacerbated by combination of high dietary fat and copper restriction. Specifically, when copper restriction and dietary fat supplementation were tested separately and together, the lowest level of cardiac cytochrome C oxidase activity was observed in copper-deficient rats on a high fat diet (63).

3.2. Fructose, lipids, and copper metabolism

The influence of dietary sugar consumption on lipid metabolism may be mediated, in part, by exacerbation of copper deficiency. Copper-deficient rats fed a sucrose-based or starch-based diets all had increased plasma cholesterol and lower plasma ceruloplasmin levels, as observed in copper deficiency alone (64). However, feeding sucrose rather than starch greatly enhanced deleterious effects of copper deficiency, such that those animals showed 60% mortality in the 9-week study. The copper deficient sucrose fed rats had a 3-fold lower hepatic copper level compared to starch-fed copper deficient rats. These results suggested a sucrose-dependent change in copper mobilization or retention within the liver (64). Cardiac abnormalities consistent with copper deficiency were also observed. Follow-up work indicated that when diets with fructose, glucose or starch were combined with copper deficiency, both glucose and fructose raised plasma cholesterol levels. However, severity of copper deficiency and mortality were much greater with fructose as opposed to glucose feeding (65), suggesting that the exacerbation of copper deficiency by sucrose was due to the fructose component. More recent work (66) indicates that the effect of fructose may be at the level of absorption, whereby copper deficiency induces upregulation of the copper transporter Ctr1, but this effect is eliminated by high fructose feeding (Figure 1).

Dietary fructose consumption and dietary copper deficiency independently alter fatty-acid metabolism; in combination, the effect is enhanced (66-69). Feeding weanling rats for three weeks on a diet adequate or deficient in copper along with either fructose or corn starch as a carbohydrate source (62% carbohydrate) revealed that fructose feeding enhanced indicators of copper deficiency, such as enhanced heart/body weight ratio and reduced hepatic copper (70). Analysis of hepatic enzymes involved in the lipid and carbohydrate metabolism also indicated that a diet deficient in copper had greatest metabolic effects in combination with fructose, less with glucose and least with starch (71). Glucose-6-phosphate dehydrogenase, malic enzyme, L-alpha-glycerophosphate dehydrogenase and fructose 1-6-diphosphatase were all unaffected by Cu deficiency, but their activities were enhanced most in combination with fructose, suggesting a complementary rather than direct role for fructose in exacerbating copper deficiency (71).

Copper deficiency in combination with fructose feeding alters the fatty acid composition of triacylglycerol in the heart and the liver. Cardiac phosphatidylinositol and phosphatidylserine were shown to increase nearly two-fold and arachidonic acid and docosapentaenoic acid to be elevated more than two-fold in copper deficient, fructose fed animals (70). A change in cardiac phospholipids may explain the increased mortality observed in copper deficient/fructose fed rats and suggest a potentially significant role for these dietary factors in ischemic heart disease. However, the observed changes in the lipid composition could not be correlated with the extent of copper deficiency, illustrating once again that a detailed mechanistic understanding of these dietary interactions could be highly beneficial.

Western diet is characterized by high fructose and high fat. In combination with a likely mild copper deficiency (see above), it stands to reason that these factors may all interact to induce changes in whole body metabolism, especially lipid metabolism, producing deleterious hepatic and cardiovascular effects. When this idea is tested in rats by combining high fat and fructose, or low fat and fructose with copper deficiency, liver metabolism is most significantly affected by the fat and fructose combination (28). Sugars mobilize copper from the liver to other tissues (64), possibly causing a change in liver physiology. Recent work also indicates that the mobilization of copper from the liver may be driven by heart-specific copper deficiency (10). Thus, in addition to interaction during absorption, an important inter-organ communication exists that jointly modulates levels of copper and lipids in various tissues

4. Copper misbalance and lipid metabolism in human disease

4.1. Lipid metabolism in Menkes disease

The studies discussed above were focused on the effects of dietary copper deficiency. In humans and in animals, genetic inactivation of the copper transporting ATPase ATP7A impairs copper export from the intestine, effectively limiting copper supply to many tissues and causing lethal pathology known as Menkes disease, MND (72). Depending on the type of mutation in ATP7A, severity of copper deficiency as well as disease manifestations vary between MND patients. Lipid profiles have been explored in some patients and found affected, but inconsistently, with the exception of a higher neutral lipid content of VLDL in all tested MND patients compared to controls. Interestingly, although ApoB in patients appeared normal, it degraded faster during storage suggesting lower stability (73). Variations in lipid profiles could also be age-related. Studies in animals (including an animal model for Menkes disease) demonstrate that unlike adults, copper deficient young animals do not show elevated cholesterol in the serum (74). The resistance of young mice and rats to hypercholesterolemia could be due to insufficient depletion of copper in the liver, which serves as a major store of copper in neonatal animals, or/and insufficiently progressed functional defects in the liver at young age (74).

ATP7A plays an important role in the development and maintenance of vasculature by supplying copper for functional maturation of lysyl oxidase. Recent studies also suggested the important role for ATP7A in the pathogenesis of atherosclerosis (75). ATP7A was detected in atherosclerotic lesions of mice with genetically inactivated LDL receptor where it colocalized with macrophages. Down-regulation of ATP7A in a macrophage-derived cell culture by siRNA resulted in decreased expression and enzymatic activity of cytosolic phospholipase A(2) alpha, an important enzyme involved in LDL oxidation (75). Furthermore, only cell-mediated LDL oxidation was reduced following down-regulation of ATP7A, whereas conditioned medium from either control or ATP7A down-regulated cells was without such effect (75). This result indicates that the reduced LDL oxidation is not simply due to a diminished copper export from cells with down-regulated ATP7A, but rather due to complex metabolic interactions between copper misbalance and lipid metabolism

4.2. Copper overload in Wilson's disease markedly alters lipid metabolism.

Direct evidence for the important role of copper in modulating hepatic lipid metabolism and serum lipid profiles has been produced by studies using *Atp7b-/-* mice (an animal model of Wilson's disease, WD) and, subsequently, samples from WD patients. Wilson's disease is a severe genetic disorder of copper overload, caused by inactivating mutations of copper transporting ATPase ATP7B and inability to excrete excess copper from hepatocytes (76). Despite massive accumulation of copper in a cytosol, copper incorporation into ceruloplasmin is impaired and serum levels and activity of ceruloplasmin are greatly diminished (phenotypically resembling consequences of copper deficiency, Figure 2). The genetically engineered knockouts of Atp7b (*Atp7b-/-* mice) accurately reproduce these key features of WD (77). Consequently, these animals have been used to investigate consequences of copper overload at the molecular level.

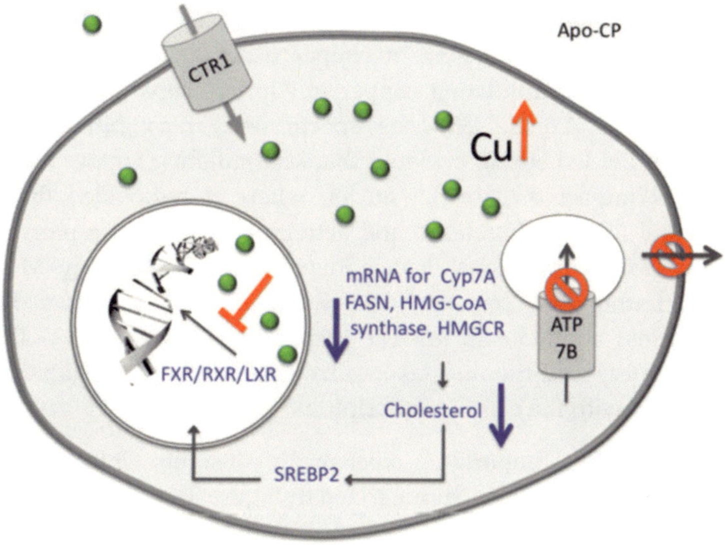

Figure 2. Elevated copper in *Atp7b-/-* hepatocytes inhibits activities of nuclear receptors and dysregulates lipid metabolism. In Wilson's disease, genetic inactivation of the copper transporting ATPase ATP7B results in an impaired copper export from hepatocytes, loss of copper incorporation into ceruloplasmin, CP, (and a secretion of Apo-CP into the serum) along with massive copper accumulation in hepatocytes. Copper concentrates preferentially in the cytosol and nuclei. Cytosolic copper does not prevent sensing of cholesterol levels, allowing SREBP-2 cleavage and entry into the nucleus in response to low cholesterol. However, high copper in the nucleus blocks activity of nuclear receptors, presumably through binding or oxidation. Impaired function of nuclear proteins is associated with a decrease in the mRNA levels for several enzymes, including HMG-CoA reductase (HMGCR) and HMG-CoA synthase, and low total cholesterol in the liver.

Studies at the early stage of pathology development in *Atp7b-/-* mice (prior to the onset of visible morphologic changes in the liver) were particularly informative. The analysis of liver transcriptome revealed that copper accumulation is associated with distinct metabolic changes: upregulation of genes involved in cell cycle and chromosome maintenance and down-regulation of lipid metabolism, especially cholesterol biosynthesis (78, 79). The mRNA studies were complemented by the analysis of metabolites, which confirmed significant (30-40%) decrease of cholesterol in the liver, and the lower levels of VLDL cholesterol in the serum (79). These early changes in lipid metabolism are maintained throughout the course of the disease as indicated by the analysis of the mRNA levels and serum lipid profiles at the later stages of the disease (80). Follow-up studies revealed that the sterol metabolism in a brain of young *Atp7b-/-* mice was also dysregulated, with cholesterol, 8-dehydrocholesterol, desmosterol, 7-dehydrocholesterol, and lathosterol all being highly increased (81, 82). It should be noted that the main cholesterol-sensing pathway that involves proteolysis and nuclear localization of SREBP2 transcription factor is not impaired in *Atp7b*$^{-/-}$ hepatocytes (79).

These important observations necessitated further mechanistic studies. Such work has recently been done using systems biology approach and biochemical/biophysical measurements. Direct *in situ* imaging of copper using X-fluorescence revealed the non-uniform distribution of accumulating copper in *Atp7b-/-* hepatocytes with a predominant increase in the cytosol and nuclei (80). Mass-spectrometry in combination with generation of protein networks provided strong evidence that accumulating copper had a significant and specific functional impact on *Atp7b-/-* nuclei, where it remodeled the RNA-processing machinery (83) and altered abundance and activity of nuclear receptors (84). Specifically, using quantitative Multidimensional Protein Identification Technology (MuDPIT), Wilmarth and colleagues found that the ligand-activated nuclear receptors FXR/NR1H4 and GR/NR3C1 were less abundant in nuclear preparations from *Atp7b-/-* liver, whereas the DNA repair machinery and the nucleus-localized glutathione peroxidase SelH were more abundant, consistent with the earlier transcriptome studies (79).

These findings provide important mechanistic insights into a copper-dependent dysregulation of lipid metabolism (summarized in Figure 2). It seems that hepatic nuclei are the primary sites of action for elevated copper. In WD, the local copper concentration in the nuclei can increase up to 50-100 fold (80). Copper is a redox active metal, and such marked elevation is likely to alter the nuclear redox environment, as also suggested by the upregulation of nuclear glutathione peroxidase SelH. Oxidation of sensitive cysteine residues and/or competition between copper and zinc in zinc fingers (which are common structural features in nuclear proteins) are likely mechanisms that impair activity of nuclear factors, such as transcription factors and/or components of the RNA splicing machinery (Figure 2). Current data suggest that neither potential cysteine oxidation nor copper-zinc competition are wide spread (83) and that nuclear proteins regulating lipid metabolism are preferentially affected by elevated copper. Thus, further studies are needed to understand the molecular basis of this increased sensitivity to copper levels.

The identification of FXR/LXR/RXR as important players in pathology development of WD (85) opens a new avenue for studies aimed on better understanding of the role of a diet (especially cholesterol and fat components) in the time-of-onset and severity of WD. It is important to emphasize that the effect of high copper on lipid metabolism is conserved between species, as evidenced by down-regulation of the same key enzymes in the lipid biosynthesis pathways in mice and human liver in response to copper overload (79). Recent studies of serum samples in the cohort of WD patient revealed differences in cholesterol metabolism that diminished with a copper-chelation therapy (82). These observations further supports high metabolic significance of copper:lipid interactions.

A marked effect of elevated copper on lipid metabolism was also reported in Long-Evans Cinnamon (LEC) rat, another murine model of WD (86). Analysis of the liver and serum lipid profiles in these animals showed that copper overload was associated with a higher content of triglycerides, free cholesterol and cholesteryl ester when compared to controls. The effect is actually opposite to that reported in *Atp7b-/-* mice. At present, the reason for this discrepancy is not clear. In LEC rat, liver disease is more severe compared to *Atp7b-/-* mice, invariably leading to animals death, which is not the case in mice. The mitochondrial function in these rats is more significantly affected (87), perhaps contributing to metabolic differences. Nevertheless, similarly to *Atp7b-/-* mice, the LEC serum is characterized by hypotriglyceridemia, hypocholesterolemia and abnormalities in the composition and size of circulating lipoproteins. Also similarly to *Atp7b-/-* and human liver, the activity of hepatic 3-hydroxy-3-methylglutaryl coenzyme A reductase is reduced in LEC rats, along with other important enzyme involved in lipid biosynthesis (Figure 2) (86).

4.3. Copper and NAFLD

The earlier studies of copper misbalance were focused mostly on the effects of copper deficiency and resulting dyslipidemia on cardiovascular disease. The liver, however, is the central organ of copper homeostasis and, as discussed above, it is greatly affected in WD. It may also be functionally affected in copper deficiency (88). Caloric excess associated with the modern Western diet is implicated in NAFLD, however caloric excess does not compensate for copper deficiency. Furthermore, copper deficiency can still be experienced by the liver, even when serum copper levels are maintained or increased due to factors such as dietary cholesterol.

Although numerous studies clearly link copper deficiency to altered lipid metabolism in animal models (12, 22, 24, 89-92) and human volunteers (29), only recently has low dietary copper been implicated in liver dyslipidemia pathology, including non-alcoholic fatty-liver disease (NAFLD) and non-alcoholic steatohepatitis (NASH). In a recent groundbreaking study, hepatic copper content in biopsy specimens was inversely correlated with the severity of fatty liver disease, and copper deficiency in a rodent model was found sufficient to induce NAFLD and metabolic syndrome (12). Hepatic iron accumulation, a known consequence of copper deficiency, is also observed in NAFLD (93). Iron accumulation likely results from the loss of holoceruloplasmin, a copper-dependent ferroxidase instrumental in iron distribution (94). This, in turn, results in lower levels of ferroportin in copper deficient rats; coincidentally, NAFLD patients show less ferroportin expression than controls (93). Copper supplementation has been suggested as a therapy for NAFLD based on study in which a diet-induced (high carbohydrate fat-free diet) NAFLD in rats was improved by treatment with a Cu(I)-nicotinate complex (95).

Studies of NAFLD also reflect the intersection of copper deficiency, hepatic lipid metabolism and consumption of fructose as causative agents in NAFLD. High dietary sugars, particularly fructose, have been implicated in development of NAFLD and NASH (96, 97). As discussed above, there is evidence that dietary fructose contributes to copper deficiency (66, 69), indicating cross talk between these dietary factors. Sucrose and fructose may have similar effects, as the enzyme sucrase acts in the digestive system to convert the disaccharide sucrose into fructose and glucose for transport in the bloodstream. High dietary fructose results in decreased CuZnSOD expression (98), lowering resistance of oxidative damage. A diet of 60% fructose affects lipid metabolism as well as antioxidant status, including CuZnSOD, in the liver of rats after 13 weeks of treatment (68). It is clear these high fructose diets induce NAFLD in rodent models, however these diets are typically 60-70% fructose and may not accurately reflect human fructose consumption (for review see (99)).

It is proposed that fructose metabolism induces oxidative stress, and this may trigger NAFLD. A copper-fructose feeding study indicated that lipid peroxidation due to copper deficiency and a 62% fructose diet could be reduced by supplementing vitamin E to 1 g/kg, however copper deficiency remained, indicating that copper deficiency with fructose feeding may not be entirely a result of oxidative stress (100). Nevertheless, hepatic lipid peroxidation is enhanced significantly in copper deficiency with fructose feeding, supporting the role for oxidative stress in liver disease through the impairment of hepatic antioxidant systems (66).

Tissue	Increase	Decrease	Other observation
Erythrocytes	cholesterol, phospholipid, stearic acid, docosadienoic acid	cholesterol:phospholipid ratio, cholesterol: mebmbrane protein ratio, linoleic acid, oleic acid	membrane fluidity?
Plasma and serum	triglycerides, phospholipids and cholesterol in lipoproteins; apoA, apoB, apoE; plasma volume	N/A	hematocrit
Liver	apolipoprotein secretion, cholesterol synthesis and secretion, fatty acid syntase expression	apoE-free HDL binding; monounsaturated:saturate d fatty acids ratio	no change in apolipoprotein transcript levels
Heart	stearic acid; docosahexaenoic acid; total phospholipid	elastic fibers; palmitic acid; oleic acid	hypertrophy; inflammation; distorted elastic fibers
Small intestine	transcripts in cholesterol transport	transcripts in fatty-acid beta-oxidation	NA
Kidney	NA	triacylglycrol and phospholipid	NA

Table 1. Tissue-specific effects of copper deficiency on lipid metabolism

5. Conclusions

Copper deficiency and copper overload have multiple and significant effects on systemic and cellular lipid metabolism. Recent studies indicate that copper misbalance is an emerging factor in dyslipidemia and/or fatty-liver disease. In turn, lipid metabolism could be an important modifier of the time-of-onset and severity in Wilson's disease. Work over several decades has yielded physiological and biochemical data on the consequences of copper deficiency, particularly with respect to lipid metabolism, in rodent models. Understanding of human disease would greatly benefit from further analysis of copper levels and lipid profiles in human clinical specimens, as well as assessment of the influence of other nutrients at the molecular level. Animal models will remain important. As much as has already been learned, further mechanistic studies are bound to yield molecular level understanding of the important copper:lipid relationship. It is still not clear how copper deficiency alters gene expression and protein expression/function to produce observed pathologies. Transcript profiling, proteomic analysis, and metabolite profiling, in both data-driven and targeted formats, promise to provide more mechanistic details in animal models that can be tested in human pathology.

Author details

Jason L. Burkhead
Department of Biological Sciences, University of Alaska Anchorage, Anchorage, AK, USA

Svetlana Lutsenko
Department of Physiology, Johns Hopkins University, Baltimore, MD, USA

6. References

[1] Nose Y, Kim BE, Thiele DJ. Ctr1 drives intestinal copper absorption and is essential for growth, iron metabolism, and neonatal cardiac function. Cell Metab. 2006 Sep;4(3):235-44.

[2] Vulpe CD, Packman S. Cellular copper transport. Annu Rev Nutr. 1995;15:293-322.

[3] Lee J, Prohaska JR, Thiele DJ. Essential role for mammalian copper transporter Ctr1 in copper homeostasis and embryonic development. Proc Natl Acad Sci U S A. 2001 Jun 5;98(12):6842-7.

[4] Kuo YM, Zhou B, Cosco D, Gitschier J. The copper transporter CTR1 provides an essential function in mammalian embryonic development. Proc Natl Acad Sci U S A. 2001 Jun 5;98(12):6836-41.

[5] Mercer JF, Ambrosini L, Horton S, Gazeas S, Grimes A. Animal models of Menkes disease. Adv Exp Med Biol. 1999;448:97-108.

[6] Lutsenko S, Gupta A, Burkhead JL, Zuzel V. Cellular multitasking: the dual role of human Cu-ATPases in cofactor delivery and intracellular copper balance. Arch Biochem Biophys. 2008 Aug 1;476(1):22-32.

[7] Gupta A, Lutsenko S. Human copper transporters: mechanism, role in human diseases and therapeutic potential. Future Med Chem. 2009 Sep;1(6):1125-42.

[8] Lutsenko S, Barnes NL, Bartee MY, Dmitriev OY. Function and regulation of human copper-transporting ATPases. Physiol Rev. 2007 Jul;87(3):1011-46.

[9] Gerbasi V, Lutsenko S, Lewis EJ. A mutation in the ATP7B copper transporter causes reduced dopamine beta-hydroxylase and norepinephrine in mouse adrenal. Neurochem Res. 2003 Jun;28(6):867-73.

[10] Kim B, Turski M, Nose Y, Casad M, Rockman H, Thiele D. Cardiac copper deficiency activates a systemic signaling mechanism that communicates with the copper acquisition and storage organs. Cell Metab. 2010 May 5;11(5):353-63.

[11] Kegley KM, Sellers MA, Ferber MJ, Johnson MW, Joelson DW, Shrestha R. Fulminant Wilson's disease requiring liver transplantation in one monozygotic twin despite identical genetic mutation. Am J Transplant. 2010 May;10(5):1325-9.

[12] Aigner E, Strasser M, Haufe H, Sonnweber T, Hohla F, Stadlmayr A, et al. A role for low hepatic copper concentrations in nonalcoholic Fatty liver disease. Am J Gastroenterol. 2010 Sep;105(9):1978-85.

[13] Lampon N, Tutor JC. Effect of valproic acid treatment on copper availability in adult epileptic patients. Clin Biochem. 2010 Sep;43(13-14):1074-8.

[14] Lampon N, Tutor JC. A preliminary investigation on the possible association between diminished copper availability and non-alcoholic fatty liver disease in epileptic patients treated with valproic acid. Ups J Med Sci. 2011 May;116(2):148-54.

[15] Stemmer KL, Petering HG, Murthy L, Finelli VN, Menden EE. Copper deficiency effects on cardiovascular system and lipid metabolism in the rat; the role of dietary proteins and excessive zinc. Ann Nutr Metab. 1985;29(6):332-47.

[16] Ernst B, Thurnheer M, Schultes B. Copper deficiency after gastric bypass surgery. Obesity (Silver Spring). 2009 Nov;17(11):1980-1.

[17] Gletsu-Miller N, Broderius M, Frediani J, Zhao V, Griffith D, Davis SJ, et al. Incidence and prevalence of copper deficiency following roux-en-y gastric bypass surgery. Int J Obes (Lond). 2012 Mar;36(3):328-35.

[18] Medeiros D. Gastric bypass and copper deficiency: a possible overlooked consequence. Obes Surg. 2011 Sep;21(9):1482-3; author reply 4-5.

[19] Evans J, Newman S, Sherlock S. Liver copper levels in intrahepatic cholestasis of childhood. Gastroenterology. 1978 Nov;75(5):875-8.

[20] Chambers A, Krewski D, Birkett N, Plunkett L, Hertzberg R, Danzeisen R, et al. An exposure-response curve for copper excess and deficiency. J Toxicol Environ Health B Crit Rev. 2010 Oct;13(7-8):546-78.

[21] Reiser S, Smith JJ, Mertz W, Holbrook J, Scholfield D, Powell A, et al. Indices of copper status in humans consuming a typical American diet containing either fructose or starch. Am J Clin Nutr. 1985 Aug;42(2):242-51.

[22] Lei K. Alterations in plasma lipid, lipoprotein and apolipoprotein concentrations in copper-deficient rats. J Nutr. 1983 Nov;113(11):2178-83.

[23] Saari J. Copper deficiency and cardiovascular disease: role of peroxidation, glycation, and nitration. Can J Physiol Pharmacol. 2000 Oct;78(10):848-55.

[24] Tang Z, Gasperkova D, Xu J, Baillie R, Lee J, Clarke S. Copper deficiency induces hepatic fatty acid synthase gene transcription in rats by increasing the nuclear content of mature sterol regulatory element binding protein 1. J Nutr. 2000 Dec;130(12):2915-21.

[25] Klevay L. Is the Western diet adequate in copper? J Trace Elem Med Biol. 2011 Oct 5.

[26] Klevay L. Ischemic heart disease as deficiency disease. Cell Mol Biol (Noisy-le-grand). 2004 Dec;50(8):877-84.

[27] Aliabadi H. A deleterious interaction between copper deficiency and sugar ingestion may be the missing link in heart disease. Med Hypotheses. 2008;70(6):1163-6.

[28] Wapnir R, Devas G. Copper deficiency: interaction with high-fructose and high-fat diets in rats. Am J Clin Nutr. 1995 Jan;61(1):105-10.

[29] Klevay L, Inman L, Johnson L, Lawler M, Mahalko J, Milne D, et al. Increased cholesterol in plasma in a young man during experimental copper depletion. Metabolism. 1984 Dec;33(12):1112-8.

[30] Disilvestro R, Joseph E, Zhang W, Raimo A, Kim Y. A randomized trial of copper supplementation effects on blood copper enzyme activities and parameters related to cardiovascular health. Metabolism. 2012 Mar 21.

[31] Allen K, Klevay L. Cholesterolemia and cardiovascular abnormalities in rats caused by copper deficiency. Atherosclerosis. 1978 Jan;29(1):81-93.

[32] Carr T, Lei K. High-density lipoprotein cholesteryl ester and protein catabolism in hypercholesterolemic rats induced by copper deficiency. Metabolism. 1990 May;39(5):518-24.

[33] al-Othman A, Rosenstein F, Lei K. Pool size and concentration of plasma cholesterol are increased and tissue copper levels are reduced during early stages of copper deficiency in rats. J Nutr. 1994 May;124(5):628-35.

[34] Carr T, Lei K. In vivo apoprotein catabolism of high density lipoproteins in copper-deficient, hypercholesterolemic rats. Proc Soc Exp Biol Med. 1989 Sep;191(4):370-6.

[35] Hoogeveen R, Reaves S, Lei K. Copper deficiency increases hepatic apolipoprotein A-I synthesis and secretion but does not alter hepatic total cellular apolipoprotein A-I mRNA abundance in rats. J Nutr. 1995 Dec;125(12):2935-44.

[36] Mazur A, Nassir F, Gueux E, Cardot P, Bellanger J, Lamand M, et al. The effect of dietary copper on rat plasma apolipoprotein B, E plasma levels, and apolipoprotein gene expression in liver and intestine. Biol Trace Elem Res. 1992 Aug;34(2):107-13.

[37] Nassir F, Mazur A, Serougne C, Gueux E, Rayssiguier Y. Hepatic apolipoprotein B synthesis in copper-deficient rats. FEBS Lett. 1993 May 3;322(1):33-6.

[38] Nassir F, Giannoni F, Mazur A, Rayssiguier Y, Davidson N. Increased hepatic synthesis and accumulation of plasma apolipoprotein B100 in copper-deficient rats does not result from modification in apolipoprotein B mRNA editing. Lipids. 1996 Apr;31(4):433-6.

[39] Norn M. Pemphigoid related to epinephrine treatment. Am J Ophthalmol: United States; 1977. p. 138.

[40] Wu J, Lei K. Copper deficiency increases total protein and apolipoprotein A-I synthesis in the rat small intestine. Proc Soc Exp Biol Med. 1996 Sep;212(4):369-77.

[41] Hassel C, Lei K, Carr T, Marchello J. Lipoprotein receptors in copper-deficient rats: apolipoprotein E-free high density lipoprotein binding to liver membranes. Metabolism. 1987 Nov;36(11):1054-62.

[42] Yount N, McNamara D, Al-Othman A, Lei K. The effect of copper deficiency on rat hepatic 3-hydroxy-3-methylglutaryl coenzyme A reductase activity. J Nutr Biochem. 1990 Jan;1(1):21-7.

[43] Gold J, Phillips M. Effects of membrane lipids and -proteins and cytoskeletal proteins on the kinetics of cholesterol exchange between high density lipoprotein and human red blood cells, ghosts and microvesicles. Biochim Biophys Acta. 1992 Oct 19;1111(1):103-10.

[44] Nikolic M, Stanic D, Baricevic I, Jones D, Nedic O, Niketic V. Efflux of cholesterol and phospholipids derived from the haemoglobin-lipid adduct in human red blood cells into plasma. Clin Biochem. 2007 Mar;40(5-6):305-9.

[45] Schick B, Schick P. Cholesterol exchange in platelets, erythrocytes and megakaryocytes. Biochim Biophys Acta. 1985 Feb 8;833(2):281-90.

[46] Jain S, Williams D. Copper deficiency anemia: altered red blood cell lipids and viscosity in rats. Am J Clin Nutr. 1988 Sep;48(3):637-40.

[47] Abu-Salah K, al-Othman A, Lei K. Lipid composition and fluidity of the erythrocyte membrane in copper-deficient rats. Br J Nutr. 1992 Sep;68(2):435-43.

[48] Lei K, Rosenstein F, Shi F, Hassel C, Carr T, Zhang J. Alterations in lipid composition and fluidity of liver plasma membranes in copper-deficient rats. Proc Soc Exp Biol Med. 1988 Jul;188(3):335-41.

[49] Rock E, Gueux E, Mazur A, Motta C, Rayssiguier Y. Anemia in copper-deficient rats: role of alterations in erythrocyte membrane fluidity and oxidative damage. Am J Physiol. 1995 Nov;269(5 Pt 1):C1245-9.

[50] Motta C, Gueux E, Mazur A, Rayssiguier Y. Lipid fluidity of triacylglycerol-rich lipoproteins isolated from copper-deficient rats. Br J Nutr. 1996 May;75(5):767-73.

[51] Cunnane S, McAdoo K, Prohaska J. Lipid and fatty acid composition of organs from copper-deficient mice. J Nutr. 1986 Jul;116(7):1248-56.

[52] Wahle E, Davies N. Effect of dietary copper deficiency. in the rat on fatty acid composition of adipose tissue and desaturase activity of liver microsomes. Br J Nutr. 1975 Jul;34(1):105-12.

[53] Cornatzer W, Haning J, Klevay L. The effect of copper deficiency on heart microsomal phosphatidylcholine biosynthesis and concentration. Int J Biochem. 1986;18(12):1083-7.

[54] Hoogeveen R, Reaves S, Reid P, Reid B, Lei K. Copper deficiency shifts energy substrate utilization from carbohydrate to fat and reduces fat mass in rats. J Nutr. 1994 Sep;124(9):1660-6.

[55] Wildman R, Mao S. Tissue-specific alterations in lipoprotein lipase activity in copper-deficient rats. Biol Trace Elem Res. 2001 Jun;80(3):221-9.

[56] Lynch S, Strain J. Dietary saturated or polyunsaturated fat and copper deficiency in the rat. Biol Trace Elem Res. 1989 Nov;22(2):131-9.

[57] Tosco A, Fontanella B, Danise R, Cicatiello L, Grober O, Ravo M, et al. Molecular bases of copper and iron deficiency-associated dyslipidemia: a microarray analysis of the rat intestinal transcriptome. Genes Nutr. 2010 Mar;5(1):1-8.

[58] Lau B, Klevay L. Plasma lecithin: cholesterol acyltransferase in copper-deficient rats. J Nutr. 1981 Oct;111(10):1698-703.

[59] Mozaffarian D, Micha R, Wallace S. Effects on coronary heart disease of increasing polyunsaturated fat in place of saturated fat: a systematic review and meta-analysis of randomized controlled trials. PLoS Med. 2010 Mar;7(3):e1000252.

[60] Wapnir R, Sia M. Copper intestinal absorption in the rat: effect of free fatty acids and triglycerides. Proc Soc Exp Biol Med. 1996 Apr;211(4):381-6.

[61] Klevay L. Dietary cholesterol lowers liver copper in rabbits. Biol Trace Elem Res. 1988 Jun;16(1):51-7.

[62] Lamb D, Reeves G, Taylor A, Ferns G. Dietary copper supplementation reduces atherosclerosis in the cholesterol-fed rabbit. Atherosclerosis. 1999 Sep;146(1):33-43.

[63] Jalili T, Medeiros D, Wildman R. Aspects of cardiomyopathy are exacerbated by elevated dietary fat in copper-restricted rats. J Nutr. 1996 Apr;126(4):807-16.

[64] Fields M, Ferretti R, Smith JJ, Reiser S. Effect of copper deficiency on metabolism and mortality in rats fed sucrose or starch diets. J Nutr. 1983 Jul;113(7):1335-45.

[65] Fields M, Ferretti R, Smith JJ, Reiser S. The interaction of type of dietary carbohydrates with copper deficiency. Am J Clin Nutr. 1984 Feb;39(2):289-95.

[66] Song M, Schuschke D, Zhou Z, Chen T, Pierce W, Wang R, et al. High Fructose Feeding Induces Copper Deficiency in Sprague-Dawley rats: A Novel Mechanism for Obesity Related Fatty Liver. J Hepatol. 2011 Jul 19.

[67] Fields M, Lewis C. Dietary fructose but not starch is responsible for hyperlipidemia associated with copper deficiency in rats: effect of high-fat diet. J Am Coll Nutr. 1999 Feb;18(1):83-7.

[68] Girard A, Madani S, Boukortt F, Cherkaoui-Malki M, Belleville J, Prost J. Fructose-enriched diet modifies antioxidant status and lipid metabolism in spontaneously hypertensive rats. Nutrition. 2006 Jul-Aug;22(7-8):758-66.

[69] Redman R, Fields M, Reiser S, Smith JJ. Dietary fructose exacerbates the cardiac abnormalities of copper deficiency in rats. Atherosclerosis. 1988 Dec;74(3):203-14.

[70] Cunnane S, Fields M, Lewis C. Dietary carbohydrate influences tissue fatty acid and lipid composition in the copper-deficient rat. Biol Trace Elem Res. 1989 -1990 Winter;23:77-87.

[71] Fields M, Ferretti R, Judge J, Smith J, Reiser S. Effects of different dietary carbohydrates on hepatic enzymes of copper-deficient rats. Proc Soc Exp Biol Med. 1985 Mar;178(3):362-6.

[72] Gasch AT, Kaler SG, Kaiser-Kupfer M. Menkes disease. Ophthalmology. 1999 Mar;106(3):442-3.

[73] Blackett PR, Lee DM, Donaldson DL, Fesmire JD, Chan WY, Holcombe JH, et al. Studies of lipids, lipoproteins, and apolipoproteins in Menkes' disease. Pediatr Res. 1984 Sep;18(9):864-70.

[74] Prohaska JR, Korte JJ, Bailey WR. Serum cholesterol levels are not elevated in young copper-deficient rats, mice or brindled mice. J Nutr. 1985 Dec;115(12):1702-7.

[75] Qin Z, Konaniah ES, Neltner B, Nemenoff RA, Hui DY, Weintraub NL. Participation of ATP7A in macrophage mediated oxidation of LDL. J Lipid Res. 2010 Jun;51(6):1471-7.

[76] Das SK, Ray K. Wilson's disease: an update. Nat Clin Pract Neurol. 2006 Sep;2(9):482-93.

[77] Lutsenko S. Atp7b-/- mice as a model for studies of Wilson's disease. Biochem Soc Trans. 2008 Dec;36(Pt 6):1233-8.

[78] Huster D, Lutsenko S. Wilson disease: not just a copper disorder. Analysis of a Wilson disease model demonstrates the link between copper and lipid metabolism. Mol Biosyst. 2007 Dec;3(12):816-24.

[79] Huster D, Purnat TD, Burkhead JL, Ralle M, Fiehn O, Stuckert F, et al. High copper selectively alters lipid metabolism and cell cycle machinery in the mouse model of Wilson disease. J Biol Chem. 2007 Mar 16;282(11):8343-55.

[80] Ralle M, Huster D, Vogt S, Schirrmeister W, Burkhead JL, Capps TR, et al. Wilson disease at a single cell level: intracellular copper trafficking activates compartment-specific responses in hepatocytes. J Biol Chem. 2010 Oct 1;285(40):30875-83.

[81] Sauer SW, Merle U, Opp S, Haas D, Hoffmann GF, Stremmel W, et al. Severe dysfunction of respiratory chain and cholesterol metabolism in Atp7b(-/-) mice as a model for Wilson disease. Biochim Biophys Acta. 2011 Dec;1812(12):1607-15.

[82] Seessle J, Gohdes A, Gotthardt DN, Pfeiffenberger J, Eckert N, Stremmel W, et al. Alterations of lipid metabolism in Wilson disease. Lipids Health Dis. 2011;10:83.

[83] Burkhead JL, Ralle M, Wilmarth P, David L, Lutsenko S. Elevated copper remodels hepatic RNA processing machinery in the mouse model of Wilson's disease. J Mol Biol. 2011 Feb 11;406(1):44-58.

[84] Wilmarth PA, Short KK, Fiehn O, Lutsenko S, David LL, Burkhead JL. A systems approach implicates nuclear receptor targeting in the Atp7b(-/-) mouse model of Wilson's disease. Metallomics. 2012 Jul 28;4(7):660-8.

[85] Burkhead JL, Gray LW, Lutsenko S. Systems biology approach to Wilson's disease. Biometals. 2011 Jun;24(3):455-66.

[86] Levy E, Brunet S, Alvarez F, Seidman E, Bouchard G, Escobar E, et al. Abnormal hepatobiliary and circulating lipid metabolism in the Long-Evans Cinnamon rat model of Wilson's disease. Life Sci. 2007 Mar 27;80(16):1472-83.

[87] Zischka H, Lichtmannegger J, Schmitt S, Jagemann N, Schulz S, Wartini D, et al. Liver mitochondrial membrane crosslinking and destruction in a rat model of Wilson disease. J Clin Invest. 2011 Apr;121(4):1508-18.

[88] Roberts E, Sarkar B. Liver as a key organ in the supply, storage, and excretion of copper. Am J Clin Nutr. 2008 Sep;88(3):851S-4S.

[89] al-Othman A, Rosenstein F, Lei K. Copper deficiency increases in vivo hepatic synthesis of fatty acids, triacylglycerols, and phospholipids in rats. Proc Soc Exp Biol Med. 1993 Oct;204(1):97-103.

[90] Cunnane S, Horrobin D, Manku M. Contrasting effects of low or high copper intake on rat tissue lipid essential fatty acid composition. Ann Nutr Metab. 1985;29(2):103-10.

[91] Petering H, Murthy L, O'Flaherty E. Influence of dietary copper and zinc on rat lipid metabolism. J Agric Food Chem. 1977 Sep-Oct;25(5):1105-9.

[92] Stemmer K, Petering H, Murthy L, Finelli V, Menden E. Copper deficiency effects on cardiovascular system and lipid metabolism in the rat; the role of dietary proteins and excessive zinc. Ann Nutr Metab. 1985;29(6):332-47.

[93] Aigner E, Theurl I, Haufe H, Seifert M, Hohla F, Scharinger L, et al. Copper availability contributes to iron perturbations in human nonalcoholic fatty liver disease. Gastroenterology. 2008 Aug;135(2):680-8.

[94] Miyajima H, Takahashi Y, Kono S. Aceruloplasminemia, an inherited disorder of iron metabolism. Biometals. 2003;16(1):205-13.

[95] Salama R, Nassar A, Nafady A, Mohamed H. A novel therapeutic drug (copper nicotinic acid complex) for non-alcoholic fatty liver. Liver Int. 2007 May;27(4):454-64.

[96] Alisi A, Manco M, Pezzullo M, Nobili V. Fructose at the center of necroinflammation and fibrosis in nonalcoholic steatohepatitis. Hepatology. 2011 Jan;53(1):372-3.

[97] Sanchez-Lozada L, Mu W, Roncal C, Sautin Y, Abdelmalek M, Reungjui S, et al. Comparison of free fructose and glucose to sucrose in the ability to cause fatty liver. Eur J Nutr. 2010 Feb;49(1):1-9.

[98] Francini F, Castro M, Schinella G, Garcia M, Maiztegui B, Raschia M, et al. Changes induced by a fructose-rich diet on hepatic metabolism and the antioxidant system. Life Sci. 2010 Jun 19;86(25-26):965-71.

[99] Yilmaz Y. Review article: fructose in non-alcoholic fatty liver disease. Aliment Pharmacol Ther. 2012 Apr 2.

[100] Silverman S, Fields M, Lewis C. The effect of vitamin E on lipid peroxidation in the copper-deficient rat. J Nutr Biochem. 1990 Feb;1(2):98-101.

Chapter 4

The Role of Liver X Receptor in Hepatic *de novo* Lipogenesis and Cross-Talk with Insulin and Glucose Signaling

Line M. Grønning-Wang, Christian Bindesbøll and Hilde I. Nebb

Additional information is available at the end of the chapter

http://dx.doi.org/10.5772/51357

1. Introduction

Regulation of nutrient balance by the liver is important to ensure whole body metabolic control. Hepatic expression of genes involved in lipid and glucose metabolism is tightly regulated in response to nutritional cues, such as glucose and insulin. In response to dietary carbohydrates, the liver converts excess glucose into fat for storage through *de novo* lipogenesis. The liver X receptors (LXRα and LXRβ) are important transcriptional regulators of this process. LXRs are classically known as oxysterol sensing nuclear receptors that heterodimerize with the retinoic X receptor (RXR) family and activate transcription of nutrient sensing transcription factors such as sterol regulatory element-binding protein 1c (SREBP1c) (Repa et al., 2000; Yoshikawa et al., 2002; Liang et al., 2002) and carbohydrate response element-binding protein (ChREBP) (Cha & Repa, 2007). LXR also induces the transcription of the lipogenic enzyme genes fatty acid synthase (FAS), stearoyl-Coenzyme A desaturase (SCD1) and Acetyl CoA carboxylase (ACC), alone or in concert with SREBP1c and/or ChREBP (Chu et al., 2006; Joseph et al., 2002; Talukdar & Hillgartner, 2006). LXR activate transcription of hepatic lipogenic genes in response to feeding, which is believed to be mediated by insulin (Tobin et al., 2002). The mechanisms by which insulin activates LXR-mediated gene expression is not clearly understood, but may involve production of endogenous ligand for LXRs and/or act by signal transduction mechanisms downstream of the insulin receptor (IR). Both glucose and insulin regulate *de novo* lipogenesis, however, some lipogenic genes can be regulated by glucose without the need of insulin which has been shown for SREBP1c (Hasty et al., 2000; Matsuzaka et al., 2004). A well known glucose-mediator in liver is ChREBP, an important regulator of *de novo* lipogenesis in response to glucose (Yamashita et al., 2001). ChREBP is activated by glucose via hexose- and pentose-phosphate-dependent mechanisms involving dephosphorylation of ChREBP and translocation to the nucleus (Havula & Hietakangas, 2012). Interestingly, both LXR and ChREBP were recently shown to be post-translationally modified by O-linked β-N-acetylglucosamine (O-GlcNAc) in response to glucose potentiating their lipogenic capacity (Anthonisen et al., 2010; Guinez et al., 2011). Glucose flux through the hexosamine signaling pathway generates UDP-N-acetyl-glucosamine (UDP-GlcNAc), a substrate for O-GlcNAc modification of nucleocytoplasmic proteins by the enzyme O-GlcNAc transferase (OGT). We have shown that O-GlcNAcylation of LXR is increased in mouse livers in response to feeding and in livers from hyperglycemic diabetic mice potentiating SREBP1c expression (Anthonisen et al., 2010). Furthermore, preliminary studies in our laboratory indicate that LXR potentiate ChREBP activity under hyperglycemic conditions establishing a link between glucose metabolism, LXR and ChREBP. These observations suggest that LXR, SREBP1c and ChREBP contribute to converting carbohydrates into fat in a cooperative manner in response to high circulating glucose levels and that O-GlcNAc signaling plays a role in this process. As O-GlcNAc cycling appear to be essential for proper insulin signaling and the sensitivity of OGT to glucose increases with decreasing insulin signaling (Mondoux et al., 2011; Hanover et al., 2010) the relative roles of LXR, SREBP1c and ChREBP in regulating *de novo* lipogenesis in response to feeding and modification by O-GlcNAc signaling under insulin sensitive and insulin resistant conditions will be discussed.

2. Liver X Receptors (LXR)

2.1. LXR structure and function

LXRα (NR1H3) and LXRβ (NR1H2) are ligand-activated transcription factors belonging to the nuclear receptor (NR) superfamily (Lehmann JM (Lehmann et al., 1997; Willy et al., 1995; Janowski et al., 1996). LXRα is primarily expressed in metabolically active tissues, such as liver, intestine, adipose tissue, kidney and macrophages, whereas LXRβ is ubiquitously expressed (Apfel et al., 1994; Teboul et al., 1995; Teboul et al., 1995). LXRs are intracellular sensors of cholesterol and oxidized cholesterol derivatives (oxysterols) have been identified as their endogenous ligands (Janowski et al., 1996; Lehmann et al., 1997). The two isotypes originates from two different genes on separate chromosomes, but share the same modular structure, which is characteristic of most NRs (Fig. 1).

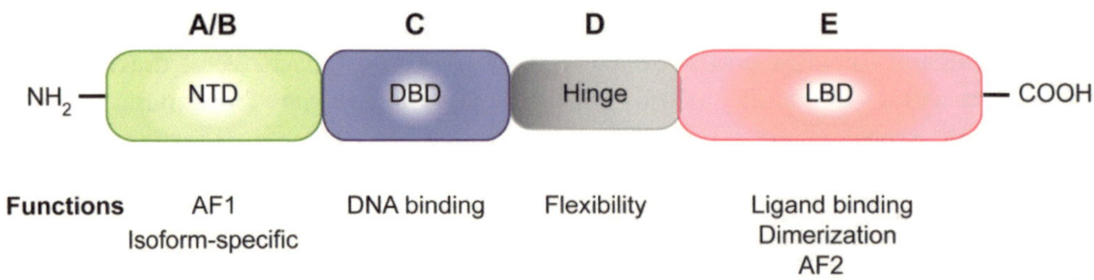

Figure 1. Structure of the LXRs

The DNA-binding domain (DBD) and the ligand binding domain (LBD) are highly structured domains. LXRα and LXRβ share 78 % amino acid sequence identity in these regions, while the N-terminal domain (NTD) and the hinge domain are far more disordered and less conserved. DNA binding requires dimerization with RXR. Transactivation by the LXRs is mediated through the ligand independent activation function (AF1) in NTD and the ligand dependent activation function 2 (AF2) in the LBD. Binding of a ligand to the hydrophobic ligand binding pocket leads to a conformational change that releases corepressors (CR) and exposes binding sites for coactivators (CA), recruiting the general transcription machinery and RNA polymerase II (RNA Pol II) (Fig. 2). This leads to changes in LXR dependent gene expression. The interactions with coregulators can also occur independently of ligand to AF1, however this is far less characterized. Upon activation, LXRs regulate a number of genes involved in lipid, cholesterol and glucose metabolism by binding to LXR response elements (LXREs) in their promoter region. These consist of a direct repeat of the nucleotide hexamer AGGTCA spaced by four nucleotides. Insights into LXR function in metabolism was provided by the generation of LXR mutant mice. These mice accumulate hepatic cholesterol, ultimately causing liver dysfunction (Peet et al., 1998; Ulven et al., 2005). It was found that LXRα controls cholesterol metabolism by conversion of cholesterol to bile acid by induction of the cholesterol 7 alpha-hydroxylase (Cyp7A1) gene, biliary cholesterol excretion and cholesterol efflux via induction of ABCG5/8 and ABCA1/ABCG1, respectively (Lehmann et al., 1997; Chiang et al., 2001; Yu et al., 2003; Repa et al., 2002; Graf et al., 2002; Costet et al., 2000; Sabol et al., 2005; Venkateswaran et al., 2000; Venkateswaran et al., 2000). LXRs are strongly implicated in the development of metabolic disorders and associated pathologies, notably, hyperlipidemia and atherosclerosis (Peet et al., 1998; Calkin & Tontonoz, 2010). Thus, LXRs are key players in maintaining metabolic homeostasis in health and disease by regulating inflammation and lipid/carbohydrate metabolism.

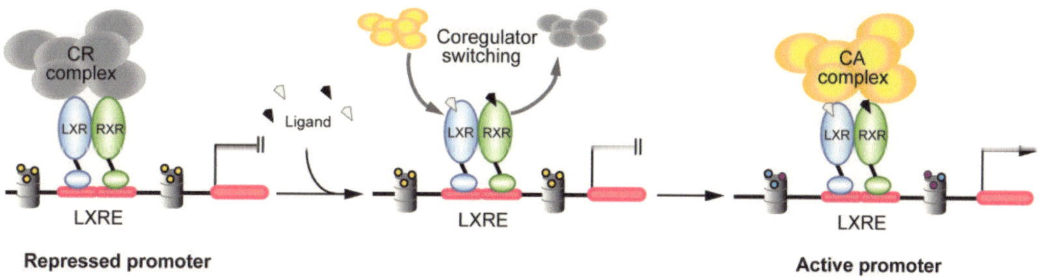

Figure 2. Activation of LXR by coregulator switching

2.2. Modulation of LXR activity by coregulators and PTMs

The transcriptional activity of LXRs is highly dependent on the presence of coregulators which has been linked to several metabolic processes (Jakobsson et al., 2009; Kim et al., 2003; Huuskonen et al., 2004; Kim et al., 2008; Oberkofler et al., 2003). Coregulators constitutes large multisubunit protein complexes containing chromatin-remodelling and/or –modifying enzymes with intrinsic histone acetylase (HAT)/ deacetylase (HDAC) and histone methylase (HMT)/demethylase (HDM) activities, depending on whether they act as activators or repressors, respectively (Kato et al., 2011). It has been assumed that that the unliganded LXRs are localized in the nucleus and interact with CRs, including nuclear receptor corepressor/silencing mediator of retinoic acid and thyroid receptor (NcoR/SMRT) (Wagner et al., 2003). However, recent chromatin immunoprecipitation (ChIP) studies, including ChIP-sequencing (ChIP-Seq), have challenged this classical model. These studies put forward a more complex view, that ligands, pioneer factors, coregulators and posttranslational modifications (PTMs) play different roles in determining the LXR binding sites and actions *in vivo* (Boergesen et al., 2012; Heinz et al., 2010; Pehkonen et al., 2012). Furthermore, some coregulators have been shown to act as dual function activators/repressors, such as the coregulator protein receptor interacting protein 140 (RIP140). RIP140 has been shown to serve as a CA for LXR in lipogenesis but as a CR in gluconeogenesis independent of ligand activation (Herzog et al., 2007). General mechanisms of coregulator actions are assumed to be conserved between LXRs, but based on the low amino acid sequence identity in the NTD (32%) and the hinge domain (25%) it is possible that they contain novel isotype specific interaction surfaces. Also, the specific coregulator requirement to lipogenic LXR target genes in response to different feeding regiments under normal and diabetic conditions remain largely unexplored. In addition to ligand binding, LXRs can be posttranslationally modified by phosphorylation, acetylation, and sumoylation, affecting their target gene specificity, stability, and transactivating and transrepressional activity, respectively (Li et al., 2007; Ghisletti et al., 2007; Chen et al., 2006; Yamamoto et al., 2007). We have recently shown that LXR can be modified by O-GlcNAcylation in response to glucose (see section 4.3), increasing its transactivation of the SREBP1c promoter (Anthonisen et al., 2010). PTMs may alter the structural conformation of LXR thereby modifying the affinity of coregulators that determines whether a target gene is induced or suppressed. Modulation by PTMs can occur both in the absence and presence of natural ligand tuning LXR activities in a cell- and gene-specific manner (Rosenfeld et al., 2006) depending on the nutritional stimuli.

3. LXR in hepatic *de novo* lipogenesis

3.1. LXR lipogenic target genes

In addition to being central regulators of cholesterol metabolism, the LXRs are involved in induction of fatty acid and triglyceride (TG) biosynthesis in response to feeding. *De novo* lipogenesis ensures that excess acetyl-CoA, which is an intermediate product of glucose metabolism, is converted into fats and subsequent TGs. LXRs are involved in hepatic lipogenesis through direct regulation of SREBP1c and ChREBP expression (Repa et al., 2000; Cha & Repa, 2007; Shimano, 2001). SREBP1c is a well described transcriptional regulator of hepatic lipogenesis (Shimano, 2001), and together with LXR and glucose-regulated ChREBP (see section 4.1), it controls expression of essential enzymes in lipogenesis, lipid storage and secretion (Fig. 3). SREBP1c deficiency does not fully abolish the expression of genes involved

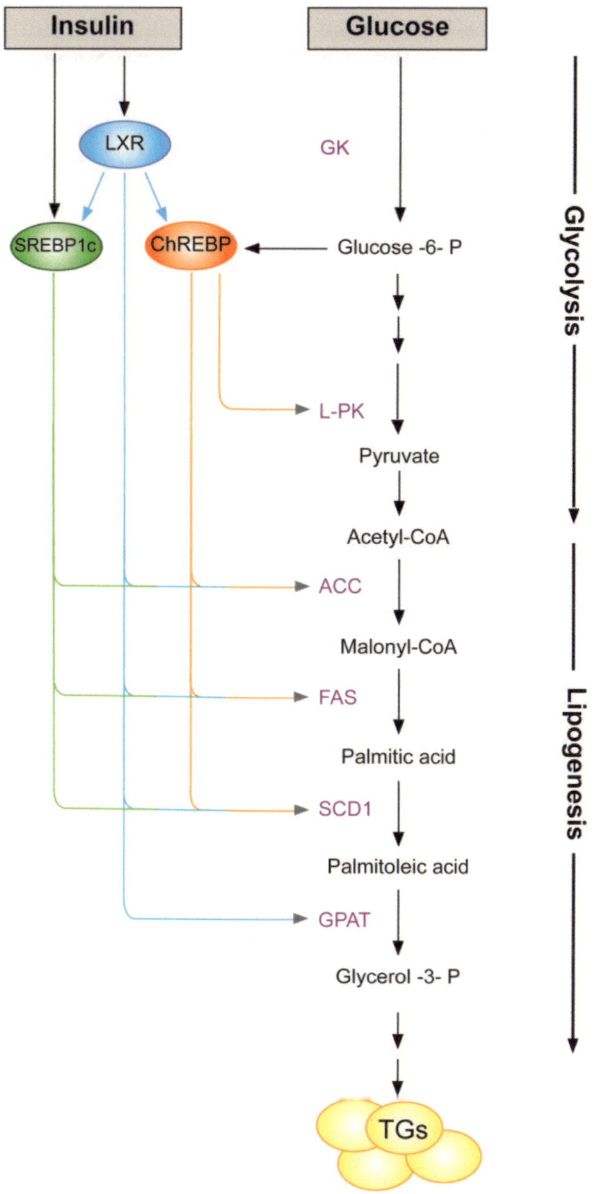

Figure 3. Regulation of hepatic lipogenesis by LXR, SREBP1c and ChREBP.

in hepatic lipogenesis. SREBP1c null mice treated with an LXR agonist results in induction of a subset of lipogenic genes and a modest increase in fatty acid synthesis (Liang et al., 2002), which implies that LXR can act independently of SREBP1c. In particular, the SCD1 gene is directly regulated by LXRα in response to synthetic ligands, also in the absence of SREBP1c (Chu et al., 2006). SCD1 is central in desaturation of saturated fatty acyl-CoAs important for formation of cholesterol esters (CEs) and TGs. Thus, specific LXR-mediated regulation of SCD1 can be explained by the essential role of LXR in limiting toxic free cholesterol in response to diets rich in cholesterol and saturated fat. The expression of LXRα in liver is rapidly upregulated by insulin *in vivo*, increasing mRNA expression of SREBP1c, malic enzyme (ME), ACC and FAS. Furthermore, expression of these lipogenic genes was abolished in insulin-injected LXRα/β double knock out mice (Tobin et al., 2002), indicating an essential role for LXR in insulin-mediated regulation of hepatic lipogenesis. The mechanisms by which insulin activate LXR-mediated gene expression is not clearly understood, but may involve production of endogenous ligand for LXRα/β (Chen et al., 2004) and/or by signal transduction mechanisms downstream of the IR affecting CA recruitment to LXRs and/or PTMs of LXRs. This will be discussed in more detail below. Of note, PKA-induced phosphorylation of LXRα has been shown to inhibit the expression of SREBP1c in liver from mice via reduced DNA binding and CA recruitment (Yamamoto et al., 2007). Since glucagon/cAMP/PKA signaling may, at least in part, explain down-regulation of SREBP1c expression in response to fasting, it is likely that PKA-mediated phosphorylation of LXR contributes to the fasting signal on SREBP1c.

3.2. Putative mechanisms regulating LXR-mediated *de novo* lipogenesis in response to insulin

Insulin is the most important anabolic hormone in the body, regulating many processes important for cellular growth and energy storage such as glucose uptake and metabolism, glycogen and lipid synthesis, gene transcription and translation. A classic action of insulin is to mediate a metabolic switch from fatty acid oxidation to synthesis and suppress hepatic glycogenolysis and gluconeogenesis in response to carbohydrate excess, a process that is largely regulated at the transcriptional level. In this way, hepatic insulin signaling maintains whole body energy homeostasis. In the insulin-resistant state, only the ability of insulin to suppress hepatic gluconeogenesis is lost, while its ability to activate lipogenesis is retained (Shimomura et al., 2000; Matsumoto et al., 2006; Brown & Goldstein, 2008). This bifurcated insulin resistance can be explained by failure of insulin to inhibit the gluconeogenic transcription factor Forkhead box protein O1 (FoxO1), but maintaining signaling to lipogenic transcriptional regulators including LXR and SREBP1c.

3.2.1. The insulin signaling cascade

The insulin signaling cascade is initiated by the binding of insulin to the extracellular β-subunits of the dimerized IR followed by autophosphorylation on several intracellular tyrosine residues on the IR. Insulin receptor substrate (IRS) is an essential protein docking onto the phosphorylated IR which in turn is phosphorylated itself on multiple tyrosine residues. This creates docking sites for src homology 2 (SH2) domain containing proteins. The best studied SH2 protein that binds to tyrosine phosphorylated IRS proteins is the regulatory subunit of the phosphoinositide 3-kinase (PI3K). PI3K catalyzes the formation of the lipid second messenger phosphatidylinositol (3,4,5) trisphosphate (PIP3), which is necessary to recruit downstream kinases. PIP3 generates a binding site for proteins containing Pleckstrin homology (PH) domains, such as 3′-phosphoinositide-dependent protein kinase (PDK1), the serine/threonine kinase Akt/protein kinase B and possibly also mammalian target of rapamycin complex 2 (mTORC2). PDK and mTORC2 are both necessary for full activation of Akt downstream of the insulin receptor via PDK1-mediated phosphorylation of Akt on threonine 308 and mTORC2-mediated phosphorylation on serine 472 (Saltiel & Kahn, 2001; White, 2003; Jacinto et al., 2006). All these events occur transiently in specific cholesterol rich plasma membrane microdomains called caveolae, generating a specific signaling unit for proper downstream insulin signaling where Akt plays a central role.

3.2.2. Regulation by mTOR

One of the targets of Akt is mTORC1 (Zoncu et al., 2011). Recent evidence suggests that mTORC1 is involved in LXR-mediated lipogenic gene transcription including induction of SREBP1c, FAS and ACC in liver from mice subjected to a high fat diet (Hwahng et al., 2009). The authors show that the mechanism by which mTORC1 activates LXR is via p70 S6 kinase (S6K)-mediated phosphorylation of LXR. Conversely, in the fasted state, LXR was shown to be inhibited by AMPK-mediated phosphorylation. In agreement with these observations, Li et al (Li et al., 2010) showed that insulin-activated hepatic transcription of SREBP1c, FAS and SCD1 is mediated by mTORC1, however independent of S6K. As both LXR and SREBP1c induce lipogenic promoters in response to insulin, this might suggest that activation of LXR in response to insulin/nutrients is mediated, at least in part, by mTORC1 and S6K, whereas insulin-signaling to SREBP1c requires mTORC2 independently of S6K, possibly via Akt-mediated inhibition of glycogen synthase kinase-3 (GSK3) (Hagiwara et al., 2012). In this way, GSK3-mediated phosphorylation and degradation of SREBP1c is prevented by insulin signaling to mTORC2 and Akt. Of note, insulin has primarily been shown to act on the SREBP1c promoter by activating LXRs and not SREBP1c (Chen et al., 2004) and the effect of insulin on SREBP1c is mainly at the posttranslational level. In a recent publication, mTORC1 was shown to phosphorylate a phosphatidic acid phosphatase, Lipin 1, preventing its nuclear entry and subsequent inhibition of SREBP1c-mediated activation of the FAS promoter (Peterson et al., 2011). Furthermore, Yecies JL et al (Yecies et al., 2011) showed that Akt2 independently of mTORC1 downregulate the mRNA expression of insulin induced gene 2 (Insig2a), an inhibitor of SREBP1c. This finding has been debated by Wan M et al (Wan et al., 2011), who could not observe any downregulation of Insig2a by Akt2. They postulate that Akt2 acts independently of mTORC1 and SREBP1c, possibly via posttranslational mechanisms, and that nutrients have a direct role in the liver to promote lipogenesis by a process dependent on both mTORC1 and other insulin-dependent signaling pathways. In light of the above mentioned studies, both mTORC1 and mTORC2 (Soukas et al., 2009; Guertin et al., 2006; Lamming et al., 2012; Hagiwara et al., 2012) appear to play important roles in lipid synthesis and storage in hepatocytes. Further studies will reveal the relative roles of Akt1, Akt2, mTORC1/C2 and S6kinase on activation of LXR and SREBP1c in this regulation under insulin sensitive and insulin resistant conditions and cross-talk with glucose metabolism and signaling (Fig.4).

3.2.3. Regulation by FoxO1

Another mechanism by which insulin may promote LXR-mediated SREBP1c transcription is through the transcription factor FoxO1. FoxO1, generally known as an activator of gluconeogenic genes during fasting, can repress the transactivating ability of LXR and cooperating transcription factors SREBP1c and Specificity protein 1 (Sp1) to activate SREBP1c transcription during fasting (Liu et al., 2010; Deng et al., 2012). FoxO1 does not seem to bind directly to the SREBP1c promoter, but appears to act as a repressor through protein-protein interactions, possibly by recruiting CR proteins (Deng et al., 2012). Upon feeding, FoxO1 is inhibited by insulin via PI3-kinase activation and phosphorylation by Akt, which excludes phosphorylated FoxO1 from the nucleus via association with the 14-3-3 protein (reviewed in (Tzivion et al., 2011)). In this way, at least under insulin sensitive conditions, inhibition mediated by FoxO1 and associating CRs is relieved, enabling LXR, Sp1 and SREBP1c to activate the SREBP1c promoter in a cooperative fashion. Of note, an important role for the E-box transcription factor Upstream Stimulatory Factor (USF) in mediating insulin activation of the SREBP1c promoter has also been reported (Wong & Sul, 2010). The relative roles of LXR, SREBP1c and cooperating transcription factors in regulation of the SREBP1c promoter after high-carbohydrate feeding under normal and insulin resistant conditions and the role of FoxO1 in this process in insulin resistance is currently not known. Recently, the role of Akt as a central regulator of both gluconeogenesis, through inhibition of FoxO1, and lipogenesis, through activation of mTORC1/2 in hepatic insulin signaling, was debated as the insulin resistant phenotype of mice lacking hepatic Akt1/2 were normalized in mice with concomitant liver-specific deletion of FoxO1 (Lu et al., 2012). This work suggests that a major role for Akt as a metabolic regulator in response to insulin is largely to restrain FoxO1 activity, at least for suppression of liver glucose output.

3.2.4. Regulation by insulin-mediated oxysterol production

Considering the bifurcated nature of insulin resistance and the postulated central role of Akt in this process, a very recent work by Wu and Williams (Wu & Williams, 2012), put forward an interesting theory. They suggest that disturbance of a single molecule, NAD(P)H oxidase 4 (NOX4), is sufficient to induce the key harmful features of insulin resistance. NOX4 is activated upon IR activation, generating a transient burst of superoxide (O_2^-) and its byproduct H_2O_2. This enhances signal transduction by disabling enzymes in the protein-tyrosine phosphatase gene family. In this way, essential inhibiting enzymes in the insulin signaling cascade is blocked, notably the PI3K inhibitor PTEN and protein-tyrosine phosphatase-1B (PTP1B) (Wu & Williams, 2012). Intriguingly, NOX4 may also be the link between insulin signaling and production of oxysterol ligand for LXR, as NOX4 through its superoxide producing activity may mediate the production of oxygenated cholesterol. The evidence for this is that pharmacological inhibition of NOX4 blocked insulin-induction of SREBP1c mRNA in rat primary hepatocytes, even though phosphorylations upstream and downstream of mTORC1 remained responsive (Wu & Williams, 2012). Furthermore, NOX4 is transiently localized to caveolae (Han et al., 2012), possibly via recruitment to the IR, placing the enzyme in close proximity to cholesterol-rich areas of the plasma membrane. A complete summary of putative mechanisms of insulin-mediated signaling to LXR, SREBP1c and lipogenesis is depicted in Fig. 4.

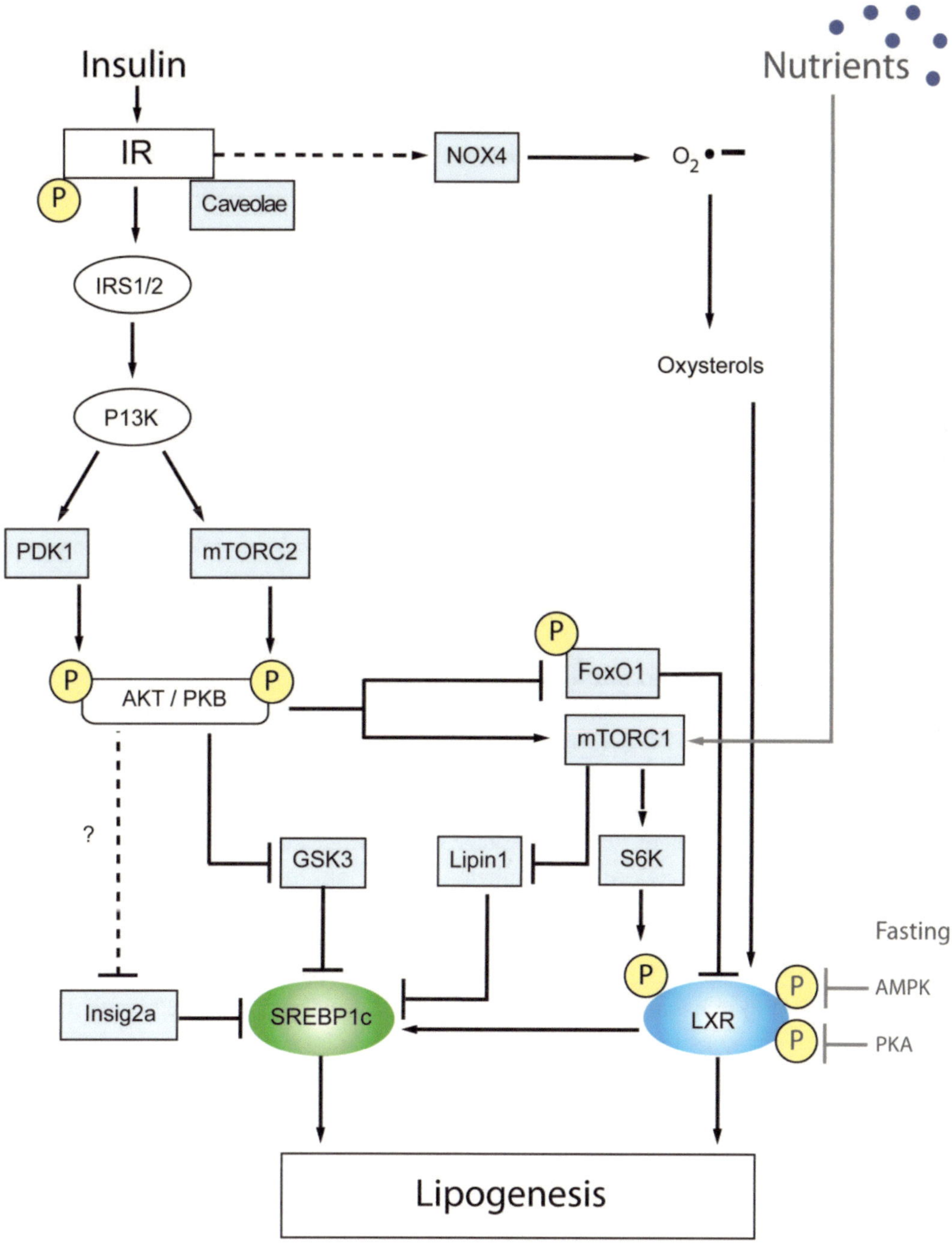

Figure 4. Insulin-mediated regulation of hepatic lipogenesis

4. Lipogenic gene expression in response to glucose metabolism

Hepatic glucose metabolism activates the transcription of various genes encoding enzymes of glycolysis and lipogenesis independently of insulin. However, the initial modification of glucose into Glucose-6-phosphate (G6P) by the enzyme Glucokinase (GK; Hexokinase 4) required for transcriptional regulation by glucose is highly dependent on insulin (Bosco et al., 2000), possibly via SREBP1c (Foretz et al., 1999; Kim et al., 2004) in concert with LXR and Peroxisome Proliferator-Activated Receptor gamma (PPARγ) (Kim et al., 2009). Thus the actions of glucose and insulin may be considered interdependent and that regulation of gene expression in response to glucose seems to require active LXR, SREBP1c and/or PPARγ.

4.1. Glucose regulation via ChREBP

A majority of hepatic glucose-responsive genes is thought to be regulated by the transcription factor ChREBP (Yamashita et al., 2001; Ishii et al., 2004). ChREBP mediates transcriptional regulation of glycolytic and lipogenic enzymes and is particularly important for the induction of liver-pyruvate kinase (L-PK), one of the rate limiting enzymes of glycolysis, which is exclusively dependent on glucose (Matsuda et al., 1990; Dentin et al., 2004). Furthermore, ChREBP is involved in regulating ACC and FAS in concert with LXR and SREBP1c in response to glucose and insulin, respectively, suggesting its involvement of the conversion of carbohydrates into fat (Joseph et al., 2002; Talukdar & Hillgartner, 2006). Moreover, stimulation by a synthetic LXR ligand, induces hepatic expression and activity of ChREBP (Cha & Repa, 2007). However, ChREBP is apparently not dependent on LXR for its hepatic expression and activity in mice fed a high carbohydrate/high fat diet (Denechaud et al., 2008), suggesting that ChREBP activity is reinforced by upstream LXR under certain nutritional conditions. At low glucose concentrations, the ChREBP protein is retained as an inactive phosphoprotein in the cytoplasm (reviewed in (Havula & Hietakangas, 2012)). The mechanisms by which glucose activate ChREBP is not clear, but involves induction of the ChREBP mRNA, dephosphorylation of the protein, shuttling to the nucleus and binding to the ChREBP response element at the promoter of its target genes (Uyeda & Repa, 2006). Early studies pointed to xylose 5-phosphate (Xu5P), an intermediate of the pentose phosphate pathway (PPP), as an activating signal through its ability to activate protein phosphatase 2A (PP2A) and subsequent dephosphorylation of ChREBP (Havula & Hietakangas, 2012). Recently, ChREBP was shown to be activated by fructose 2,6-biphosphate (F2,6BP) in hepatocytes (Arden et al., 2012). The level of F2,6BP is regulated by the bifunctional enzyme 6-phosphofructokinase-2-kinase/fructose-2,6-biphosphatase (PFK2/FBP2). Thus, PFK2 catalyzes the synthesis and degradation of F2,6BP and as a result, the enzyme is involved in both glycolysis and gluconeogenesis. In the fed state, insulin and carbohydrates dephosphorylate PFK2 in the liver making the enzyme kinase dominant. Subsequently, F6P is converted to F2,6BP that activates PFK1, which in turn stimulates glycolysis (Fig. 6). Interestingly, LXRα was recently shown to be a central regulator of hepatic PFK2 mRNA expression (Zhao et al., 2012). Activation of ChREBP in response to glucose appears to depend on multiple glucose metabolites, including G6P, X5P and F2,6BP. As LXRα is involved in regulation GK- and PFK2-expression in response to insulin, this may suggest that ChREBP is dependent on insulin signaling via LXR for proper substrate availability.

4.2. Glucose metabolism via the hexosamine biosynthetic pathway and O-GlcNAc signaling

Glucose metabolism from F6P can follow the alternative hexosamine biosynthetic pathway (HBP) where the enzyme glutamine fructose-6-phosphate amidotransferase (GFAT) controls the first and rate limiting step (Fig. 5).

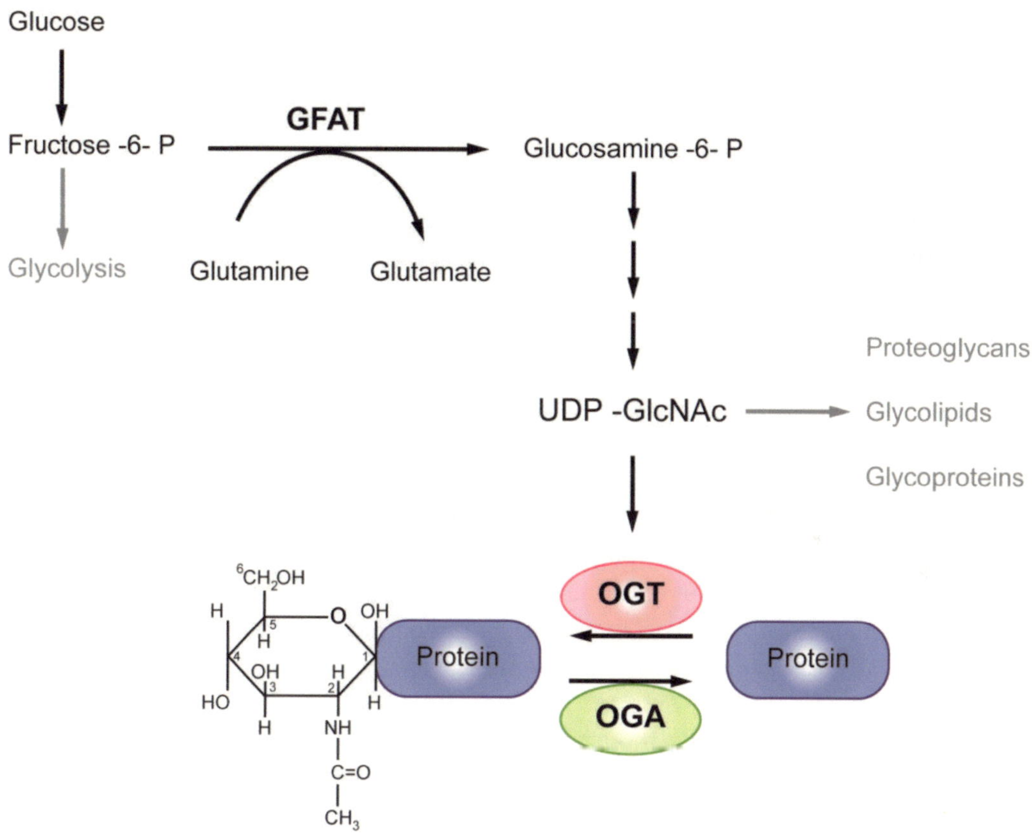

Figure 5. Nutrient flux and O-GlcNAc modification of nucleocytoplasmatic proteins through the HBP

The end product of this pathway is Uridine diphosphate *N*-acetylglucosamine (UDP-GlcNAc), an essential building block for N-and O-linked glycosylation of proteins and lipids. Cytoplasmic and nuclear proteins can be dynamically modified by O-linked β-N-acetylglucosamine (*O*-GlcNAc) on serine and threonine residues by the enzyme O-GlcNAc transferase (OGT) using UDP-GlcNAc as substrate. OGT is an essential enzyme as targeted deletion of this gene is lethal (Shafi et al., 2000). The enzyme O-GlcNAc transferase (OGA) hydrolyses the sugar analogous to protein dephosphorylation of phosphorylated proteins by phosphatases (Hart et al., 2007; Love, 2005). Because *O*-GlcNAc levels on proteins appear to be sensitive to increasing flux through this pathway in response to nutrient excess, OGT can be considered as a general sensor of glucose availability that modifies proteins according to changes in UDP-GlcNAc levels. There is no identified consensus sequence for GlcNAcylation, and unlike the multiple genes encoding kinases, there is only a single X-linked gene encoding the catalytic subunit of OGT in mammals (Shafi et al., 2000). For this reason, it has been hypothesized that OGT is the catalytic subunit in large transient enzyme complexes where interacting proteins are able to target OGT to its many substrates. Many transcription factors are modified by O-GlcNAc in the liver (Dentin et al., 2008; Housley et al., 2008; Kuo et al., 2008; Ozcan et al., 2010). Interestingly, FoxO1 has been shown to be a target for O-GlcNAcylation in hepatocytes in response to hyperglycemia in the insulin resistant state, resulting in elevated transactivating capacity for FoxO1 against its gluconeogenic targets phosphoenolpyruvate carboxykinase (PEPCK) and glucose-6-phosphatase (G6Pase) reinforcing hepatic glucose production (Housley et al., 2008; Kuo et al., 2008). Moreover, this activation was later shown to be dependent on targeting of OGT to FoxO1 via interaction with the coactivator PGC1α, which itself was shown to be modified by O-GlcNAc upon interaction with OGT (Housley et al., 2009). As PGC1α have been shown to significantly amplify LXRα-mediated activation of the SREBP1c promoter (Oberkofler et al., 2003; Kim et al., 2008), a possible recruitment of an OGT/PGC1α-complex to LXR on lipogenic target genes under insulin resistant conditions remains to be explored. Recently, ChREBP was also shown to be a target for O-GlcNAcylation in response to hyperglycemia (Guinez et al., 2011). Adenoviral overexpression of OGT in liver increased ChREBP O-GlcNAc modification, protein stability and transactivating activity of L-PK, as well as potentiating expression of ACC, FAS and SCD1 mRNA expression in response to refeeding (Guinez et al., 2011). In contrast, hepatic overexpression of OGA reduced lipogenic protein content (ACC and FAS) and hepatic steatosis (excessive accumulation of TGs and CEs) in db/db mice, suggesting that enhanced OGT signaling to ChREBP and cooperating transcription factors/coregulators contributes to hepatic steatosis under insulin resistant conditions.

4.3. O-GlcNAc signaling activates LXR and hepatic lipogenesis

In 2007, glucose was reported as an endogenous ligand for LXR (Mitro et al., 2007). This has, however, been debated considering the hydrophobic nature of the ligand binding pocket (Lazar & Willson, 2007). Instead, we asked the question whether glucose exert its effect via hexosamine signaling and posttranslational O-GlcNAc modification of LXR. In a recent publication, we show that LXR is O-GlcNAc modified in response to high glucose (25 mM) in absence of insulin (cells cultured in 2 % serum, approximately 1-2 pmol/l insulin) and synthetic LXR-ligand in Huh7 cells, a human hepatoma cell line (Anthonisen et al., 2010). By pharmacological inhibition we demonstrated that hexosamine signaling and O-GlcNAc cycling mediates LXR dependent activation of the SREBP1c promoter in response to glucose. Furthermore, we observed increased O-GlcNAc modification of LXR in livers from refed mice and streptozotosin (STZ) treated diabetic mice corresponding with increased SREBP1c mRNA expression. Moreover, general protein O-GlcNAcylation was increased in STZ-treated hyperglycemic mice compared to control mice. Our results suggest that LXR is regulated by O-GlcNAc modification, thereby increasing its lipogenic potential. Whether O-GlcNAc-LXR is able to transactivate other lipogenic genes in addition to SREBP1c, is currently under investigation in our laboratory. Our preliminary studies point to a role for O-GlcNAc-LXR in upregulating ChREBP, FAS, ACC and SCD1 expression (Bindesbøll et al, unpublished). Furthermore, preliminary reChIP experiments in our laboratory (LXR ChIP followed by O-GlcNAc ChIP), show a strong induction of O-GlcNAc-associated LXR binding to LXRE on the promoters of SREBP1c, ChREBP, FAS and SCD1 in response to feeding both in control mice and STZ treated mice. Our study is supported by the observation that the SREBP1c promoter activity and protein levels of SREBP1c are increased in response to elevated glucose concentration in the mouse hepatocyte cell line H2-35 (Hasty et al., 2000). Furthermore, treatment with azaserine, an inhibitor of GFAT, completely suppressed expression of both cytoplasmic and nuclear SREBP1c protein, suggesting that hexosamine-dependent O-GlcNAc signaling indeed is involved in glucose-induced SREBP1c mRNA expression, possibly via activation of LXR and/or cooperating transcription factors/CAs.

In our *in vitro* studies, we observed only modest LXR/RXR transactivation of the SREBP1c promoter in high glucose/low insulin-treated cells. This might be explained by constitutive phosphorylation competing for the same site(s) as GlcNAc on LXR and/or inhibitory phosphorylation occurring on adjacent GlcNAc sites. Housley et al. (Housley et al., 2008) reported elevated *O*-GlcNAc on FoxO1 by high glucose and a subsequent reduction by insulin. They further showed that *O*-GlcNAc modification increased substantially on the insulin-insensitive mutant FoxO1 lacking three AKT phosphorylation sites (T24A, S256A, S319A), resulting in increased FoxO1-dependent luciferase reporter activity. These observations imply overlapping and/or adjacent phosphorylation and GlcNAc sites on FoxO1. Indeed, the authors also identified several O-GlcNAc sites on FoxO1, one of which is adjacent to an Akt phosphorylation site (Thr^{317}). In the case of LXR, which is activated by insulin, apparently in part via S6K-mediated phosphorylation (Hwahng et al., 2009), GlcNAcylation and phosphorylation might act synergistically on LXR in response to glucose and insulin. In fact, extensive cross-talk between O-GlcNAcylation and phosphorylation appear to contribute to the pathology of various diseases (Hart et al., 2011). In addition, GlcNAc and inhibiting phosphate (in response to fasting via PKA and/or AMPK) may compete for the same sites or are situated at different serines and/or threonines on LXR. Furthermore, GlcNAcylation and phosphorylation of LXR might be affected by ligand binding, which has been shown for SUMOylation and acetylation of LXR (Venteclef et al., 2010; Lee et al., 2009). A study by Torra et al. (Torra et al., 2008) reported that Ser^{198} phosphorylation of LXRα in RAW macrophages was induced by both synthetic and natural oxysterol LXR ligands and reduced by the RXR ligand 9-*cis*-retinoc acid. As such, we cannot exclude the possibility that LXR O-GlcNAcylation may be positively or negatively regulated by LXR and/or RXR ligands. From our *in vitro* GlcNAcylation results (Anthonisen et al., 2010) we believe that the major O-GlcNAc site(s) on LXRα and LXRβ resides in the N-terminal region containing the AF1 and DBD, indicating that O-GlcNAcylation occur independently of ligand. However, under hyperglycemic conditions, ligand binding may recruit OGT to LXR via CAs, possibly PGC1α as reported for FoxO1 (Housley et al., 2009). A more detailed mapping of the GlcNAc sites on LXR and site-directed mutagenesis as well as identification of coregulators of LXR under hyperglycemic conditions, are under way in our laboratory to elucidate the biological role of O-GlcNAc on LXR. A complete summary of putative mechanisms of glucose-signaling to LXR, ChREBP and lipogenesis is depicted in Figure 6.

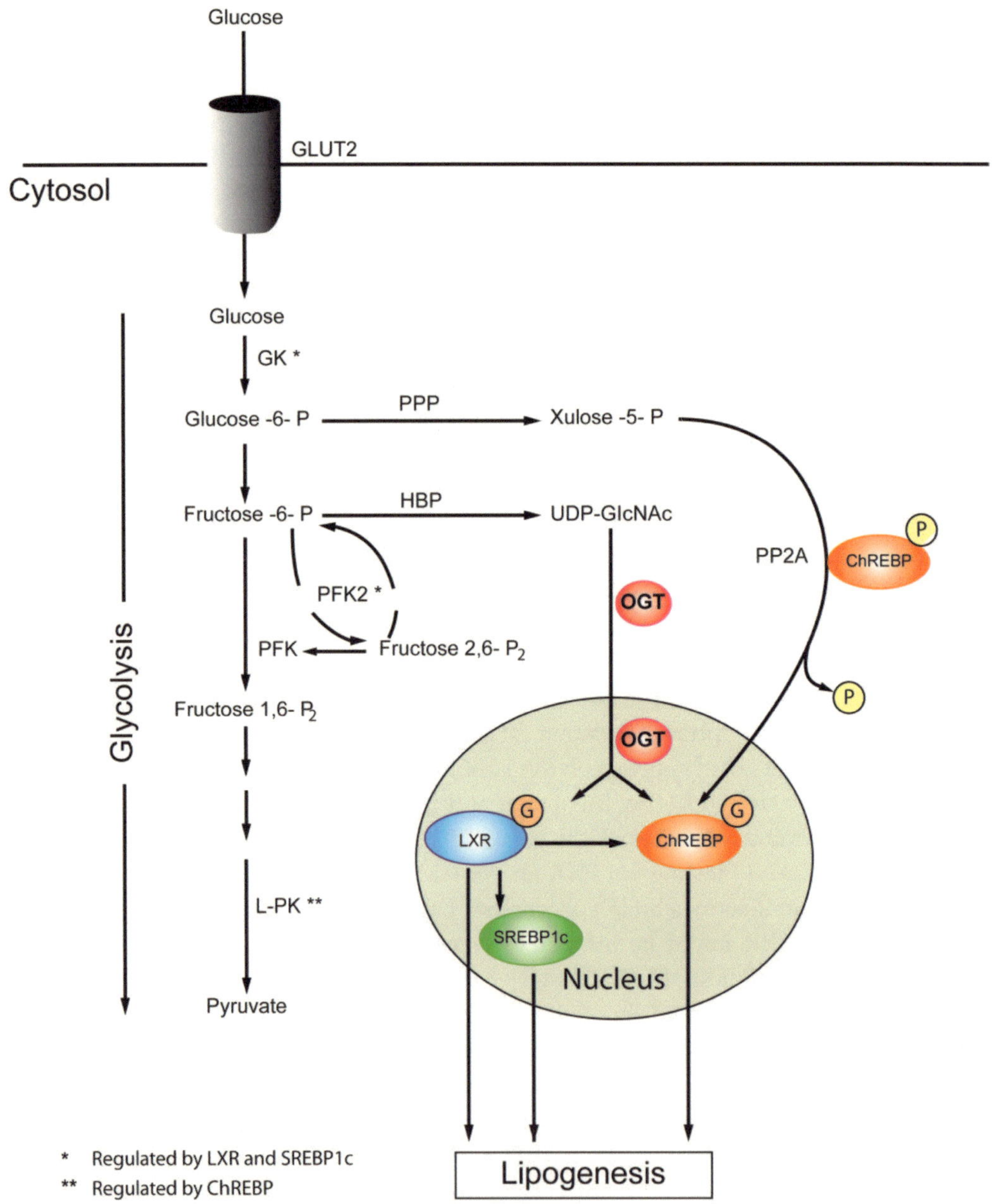

Figure 6. Glucose-mediated regulation of hepatic lipogenesis

5. Cross-talk between O-GlcNAc- and insulin signaling

Studies in *C.elegans* demonstrate that O-GlcNAc cycling phenotypes are very sensitive to insulin as well as nutrient composition and that levels of insulin and nutrients influence the role of O-GlcNAc cycling and vice versa (Mondoux et al., 2011; Hanover et al., 2010; Hanover et al., 2010; Whelan et al., 2008). Intriguingly, O-GlcNAc-marked promoters in *C.elegans* are biased toward genes associated with PIP3 signaling, hexosamine biosynthesis, and lipid/carbohydrate metabolism (Love et al., 2010a). Defects in O-GlcNAc cycling results in deregulation of genes necessary for carbohydrate and lipid metabolism in response to insulin (Forsythe et al., 2006; Hanover et al., 2010) suggesting that both O-GlcNAc cycling and insulin-signaling are required for a robust and adaptable response to hyperglycemia. Several studies have implicated O-GlcNAc cycling in the development of insulin resistance (reviewed in (Mondoux et al., 2011)). Mice overexpressing OGT in muscle or fat and mammalian cells overexpressing OGA develop insulin resistance (McClain, 2002; Arias et al., 2004; Vosseller et al., 2002). Later studies revealed that a subset of OGT was able to transiently translocate to the plasma membrane via association with PIP3 generated by insulin-activated PI3K (Yang et al., 2008). In response to increased glucose metabolism, PIP3-associated OGT can O-GlcNAcylate IR, IRS and Akt antagonizing insulin signaling (Yang et al., 2008; Whelan et al., 2010). Moreover, OGT may also interact with the mTOR pathway (Hanover et al., 2010). As mentioned in section 3.2.3, the downstream target for insulin signaling, FoxO1, is also modified by O-GlcNAc, apparently via OGT recruitment to PGC1α, providing another mechanism for OGT to contribute to insulin resistance, at least for sustained hepatic glucose production in response to hyperglycemia (Housley et al., 2009). Directing OGT to transcriptional targets implies that PGC1α can integrate multiple nutrient signals to regulate gene expression. Whether OGT via PGC1α or other CAs is also recruited to ChREBP- and LXR-regulated promoters is currently not known. OGT is recruited to and O-GlcNAcylate several coregulators and histone modifying enzymes (acetylases/deacetylases, metylases/demetylases) and even histones themselves (Fujiki et al., 2009; Hanover et al., 2012; Fujiki et al., 2011; Sakabe et al., 2010). Depending on the nutritional stimuli, all components of the transciptional machinery from specific transcription factors to coregulators, histones and RNA polymerase II are subject to epigenetic regulation by acetylation, ubiquitinylation, SUMOylation, phosphorylation and/or O-GlcNAcylation (Rosenfeld et al., 2006; Venteclef et al., 2011; Love et al., 2010b; Kato et al., 2011). The fine-tuning of these modifications determines whether a gene is activated or repressed. Furthermore, as the substrate specificity of OGT is believed to be spatio-temporally regulated by transient interactions with large enzyme complexes, its binding to PIP3 may not occur solely at the plasma membrane, as PI3K is also active in the nucleus where it is involved in regulation of protein-chromatin interactions, transcription and mRNA export (Viiri et al., 2012; Kebede et al., 2012; Okada & Ye, 2009). As protein O-GlcNAcylation is rapidly increased at both the plasma membrane and the nucleus in response to serum-stimulation (Carrillo et al., 2011), OGT-binding to nuclear PIP3 may also be instrumental in transcriptional regulation in response to feeding. Interestingly, nonalcoholic fatty liver disease is often accompanied by hepatic insulin resistance, metabolic syndrome, and diabetes (reviewed in (Scorletti et al., 2011)) and the sensitivity of OGT to glucose increases with decreasing insulin signaling (Mondoux et al., 2011). These findings suggest that elevated O-GlcNAc cycling on key nuclear proteins contributes to the development of hepatic steatosis. This notion is also in line with the above mentioned observation by Guinez et al (Guinez et al., 2011), where overexpression of OGA reduced hepatic steatosis in db/db mice. A complete summary of a putative glucose-insulin cross-talk in regulation of hepatic *de novo* lipogenesis is depicted in Fig. 7.

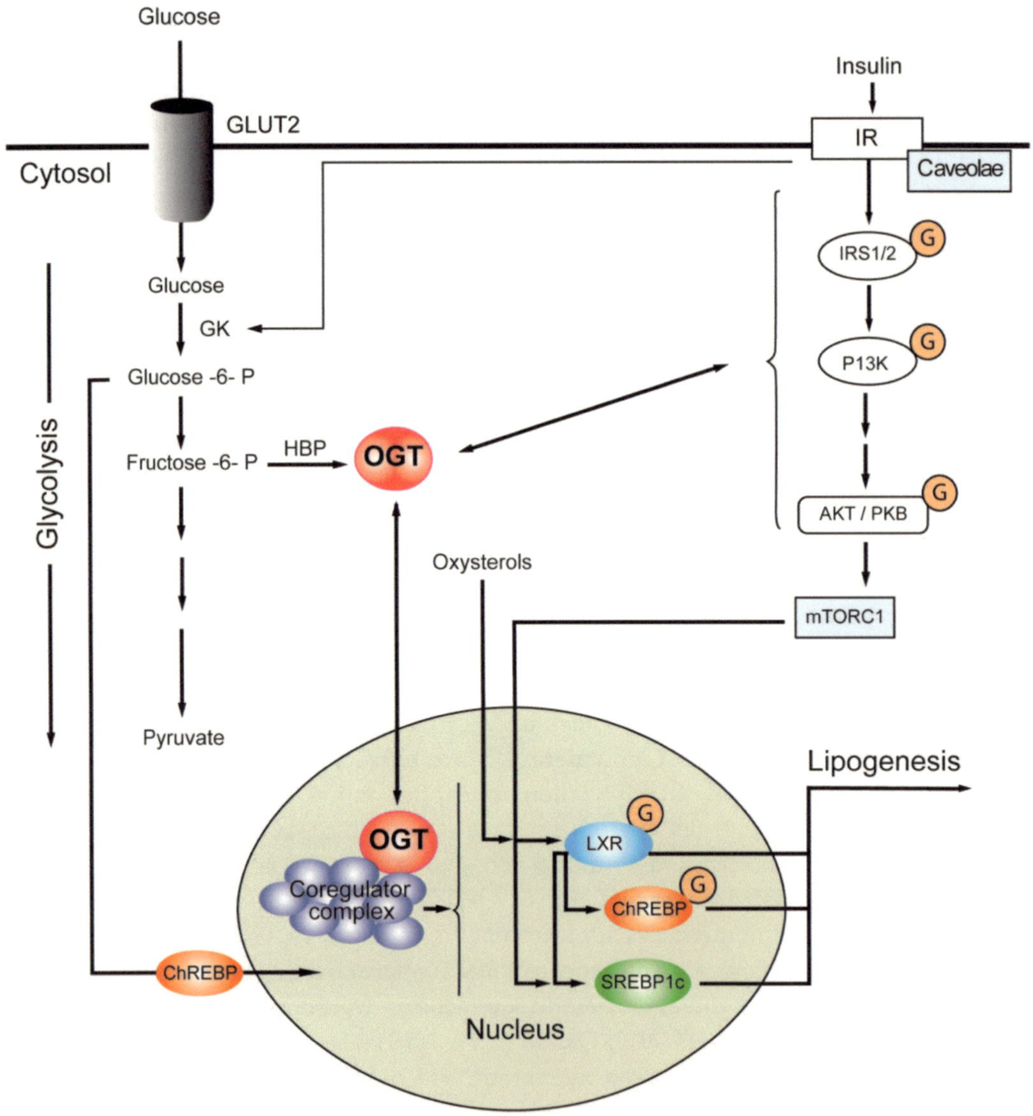

Figure 7. Glucose-insulin cross-talk in regulation of hepatic lipogenesis

6. Concluding remarks

In mice and humans, hepatic *de novo* lipogenesis is activated by a high intake of both glucose and fructose (Scorletti et al., 2011; Schwarz et al., 1995; Schwarz et al., 2003). Fructose increase hepatic hexosamine signaling (Hirahatake et al., 2011) and induce SREBP1c and ChREBP expression in hepatic cells (Matsuzaka et al., 2004; Haas et al., 2012; Koo et al., 2009), which may, in part be mediated by LXR. The response of LXR to glucose has been debated (Lazar & Willson, 2007), but a recent study support the notion of LXR as a glucose/fructose sensor as high sucrose fed mice exhibit elevated hepatic expression of SREBP1c and increased TG levels, which was not observed in LXRα/β double knock out mice (Korach-Andre et al., 2011). LXR increases lipogenesis, in part by activating SREBP1c and ChREBP proteins. Thus, in response to feeding, they can cooperately activate most of the genes required for hepatic lipogenesis and TG secretion. Whether hepatic LXR drives the expression of SREBP1c and/or ChREBP to the same degree under different nutritional conditions is currently not known, as most studies have been performed using synthetic LXR agonists. We have preliminary results showing that hepatic expression of SREBP1c and ChREBP is upregulated in refed control mice and to a lesser extent in STZ-treated hyperglycemic mice, which is not observed in LXRα/β double knock out mice (Bindesbøll et al, unpublished). O-GlcNAc modification of LXR is increased in STZ-treated mice (Anthonisen et al., 2010) and we postulate that O-GlcNAc modification of LXR in response to glucose activates LXR and drives the expression of ChREBP and SREBP1c and in particular the lipogenic genes, ACC and SCD1. Furthermore, RNA Pol II ChIP-Seq data show reduced binding of RNA Pol II to the L-PK promoter and no binding of RNA Pol II to the SCD1 promoter in LXR α/β double knock out mice compared to control mice. Moreover, a novel LXRE immediately downstream of SCD1 was found, to which LXR bound more strongly than the previously published upstream LXR binding site (Boergesen et al., 2012). This suggests an important role for LXR as an upstream activator of ChREBP-mediated transcription and argues for LXR acting independently on the SCD1 promoter, at least under certain nutritional conditions. Previous studies have demonstrated that LXR directly activates key lipogenic genes (Joseph et al., 2002), most notably SCD1 in the liver of SREBP1c knockout mice (Liang et al., 2002; Chu et al., 2006). Why there would be a need for LXR to activate lipogenic genes directly, may be explained by the nutritional conditions and redundancy in the system. Oxysterols bind the endoplasmic reticulum resident Insig protein and could inhibit the proteolytic maturation of SREBP1c (Radhakrishnan et al., 2007). This would limit transcription by SREBP1c, and direct activation by LXR would be required to stimulate lipogenesis. In the absence of active SREBP1c, however, LXR may act in concert with ChREBP in regulating lipogenic expression. A recent study show that hepatic overexpression of ChREBP induces SCD1 expression and hepatic steatosis, but not insulin resistance (Benhamed et al., 2012). Whether overexpression of ChREBP affected LXR protein expression and transactivation of the SCD1 promoter was not investigated in this study. In later studies, it would be interesting to investigate the SCD1 expression and activity in livers or hepatocytes with targeted deletion of ChREBP. Benhamed et al (Benhamed et al., 2012) also showed that ChREBP expression was increased in liver biopsies from patients with steatosis and decreased in liver of patients with severe insulin resistance, suggesting that ChREBP, alone or in combination with LXR, drives SCD1 expression and steatosis independent of insulin resistance. This is in line with recent human studies showing no relationship between hepatic TG accumulation and insulin resistance (Cohen et al., 2011; Hooper et al., 2011). Thus, hepatic steatosis can either be the result or cause of hepatic insulin resistance. The mechanisms of hepatic insulin resistance is still not clear (Farese, Jr. et al., 2012), but may involve specific lipids, nutrition-induced metabolites and PTMs including O-GlcNAc. Hepatic TG synthesis may be a protective mechanism to limit accumulation of toxic free fatty acids, liver damage and fibrosis (Choi & Diehl, 2008) where particularly SCD1 seem to play a protective role (Li et al., 2009).

As LXR is shown also to act anti-inflammatory in liver (Wouters et al., 2008; Venteclef et al., 2010), LXR activation may be an important compensative mechanism in response to excess nutrients to limit liver damage, inflammation and fibrosis. SUMOylation is an important ligand-activated transrepressional PTM of LXR on inflammatory genes (Venteclef et al., 2011) and future studies in our laboratory aim to elucidate a putative cross-talk between OGT and E3 ligases (SUMO conjugating enzymes) in liver in response to excess nutrients, especially high sugar levels (glucose and fructose). The relative roles of LXR, SREBP1c and ChREBP in driving lipogenesis is clearly dependent on both insulin and glucose signaling and cross-talk between these pathways. Both phosphorylation and GlcNAcylation appear instrumental in hepatic lipogenesis and future focus in our laboratory will be to elucidate a possible cross-talk between these PTMs, endogenous LXR ligands and interacting CAs in response to various feeding conditions (high glucose, fructose and/or fatty acids, cholesterol) and the impact on downstream ChREBP, SREBP1c and lipogenic enzyme expression and activity. ChIP and reChIP analysis in combination with loss of function studies have become powerful tools to analyze activation of specific genes by specific transcription factors in response to extracellular stimuli. By these methods, we anticipate that the signaling mechanisms and relative roles of LXR, ChREBP, SREBP1c and cooperating transcription factors in driving hepatic *de novo* lipogenesis will be revealed in the not too distant future.

Author details

Line M. Grønning-Wang, Christian Bindesbøll and Hilde I. Nebb
The Medical Faculty, Institute of Basic Medical Sciences,
Department of Nutrition, University of Oslo, Norway

7. References

Anthonisen, E.H., Berven, L., Holm, S., Nygard, M., Nebb, H.I., & Gronning-Wang, L.M. (2010). Nuclear receptor liver X receptor is O-GlcNAc-modified in response to glucose. *J.Biol.Chem.*, Vol. 285, No. 3, pp. 1607-1615, PM:19933273

Apfel, R., Benbrook, D., Lernhardt, E., Ortiz, M.A., Salbert, G., & Pfahl, M. (1994). A novel orphan receptor specific for a subset of thyroid hormone-responsive elements and its interaction with the retinoid/thyroid hormone receptor subfamily. *Mol.Cell Biol.,* Vol. 14, No. 10, pp. 7025-7035, PM:7935418

Arden, C., Tudhope, S.J., Petrie, J.L., Al-Oanzi, Z.H., Cullen, K.S., Lange, A.J., Towle, H.C., & Agius, L. (2012). Fructose 2,6-bisphosphate is essential for glucose-regulated gene transcription of glucose-6-phosphatase and other ChREBP target genes in hepatocytes. *Biochem.J.,* Vol. 443, No. 1, pp. 111-123, PM:22214556

Arias, E.B., Kim, J., & Cartee, G.D. (2004). Prolonged incubation in PUGNAc results in increased protein O-Linked glycosylation and insulin resistance in rat skeletal muscle. *Diabetes,* Vol. 53, No. 4, pp. 921-930, PM:15047606

Benhamed, F., Denechaud, P.D., Lemoine, M., Robichon, C., Moldes, M., Bertrand-Michel, J., Ratziu, V., Serfaty, L., Housset, C., Capeau, J., Girard, J., Guillou, H., & Postic, C. (2012). The lipogenic transcription factor ChREBP dissociates hepatic steatosis from insulin resistance in mice and humans. *J.Clin.Invest,* Vol. 122, No. 6, pp. 2176-2194, PM:22546860

Boergesen, M., Pedersen, T.A., Gross, B., van Heeringen, S.J., Hagenbeek, D., Bindesboll, C., Caron, S., Lalloyer, F., Steffensen, K.R., Nebb, H.I., Gustafsson, J.A., Stunnenberg, H.G., Staels, B., & Mandrup, S. (2012). Genome-wide profiling of liver X receptor, retinoid X receptor, and peroxisome proliferator-activated receptor alpha in mouse liver reveals extensive sharing of binding sites. *Mol.Cell Biol.,* Vol. 32, No. 4, pp. 852-867, PM:22158963

Bosco, D., Meda, P., & Iynedjian, P.B. (2000). Glucokinase and glucokinase regulatory protein: mutual dependence for nuclear localization. *Biochem.J.,* Vol. 348 Pt 1, No.pp. 215-222, PM:10794734

Brown, M.S., & Goldstein, J.L. (2008). Selective versus total insulin resistance: a pathogenic paradox. *Cell Metab,* Vol. 7, No. 2, pp. 95-96, PM:18249166

Calkin, A.C., & Tontonoz, P. (2010). Liver x receptor signaling pathways and atherosclerosis. *Arterioscler.Thromb.Vasc.Biol.,* Vol. 30, No. 8, pp. 1513-1518, PM:20631351

Carrillo, L.D., Froemming, J.A., & Mahal, L.K. (2011). Targeted in vivo O-GlcNAc sensors reveal discrete compartment-specific dynamics during signal transduction. *J.Biol.Chem.,* Vol. 286, No. 8, pp. 6650-6658, PM:21138847

Cha, J.Y., & Repa, J.J. (2007). The liver X receptor (LXR) and hepatic lipogenesis. The carbohydrate-response element-binding protein is a target gene of LXR. *J.Biol.Chem.,* Vol. 282, No. 1, pp. 743-751, PM:17107947

Chen, G., Liang, G., Ou, J., Goldstein, J.L., & Brown, M.S. (2004). Central role for liver X receptor in insulin-mediated activation of Srebp-1c transcription and stimulation of fatty acid synthesis in liver. *Proc.Natl.Acad.Sci.U.S.A,* Vol. 101, No. 31, pp. 11245-11250, PM:15266058

Chen, M., Bradley, M.N., Beaven, S.W., & Tontonoz, P. (2006). Phosphorylation of the liver X receptors. *FEBS Lett.,* Vol. 580, No. 20, pp. 4835-4841, PM:16904112

Chiang, J.Y., Kimmel, R., & Stroup, D. (2001). Regulation of cholesterol 7alpha-hydroxylase gene (CYP7A1) transcription by the liver orphan receptor (LXRalpha). *Gene,* Vol. 262, No. 1-2, pp. 257-265, PM:11179691

Choi, S.S., & Diehl, A.M. (2008). Hepatic triglyceride synthesis and nonalcoholic fatty liver disease. *Curr.Opin.Lipidol.,* Vol. 19, No. 3, pp. 295-300, PM:18460922

Chu, K., Miyazaki, M., Man, W.C., & Ntambi, J.M. (2006). Stearoyl-coenzyme A desaturase 1 deficiency protects against hypertriglyceridemia and increases plasma high-density lipoprotein cholesterol induced by liver X receptor activation. *Mol.Cell Biol.,* Vol. 26, No. 18, pp. 6786-6798, PM:16943421

Cohen, J.C., Horton, J.D., & Hobbs, H.H. (2011). Human fatty liver disease: old questions and new insights. *Science,* Vol. 332, No. 6037, pp. 1519-1523, PM:21700865

Costet, P., Luo, Y., Wang, N., & Tall, A.R. (2000). Sterol-dependent transactivation of the ABC1 promoter by the liver X receptor/retinoid X receptor. *J.Biol.Chem.,* Vol. 275, No. 36, pp. 28240-28245, PM:10858438

Denechaud, P.D., Bossard, P., Lobaccaro, J.M., Millatt, L., Staels, B., Girard, J., & Postic, C. (2008). ChREBP, but not LXRs, is required for the induction of glucose-regulated genes in mouse liver. *J.Clin.Invest,* Vol. 118, No. 3, pp. 956-964, PM:18292813

Deng, X., Zhang, W., Sullivan, I., Williams, J.B., Dong, Q., Park, E.A., Raghow, R., Unterman, T.G., & Elam, M.B. (2012). FoxO1 Inhibits Sterol Regulatory Element-binding Protein-1c (SREBP-1c) Gene Expression via Transcription Factors Sp1 and SREBP-1c. *J.Biol.Chem.,* Vol. 287, No. 24, pp. 20132-20143, PM:22511764

Dentin, R., Hedrick, S., Xie, J., Yates, J., III, & Montminy, M. (2008). Hepatic glucose sensing via the CREB coactivator CRTC2. *Science,* Vol. 319, No. 5868, pp. 1402-1405, PM:18323454

Dentin, R., Pegorier, J.P., Benhamed, F., Foufelle, F., Ferre, P., Fauveau, V., Magnuson, M.A., Girard, J., & Postic, C. (2004). Hepatic glucokinase is required for the synergistic action of ChREBP and SREBP-1c on glycolytic and lipogenic gene expression. *J.Biol.Chem.,* Vol. 279, No. 19, pp. 20314-20326, PM:14985368

Farese, R.V., Jr., Zechner, R., Newgard, C.B., & Walther, T.C. (2012). The problem of establishing relationships between hepatic steatosis and hepatic insulin resistance. *Cell Metab,* Vol. 15, No. 5, pp. 570-573, PM:22560209

Foretz, M., Pacot, C., Dugail, I., Lemarchand, P., Guichard, C., Le Liepvre, X., Berthelier-Lubrano, C., Spiegelman, B., Kim, J.B., Ferre, P., & Foufelle, F. (1999). ADD1/SREBP-1c is required in the activation of hepatic lipogenic gene expression by glucose. *Molecular and Cellular Biology,* Vol. 19, No. 5, pp. 3760-3768, ISI:000079821100052

Forsythe, M.E., Love, D.C., Lazarus, B.D., Kim, E.J., Prinz, W.A., Ashwell, G., Krause, M.W., & Hanover, J.A. (2006). Caenorhabditis elegans ortholog of a diabetes susceptibility locus: oga-1 (O-GlcNAcase) knockout impacts O-GlcNAc cycling, metabolism, and dauer. *Proc.Natl.Acad.Sci.U.S.A,* Vol. 103, No. 32, pp. 11952-11957, PM:16882729

Fujiki, R., Chikanishi, T., Hashiba, W., Ito, H., Takada, I., Roeder, R.G., Kitagawa, H., & Kato, S. (2009). GlcNAcylation of a histone methyltransferase in retinoic-acid-induced granulopoiesis. *Nature,* Vol. 459, No. 7245, pp. 455-459, PM:19377461

Fujiki, R., Hashiba, W., Sekine, H., Yokoyama, A., Chikanishi, T., Ito, S., Imai, Y., Kim, J., He, H.H., Igarashi, K., Kanno, J., Ohtake, F., Kitagawa, H., Roeder, R.G., Brown, M., & Kato, S. (2011). GlcNAcylation of histone H2B facilitates its monoubiquitination. *Nature,* Vol. 480, No. 7378, pp. 557-560, PM:22121020

Ghisletti, S., Huang, W., Ogawa, S., Pascual, G., Lin, M.E., Willson, T.M., Rosenfeld, M.G., & Glass, C.K. (2007). Parallel SUMOylation-dependent pathways mediate gene- and signal-specific transrepression by LXRs and PPARgamma. *Mol.Cell,* Vol. 25, No. 1, pp. 57-70, PM:17218271

Graf, G.A., Li, W.P., Gerard, R.D., Gelissen, I., White, A., Cohen, J.C., & Hobbs, H.H. (2002). Coexpression of ATP-binding cassette proteins ABCG5 and ABCG8 permits their transport to the apical surface. *J.Clin.Invest,* Vol. 110, No. 5, pp. 659-669, PM:12208867

Guertin, D.A., Stevens, D.M., Thoreen, C.C., Burds, A.A., Kalaany, N.Y., Moffat, J., Brown, M., Fitzgerald, K.J., & Sabatini, D.M. (2006). Ablation in mice of the mTORC components raptor, rictor, or mLST8 reveals that mTORC2 is required for signaling to Akt-FOXO and PKCalpha, but not S6K1. *Dev.Cell,* Vol. 11, No. 6, pp. 859-871, PM:17141160

Guinez, C., Filhoulaud, G., Rayah-Benhamed, F., Marmier, S., Dubuquoy, C., Dentin, R., Moldes, M., Burnol, A.F., Yang, X., Lefebvre, T., Girard, J., & Postic, C. (2011). O-GlcNAcylation increases ChREBP protein content and transcriptional activity in the liver. *Diabetes,* Vol. 60, No. 5, pp. 1399-1413, PM:21471514

Haas, J.T., Miao, J., Chanda, D., Wang, Y., Zhao, E., Haas, M.E., Hirschey, M., Vaitheesvaran, B., Farese, R.V., Jr., Kurland, I.J., Graham, M., Crooke, R., Foufelle, F., & Biddinger, S.B. (2012). Hepatic Insulin Signaling Is Required for Obesity-Dependent Expression of SREBP-1c mRNA but Not for Feeding-Dependent Expression. *Cell Metab,* Vol. 15, No. 6, pp. 873-884, PM:22682225

Hagiwara, A., Cornu, M., Cybulski, N., Polak, P., Betz, C., Trapani, F., Terracciano, L., Heim, M.H., Ruegg, M.A., & Hall, M.N. (2012). Hepatic mTORC2 activates glycolysis and lipogenesis through Akt, glucokinase, and SREBP1c. *Cell Metab,* Vol. 15, No. 5, pp. 725-738, PM:22521878

Han, C.Y., Umemoto, T., Omer, M., Den Hartigh, L.J., Chiba, T., LeBoeuf, R., Buller, C.L., Sweet, I.R., Pennathur, S., Abel, E.D., & Chait, A. (2012). NADPH oxidase-derived reactive oxygen species increases expression of monocyte chemotactic factor genes in cultured adipocytes. *J.Biol.Chem.,* Vol. 287, No. 13, pp. 10379-10393, PM:22287546

Hanover, J.A., Krause, M.W., & Love, D.C. (2010). The hexosamine signaling pathway: O-GlcNAc cycling in feast or famine. *Biochim.Biophys.Acta,* Vol. 1800, No. 2, pp. 80-95, PM:19647043

Hanover, J.A., Krause, M.W., & Love, D.C. (2012). Bittersweet memories: linking metabolism to epigenetics through O-GlcNAcylation. *Nat.Rev.Mol.Cell Biol.,* Vol. 13, No. 5, pp. 312-321, PM:22522719

Hart, G.W., Housley, M.P., & Slawson, C. (2007). Cycling of O-linked beta-N-acetylglucosamine on nucleocytoplasmic proteins. *Nature,* Vol. 446, No. 7139, pp. 1017-1022, PM:17460662

Hart, G.W., Slawson, C., Ramirez-Correa, G., & Lagerlof, O. (2011). Cross talk between O-GlcNAcylation and phosphorylation: roles in signaling, transcription, and chronic disease. *Annu.Rev.Biochem.,* Vol. 80, No.pp. 825-858, PM:21391816

Hasty, A.H., Shimano, H., Yahagi, N., Amemiya-Kudo, M., Perrey, S., Yoshikawa, T., Osuga, J., Okazaki, H., Tamura, Y., Iizuka, Y., Shionoiri, F., Ohashi, K., Harada, K., Gotoda, T., Nagai, R., Ishibashi, S., & Yamada, N. (2000). Sterol regulatory element-binding protein-1 is regulated by glucose at the transcriptional level. *J.Biol.Chem.,* Vol. 275, No. 40, pp. 31069-31077, PM:10913129

Havula, E., & Hietakangas, V. (2012). Glucose sensing by ChREBP/MondoA-Mlx transcription factors. *Semin.Cell Dev.Biol.,* PM:22406740

Heinz, S., Benner, C., Spann, N., Bertolino, E., Lin, Y.C., Laslo, P., Cheng, J.X., Murre, C., Singh, H., & Glass, C.K. (2010). Simple combinations of lineage-determining transcription factors prime cis-regulatory elements required for macrophage and B cell identities. *Mol.Cell,* Vol. 38, No. 4, pp. 576-589, PM:20513432

Herzog, B., Hallberg, M., Seth, A., Woods, A., White, R., & Parker, M.G. (2007). The nuclear receptor cofactor, receptor-interacting protein 140, is required for the regulation of hepatic lipid and glucose metabolism by liver X receptor. *Mol.Endocrinol.,* Vol. 21, No. 11, pp. 2687-2697, PM:17684114

Hirahatake, K.M., Meissen, J.K., Fiehn, O., & Adams, S.H. (2011). Comparative effects of fructose and glucose on lipogenic gene expression and intermediary metabolism in HepG2 liver cells. *PLoS.One.,* Vol. 6, No. 11, pp. e26583, PM:22096489

Hooper, A.J., Adams, L.A., & Burnett, J.R. (2011). Genetic determinants of hepatic steatosis in man. *J.Lipid Res.,* Vol. 52, No. 4, pp. 593-617, PM:21245030

Housley, M.P., Rodgers, J.T., Udeshi, N.D., Kelly, T.J., Shabanowitz, J., Hunt, D.F., Puigserver, P., & Hart, G.W. (2008). O-GlcNAc regulates FoxO activation in response to glucose. *J.Biol.Chem.,* Vol. 283, No. 24, pp. 16283-16292, PM:18420577

Housley, M.P., Udeshi, N.D., Rodgers, J.T., Shabanowitz, J., Puigserver, P., Hunt, D.F., & Hart, G.W. (2009). A PGC-1alpha-O-GlcNAc transferase complex regulates FoxO transcription factor activity in response to glucose. *J.Biol.Chem.,* Vol. 284, No. 8, pp. 5148-5157, PM:19103600

Huuskonen, J., Fielding, P.E., & Fielding, C.J. (2004). Role of p160 coactivator complex in the activation of liver X receptor. *Arterioscler.Thromb.Vasc.Biol.,* Vol. 24, No. 4, pp. 703-708, PM:14764426

Hwahng, S.H., Ki, S.H., Bae, E.J., Kim, H.E., & Kim, S.G. (2009). Role of adenosine monophosphate-activated protein kinase-p70 ribosomal S6 kinase-1 pathway in repression of liver X receptor-alpha-dependent lipogenic gene induction and hepatic steatosis by a novel class of dithiolethiones. *Hepatology,* Vol. 49, No. 6, pp. 1913-1925, PM:19378344

Ishii, S., Iizuka, K., Miller, B.C., & Uyeda, K. (2004). Carbohydrate response element binding protein directly promotes lipogenic enzyme gene transcription. *Proc.Natl.Acad.Sci.U.S.A,* Vol. 101, No. 44, pp. 15597-15602, PM:15496471

Jacinto, E., Facchinetti, V., Liu, D., Soto, N., Wei, S., Jung, S.Y., Huang, Q., Qin, J., & Su, B. (2006). SIN1/MIP1 maintains rictor-mTOR complex integrity and regulates Akt phosphorylation and substrate specificity. *Cell,* Vol. 127, No. 1, pp. 125-137, PM:16962653

Jakobsson, T., Venteclef, N., Toresson, G., Damdimopoulos, A.E., Ehrlund, A., Lou, X., Sanyal, S., Steffensen, K.R., Gustafsson, J.A., & Treuter, E. (2009). GPS2 is required for cholesterol efflux by triggering histone demethylation, LXR recruitment, and coregulator assembly at the ABCG1 locus. *Mol.Cell,* Vol. 34, No. 4, pp. 510-518, PM:19481530

Janowski, B.A., Willy, P.J., Devi, T.R., Falck, J.R., & Mangelsdorf, D.J. (1996). An oxysterol signalling pathway mediated by the nuclear receptor LXR alpha. *Nature,* Vol. 383, No. 6602, pp. 728-731, PM:8878485

Joseph, S.B., Laffitte, B.A., Patel, P.H., Watson, M.A., Matsukuma, K.E., Walczak, R., Collins, J.L., Osborne, T.F., & Tontonoz, P. (2002). Direct and indirect mechanisms for regulation of fatty acid synthase gene expression by liver X receptors. *J.Biol.Chem.,* Vol. 277, No. 13, pp. 11019-11025, PM:11790787

Kato, S., Yokoyama, A., & Fujiki, R. (2011). Nuclear receptor coregulators merge transcriptional coregulation with epigenetic regulation. *Trends Biochem.Sci.,* Vol. 36, No. 5, pp. 272-281, PM:21315607

Kebede, M., Ferdaoussi, M., Mancini, A., Alquier, T., Kulkarni, R.N., Walker, M.D., & Poitout, V. (2012). Glucose activates free fatty acid receptor 1 gene transcription via phosphatidylinositol-3-kinase-dependent O-GlcNAcylation of pancreas-duodenum homeobox-1. *Proc.Natl.Acad.Sci.U.S.A,* Vol. 109, No. 7, pp. 2376-2381, PM:22308370

Kim, K., Kim, K.H., Kim, H.H., & Cheong, J. (2008). Hepatitis B virus X protein induces lipogenic transcription factor SREBP1 and fatty acid synthase through the activation of nuclear receptor LXRalpha. *Biochem.J.,* Vol. 416, No. 2, pp. 219-230, PM:18782084

Kim, S.W., Park, K., Kwak, E., Choi, E., Lee, S., Ham, J., Kang, H., Kim, J.M., Hwang, S.Y., Kong, Y.Y., Lee, K., & Lee, J.W. (2003). Activating signal cointegrator 2 required for liver lipid metabolism mediated by liver X receptors in mice. *Mol.Cell Biol.,* Vol. 23, No. 10, pp. 3583-3592, PM:12724417

Kim, S.Y., Kim, H.I., Kim, T.H., Im, S.S., Park, S.K., Lee, I.K., Kim, K.S., & Ahn, Y.H. (2004). SREBP-1c mediates the insulin-dependent hepatic glucokinase expression. *J.Biol.Chem.,* Vol. 279, No. 29, pp. 30823-30829, PM:15123649

Kim, T.H., Kim, H., Park, J.M., Im, S.S., Bae, J.S., Kim, M.Y., Yoon, H.G., Cha, J.Y., Kim, K.S., & Ahn, Y.H. (2009). Interrelationship between liver X receptor alpha, sterol regulatory element-binding protein-1c, peroxisome proliferator-activated receptor gamma, and small heterodimer partner in the transcriptional regulation of glucokinase gene expression in liver. *J.Biol.Chem.,* Vol. 284, No. 22, pp. 15071-15083, PM:19366697

Koo, H.Y., Miyashita, M., Cho, B.H., & Nakamura, M.T. (2009). Replacing dietary glucose with fructose increases ChREBP activity and SREBP-1 protein in rat liver nucleus. *Biochem.Biophys.Res.Commun.,* Vol. 390, No. 2, pp. 285-289, PM:19799862

Korach-Andre, M., Archer, A., Gabbi, C., Barros, R.P., Pedrelli, M., Steffensen, K.R., Pettersson, A.T., Laurencikiene, J., Parini, P., & Gustafsson, J.A. (2011). Liver X receptors regulate de novo lipogenesis in a tissue-specific manner in C57BL/6 female mice. *Am.J.Physiol Endocrinol.Metab,* Vol. 301, No. 1, pp. E210-E222, PM:21521718

Kuo, M., Zilberfarb, V., Gangneux, N., Christeff, N., & Issad, T. (2008). O-glycosylation of FoxO1 increases its transcriptional activity towards the glucose 6-phosphatase gene. *FEBS Lett.,* Vol. 582, No. 5, pp. 829-834, PM:18280254

Lamming, D.W., Ye, L., Katajisto, P., Goncalves, M.D., Saitoh, M., Stevens, D.M., Davis, J.G., Salmon, A.B., Richardson, A., Ahima, R.S., Guertin, D.A., Sabatini, D.M., & Baur, J.A. (2012). Rapamycin-induced insulin resistance is mediated by mTORC2 loss and uncoupled from longevity. *Science,* Vol. 335, No. 6076, pp. 1638-1643, PM:22461615

Lazar, M.A., & Willson, T.M. (2007). Sweet dreams for LXR. *Cell Metab,* Vol. 5, No. 3, pp. 159-161, PM:17339022

Lee, J.H., Park, S.M., Kim, O.S., Lee, C.S., Woo, J.H., Park, S.J., Joe, E.H., & Jou, I. (2009). Differential SUMOylation of LXRalpha and LXRbeta mediates transrepression of STAT1 inflammatory signaling in IFN-gamma-stimulated brain astrocytes. *Mol.Cell,* Vol. 35, No. 6, pp. 806-817, PM:19782030

Lehmann, J.M., Kliewer, S.A., Moore, L.B., Smith-Oliver, T.A., Oliver, B.B., Su, J.L., Sundseth, S.S., Winegar, D.A., Blanchard, D.E., Spencer, T.A., & Willson, T.M. (1997). Activation of the nuclear receptor LXR by oxysterols defines a new hormone response pathway. *J.Biol.Chem.,* Vol. 272, No. 6, pp. 3137-3140, PM:9013544

Li, S., Brown, M.S., & Goldstein, J.L. (2010). Bifurcation of insulin signaling pathway in rat liver: mTORC1 required for stimulation of lipogenesis, but not inhibition of gluconeogenesis. *Proc.Natl.Acad.Sci.U.S.A,* Vol. 107, No. 8, pp. 3441-3446, PM:20133650

Li, X., Zhang, S., Blander, G., Tse, J.G., Krieger, M., & Guarente, L. (2007). SIRT1 deacetylates and positively regulates the nuclear receptor LXR. *Mol.Cell,* Vol. 28, No. 1, pp. 91-106, PM:17936707

Li, Z.Z., Berk, M., McIntyre, T.M., & Feldstein, A.E. (2009). Hepatic lipid partitioning and liver damage in nonalcoholic fatty liver disease: role of stearoyl-CoA desaturase. *J.Biol.Chem.,* Vol. 284, No. 9, pp. 5637-5644, PM:19119140

Liang, G.S., Yang, J., Horton, J.D., Hammer, R.E., Goldstein, J.L., & Brown, M.S. (2002). Diminished hepatic response to fasting/refeeding and liver X receptor agonists in mice with selective deficiency of sterol regulatory element-binding protein-1c. *Journal of Biological Chemistry,* Vol. 277, No. 11, pp. 9520-9528, ISI:000174400600105

Liu, X., Qiao, A., Ke, Y., Kong, X., Liang, J., Wang, R., Ouyang, X., Zuo, J., Chang, Y., & Fang, F. (2010). FoxO1 represses LXRalpha-mediated transcriptional activity of SREBP-1c promoter in HepG2 cells. *FEBS Lett.,* Vol. 584, No. 20, pp. 4330-4334, PM:20868688

Love, D.C., Ghosh, S., Mondoux, M.A., Fukushige, T., Wang, P., Wilson, M.A., Iser, W.B., Wolkow, C.A., Krause, M.W., & Hanover, J.A. (2010a). Dynamic O-GlcNAc cycling at promoters of Caenorhabditis elegans genes regulating longevity, stress, and immunity. *Proc.Natl.Acad.Sci.U.S.A,* Vol. 107, No. 16, pp. 7413-7418, PM:20368426

Love, D.C., Krause, M.W., & Hanover, J.A. (2010b). O-GlcNAc cycling: emerging roles in development and epigenetics. *Semin.Cell Dev.Biol.,* Vol. 21, No. 6, pp. 646-654, PM:20488252

Love, D.C.a.H.J.A. (2005). The Hexosamine Signaling Pathway: Deciphering the "O-GlcNAc Code". *Sci.STKE,* Vol. 312, No. re13, pp. 1-14,

Lu, M., Wan, M., Leavens, K.F., Chu, Q., Monks, B.R., Fernandez, S., Ahima, R.S., Ueki, K., Kahn, C.R., & Birnbaum, M.J. (2012). Insulin regulates liver metabolism in vivo in the absence of hepatic Akt and Foxo1. *Nat.Med.,* Vol. 18, No. 3, pp. 388-395, PM:22344295

Matsuda, T., Noguchi, T., Yamada, K., Takenaka, M., & Tanaka, T. (1990). Regulation of the gene expression of glucokinase and L-type pyruvate kinase in primary cultures of rat hepatocytes by hormones and carbohydrates. *J.Biochem.,* Vol. 108, No. 5, pp. 778-784, PM:1964454

Matsumoto, M., Han, S., Kitamura, T., & Accili, D. (2006). Dual role of transcription factor FoxO1 in controlling hepatic insulin sensitivity and lipid metabolism. *J.Clin.Invest,* Vol. 116, No. 9, pp. 2464-2472, PM:16906224

Matsuzaka, T., Shimano, H., Yahagi, N., Amemiya-Kudo, M., Okazaki, H., Tamura, Y., Iizuka, Y., Ohashi, K., Tomita, S., Sekiya, M., Hasty, A., Nakagawa, Y., Sone, H., Toyoshima, H., Ishibashi, S., Osuga, J., & Yamada, N. (2004). Insulin-independent induction of sterol regulatory element-binding protein-1c expression in the livers of streptozotocin-treated mice. *Diabetes,* Vol. 53, No. 3, pp. 560-569, PM:14988238

McClain, D.A. (2002). Hexosamines as mediators of nutrient sensing and regulation in diabetes. *Journal of Diabetes and Its Complications,* Vol. 16, No. 1, pp. 72-80, ISI:000174300400016

Mitro, N., Mak, P.A., Vargas, L., Godio, C., Hampton, E., Molteni, V., Kreusch, A., & Saez, E. (2007). The nuclear receptor LXR is a glucose sensor. *Nature,* Vol. 445, No. 7124, pp. 219-223, PM:17187055

Mondoux, M.A., Love, D.C., Ghosh, S.K., Fukushige, T., Bond, M., Weerasinghe, G.R., Hanover, J.A., & Krause, M.W. (2011). O-linked-N-acetylglucosamine cycling and insulin signaling are required for the glucose stress response in Caenorhabditis elegans. *Genetics,* Vol. 188, No. 2, pp. 369-382, PM:21441213

Oberkofler, H., Schraml, E., Krempler, F., & Patsch, W. (2003). Potentiation of liver X receptor transcriptional activity by peroxisome-proliferator-activated receptor gamma co-activator 1 alpha. *Biochem.J.,* Vol. 371, No. Pt 1, pp. 89-96, PM:12470296

Okada, M., & Ye, K. (2009). Nuclear phosphoinositide signaling regulates messenger RNA export. *RNA.Biol.,* Vol. 6, No. 1, pp. 12-16, PM:19106628

Ozcan, S., Andrali, S.S., & Cantrell, J.E. (2010). Modulation of transcription factor function by O-GlcNAc modification. *Biochim.Biophys.Acta,* Vol. 1799, No. 5-6, pp. 353-364, PM:20202486

Peet, D.J., Turley, S.D., Ma, W., Janowski, B.A., Lobaccaro, J.M., Hammer, R.E., & Mangelsdorf, D.J. (1998). Cholesterol and bile acid metabolism are impaired in mice lacking the nuclear oxysterol receptor LXR alpha. *Cell,* Vol. 93, No. 5, pp. 693-704, PM:9630215

Pehkonen, P., Welter-Stahl, L., Diwo, J., Ryynanen, J., Wienecke-Baldacchino, A., Heikkinen, S., Treuter, E., Steffensen, K.R., & Carlberg, C. (2012). Genome-wide landscape of liver X receptor chromatin binding and gene regulation in human macrophages. *BMC.Genomics,* Vol. 13, No.pp. 50, PM:22292898

Peterson, T.R., Sengupta, S.S., Harris, T.E., Carmack, A.E., Kang, S.A., Balderas, E., Guertin, D.A., Madden, K.L., Carpenter, A.E., Finck, B.N., & Sabatini, D.M. (2011). mTOR complex 1 regulates lipin 1 localization to control the SREBP pathway. *Cell,* Vol. 146, No. 3, pp. 408-420, PM:21816276

Radhakrishnan, A., Ikeda, Y., Kwon, H.J., Brown, M.S., & Goldstein, J.L. (2007). Sterol-regulated transport of SREBPs from endoplasmic reticulum to Golgi: oxysterols block transport by binding to Insig. *Proc.Natl.Acad.Sci.U.S.A,* Vol. 104, No. 16, pp. 6511-6518, PM:17428920

Repa, J.J., Berge, K.E., Pomajzl, C., Richardson, J.A., Hobbs, H., & Mangelsdorf, D.J. (2002). Regulation of ATP-binding cassette sterol transporters ABCG5 and ABCG8 by the liver X receptors alpha and beta. *J.Biol.Chem.,* Vol. 277, No. 21, pp. 18793-18800, PM:11901146

Repa, J.J., Liang, G., Ou, J., Bashmakov, Y., Lobaccaro, J.M., Shimomura, I., Shan, B., Brown, M.S., Goldstein, J.L., & Mangelsdorf, D.J. (2000). Regulation of mouse sterol regulatory element-binding protein-1c gene (SREBP-1c) by oxysterol receptors, LXRalpha and LXRbeta. *Genes Dev.,* Vol. 14, No. 22, pp. 2819-2830, PM:11090130

Rosenfeld, M.G., Lunyak, V.V., & Glass, C.K. (2006). Sensors and signals: a coactivator/corepressor/epigenetic code for integrating signal-dependent programs of transcriptional response. *Genes Dev.,* Vol. 20, No. 11, pp. 1405-1428, PM:16751179

Sabol, S.L., Brewer, H.B., Jr., & Santamarina-Fojo, S. (2005). The human ABCG1 gene: identification of LXR response elements that modulate expression in macrophages and liver. *J.Lipid Res.,* Vol. 46, No. 10, pp. 2151-2167, PM:16024918

Sakabe, K., Wang, Z., & Hart, G.W. (2010). Beta-N-acetylglucosamine (O-GlcNAc) is part of the histone code. *Proc.Natl.Acad.Sci.U.S.A,* Vol. 107, No. 46, pp. 19915-19920, PM:21045127

Saltiel, A.R., & Kahn, C.R. (2001). Insulin signalling and the regulation of glucose and lipid metabolism. *Nature,* Vol. 414, No. 6865, pp. 799-806, PM:11742412

Schwarz, J.M., Linfoot, P., Dare, D., & Aghajanian, K. (2003). Hepatic de novo lipogenesis in normoinsulinemic and hyperinsulinemic subjects consuming high-fat, low-carbohydrate and low-fat, high-carbohydrate isoenergetic diets. *Am.J.Clin.Nutr.*, Vol. 77, No. 1, pp. 43-50, PM:12499321

Schwarz, J.M., Neese, R.A., Turner, S., Dare, D., & Hellerstein, M.K. (1995). Short-term alterations in carbohydrate energy intake in humans. Striking effects on hepatic glucose production, de novo lipogenesis, lipolysis, and whole-body fuel selection. *J.Clin.Invest*, Vol. 96, No. 6, pp. 2735-2743, PM:8675642

Scorletti, E., Calder, P.C., & Byrne, C.D. (2011). Non-alcoholic fatty liver disease and cardiovascular risk: metabolic aspects and novel treatments. *Endocrine.*, Vol. 40, No. 3, pp. 332-343, PM:21894514

Shafi, R., Iyer, S.P., Ellies, L.G., O'Donnell, N., Marek, K.W., Chui, D., Hart, G.W., & Marth, J.D. (2000). The O-GlcNAc transferase gene resides on the X chromosome and is essential for embryonic stem cell viability and mouse ontogeny. *Proc.Natl.Acad.Sci.U.S.A*, Vol. 97, No. 11, pp. 5735-5739, PM:10801981

Shimano, H. (2001). Sterol regulatory element-binding proteins (SREBPs): transcriptional regulators of lipid synthetic genes. *Prog.Lipid Res.*, Vol. 40, No. 6, pp. 439-452, PM:11591434

Shimomura, I., Matsuda, M., Hammer, R.E., Bashmakov, Y., Brown, M.S., & Goldstein, J.L. (2000). Decreased IRS-2 and increased SREBP-1c lead to mixed insulin resistance and sensitivity in livers of lipodystrophic and ob/ob mice. *Mol.Cell*, Vol. 6, No. 1, pp. 77-86, PM:10949029

Soukas, A.A., Kane, E.A., Carr, C.E., Melo, J.A., & Ruvkun, G. (2009). Rictor/TORC2 regulates fat metabolism, feeding, growth, and life span in Caenorhabditis elegans. *Genes Dev.*, Vol. 23, No. 4, pp. 496-511, PM:19240135

Talukdar, S., & Hillgartner, F.B. (2006). The mechanism mediating the activation of acetyl-coenzyme A carboxylase-alpha gene transcription by the liver X receptor agonist T0-901317. *J.Lipid Res.*, Vol. 47, No. 11, pp. 2451-2461, PM:16931873

Teboul, M., Enmark, E., Li, Q., Wikstrom, A.C., Pelto-Huikko, M., & Gustafsson, J.A. (1995). OR-1, a member of the nuclear receptor superfamily that interacts with the 9-cis-retinoic acid receptor. *Proc.Natl.Acad.Sci.U.S.A*, Vol. 92, No. 6, pp. 2096-2100, PM:7892230

Tobin, K.A., Ulven, S.M., Schuster, G.U., Steineger, H.H., Andresen, S.M., Gustafsson, J.A., & Nebb, H.I. (2002). Liver X receptors as insulin-mediating factors in fatty acid and cholesterol biosynthesis. *J.Biol.Chem.*, Vol. 277, No. 12, pp. 10691-10697, PM:11781314

Torra, I.P., Ismaili, N., Feig, J.E., Xu, C.F., Cavasotto, C., Pancratov, R., Rogatsky, I., Neubert, T.A., Fisher, E.A., & Garabedian, M.J. (2008). Phosphorylation of liver X receptor alpha selectively regulates target gene expression in macrophages. *Mol.Cell Biol.*, Vol. 28, No. 8, pp. 2626-2636, PM:18250151

Tzivion, G., Dobson, M., & Ramakrishnan, G. (2011). FoxO transcription factors; Regulation by AKT and 14-3-3 proteins. *Biochim.Biophys.Acta*, Vol. 1813, No. 11, pp. 1938-1945, PM:21708191

Ulven, S.M., Dalen, K.T., Gustafsson, J.A., & Nebb, H.I. (2005). LXR is crucial in lipid metabolism. *Prostaglandins Leukot.Essent.Fatty Acids,* Vol. 73, No. 1, pp. 59-63, PM:15913974

Uyeda, K., & Repa, J.J. (2006). Carbohydrate response element binding protein, ChREBP, a transcription factor coupling hepatic glucose utilization and lipid synthesis. *Cell Metab,* Vol. 4, No. 2, pp. 107-110, PM:16890538

Venkateswaran, A., Laffitte, B.A., Joseph, S.B., Mak, P.A., Wilpitz, D.C., Edwards, P.A., & Tontonoz, P. (2000). Control of cellular cholesterol efflux by the nuclear oxysterol receptor LXR alpha. *Proc.Natl.Acad.Sci.U.S.A,* Vol. 97, No. 22, pp. 12097-12102, PM:11035776

Venteclef, N., Jakobsson, T., Ehrlund, A., Damdimopoulos, A., Mikkonen, L., Ellis, E., Nilsson, L.M., Parini, P., Janne, O.A., Gustafsson, J.A., Steffensen, K.R., & Treuter, E. (2010). GPS2-dependent corepressor/SUMO pathways govern anti-inflammatory actions of LRH-1 and LXRbeta in the hepatic acute phase response. *Genes Dev.,* Vol. 24, No. 4, pp. 381-395, PM:20159957

Venteclef, N., Jakobsson, T., Steffensen, K.R., & Treuter, E. (2011). Metabolic nuclear receptor signaling and the inflammatory acute phase response. *Trends Endocrinol.Metab,* Vol. 22, No. 8, pp. 333-343, PM:21646028

Viiri, K., Maki, M., & Lohi, O. (2012). Phosphoinositides as regulators of protein-chromatin interactions. *Sci.Signal.,* Vol. 5, No. 222, pp. e19, PM:22550339

Vosseller, K., Wells, L., Lane, M.D., & Hart, G.W. (2002). Elevated nucleocytoplasmic glycosylation by O-GlcNAc results in insulin resistance associated with defects in Akt activation in 3T3-L1 adipocytes. *Proc.Natl.Acad.Sci.U.S.A,* Vol. 99, No. 8, pp. 5313-5318, PM:11959983

Wagner, B.L., Valledor, A.F., Shao, G., Daige, C.L., Bischoff, E.D., Petrowski, M., Jepsen, K., Baek, S.H., Heyman, R.A., Rosenfeld, M.G., Schulman, I.G., & Glass, C.K. (2003). Promoter-specific roles for liver X receptor/corepressor complexes in the regulation of ABCA1 and SREBP1 gene expression. *Mol.Cell Biol.,* Vol. 23, No. 16, pp. 5780-5789, PM:12897148

Wan, M., Leavens, K.F., Saleh, D., Easton, R.M., Guertin, D.A., Peterson, T.R., Kaestner, K.H., Sabatini, D.M., & Birnbaum, M.J. (2011). Postprandial hepatic lipid metabolism requires signaling through Akt2 independent of the transcription factors FoxA2, FoxO1, and SREBP1c. *Cell Metab,* Vol. 14, No. 4, pp. 516-527, PM:21982711

Whelan, S.A., Dias, W.B., Thiruneelakantapillai, L., Lane, M.D., & Hart, G.W. (2010). Regulation of insulin receptor substrate 1 (IRS-1)/AKT kinase-mediated insulin signaling by O-Linked beta-N-acetylglucosamine in 3T3-L1 adipocytes. *J.Biol.Chem.,* Vol. 285, No. 8, pp. 5204-5211, PM:20018868

Whelan, S.A., Lane, M.D., & Hart, G.W. (2008). Regulation of the O-linked beta-N-acetylglucosamine transferase by insulin signaling. *J.Biol.Chem.,* Vol. 283, No. 31, pp. 21411-21417, PM:18519567

White, M.F. (2003). Insulin signaling in health and disease. *Science,* Vol. 302, No. 5651, pp. 1710-1711, PM:14657487

Willy, P.J., Umesono, K., Ong, E.S., Evans, R.M., Heyman, R.A., & Mangelsdorf, D.J. (1995). LXR, a nuclear receptor that defines a distinct retinoid response pathway. *Genes Dev.,* Vol. 9, No. 9, pp. 1033-1045, PM:7744246

Wong, R.H., & Sul, H.S. (2010). Insulin signaling in fatty acid and fat synthesis: a transcriptional perspective. *Curr.Opin.Pharmacol.,* Vol. 10, No. 6, pp. 684-691, PM:20817607

Wouters, K., van Gorp, P.J., Bieghs, V., Gijbels, M.J., Duimel, H., Lutjohann, D., Kerksiek, A., van, K.R., Maeda, N., Staels, B., van, B.M., Shiri-Sverdlov, R., & Hofker, M.H. (2008). Dietary cholesterol, rather than liver steatosis, leads to hepatic inflammation in hyperlipidemic mouse models of nonalcoholic steatohepatitis. *Hepatology,* Vol. 48, No. 2, pp. 474-486, PM:18666236

Wu, X., & Williams, K.J. (2012). NOX4 pathway as a source of selective insulin resistance and responsiveness. *Arterioscler.Thromb.Vasc.Biol.,* Vol. 32, No. 5, pp. 1236-1245, PM:22328777

Yamamoto, T., Shimano, H., Inoue, N., Nakagawa, Y., Matsuzaka, T., Takahashi, A., Yahagi, N., Sone, H., Suzuki, H., Toyoshima, H., & Yamada, N. (2007). Protein kinase A suppresses sterol regulatory element-binding protein-1C expression via phosphorylation of liver X receptor in the liver. *J.Biol.Chem.,* Vol. 282, No. 16, pp. 11687-11695, PM:17296605

Yamashita, H., Takenoshita, M., Sakurai, M., Bruick, R.K., Henzel, W.J., Shillinglaw, W., Arnot, D., & Uyeda, K. (2001). A glucose-responsive transcription factor that regulates carbohydrate metabolism in the liver. *Proc.Natl.Acad.Sci.U.S.A,* Vol. 98, No. 16, pp. 9116-9121, PM:11470916

Yang, X., Ongusaha, P.P., Miles, P.D., Havstad, J.C., Zhang, F., So, W.V., Kudlow, J.E., Michell, R.H., Olefsky, J.M., Field, S.J., & Evans, R.M. (2008). Phosphoinositide signalling links O-GlcNAc transferase to insulin resistance. *Nature,* Vol. 451, No. 7181, pp. 964-969, PM:18288188

Yecies, J.L., Zhang, H.H., Menon, S., Liu, S., Yecies, D., Lipovsky, A.I., Gorgun, C., Kwiatkowski, D.J., Hotamısligil, G.S., Lee, C.H., & Manning, B.D. (2011). Akt stimulates hepatic SREBP1c and lipogenesis through parallel mTORC1-dependent and independent pathways. *Cell Metab,* Vol. 14, No. 1, pp. 21-32, PM:21723501

Yoshikawa, T., Shimano, H., Yahagi, N., Ide, T., Amemiya-Kudo, M., Matsuzaka, T., Nakakuki, M., Tomita, S., Okazaki, H., Tamura, Y., Iizuka, Y., Ohashi, K., Takahashi, A., Sone, H., Osuga, J., Gotoda, T., Ishibashi, S., & Yamada, N. (2002). Polyunsaturated fatty acids suppress sterol regulatory element-binding protein 1c promoter activity by inhibition of liver X receptor (LXR) binding to LXR response elements. *Journal of Biological Chemistry,* Vol. 277, No. 3, pp. 1705-1711, ISI:000173421300013

Yu, L., York, J., von, B.K., Lutjohann, D., Cohen, J.C., & Hobbs, H.H. (2003). Stimulation of cholesterol excretion by the liver X receptor agonist requires ATP-binding cassette transporters G5 and G8. *J.Biol.Chem.*, Vol. 278, No. 18, pp. 15565-15570, PM:12601003

Zhao, L.F., Iwasaki, Y., Nishiyama, M., Taguchi, T., Tsugita, M., Okazaki, M., Nakayama, S., Kambayashi, M., Fujimoto, S., Hashimoto, K., Murao, K., & Terada, Y. (2012). Liver X receptor alpha is involved in the transcriptional regulation of the 6-phosphofructo-2-kinase/fructose-2,6-bisphosphatase gene. *Diabetes,* Vol. 61, No. 5, pp. 1062-1071, PM:22415873

Zoncu, R., Efeyan, A., & Sabatini, D.M. (2011). mTOR: from growth signal integration to cancer, diabetes and ageing. *Nat.Rev.Mol.Cell Biol.,* Vol. 12, No. 1, pp. 21-35, PM:21157483

The 18 kDa Translocator Protein and Atherosclerosis in Mice Lacking Apolipoprotein E

Jasmina Dimitrova-Shumkovska, Leo Veenman, Inbar Roim and Moshe Gavish

Additional information is available at the end of the chapter

http://dx.doi.org/10.5772/54974

1. Introduction

1.1. Apolipoprotein E, inflammation and atherosclerosis

The inflammatory disease atherosclerosis is characterized by plaque formation in the cardiovascular system, which together with thrombosis can lead to obstruction of blood vessels, potentially leading to ischemia, stroke, and heart failure (Libby et al., 2009; Chen et al., 2010; Drake et al., 2011). Atherosclerosis is triggered and sustained by inflammation related cytokines, chemokines, adhesion molecules and by the cellular components of the immune system (Ross, 1999; Epstein et al., 2004). Cholesterol, most of it transported as a low density lipoprotein (LDL) particle in the bloodstream, supports foam cell formation in atherosclerotic plaques. In parallel, cholesterol plays an important role in steroidogenesis and bile production (Lacapere and Papadopoulos, 2003), which have been correlated with mitochondrial 18 kDa Translocator Protein (TSPO) and apolipoprotein E (apoE) expression (Fujimura et al., 2008; Gaemperli et al., 2011). Lipoproteins are lipid transport vehicles that ensure the solubility of lipids within aqueous biological environments. Apolipoproteins stabilize the surface of lipoproteins, serve as cofactors for enzymatic reactions, and present themselves as ligands for lipoprotein receptors. The soluble apolipoprotein gene family, which includes apoE, encodes proteins with amphipathic structures that allow them to exist at the water-lipid interface (Chan, 1989). ApoE is a polymorphic 229-aa, 34-kDa protein, which is present in the cell nucleus and cytosolic compartments (Mahley & Huang, 1999). The human gene, located on chromosome 19, encodes three alleles: apoE2 (frequency in the human population, 5–10%), apoE3 (60–70%), and apoE4 (15–20%). The isoforms differ only at residues 112 and 158 (Cedazo-Minguez & Cowburn, 2001). However, there is only one isoform of apoE in mouse and it behaves like human apoE3 (Strittmatter & Bova Hill, 2002). It is suggested that apoE deficiency in mice mimics the human apoE4 status, which implies reduced apoE3 levels relative to apoE4 levels (Buttini et al., 1999; Sheng et al., 1998).

ApoE is synthesized in several areas of the body, including the liver, where it is produced by hepatic parenchymal cells, and becomes a component in the surface of circulating triglyceride-rich lipoproteins [very low density lipoprotein (VLDL) and chylomicrons, or their remnants], and certain high density lipoprotein (HDL) particles (Mahley, 1988). ApoE plays a major role in the transport of lipids in the bloodstream, where it participates in the delivery and clearance of serum triglycerides, phospholipids, and cholesterol (Mahley, 1988). ApoE is also synthesized in the spleen, lungs, adrenals, ovaries, kidneys, muscle cells, and macrophages (Mahley, 1988). ApoE-containing lipoproteins are bound and internalized via receptor-mediated endocytosis by a number of proteins of the LDL receptor (LDLR) and LDLR-related protein (LRP) families (Davignon et al., 1998). ApoE is considered to be a ligand that binds to 27 clusters of negatively charged cysteine-rich repeats in the extracellular domains of all LDLR gene family members. It has been suggested that apoE made its entrance on the evolutionary stage long after the receptors to which it binds (Beffert et al., 2004). This also indicates that the original primordial functions of the LDLR family did not involve interactions with apoE. The original functions of the LDLR family may have been on the one hand transporting macromolecules between increasingly specialized cells and on the other hand serving as sensors for intercellular communication and environmental conditions (Beffert et al., 2003).

Cholesterol accumulation within atherosclerotic plaque occurs when cholesterol influx into the arterial wall (from apoB-containing lipoproteins) exceeds cholesterol efflux. Early in atherogenesis circulating monocytes are recruited to the arterial sub-endothelium where they differentiate into macrophages, ingest cholesterol, and develop into "foam cells" (Ross, 1973; 1999; Ross et al., 2001). Initially, monocytes adhere to activated endothelium on which up-regulated cell adhesion molecules (CAMs) are displayed, a dynamic process sensitive to inflammatory cytokines, shear stress, and oxidative insults (Chia, 1998). Induction of vascular cell adhesion molecule-1 (VCAM-1), a member of the immunoglobulin superfamily of CAMs, is increasingly described as the key factor in monocyte infiltration (Nakashima et al., 1998; Truskey et al., 1999). ApoE-knockout mice (apoE KO) have been extensively used to study the relation of hypercholesterolemia and lipoprotein oxidation to atherogenesis (Hoen et al., 2003; Yang et al., 2009; Kunitomo et al., 2009). ApoE-deficient mice have elevated VCAM-1 in aortic lesions (Nakashima et al., 1998), which enhances monocyte recruitment and adhesion (Ramos & Partridge, 2005), while apoE expression in the artery wall reduces early foam cell lesion formation (Hasty et al., 1999). These findings imply that apoE may influence early inflammatory responses by suppressing endothelial activation and CAM expression (Stannard et al., 2001). ApoE helps protect against atherosclerosis, in part by mediating hepatic clearance of remnant plasma lipoproteins (Weisgraber et al., 1994). When apoE is absent or dysfunctional, severe hyperlipidemia and atherosclerosis ensue (Kashyap et al., 1995; Linton & Fazio, 1999). ApoE is also abundant in atherosclerotic lesions, secreted by resident cholesterol-loaded macrophages (Linton & Fazio, 1999). This locally produced apoE is atheroprotective by contributing to reverse cholesterol transport and by inhibiting smooth muscle cell proliferation (Mahley et al., 1999; Mahley and Ji, 2006). ApoE exerts several functions regarding lipid and cholesterol transport and metabolism: 1) apoE functions as an important carrier protein in the redistribution of lipids among cells (by incorporation into HDL (as HDL-E); 2) it plays a prominent role in the transport of cholesterol (by incorporating into intestinally synthesized cholymicrons); and 3) it takes part metabolism of plasma cholesterol and triglyceride (by interaction with the LDLR and the receptor binding of apoE lipoproteins (Krul & Tikkanen, 1988; Quinn et al., 2004; Elliott et al., 2007).

ApoE has an established immune modulatory function in the peripheral immune response to bacteria and viruses (Mahley & Rall, 2000). It also modulates inflammatory responses in cell culture models *in vitro* and in *in vivo* models of brain injury, where an apoE mimetic therapeutic peptide has been shown to reduce CNS inflammation (Lynch et al., 2003; McAdoo et al., 2005; Aono et al., 2003). Involvement of apoE in injurious and inflammatory processes in the brain has attracted intensive attention (Drake et al., 2011; Potter and Wisniewski, 2012). In the brain, as well as in the cerebrospinal fluid, non-neuronal cell types, most notably astroglia and microglia, are the primary producers of apoE (Boyles et al., 1985; Quinn et al., 2004), while neurons preferentially express the receptors for apoE (Beffert et al., 2003). Regarding pathological conditions, it has been shown that human neuroblastoma cells, such as SK-N-SH, express apoE mRNA and apoE protein (Elliott et al., 2007). ApoE expression in neurons can be induced during nerve regeneration after injury and in growth and development of the CNS (Quinn et al., 2004). Moreover, Harris et al. (2004) showed that neuron-generated apoE tends to accumulate intracellularly, whereas astrocyte-generated apoE tends to be secreted. ApoE present in neurons is found in the cytoplasm (Han et al., 1994; Xu et al., 1996). The appearance of apoE in neurons may be due to neuronal synthesis under particular conditions, or by insertion into the cytoplasm of extracellular apoE (Dupont-Wallois et al., 1997). As neurons, human fibroblasts express low level of apoE under normal conditions, but under specific circumstances, such as apoptosis and nerve injury, they can produce increased levels of apoE (Do-Carmo et al., 2002; Quinn et al., 2004).

1.2. The 18kDa Translocator Protein (TSPO) and apolipoprotein E

Recent studies by us and others have indicated that the mitochondrial 18kDa Translocator Protein (TSPO), also known as peripheral-type benzodiazepine receptor (PBR) is present throughout the cardiovascular system and may be involved in cardiovascular disorders including atherosclerosis (Veenman and Gavish, 2006). The primary intracellular location of the TSPO is the outer mitochondrial membrane. Various studies over the course of the last 3 decennia have indicated that mitochondrial TSPO, potentially in relation to cardiovascular disease, is involved in the regulation of cholesterol transport into mitochondria in relation to bile production and steroidogenesis (Krueger and Papadopoulos, 1990; Papadopoulos et al., 2006). In particular, TSPO regulates cholesterol transport from the outer to the inner mitochondrial membrane which is the rate-limiting step in steroid and bile acid biosyntheses (Krueger and Papadopoulos, 1990; Lacapère and Papadopoulos, 2003; Veenman et al., 2007). Three-dimensional models of the channel formed by the five α-helices of the TSPO indicate that it can accommodate a cholesterol molecule in the space delineated by the five helices. According to these models, the inner surface of the channel formed by the TSPO molecule would present a hydrophilic but uncharged pathway, allowing amphiphilic cholesterol molecules to cross the outer mitochondrial membrane (Papadopoulos et al., 1997, 2006; Veenman et al., 2007). At cellular levels TSPO is present in virtually all of the cells of the cardiovascular system, where they appear to take part in the responses to various challenges that an organism and its cardiovascular system face (Veenman & Gavish, 2006), including atherosclerosis and accompanying symptoms (Onyimba et al., 2011; Bird et al., 2010; Dimitrova-Shumkovska et al., 2010a,b,c, 2012).

TSPO are located in various components of blood vessels, including endothelial cells where TSPO may take part in immunologic and inflammatory responses (Hollingsworth et al., 1985; Bono et al., 1999; Milner et al., 2004; Veenman & Gavish, 2006). To establish a factual correlation between atherogenic challenges and TSPO binding characteristics, we have previously assayed TSPO binding characteristics in different tissues of rats fed a high fat high cholesterol (HFHC) diet, in comparison to rats fed a normal diet (Dimitrova-Shumkovska et al., 2010a). It appeared that enhancement of oxidative stress in the aorta and liver due to the atherogenic HFHC diet was accompanied by significant reductions in TSPO binding density in these organs. Binding levels of the TSPO specific ligand [^{3}H]PK 11195 in heart appeared not to be affected by the HFHC diet in this rat model.

Previous studies have shown that TSPO as well as apoE can be associated with processes such as: cholesterol metabolism, oxidative stress, apoptosis, glial activation, inflammation, and immune responses. As a ligand for cell-surface lipoprotein receptors, apoE can prevent atherosclerosis by clearing cholesterol-rich lipoproteins from plasma (Mahley and Huang, 1999). The TSPO protein has also been shown to be present in the plasma membrane of red blood cells, as well as in the plasma membrane of neutrofils, where it was shown to stimulate NADPH-oxidase activation of these cells. The plasma membrane forms of TSPO may be involved in heme metabolism, calcium channel modulation, cell growth, and immunomodulation. Furthermore, nucleus expulsion in mature erythrocytes is inhibited by excess cellular cholesterol (Fan et al., 2009). However, the involvement of the TSPO in this process has not been investigated. A recent study in cell culture showed that TSPO is important for the regulation of mitochondrial protoporphyrin IX and heme levels (Zeno et al., 2012). Thus, the TSPO appears to take part in various stages of red blood cell formation.

Furthermore, TSPO takes part in the regulation of gene expression for proteins involved in adhesion, which potentially may play a role in platelet aggregation (Bode et al., 2012; Veenman et al., 2012). ApoE has also been found to be involved in platelet aggregation, while TSPO platelet levels have been found to be increased with various neurological disorders, in particular stress related disorders (Veenman and Gavish, 2000, 2006, 2012). It has been suggested that platelet aggregation may be affected by nitric oxide (NO) generation via apoE, while other studies suggest that NO requires the TSPO to induce collapse of the mitochondrial membrane potential ($\Delta\Psi m$), mitochondrial reactive oxygen species (ROS) generation and cell death (Shargorodsky et al., 2012). Thus, the TSPO may present one pathway whereby NO does affect platelet aggregation. Furthermore, various alteration in TSPO density in the heart as a response to stress have been reported (Gavish et al., 1992; Veenman and Gavish, 2006), suggesting one aspect of involvement of TSPO in cardiovascular diseases, including cardiac ischemia. It has also been shown that apoE is involved in cardiac ischemia (Mahley, 1988).

Apparently as a consequence of its role in steroidogenesis, TSPO typically are very abundant in steroidogenic tissues (Benavides et al., 1983; De Souza et al., 1985). Steroid hormones can affect TSPO levels, while in turn TSPO provides a modulatory function for steroid hormone production by regulation of mitochondrial cholesterol transport (Veenman et al., 2007). It is known that cholesterol affects TSPO function (Falchi et al., 2007). Interestingly, apoE is also well expressed in steroidogenic organs such as adrenal gland, ovary, and testis (Blue et al., 1983; Elshourbagy et al., 1985; Law et al., 1997). Nonetheless, studies by us suggests that elevated cholesterol levels, such as found in apoE KO mice, do not appear to affect TSPO levels in steroidogenic organs (Inbar Roim, M.Sc. Thesis, Technion – Israel Institute of Technology, 2008), even though effects in the cardiovascular system can be observed (Dimitrova-Shumkovska et al., 2010a). As has been reported, TSPO levels can be regulated by steroid hormones, which may be part of an organism's response to stress and injury (Anholt et al., 1985; Weizman et al., 1992; Gavish & Weizman, 1997; Gavish et al., 1999; Veenman et al., 2007; Mazurika et al., 2009; Veenman and Gavish, 2012). This suggests that TSPO levels may be part of a feedback control system for steroid production (responding to alterations in steroid levels), rather than be regulated by a feed forward signal provided by cholesterol (i.e. TSPO levels in relation to steroidogenesis are not being regulated by cholesterol levels *in vivo*) (Veenman and Gavish, 2012).

1.2.1. Involvement of TSPO in inflammation

Various studies have shown the presence of TSPO in all cell types of the immune system, thus proposed functional roles of the TSPO included modulation of stress-induced immunosuppression and immune cell activity (Lenfant et al., 1985; Ruff et al., 1985; Bessier et al., 1992; Marchetti et al., 1996; Bono et al., 1999; Veenman & Gavish, 2006). TSPO are present in platelets, lymphocytes, and mononuclear cells, and are also found in the endothelium, the striated cardiac muscle, the vascular smooth muscles, and the mast cells of the cardiovascular system (Veenman & Gavish, 2006). TSPO in the cardiovascular system appears to play roles in several aspects of the immune response, such as phagocytosis and the secretion of interleukin-2, interleukin-3, and immunoglobulin A (Veenman & Gavish, 2006). Mast cells are considered to be important for immune response to pathogens (Marshall, 2004) and they have also been implicated in the regulation of thrombosis and inflammation and cardiovascular disease processes such as atherosclerosis as well as in neoplastic conditions (Wojta et al., 2003). Studies have shown that benzodiazepines' inhibition of serotonin release in mast cells could reduce blood brain barrier permeability, influence pain levels, and decrease vascular smooth muscle contractions (Veenman and Gavish, 2006). Benzodiazepines have been found to bind to specific receptors constituted by the TSPO on macrophages and to modulate *in vitro* their metabolic oxidative responsiveness (Lenfant et al., 1985). TSPO in the cardiovascular system also has been associated with the development of atherosclerosis (Camici et al., 2012). It for example has been suggested that reductions in TSPO levels may act as a protective mechanisms against the development of oxidative stress in aorta and liver (Dimitrova-Shumkovska et al., 2010a, b, c; 2012).

Anti-inflammatory properties of TSPO ligands have been demonstrated in various tissues. TSPO ligands have been shown to reduce inflammation in animal models of rheumatoid arthritis (Waterfield et al., 1999), carrageenan-induced pleurisy (Torres et al., 2000), and pulmonary inflammation (Bribes et al., 2003). Taupin et al. (1993) have also demonstrated *in vivo* that the synthetic TSPO ligand Ro5-4864 increases brain IL-1, IL-6 and TNF-α production after brain trauma. These cytokines are known to play a role in the inflammatory reaction to brain injury (Heumann et al., 1987). Interestingly, one study showed that PK 11195, but not Ro5-4864, could exert anti-inflammatory actions on mononuclear phagocytes, regulating the release of IL-1b (Klegeris et al., 2000). In addition, *in vivo* studies have shown that TSPO ligands can reduce the typical inflammatory response presented by reactive microglia and reactive astroglia resulting from brain trauma (Ryu et al., 2005; Veiga et al., 2005).

1.3. Animal models and strategies for atherosclerosis study

Atherosclerotic plaques may appear early in life and might progress into severe, symptomatic plaques many decades later, dependent on the coexistence of risk factors such as age, genetic background, gender, hypercholesterolemia, hypertension, smoking, diabetes, etc. (Ross, 1999; Whitman, 2004). Rupture of lipid-rich coronary plaques can trigger an atherothrombotic event and probably is the most important mechanism inducing acute coronary syndrome (ACS) (Vilahuer et al., 2011).

Plaque rupture presents a major factor in ischemic processes associated with atherosclerosis (Zhao et al., 2008; Cheng et al., 2009; Gaemerli et al., 2011). Plaque rupture in the human condition, including the cardiovascular processes and events leading up to it, presently is virtually inaccessible for research. Therefore, animal models have been developed to study atherosclerosis, including plaque rupture and thrombus formation, and also how to take measures to prevent these from happening. Nonetheless, more sophisticated models need to be developed and tested to be able to better mimic the human condition. This is so, as mice and rats, for example, do not develop atherosclerosis without genetic manipulation, because they have a lipid physiology that is radically different from that in humans, as most of the cholesterol is being transported in HDL-like particles (Whitman, 2004; Singh et al., 2009; Vilahur et al., 2011). Furthermore, all of the existing animal models, including biological and mechanical triggering of atherogenesis, e.g., the Watanabe heritable hyperlipidemic (WHHL) rabbit model, the apolipoprotein E (ApoE) mouse model, and the LDL-receptor mouse model) suffer the drawback of lacking an end-stage atherosclerosis that would show plaque rupture accompanied by platelet and fibrin-rich occlusive thrombus at the rupture site (Singh et al., 2009). Another restriction of current models for cardiovascular disorders is that most of the studies explore only male mice to avoid effects of estrogens to the extent of lesion development and diminishing LDL oxidation (Caligiuri et al., 1999; Yang et al., 2004). As cardiovascular disorders also occur in women, it would be valuable to also study female animal research subjects. Furthermore, it would give direction to research relating hormonal conditions to atherosclerosis.

Cholesterol lowering by diet is associated with a reduction in DNA damage, at least in animal models (Singh et al., 2009). In general, modification of atherosclerotic risk factors by lipid lowering therapies, cessation of smoking, weight loss, and improved glucose control reduces circulating markers of inflammation. These and other findings suggest that inflammation is a primary process for atherosclerosis (Ziccardi et al., 2002; Rodriguez-Moran et al., 2003). Although high dietary intake of the anti-oxidant vitamin E and C has been associated with reduced risk of cardiovascular disease (CVD), well powered clinical trials in atherosclerosis-related CVD have indicated that supplements with vitamin C or vitamin E alone do not provide sufficient benefit, in comparison to, for example, statins (Kunitomo et al., 2009). Furthermore, specific antioxidants scavenge or metabolize some, but not all of the relevant oxidized molecules (Stocker and Keaney, 2004). Stocker and Keaney (2005) conclude that whenever a physiological process goes unchecked in case of disease, treatment strategies cannot simply rely on scavenging ROS. Nonetheless, drugs that have been proven to alter plaque progression have also been shown to alter vascular oxidative stress. For example, 3-hydroxy-3-methylglutaryl coenzyme A reductase (HMGCoA) inhibitors (Statins) reduce NAD(P)H oxidase activation and superoxide production *in vitro*, in part because of their capability to inhibit the membrane translocation (and thus activity) of the small GTP-binding protein Rac-1, which is a regulatory component of vascular NAD(P)H oxidase activation (Costopoulos et al., 2008). In conclusion, it appears that beneficial therapeutic treatments to prevent atherosclerosis include lowering of lipid levels and also reduction of oxidative stress. However, restricting a treatment to only reduction of oxidative stress does not appear to generate sufficient beneficial effects to counteract atherosclerosis.

2. The effects of cholesterol challenges that result in atherogenesis on TSPO binding density in aorta and heart

As apoE deficiency may increase cholesterol levels and induce NO generation, which in turn may affect TSPO function, we were interested to study whether TSPO binding characteristics may be affected in heart and aorta of apoE-knockout (B6.129P2-apoE^{tm1} N11) mice, in comparison to their C57BL/6 background mice (i.e. wild type, WT). For the present study homogenates of whole heart organ and aorta segments (aortic arch and descendending aorta) were used. For this approach, it was taken into consideration that accumulation of proatherogenic lipid affects all cells types present into vascular wall, and the response of the entire tissue to the cholesterol exposure is relevant as an indication of vascular defense as a whole (Hoen et al., 2003). All procedures with the animals were in accordance with National Institutes of Health (USA) guidelines for the care and use of experimental animals (NIH publication No. 85-23, revised 1996), and the experimental protocol was reviewed and approved by the local ethics committee. The mice were housed in polycarbonate cages in a pathogen – free facility set on a 12h light-dark cycle and given *ad libitum* access to water and standard laboratory feed. Prior to the experimental procedures, the rats were fed a commercial standard pellet feed (Filpaso, 52.11, Skopje, Republic of Macedonia), named "standard feed" hereafter.

At 16 weeks of age, animals were randomized into experimental groups: i) Two control groups (WT mice, n = 10) and (apoE KO mice, n = 10), both these control groups received standard feed for a additional period of 10 weeks; ii) Two experimental groups receiving the same feed for the same 10 weeks but supplemented with 1% cholesterol (1% WT mice, n = 10) and (1% apoE KO mice, n= 10); and iii) Two experimental groups received the same feed for the same 10 weeks but supplemented with 3% cholesterol (3% WT mice, n = 10) and (3% apoE KO mice, n = 10). After these 10 weeks, animals were sacrificed by cardiac puncture, under ketamine/xylazine anaesthesia, followed by the appropriated storage until application or procedures required for assays of TSPO binding characteristics, ROS parameters, and histopathology, as described in detail previously (Dimitrova-Shumkovska et al., 2010 a, b, c, 2012). Tissue homogenates of aorta and heart were prepared for our various assays. For TSPO binding assays, tissue homogenates were prepared in 50 mM PBS on ice with a Kinematika Polytron (Luzerne, Switzerland), as described previously (Dimitrova-Shumkovska et al., 2010 a, b, c). To prepare homogenates for assays of oxidative stress parameters, we used an Ultrasonic Homogenizer (Cole-Parmer Instrument Co., Chicago, IL) as described previously (Dimitrova-Shumkovska et al., 2010 a, b, c). For advanced oxidation protein products (AOPPs, Witko-Sarsat et al., 1996), tissue homogenates were prepared in 50 mM PBS at + 4 ºC, as described previously (Dimitrova-Shumkovska et al., 2010 a, b, c). For the other assays of oxidative stress (see below), tissue homogenates were prepared in 1.12 % KCl at + 4 ºC, as described previously (Dimitrova-Shumkovska et al., 2010 a, b, c). These later parameters of oxidative injury included: lipid peroxidation products [TBARs] (Draper and Hadley, 1990); protein carbonylation, PC (Shacter, 2000); superoxide dismutase activity (SOD assay kit, RA20408, Fluka, Biochemika, Steinheim, Germany), glutathione (GSH assay kit CS0260, Sigma-Aldrich, Steinheim, Germany), glutathione reductase (GSSG-Red), GRSA 114K4000, Sigma-Aldrich, Steinheim, Germany], Finally, aortas were prepared for anatomical observation and histopathology as described previously (Dimitrova-Shumkovska et al., 2010 a, b, c).

Effects of cholesterol supplements to the apoE KO mice on plaque formation in the aorta are shown in Figure 1. No atherosclerotic formation was found in WT mice regardless of diet (Figure 1A). Control aortas of apoE KO mice having access to standard feed are characterized by the presence of thin fibrous tissue caps i.e. encapsulations of collagen rich fibrous tissue without a necrotic core that showed only superficial accumulation of foam cells (Figure 1B). Cholesterol diet accelerated atherosclerosis in apoE KO mice, increasing the total surface area of plaque formation significantly over the intimal area (Figure 1C) compared to apoE mice receiving standard feed. In 1% cholesterol fed apoE KO mice, expansion of the necrotic core presenting an important pathogenic process contributing to plaque vulnerability was observed in comparison to standard fed apoE mice (Figure 1C). After administration of 3% cholesterol diet to apoE KO mice even more advanced lesions have developed. Initial xanthoma formation, cartilage tissue, and calcified nodules with an underlying fibrocalcific plaque with minimal or absence of necrosis occurred (Figure 1D). Furthermore, plaques become more progressive and lesions show luminal stenosis with pathologic intimal thickening. These observations are in line with other research data, where plague rupture was seen in apoE KO mice especially when exposed to western type diet

(Davignon et al., 1999; Johnson et al., 2005). ApoE KO mice can also develop interplaque hemorrhage and features of plaque instability that are accelerated by feeding westernized diet (Rosenfeld et al., 2000). "Western type diets for mice" typically utilize just one ingredient (milk fat or lard) as the primary source of energy from fat.

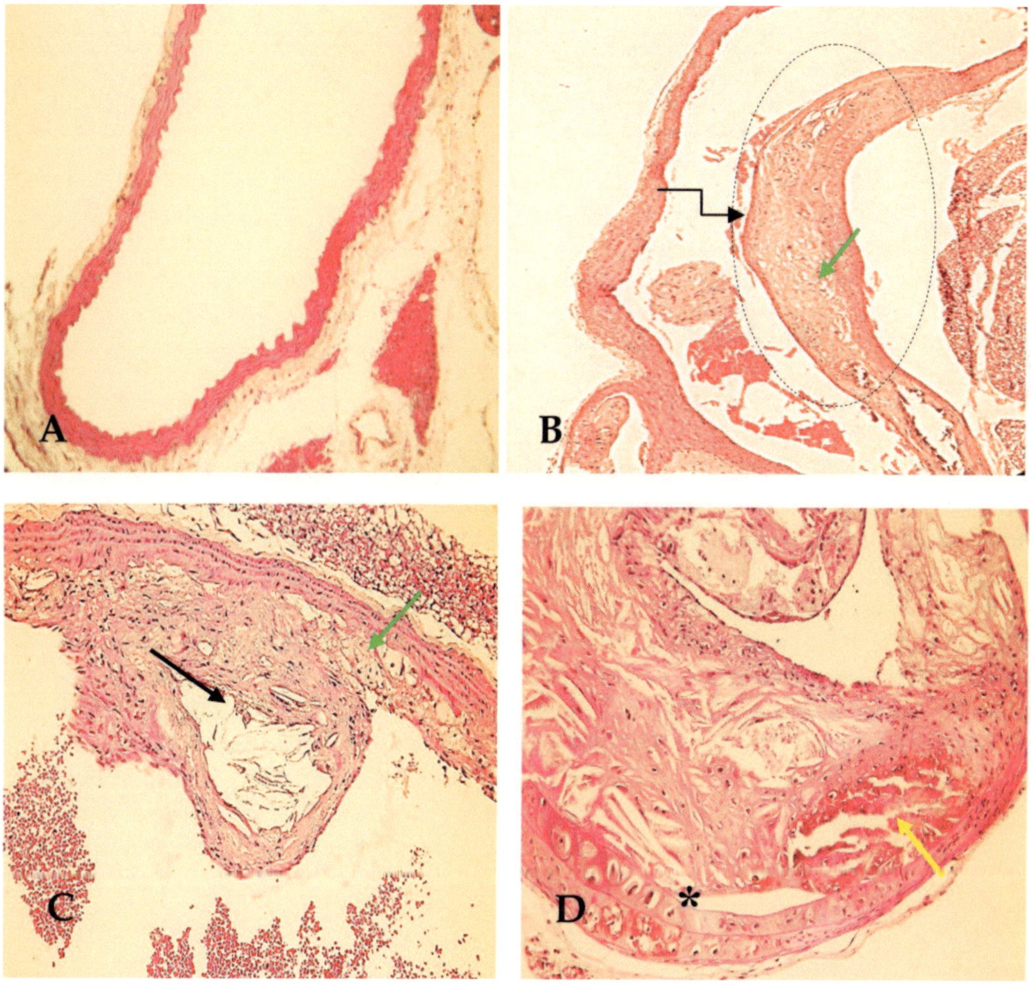

Figure 1. Representative cross-sections of mice aortas. A) No atherosclerotic lesions were found in wild-type mice regardless of the diet; B) atherosclerotic plaque (outlined) characterized by a thin fibrous tissue cap (elbow black arrow), particularly ssuperficial accumulation of foam cells (green arrow) without a necrotic core and encapsulated by collagen rich fibrous tissue in apoE KO mice given standard feed; C) accelerated atherosclerosis and deposition of cholesterol crystals (black arrow) in the endothelium of the aorta wall in 1% apoE KO; D) advanced lesions are developed in 3% apoE mice. Initial xanthoma formation, cartilage tissue (asterix) and calcified nodules (yellow arrow) with an underlying fibrocalcific plaque with minimal or absence of necrosis occur (H&E staining, microscopic magnification applied x 100).

Plasma lipoprotein levels mg/dL										
Strain		Chol			TAG			HDL		
	wk	C	1%	3%	C	1%	3%	C	1%	3%
WT	16	67.7 ± 23.3	88.07 ± 28.0	110.0 ± 27.0**	71.0 ± 18.4	71.5 ± 5.1	97.5 ± 16.2**	33.2 ± 5.1	33.6 ± 10.8	74.7 ± 10.8***

Plasma lipoprotein levels mg/dL										
Strain		Chol			TAG			HDL		
	wk	C	1%	3%	C	1%	3%	C	1%	3%
Apo E$^{(-/-)}$	16	383.7 ± 47.3	457.23 ± 62*	555.4 ± 83.3***	117.7± 24.5	105.6 ± 11.4	159.4 ± 59.0**	67.0 ± 37.5	66.6 ± 16.3	32.9 ± 11.4**

Table 1. Effects of cholesterol (Chol) supplemented diet for 10 weeks, on lipoprotein levels in apoE KO mice and their WT counterparts. Unpaired Student t-*test* was performed. Data are expressed as mean ± SD; * = $p < 0.05$, ** = $p < 0.01$, *** = $p < 0.001$.

Changes in the serum levels of total cholesterol, triglycerides and HDL-cholesterol in each group are shown in **Table 1.** Corroborating previous studies (Davignon et al., 1999; Seo et al., 2005; Zhao et al., 2008) at 16 weeks of age, even before application of the cholesterol enriched diets, apoE KO mice, already displayed approximately 5 times higher levels of total cholesterol in comparison with WT mice. At this time point, no significant differences in triglycerides (TAG) levels were observed between WT mice and apoE KO mice. However, 3% diet regimes, caused significant increases in total cholesterol level in apoE KO mice (by 44%, $p < 0.001$), compared to standard feed. The enhanced total cholesterol levels, included an almost 90% representation of non HDL – cholesterol (calculated from Friedewald formula; Friedewald et al., 1972). In contrast, 3% WT mice, showed significantly higher cholesterol levels (by 62%, $p < 0.01$), including an almost 70% representation of HDL-lipoproteins. Supplement of 3% cholesterol also provoked significantly higher triglycerides levels: by 35 % ($p < 0.01$) in apoE mice and by 36% ($p < 0.01$) in WT mice. Supplement of 1% cholesterol, resulted in slight increases in total cholesterol in apoE mice (by 20%, $p < 0.05$), but did not significantly affect the triglycerides levels. The same type of diet did not affect lipoprotein levels in WT mice.

In the aorta, 3% cholesterol diet supplement, caused significant increases in "steady-state" levels of lipid peroxides (TBARs) and oxidized proteins in WT as well as apoE KO mice (**Table 2**). In detail, regarding lipid peroxidation, TBARs production was significantly increased by 2 fold in WT and apoE KO mice subjected to 3% cholesterol supplemented diet (+100%, $p < 0.01$ for WT mice, and +125%, $p < 0.001$ for ApoE KO mice). In parallel, protein oxidation products levels (AOPP) were also significantly higher (+135%, $p < 0.01$ in 3% WT mice and +177%, $p < 0.001$, in 3% apoE KO mice). Protein carbonyls (PC) showed a slight but non-significant increase in 3% cholesterol fed WT and apoE KO mice, compared to their controls. In contrast to the 3% diet regime, 1% cholesterol supplemented diet did not affect ROS parameters in aortic tissue in both WT and apoE KO mice.

Variables / Aorta	WT Control	1% Chol	3% Chol
TBARs nmol/mg	0.16 ± 0.04 (n=8)	0.17 ± 0.06 (n=7)	0.32 ± 0.08** (n=8)
AOPP nmol/mg	37.1 ± 11.3 (n=7)	44.1 ± 19.3 (n=8)	86.8 ± 21.4** (n=8)
PC pmol/mg	45.7 ± 11.0 (n=7)	55.2 ± 22.8 (n=8)	55.3 ± 11.8 (n=8)

Variables / Aorta	Apo E Control	1% Chol	3% Chol
TBARs nmol/mg	0.24 ± 0.07 (n=8)	0.29 ± 0.11 (n=8)	0.54 ± 0.25*** (n=10)
AOPP nmol/mg	22.0 ± 17.1 (n=8)	27.9 ± 7.1 (n=8)	60.5 ± 30.6*** (n=10)
PC pmol/mg	46.6 ± 20.3 (n=8)	45.3 ± 11.3 (n=8)	52.1 ± 10.6 (n=12)

Table 2. Effects of cholesterol (Chol) supplemented diet for 10 weeks on aorta oxidative stress parameters in apoE KO mice and their WT counterparts. 1-way ANOVA followed by application of the Tukey test to assess the significance of specific intergroup differences. Data are expressed as mean ± SD; * = $p < 0.05$, ** = $p < 0.01$, *** = $p < 0.001$.

The capacity of glutathione as an electron donor to regenerate the most important antioxidants (vitamin E, glutathione peroxidase (GPx), lipid hydroperoxides), is linked with the redox state of the glutathione disulfide – glutathione couple GSSG/2GSH (Schafer and Buettner, 2001). This in turn, has a high impact on the overall redox environment in the cell. Concerning antioxidant activities in aorta tissue due to 3% cholesterol supplemented feed, significantly reduced activity of superoxide dismutase (SOD) was measured in 3% apoE KO mice compared to standard feed mice (- 41%, **Table 3**). The results also suggest a significant reverse interaction between glutathione level (GSH) and glutathione peroxidase (GPx) activity in aorta tissue. In particular, the analyzed results indicated that the glutathione content in aorta of 3% apoE animals was significantly decreased (-32%), with simultaneous slight, but significant enhancement achieved in activity of glutathione peroxidase (+10%), as compared to standard feed control ($p < 0.05$). In parallel, glutathione content in aorta was also significantly reduced in 3% WT mice for 70% ($p < 0.01$), without affecting GPx levels. Feeding the mice diet supplemented with 1% cholesterol, resulted in significantly reduced activity in SOD in apoE KO mice (by 33% $p < 0.05$) and in WT mice (by 47% $p < 0.05$).

To determine TSPO binding characteristics in this paradigm we applied binding assays with the TSPO specific ligand [^{3}H] PK 11195. The present study sought to determine whether cholesterol supplementation affects TSPO binding characteristics in aorta and heart of apoE KO mice in association with parameters for oxidative stress. Binding assays of the heart and

Variables / Aorta	WT Control	1% Chol	3% Chol
SOD U/mg	4.76 ± 1.5 (n=9)	2.5 ± 0.9* (n=7)	1.45 ± 0.6** (n=7)
GSH nmol/mg	7.8 ± 4.2 (n=9)	8.3 ± 3.7 (n=9)	3.7 ± 0.8** (n=9)
GPx mU/mg	0.261 ± 0.01 (n=8)	0.273 ± 0.01 (n=8)	0.257 ± 0.03 (n=8)

Variables / Aorta	Apo E Control	1% Chol	3% Chol
SOD U/mg	6.87 ± 1.6 (n=7)	4.6 ± 1.1* (n=6)	4.05 ± 0.88* (n=8)
GSH nmol/mg	6.7 ± 2.9 (n=9)	7.4 ± 2.7 (n=9)	4.5 ± 2.0* (n=9)
GPx mU/mg	0.242 ± 0.02 (n=9)	0.256 ± 0.01*(n=7)	0.266 ±0.03* (n=7)

Table 3. Effects of cholesterol (Chol) supplemented diet for 10 weeks on aorta antioxidant parameters in apoE KO mice and their WT counterparts. Unpaired Student t-*test* was performed. Data are expressed as mean ± SD; * = $p < 0.05$, ** = $p < 0.01$.

aorta with the TSPO specific ligand [^{3}H]PK 11195 were done to determine potential effects of cholesterol supplementation on TSPO binding characteristics, according to methods described previously (Dimitrova-Shumkovska et al., 2010 a,b,c). For representative examples, see **Figure 2.** In heart , only in WT mice significant decreases in the B_{max} of TSPO (- 42%, $p < 0.001$) was determined with [^{3}H]PK 11195 binding as a consequence of both cholesterol 1% and 3% supplemented diets, compared to control standard fed WT mice. Regarding the apoE KO mice, cholesterol supplemented diet did not induce differences in the TSPO binding characteristics in the heart **(Table 4)**. Regarding heart tissues, both in the apoE KO groups and WT groups, K_d values determined with [^{3}H] PK 11195 binding were in the nM range (0.6 – 1.6 nM) showing no significant differences between experimental and control groups.

Regarding the aorta, feeding the mice with standard feed was not accompanied by significant differences in the TSPO binding characteristics of the aorta of apoE KO mice versus WT mice (**Table 4**). Interestingly, these mouse aortas showed very TSPO binding levels, comparable to those observed in the adrenal of rats (Gavish et al., 1999). To date, the adrenal of rats is the tissue with one of highest demonstrated Bmax for TSPO ligand binding (Gavish et al., 1999). The 1% cholesterol supplemented diet significantly reduced TSPO binding capacity in aorta in both WT and apoE KO mice. In particular, reductions by 49% in WT mice and by 32% in apoE KO mice ($p < 0.001$ and $p < 0.01$, respectively) compared to their standard feed controls were observed (**Table 4**). The 3% cholesterol diet also provoked a reduction in TSPO binding density by 58% in the aorta ($p < 0.01$), but only in WT mice. In the aortas of both groups, apoE KO mice and WT mice, K_d values determined with [^{3}H] PK 11195 binding were in the nM range (1.5 – 2.6 nM), showing no significant differences between the groups.

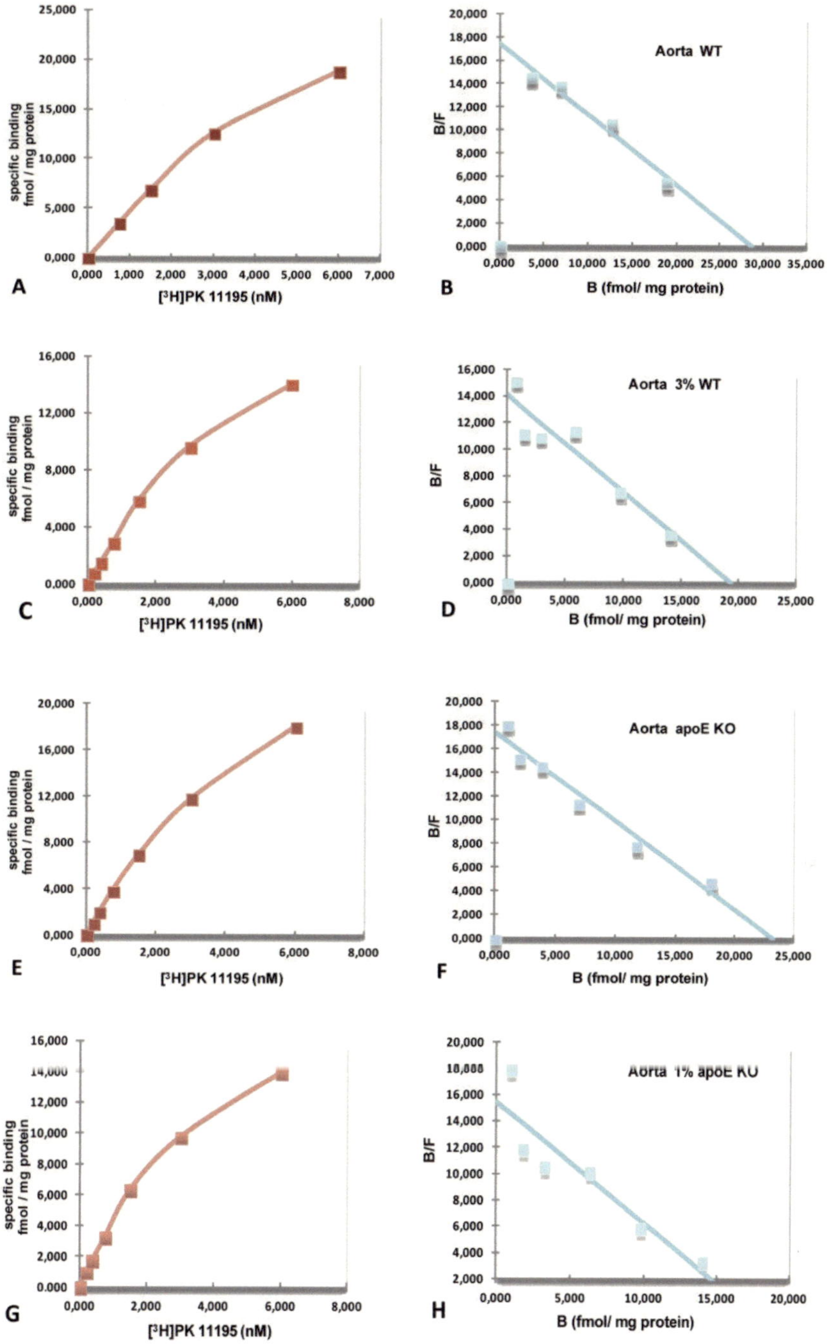

Figure 2. Representative examples of saturation curves (**A, C, E, G**) and their Scatchard plots (**B, D, F, H**) of [^{3}H]PK 11195 binding to membrane homogenates of aorta, respectively of WT mice (**A , B, C, D**) and apoE KO mice (**E, F, G, H**). Abbreviations: apoE KO = apolipoprotein deficient mice; WT- wild type mice; B: bound; B/F: bound over free.

As the effects on TSPO binding density in heart and aorta due to intake of cholesterol supplemented diet take place primarily in the WT groups, and especially not in the 3% cholesterol diet fed apoE KO mice, these data suggest that decreases of TSPO binding density in heart and aorta may serve to counteract processes typically leading to cardiovascular damage, including atherosclerosis, as explained in more detail in the Discussion.

Bb - wild type mice									
	Bb - Control			Bb - 1% Chol.			Bb - 3 % Chol.		
Tissue	B max (fmol/mg)	Kd (nmol)	n	B max (fmol/mg)	Kd (nmol)	n	B max (fmol/mg)	Kd (nmol)	n
Heart	1740 ± 180	0.65 ± 0.1	5	1005 ± 240**	1.12 ± 0.3	6	1006 ± 140 **	1.32 ± 0.5	5
Aorta	29 000 ± 9700	2.50 ± 1.2	9	14 900 ± 3370***	2.31 ± 0.8	6	12 200 ± 2920**	2.62 ± 0.5	5

Apo E KO mice									
	Apo E - Control			Apo E - 1% Chol.			Apo E - 3 % Chol.		
Tissue	B max (fmol/mg)	Kd (nmol)	n	B max (fmol/mg)	Kd (nmol)	n	B max (fmol/mg)	Kd (nmol)	n
Heart	1590 ± 390	0.92 ± 0.4	5	1260 ± 370	1.57 ± 0.8	7	2 580 ± 1890	1.62 ± 0.9	7
Aorta	24 500 ± 4100	1.9 ± 1.0	9	16 670 ± 3800 **	1.48 ± 0.5	7	20 800 ± 6850	2.68 ± 1.44	7

Table 4. Average B_{max} values **fmoles / mg** protein and K_d values (nM) of [^{3}H]PK 11195 binding to TSPO in aorta and heart homogenates of WT (Bb-Control) and apoE KO mice, fed with standard feed, and feed supplemented with 1% and 3% cholesterol (Chol). One-way analysis of variance ANOVA was used, with Mann-Whitney as the post-hoc, non-parametric test. Data are expressed as mean ± SD; * = $p < 0.05$, ** = $p < 0.01$, *** = $p < 0.001$ vs. control.

3. Discussion

There is strong evidence that accumulation of plasma derived lipoproteins in the arterial wall launches specific cell reactions that account for atherosclerosis process: enhanced NO production, amplification of the inflammatory response, apoptosis, endothelial function impairment, enhanced smooth muscle cell migration and proliferation, and macrophage foam cell formation (Steinberg et al., 2002; Whitman, 2004; Zhao et al., 2008; Singh et al., 2009). Mice lacking apoE have a substantial delay in the metabolism of lipoproteins, particularly VLDL, even fed with a regular standard chow feed (Hoen et al., 2003; Kato et al., 2009). Lesions in apoE-deficient mouse have many features in common with human atherosclerosis, even that the progression can be advantageous in many experimental situations (Dansky et al, 1999). At 26 weeks, atherosclerotic lesions are in the early stages of development, characterized by lipoprotein accumulation, leukocyte gathering, and foam cell formation. This model develops atherosclerotic lesions which progress to occlusion of coronary artery by 8th to 11 months after regular feeding (Piedrahita et al., 1992; Whitman, 2004). Aged (42-54 weeks) apoE KO mice develop intraplaque hemorrhage and plaque instability features, accelerated by feeding westernized diets (Seo et al., 2005; Singh et al., 2009). We found, similar to previous observations, advanced fibrous plaque development accompanying prolonged cholesterol feeding (Figure 1C) in apoE mice but not in WT mice. Another study by Molnar et al. (2005) showed that although high fat feeding induced endothelial cell dysfunction in WT mice, it did not enhance neointimal formation in WT mice. Also in WT rats, a high fat, high cholesterol diet does not appear to lead to atherosclerosis, although modest morphological alterations in the aortic wall could be observed (Dimitrova-Shumkovska et al., 2010a)

We also checked in blood plasma of apoE KO and WT mice the levels of total cholesterol, including triglycerides, high-density lipoprotein and low-density lipoprotein, since it can increase the risk of heart disease and atherosclerosis (Steinberg, 2002; Stocker and Keany, 2004, 2005). Mice naturally have high levels of HDL and low levels of LDL, lacking the cholesterol ester transfer protein, an enzyme responsible for trafficking cholesterol from HDL to VLDL and LDL. As reported also by others previously, we found clear cut differences in abundance of cholesterol related particles between apoE KO mice and WT mice (Table 1), (Hoen et al., 2003; Kato et al., 2009). In particular, each group of apoE KO mice had five times more plasma cholesterol than their WT counterparts. The apoE KO mice also always had higher TAG levels. HDL levels in apoE KO mice supplied with standard feed and 1% cholesterol supplemented diet was also twice as high than in WT mice. Interestingly, 3% cholesterol supplemented diet resulted in a reversal, meaning that HDL levels (i.e. "good" HDL-lipoproteins) in WT mice became twice as high as in apoE KO mice (Table 1). The generally low LDL cholesterol levels in WT mice even with cholesterol supplemented diet may be due to the capability of WT mice to efficiently suppress the percentage of dietary cholesterol absorption by increasing the excretion of gallbladder biliary cholesterol concentration (Sehayek et al., 2000).

We used this model, of apoE KO mice fed with cholesterol supplemented diet that shows well developed atherosclerosis, to assess oxidative stress in the aorta in correlation with TSPO binding density and atherosclerosis. For this purpose, homogenates of the aorta were used for ROS analysis and antioxidant enzymes activities. As accumulation of proatherogenic lipid affects all cell types present within the vascular wall, the response of the entire tissue vs. isolated cells to the hyperlipidemic conditions is relevant as an indication of vascular defense as a whole. The increase in plasma cholesterol levels was paralleled by changes in oxidative stress parameters in WT mice and ApoE KO mice, as discussed in detail below.

An indicator of cellular defence capacity against oxidative stress is the presence of reduced GSH, which we determined in the aorta homogenates after application of feed with cholesterol supplements. As seen in table 3, a reduction of GSH content in was evident compared to the corresponding controls, when 3% cholesterol diet was administered to WT as well as apoE mice. This shows that cholesterol diet regime indeed constitutes an elevated risk factor for ROS formation, due to a reduction in GSH levels in this model. It has been reported that ROS induce vascular cells to express cell adhesion molecules that trigger adhesion of leukocytes to the endothelium, which is part of the initiation atherosclerosis (Yang et al., 2009). Interestingly, it was also found that TSPO expression correlates positively with expression of adhesion molecules (Bode et al., 2012; Veenman et al., 2012). This may suggest that the reduction in TSPO levels seen in this study may counteract adhesion of leukocytes to the endothelium, and thereby prevent initiation atherosclerosis in particular in WT mice.

In accord with the observations of Hoen et al. (2003) that the mRNA levels of many antioxidant enzymes in apoE KO mice are higher (1.5 -5 fold) in the age of 6-15 weeks, compared to aged-matched wild type mice, we also saw that SOD activity were higher in aorta homogenates of apoE mice than those in age-matched WT mice (Table 3). Their hypothesis is that the aorta compensates for the oxidative stress induced by atherogenic stimuli, by stimulating the expression of antioxidant enzymes, thereby delaying the process of atheroma plaque formation. The latter was supported by Yang et al. (2004, 2009) providing evidence that over expression of catalase and superoxide dismutase delayed the development of atherosclerosis in apoE KO mice.

To determine the potential involvement of the TSPO in effects of apoE dysregulation, we studied TSPO binding density in heart and aorta of apoE KO mice (B6.129P2-apoE*tm1* N11) versus their wild type (WT) background mice, with and without inclusion of 1% and 3% cholesterol to the diet. TSPO has been detected in heart of normal mice before, and we found comparable levels in our control animals (Hashimoto et al., 1989; Weizman et al., 1992; Fares et al., 1990; Katz et al., 1994; Dumont et al., 1999). To our knowledge the present study is the first study regarding TSPO binding density in the aorta of mice, which are quite high (even comparable to TSPO levels in adrenal of rats (Gavish and Fares, 1985; Gavish et al., 1999). We found that enhanced cholesterol levels in the diet can result in reduced TSPO binding density in the aorta and heart of WT mice, as well as in the aorta of apoE mice (Table 4). The present study indicates that there is negative correlation between ROS parameters in heart tissue and TSPO binding density in cholesterol fed WT mice. Namely, in the heart of WT mice, the "steady state" levels of lipid peroxides (TBARs) showed a 2.5 fold enhancement after 3% cholesterol supplemented diet vs. a 1/3 fold enhancement in the group with 1% cholesterol supplemented diet. Regarding oxidized proteins in the heart tissues of WT mice fed with cholesterol supplements, AOPP and proteins carbonyls showed increases of 40% and 35%, respectively, regardless of the cholesterol percentage (data not shown). Such a relation between ROS parameters and TSPO binding density is not apparent in apoE mice, since in apoE mice little effect is seen on TSPO binding density.

Also in a previous study, enhanced plasma lipid levels due to HFHC diet supplied to rats, enhanced oxidative stress parameters and decreased indicators for antioxidant activity in the aorta, which were associated with reduced TSPO density in this organ (Dimitrova-Shumkovska et al., 2010a). Notably, wild type rats are not prone to develop atherosclerosis even when subjected to HFHC diet (Dimitrova-Shumkovska et al., 2010a). We have shown that reduction of TSPO expression by genetic manipulation in vitro in cell culture reduces mitochondrial ROS generation (Veenman et al., 2008, 2012; Zeno et al., 2009). We have discussed previously that the reduced TSPO levels accompanying atherogenic challenges may be a compensatory mechanism to counteract oxidative stress in the aorta and liver (Dimitrova-Shumkovska et al., 2010 a, b, c). This would be in effect similar to increased levels of SOD observed, which also counteract oxidative stress (see above). Our present study suggests that reduced TSPO binding density as observed in WT mice subjected to cholesterol supplemented diet may counteract oxidative stress as one mechanism to attenuate the development of atherosclerosis. As TSPO binding density is not affected in apoE mice subjected to cholesterol supplemented diet mentioned TSPO dependent mechanism is not available for apoE KO mice to counteract development of atherosclerosis. Presently, it is not known which components of the vascular wall, i.e. mast cells, smooth muscular, or dermal vascular endothelial cells, would be important for the potential correlation between TSPO expression, oxidative stress, and atherosclerosis (Stoebner et al., 1999; 2001; Morgan et al., 2004; Veenman and Gavish, 2006; Dimitrova-Shumkovska et al., 2010 a, b, c).

It can be assumed from the present study, that oxidative stress parameters do not absolutely correlate with the development of atherosclerotic lesions (because supplementation with 1% of cholesterol to the diet does not affect oxidative stress), but the absolute levels of cholesterol do correlate with atherosclerotic development. Nonetheless, enhancement of cholesterol percentage from 1% to 3% in the diet resulted in significant increases in ROS parameters of WT and apoE KO mice in comparison to their control groups, and also provoked advanced lesion formation in aortic intimae in apoE KO mice fed a 3% cholesterol supplemented diet (but not in WT mice). TSPO binding density is reduced due to cholesterol intake in particular in WT mice and such changes in TSPO binding density in WT mice are in negative correlation with oxidative stress measured in heart and aorta. We believe the reductions in TSPO binding density in WT mice are compensatory for oxidative stress and atherosclerotic development. Thus, the lack of a significant decrease in TSPO binding density in the aorta of 3% cholesterol fed apoE KO mice may actually correlate with the enhanced atherosclerosis in this model. The capability of apoE KO mice fed with 1% cholesterol to reduce TSPO binding density in the aorta may present a rudimentary anti-atherosclerosis protective capacity. In conclusion, this study is in accord with previous studies suggesting that reductions in arterial TSPO binding density are part of a mechanism counteracting the development of atherosclerosis. A question is how the presence of apoE, in combination with enhanced dietary cholesterol levels, can result in suppression of TSPO binding density. It is also important to find out how in a mechanistic sense a reduction in TSPO levels can contribute to self protection against the development of atherosclerosis.

Explanation of abbreviations and symbols: ACS, acute coronary syndrome; ANOVA, analysis of variance; (AOPPs), advanced oxidation protein products; ApoE-/- KO, apolipoprotein E knockout mice; cAMP, adenosine 3,5-cyclic monophosphate; CBR, central-type benzodiazepine receptor; DBI, Diazepam Binding Inhibitor; CAM, cell adhesion molecule; CVD, cardiovascular disease; HDL, high-density lipoprotein; HFHC- high fat high cholesterol diet; HMGCoA, 3-hydroxy-3-methylglutaryl coenzyme A reductase; H_2O_2, hydrogen peroxide; Hb, hemoglobin; IL-1, interleukin-1 (IL-2, etc.); kDa, kilodalton; Kd, equilibrium dissociation constant; *Km*, equilibrium constant related to Michaelis-Menten kinetics (similarly, *Kd*, *Ka*, *Keq*, *Ks*); LDL, low density lipoproteins; mPTP, mitochondrial permeability transition pore; MCP-1, monocyte chemoatractant proteins-1; NADP, nicotinamide adenine dinucleotide phosphate; NADH, reduced nicotinamide adenine dinucleotide; PBR, peripheral-type benzodiazepine receptor; PC protein carbonyls; PK 11195, 1-(2- chlorophenyl)-N-methyl-N-(1-methyl-prop1)-3 isoquinolinecarboxamide; $ONOO^-$, peroxinitrite ; Ro5-4864, (4'- chlorodiazepam); ROS , reactive oxygen species; SOD, superoxide dismutase activity; TBARs, thiobarbituric acid reactive substances; TNF, tumor necrosis factor; TSPO, 18 kDa translocator protein; VCAM-1, vascular cell adhesion molecule; VSMCs, vascular smooth muscle cells.

Author details

Jasmina Dimitrova-Shumkovska*
Institute of Biology, Department of Experimental Biochemistry and Physiology, Faculty of Natural Sciences and Mathematics, Ss. Cyril and Methodius University - Skopje, Republic of Macedonia

Leo Veenman, Inbar Roim and Moshe Gavish
Rappaport Family Institute for Research in the Medical Sciences, Technion-Israel Institute of Technology, Department of Molecular Pharmacology, Haifa, Israel

4. References

Anholt, R.R., De Souza, E.B., Kuhar, M.J., & Snyder, S.H. (1985). Depletion of peripheral-type benzodiazepine receptors after hypophysectomy in rat adrenal gland and testis. *Eur J Pharmacol.* 110:41-6.

Aono, M., Bennett, E.R., Kim, K.S., Lynch, J.R., Myers, J., Pearlstein, R.D., Warner, D.S., & Laskowitz, D.T. (2003). Protective effect of apolipoprotein E-mimetic peptides on N-methyl-D-aspartate excitotoxicity in primary rat neuronal-glial cell cultures. *Neuroscience.* 116:437-45.

Banati, R.B., Myers, R., & Kreutzberg, G.W. (1997). PK ('peripheral benzodiazepine')--binding sites in the CNS indicate early and discrete brain lesions: microautoradiographic detection of [3H] PK11195 binding to activated microglia. *J Neurocytol.* 26:77-82.

Beffert, U., Stolt, P.C., & Herz, J. (2004). Functions of lipoprotein receptors in neurons. *J Lipid Res.* 45:403-9.

Benavides, J., Malgouris, C., Imbault, F., Begassat, F., Uzan, A., Renault, C., Dubroeucq, M.C., Gueremy, C., & Le Fur, G. (1983). "Peripheral type" benzodiazepine binding sites in rat adrenals: binding studies with [3H] PK 11195 and autoradiographic localization. *Arch Int Pharmacodyn Ther.* 266:38-49.

Bird, J.L., Izquierdo-Garcia, D., Davies, J.R., Rudd, J.H., Probst, K.C., Figg, N, Clark, J.C., Weissberg, P.L., Davenport, A.P., & Warburton, E.A. (2010). Evaluation of translocator

* Jasmina Dimitrova-Shumkovska and Leo Veenman contributed equally to this book chapter.

protein quantification as a tool for characterising macrophage burden in human carotid atherosclerosis. *Atherosclerosis.* 210(2):388-91.

Blue, M.L., Williams, D.L., Zucker, S., Khan, S.A., & Blum, C.B. (1983). Apolipoprotein E synthesis in human kidney, adrenal gland, and liver. *Proc Natl Acad Sci* U S A. 80:283-7.

Bode, J., Veenman, L., Caballero, B., Lakomek, M., Kugler, W., Gavish, M. (2012). The 18 kDa translocator protein influences angiogenesis, as well as aggressiveness, adhesion, migration, and proliferation of glioblastoma cells. *Pharmacogenet Genomics.* 22:538-50.

Bono, F., Lamarche, I., Prabonnaud, V., Le Fur, G., & Herbert, J.M. (1999). Peripheral benzodiazepine receptor agonists exhibit potent antiapoptotic activities. *Biochem Biophys Res Commun*. 265:457-61.

Boyles, J.K., Pitas, R.E., Wilson, E., Mahley, R.W., & Taylor, J.M. (1985). Apolipoprotein E associated with astrocytic glia of the central nervous system and with nonmyelinating glia of the peripheral nervous system. *J Clin Invest*. 76:1501-13.

Bribes, E., Bourrie, B., & Casellas, P. (2003). Ligands of the peripheral benzodiazepine receptor have therapeutic effects in pneumopathies in vivo. *Immunol Lett.* 88:241-7.

Buttini, M., Orth, M., Bellosta, S., Akeefe, H., Pitas, R.E., Wyss-Coray, T., Mucke, L., & Mahley, R.W. (1999). Expression of human apolipoprotein E3 or E4 in the brains of Apoe-/- mice: isoform-specific effects on neurodegeneration. *J Neurosci.* 19:4867-80.

Caliguiri, G., Nicoletti, A., Zhou, X., Tornberg, I. &Hansson, G.K. (1999). Effects of sex and age on atherosclerosis and autoimmunity in apoE-deficient mice. *Atheroscler.* 145(2). 301-8.

Camici PG, Rimoldi OE, Gaemperli

O, Libby P. (2012). Non-invasive anatomic and functional imaging of vascular inflammation and unstable plaque. *Eur Heart J.* 33(11):1309-17.

Cedazo-Minquez, A. & Cowburn, R.F. (2001). Apolipoprotein E: a major piece in the Alzheimer's disease puzzle. *J CellMolMed*. 5(3): 254-66.

Chan, L. (1989). The apolipoprotein multigene family: structure, expression, evolution, and molecular genetics. *Klin Wochenschr.* 67:225-37.

Cheng, C., Tempel, D., Van Haperen, R., Van Damme, L., Algur, M., Krams, R., & De Crom, R. (2009). Activation of MMP8 and MMP13 by angiotensin II correlates to severe intra-plaque hemorrages and collagen breakdown in atherosclerotic lesions with a vulnerable phenotype. *Atheroclerosis*. 204, 26-33.

Chia, M.C. (1998). The role of adhesion molecules in atherosclerosis. *Crit Rev Clin Lab Sci.* 35:573-602.

Costopoulos, C., Liew, T.V., & Bennet, M. (2008). Ageing and Atherosclerosis: Mechanisms and Therapeutic Options. *Biochem Pharmacol.* 75, 1251- 1261.

Csont, T., Bereczki, E., Bencsik, P., Fodor, G., Gorbe, A., Zvara, A., Csonka, C., Puskas, L.G., Santha, M., & Ferdinandy, P. (2007). Hypercholesterolemia inceases myocardial oxidative and nitrosative stress thereby leading to cardiac dysfunction in apoB-100 transgenic mice. *Cardiovasc Res*. 76, 100-109.

Cullen, P., Athanasopoulos, T., Dickson, G., & Owen, J.S. (2001). Cell-derived apolipoprotein E (ApoE) particles inhibit vascular cell adhesion molecule-1 (VCAM-1) expression in human endothelial cells. *J Biol Chem*. 276:46011-6.

Dansky, H., Sherri, A., Charlton, S.A., Sikes, J., Heath, S., Simantov, R., Levin, L., Shu, P., Moore,K., Breslow, J., Smith, J.(1999). Genetic background determines the extent of atherosclerosis in ApoE deficient mice. *Arterioscler.Thromb.Vasc.Biol.* 19:1960-1968.

Davignon, J., Gregg, R.E., & Sing, C.F. (1988). Apolipoprotein E polymorphism and atherosclerosis. *Arteriosclerosis.* 8:1-21. 1988.

Davignon, J., Cohn, J.S., Mabile, L., & Bernier, L. (1999). Apolipoprotein E and atherosclerosis:insight from animal to human studies. 286:115-143.

Dimitrova-Shumkovska, J., Veenman, L., Ristoski, T., Leschiner, S., & Gavish, M. (2010a). Chronic High Fat, High Cholesterol Supplementation Decreases 18 kDa Translocator Protein Binding Capacity in Association with Increased Oxidative Stress in Rat Liver and Aorta. *Food and Chem. Toxicol.* 48, 910-921.

Dimitrova-Shumkovska, J., Veenman, L., Ristoski, T., Leschiner, S., & Gavish, M. (2010b). Dimethylbenz [alpha] anthracene induces oxidative stress and reduces the binding capacity of the mitochondrial 18-kDa translocator protein in rat aorta. *Drug Chem. Toxicol.* 33, 337-47.

Dimitrova-Shumkovska, J., Veenman, L., Ristoski, T., Leschiner, S., & Gavish, M. (2010c). Decreases in Binding Capacity of the Mitochondrial 18 kDa Translocator Protein Accompany Oxidative Stress and Pathological Signs in Rat Liver after DMBA Exposure. *Toxicol Pathol.*, 38:957-68.

Dimitrova-Shumkovska, J., Veenman, & Gavish, M. (2012). The 18kDa Translocator Protein as a Potential Participant in Atherosclerosis, in the book : „Atherogenesis", edited by Parthasarathy, S., INTECH, ISBN 978-953-307-992-9

Do Carmo, S., Seguin, D., Milne, R. & Rassart, E. (2002). Modulation of apolipoprotein D and apolipoprotein E mRNA expression by growth arrest and identification of key elements in the promoter. *J Biol Chem.* 277: 5514-23

Dumont , F., De Vos, F., Versijpt, J., Jansen, H.M., Korf, J., Dierckx, R.A., & Slegers, G. (1999). In vivo evaluation in mice and metabolism in blood of human volunteers of [123I]iodo-PK11195: a possible single-photon emission tomography tracer for visualization of inflammation. *Eur J Nucl Med.* 26:194-200.

Dupont-Wallois, L., Soulié, C., Sergeant, N., Wavrant-de Wrieze, N., Chartier-Harlin, M.C., Delacourte, A.,& Caillet-Boudin, M.L. (1997). ApoE synthesis in human neuroblastoma cells. *Neurobiol Dis.* 4:356-64.

Elliot, A.J., Maier, M.A., Moller, A.C., Friedman, R. & Meinhardt, J. (2007). Color and psychological functioning: the effect of red on performance attainment. *J Exp Psychol Gen.* 136(1): 154-68.

Elliott, D.A., Kim, W.S., Jans, D.A., & Garner, B. (2007). Apoptosis induces neuronal apolipoprotein-E synthesis and localization in apoptotic bodies. *Neurosci Lett.* 416:206-10.

Elshourbagy N.A., Liao W.S., Mahley R.W., & Taylor J.M. (1985). Apolipoprotein E mRNA is abundant in the brain and adrenals, as well as in the liver, and is present in other peripheral tissues of rats and marmosets. *Proc Natl Acad Sci* U S A. 82:203-7.

Epstein, S.E., Stabile, E., Kinnaird, T., Lee, C.W., Clavijo, L. & Burnett, M.S. (2004). Janus phenomenon: the interrelated tradeoffs inherent in therapies designed to enhance collateral formation and those designed to inhibit atherogenesis. *Circulation.* 109(23): 2826-31.

Falchi AM, Battetta B, Sanna F, Piludu M, Sogos V, Serra M, Melis M, Putzolu M, & Diaz, G. (2007). Intracellular cholesterol changes induced by translocator protein (18 kDa) TSPO/PBR ligands. *Neuropharmacology.* 53:318-29.

Fares, F., Weizman, A., Pick, C.G. & Gavish, M. (1990). Effect of prenatal and neonatal chronic exposure to phenobarbital on central and peripheral benzodiazepine receptors. *Brain Res.* 506(1): 115-9.

Finsen, B. (2006). Up-regulation of PK11195 binding in areas of axonal degeneration coincides with early microglial activation in mouse brain. *Eur J Neurosci.* 24:991-1000.

Friedewald WT, Levy RI, & Fredrickson DS. (1972). Estimation of the concentration of low-density lipoprotein cholesterol in plasma, without use of the preparative centrifuge. *Clin Chem*; 18:499—500.

Gaemperli, O., Shalhoub, J., Owen, D. R.J., Lamare, F., Johansson, S., Fouladi, N., Davies, A.H., Rimoldi, O.E., Camici, P.G. (2011). Imaging intraplaque inflammation in carotid atherosclerosis with 11C-PK11195 positron emission tomography/computed tomography. *Eur Heart J.* 33(15):1902-1910.

Gaemperli, O., Shalhoub,J., Owen, D.R.J, Lamare,D., Johansson, S., Fouladi, N., Davies, A., Ornella, E., Rimoldi, O.E.,& Camici, P., (2012). Imaging intraplaque inflammation in carotid atherosclerosis with 11C-PK11195 positron emission tomography/computed tomography. *Eur Heart J.* 33(15): 1902-1910.

Gavish, M. & Fares, F. (1985).Solubilization of peripheral benzodiazepine-binding sites from rat kidney. *J Neurosci.* 5:2889-93.

Gavish, M., Bar-Ami, S., & Weizman, R. (1992). The endocrine system and mitochondrial benzodiazepine receptors. *Mol Cell Endocrinol.* 88, 1-13.

Gavish, M. & Weizman, R. (1997). Role of peripheral-type benzodiazepine receptors in steroidogenesis. *Clin Neuropharmacol.* 20:473-81.

Gavish, M., Bachman, I., Shoukrun, R., Katz, Y., Veenman, L., Weisinger, G. & Weizman, A. (1999). Enigma of the peripheral benzodiazepine receptor. *Pharmacol. Review.* 51, 630-646.

Gunten, A.V., Ebbing, K., Imhof, A., Giannakopoulos, P., Kovari, E. (2010). Brain aging in the Oldest-Old. *Curr. Gerontol Geriatr. Res.* 358531.

Han, S.H., Einstein, G., Weisgraber, K.H., Strittmatter, W.J., Saunders, A.M., Pericak-Vance, M., Roses, A.D., & Schmechel, D.E. (1994). Apolipoprotein E is localized to the cytoplasm of human cortical neurons: a light and electron microscopic study. *J Neuropathol Exp Neurol.* 53:535-44.

Harris, F.M., Tesseur, I., Brecht, W.J., Xu, Q., Mullendorff, K., Chang, S., Wyss-Coray, T., Mahley, R.W., & Huang, Y. (2004). Astroglial regulation of apolipoprotein E expression in neuronal cells. Implications for Alzheimer's disease. *J Biol Chem.* 279:3862-8.

Hashimoto, K., Inoue, O., Suzuki, K., Yamasaki, T., & Kojima, M. (1989). Synthesis and evaluation of 11C-PK 11195 for in vivo study of peripheral-type benzodiazepine receptors using positron emission tomography. *Ann Nucl Med.* 3:63-71.

Hasty, A.H., Linton, M.F., Brandt, S.J., Babaev, V.R., Gleaves, L.A., & Fazio, S. (1999). Retroviral gene therapy in ApoE-deficient mice: ApoE expression in the artery wall reduces early foam cell lesion formation. *Circulation*. 99:2571-6.

Heumann, R., Lindholm, D., Bandtlow, C., Meyer, M., Radeke, M.J., Misko, T.P., Shooter, E.,

Hoen, P.A., Van der Lans, C.A., Van Eck, M., Bijsterbosch, M.K., Van Berkel, T.J. & Twisk, J. (2003). Aorta of ApoE-deficient mice responds to atherogenic stimuli by a prelesional increase and subsequent decrease in the expression of antioxidant enzymes. *Circ Res*. 93(3): 262-9.

Hoen, P.A.C., Van der Lans, C.A.C., Van Eck, M., Bijsterbosch, M.K., Van Berkel & T.J.C., Twisk, J. (2003). Aorta of ApoE – deficient mice responds to atherogenic stimuli by a prelesional increase and subsequent decrease in the expression of antioxidant enzymes. *Circ Res*. 93, 262-269.

Hollingsworth, E.B., McNeal, E.T., Burton, J.L., Williams, R.J., Daly, J.W., & Creveling, C.R. (1985). Biochemical characterization of a filtered synaptoneurosome preparation from guinea pig cerebral cortex: cyclic adenosine 3':5'-monophosphate-generating systems, receptors, and enzymes. *J Neurosci*. 5:2240-53.

Insull, W.Jr. (2009). The pathology of atherosclerosis: Plaque development and plaque responses to medical treatment. *Am J Med*. 122:S3-S14.

Johnson, J., Carson,K., Williams, H., Karanam, S., Newby, A., & Angelini, G. (2005). Plaque rupture after short periods of fat feeding in the apolipoprotein E-knockout mouse:model characterization and effects of pravastatin treatment. *Circulation*.111:1422-1430.

Kashyap, V.S., Santamarina-Fojo, S., Brown, D.R., Parrott, C.L., Applebaum-Bowden, D., Meyn, S., Talley, G., Paigen, B., Maeda, N., & Brewer, H.B. Jr. (1995). Apolipoprotein E deficiency in mice: gene replacement and prevention of atherosclerosis using adenovirus vectors. *J Clin Invest*. 96:1612-20.

Kato R, Mori C, Kitazato K, Arata S, Obama T, Mori M, Takahashi K, Aiuchi T, & Takano T. (2009). Transient increase in plasma oxidized LDL during the progression of atherosclerosis in apolipoprotein E knockout mice. *Arterioscler Thromb Vasc Biol*. 29: 33–9.

Klegeris, A., McGeer, E.G., & McGeer, P.L. (2000). Inhibitory action of 1-(2-chlorophenyl)-N-methyl-N-(1-methylpropyl)-3-isoquinolinecarboxam ide (PK 11195) on some mononuclear phagocyte functions. *Biochem Pharmacol*. 59:1305-14.

Kmieć Z. (2001). Cooperation of liver cells in health and disease. *Adv Anat Embryol Cell Biol*. 161:1-151.

Knight-Lozano, C.A., Young, C.G., Burow, D.L., Hu, Z.Y., Uyeminami, D., Pinkerton, K.E., Ischiropulos, H., & Ballinger, S.W. (2002). Cigarette smoke exposure and hypercholesterolemia increase mitochondrial damage in cardiovascular tissues. *Circ Res*. 105, 849-854.

Ko, K.W.S., Paul, A., Ma, K., Li, L., Chan, L. (2005) Endothelial lipase modulates plasma lipoprotein profiles but has no effect on the development od atherosclerosis in $ApoE^{-/-}$ and $LDLR^{-/-}$ mice. *J Lipid Res*. 46:2586-2594.

Krueger, K.E & Papadopoulos, V. (1990). Peripheral-type benzodiazepine receptors mediate translocation of cholesterol from outer to inner mitochondrial membranes in adrenocortical cells. *J Biol Chem.* 265:15015-22.

Krul, E.S., Tikkanen, M.J., & Schonfeld, G. (1988). Heterogeneity of apolipoprotein E epitope expression on human lipoproteins:importance for apolipoprotein E function. *J Lipid Res.* 29:1309-25.

Kunitomo, M., Yamaguchi, Y., Kagota, S., Yoshikawa, N., Nakamura, K., & Shinozuka, K. (2009). Biochemical Evidence of Atherosclerosis Progression Mediated by Increased Oxidative Stress in Apolipoprotein E-Deficient Spontaneously Hyperlipidemic Mice Exposed to Chronic Cigarette Smoke. *J Pharmacol. Sci.* 110, 354-361

Lacapère, J.J. & Papadopoulos, V. (2003). Peripheral-type benzodiazepine receptor: structure and function of a cholesterol-binding protein in steroid and bile acid biosynthesis. *Steroids.* 68:569-85.

Laskowitz, D. T. (2003). APOE genotype and an ApoE-mimetic peptide modify the systemic and central nervous system inflammatory response. *J Biol Chem.* 278:48529-33.

Law, G.L., McGuinness, M.P., Linder, C.C., & Griswold, M.D. (1997). Expression of apolipoprotein E mRNA in the epithelium and interstitium of the testis and the epididymis. *J Androl.* 18:32-42.

Lenfant, M., Zavala, F., Haumont, J., & Potier, P. (1985). [Presence of a peripheral type benzodiazepine binding site on the macrophage; its possible role in immunomodulation] *C R Acad Sci* III. 300:309-14.

Levine, R. L., Garland, D., Oliver, C.N., Amici, A., Climent, I., Lenz, A.G., Ahn, B.W., Shaltiel, S., & Stadman, E.R. (1990). Determination of carbonyl content in oxidatively modified proteins. *Methods in Enzymol.* 186, 464-478.

Libby, P., Ridker, P.M. & Hansson, G.K. (2011). Progress and challenges in translating the biology of atherosclerosis. Review. *Nature* 473:317-325

Linton, MF. & Fazio, S. (1999). Macrophages, lipoprotein metabolism, and atherosclerosis: insights from murine bone marrow transplantation studies. *Curr Opin Lipidol.* 10:97-105.

Liu S.X., Hou, F.F., Guo, Z. J., Nagai, R., Zhang, W.R., Liu, Z.Q., Zhou, Z.M., Di Xie, Wang, G.B., & Zhang, X. (2006). Advanced Oxidation Protein Products Accelerate Atherosclerosis Through Promoting Oxidative Stress and Inflammation. *Arterioscler Thromb Vasc Biol.* 26, 1156-1162.

Lynch, J.R., Tang, W, Wang, H., Vitek, M.P., Bennett ,E.R., Sullivan, P.M., Warner, D.S.,

Mahley, R.W. (1988). Apolipoprotein E: cholesterol transport protein with expanding role in cell biology. *Science.* 240(4582): 622-30.

Mahley, R.W., & Huang, Y. (1999a). Apolipoprotein E: from atherosclerosis to Alzheimer's disease and beyond. *Curr Opin Lipidol.* 10:207-17.

Mahley, R.W. & Ji, Z.S. (1999b). Remnant lipoprotein metabolism: key pathways involving cell-surface heparan sulfate proteoglycans and apolipoprotein E. *J Lipid Res.* 40:1-16.

Mahley, R.W. & Rall, S.C. Jr. (2000). Apolipoprotein E: far more than a lipid transport protein. *Annu Rev Genomics Hum Genet.* 1:507-37.

Mahley, R.W., Huang, Y., & Weisgraber, K.H. (2006).Putting cholesterol in its place: apoE and reverse cholesterol transport. *J Clin Invest.* 116:1226-9.

Marchetti, P., Trincavelli, L., Giannarelli, R., Giusti, L., Coppelli, A., Martini, C., & Marshall, J.S. (2004). Mast-cell responses to pathogens. *Nat Rev Immunol.* 4:787-99.

Mazurika, C., Veenman, L., Weizman, R., Bidder, M., Leschiner ,S., Golani, I., Spanier, I., Weisinger, G., & Gavish, M. (2009). Estradiol modulates uterine 18 kDa translocator protein gene expression in uterus and kidney of rats. *Mol Cell Endocrinol.* 307, 43-49.

McAdoo, J.D., Warner, D.S., Goldberg, R.N., Vitek, M.P., Pearlstein, R., & Laskowitz, D.T. (2005). Intrathecal administration of a novel apoE-derived therapeutic peptide improves outcome following perinatal hypoxic-ischemic injury. *Neurosci Lett.* 381:305-8.

Milner, P., Bodin, P., Guiducci, S., Del Rosso, A., Kahaleh, M.B., Matucci-Cerinic, M., & Burnstock, G. (2004). Regulation of substance P mRNA expression in human dermal microvascular endothelial cells. *Clin Exp Rheumatol.* 22:S24-7.

Morgan, J., Oseroff, A.R., & Cheney, R.T. (2004). Expression of the peripheral benzodiazepine receptor is decreased in skin cancers in comparison with normal skin. *Br J Dermatol.* 151, 846-56.

Nakashima, Y., Raines, E.W., Plump, A.S., Breslow, J.L., & Ross, R. (1998). Upregulation of VCAM-1 and ICAM-1 at atherosclerosis-prone sites on the endothelium in the ApoE-deficient mouse. *Arterioscler Thromb Vasc Biol.* 18:842-51.

Navalesi, R. & Lucacchini, A. (1996). Characterization of peripheral benzodiazepine receptors in purified large mammal pancreatic islets. *Biochem Pharmacol.* 51:1437-42.

Noeman, S.A., Hamooda, H.E., & Baalash, A.A. (2011). Biochemical study of oxidative stress markers in the liver, kidney and heart of high fat diet induced obesity in rats. *Diabetol Metab Syndr.* 3(1), 17.

Onyimba, J.A., Coronado, M.J., Garton, A.E., Kim, J.B., Bucek, A., Bedja, D., Gabrielson, K.L., Guilarte, T.R., & Fairweather, D. (2011). The innate immune response to coxsackievirus B3 predicts progression to cardiovascular disease and heart failure in male mice. *Biol Sex Differ.* 21; 2:2.

Papadopoulos, V., Baraldi, M., Guilarte, T.R., Knudsen, T.B., Lacapère, J.J., Lindemann, P., Norenberg, M.D., Nutt, D., Weizman, A., Zhang, M.R., & Gavish, M. (2006). Translocator protein (18kDa). New nomenclature for the peripheral-type benzodiazepine receptor based on its structure and molecular function. *Trends Pharmacol Sci.* 27, 402-9.

Papadopoulos, V., Berkovich, A., Krueger, K.E., Costa, E., & Guidotti, A. (1991). Diazepam binding inhibitor and its processing products stimulate mitochondrial steroid biosynthesis via an interaction with mitochondrial benzodiazepine receptors. *Endocrinology.* 129:1481-8.

Pedersen, M.D., Minuzzi, L., Wirenfeldt ,M., Meldgaard, M., Slidsborg, C., Cumming, P.,

Potter, H., Wisniewski, T. (2012). Apolipoprotein E: Essential catalyst of the Alzheimer amyloid cascade. *Int J Alzheimers Dis.* 489428.

Quinn, C.M., Kågedal, K., Terman, A., Stroikin U., Brunk, U.T., Jessup, W., & Garner, B. (2004). Induction of fibroblast apolipoprotein E expression during apoptosis, starvation-induced growth arrest and mitosis. *Biochem J.* 378:753-61. 2004.

Rosenfeld, M.E., Polinsky, P., Virmani, R., Kauser, K., Rubanyi,G., Schwartz, S.M. (2000). Advanced atherosclerotic lesions in the innominate artery of the ApoE knockout mouse. *Arterioscler. Thromb. Vasc. Biol.*20:2587-2592.

Ross, J.S., Stagliano, N.E., Donovan, M.J., Breitbart, R.E., & Ginsburg, G.S. (2001). Atherosclerosis And Cancer: Common Molecular Pathways Of Disease Development And Progression. *Ann NY Acad Sci.* 947, 271–292Ruff, M.R., Wahl S.M., Mergenhagen, S., & Pert, C.B. (1985). Opiate receptor-mediated chemotaxis of human monocytes. *Neuropeptides*. 5:363-6.

Ross, R & Glomset, J.A. (1973). Atherosclerosis and the arterial smooth muscle cell: Proliferation of smooth muscle is a key event in the genesis of the lesions of atherosclerosis. *Science* 180: 1332-1339.

Ross, R., (1999). Atherosclerosis an Inflammatory Disease. *N Engl J Med*. 340, 115-26.

Ryu, J.K., Choi, H.B., & McLarnon, J.G. (2005). Peripheral benzodiazepine receptor ligand PK11195 reduces microglial activation and neuronal death in quinolinic acid-injected rat striatum. *Neurobiol Dis.* 20:550-61.

Schafer, F.Q., Buettner, G.R. (2001) . Redox environment of the cell as viewed through the redox state of the glutathione disulfide/glutathione couple. *Free Radic Biol Med.* 30:1191-212.

Sehayek, E., Shefer, S., Nguyen, L.B., Ono, J.G., Merkel, M., & Breslow, J.L. (2000). Apolipoprotein E regulates dietary cholesterol absorption and biliary cholesterol excretion: studies in C57BL/6 apolipoprotein E knockout mice. *Proc Natl Acad Sci* U S A. 97:3433-7.

Seo, T., Qi, K., Chang, C., Liu, Y., Worgall, T.S., Ramakrishan, R., & Deckelbaum, R.J. (2005). Saturated fat-rich diet enhances selective uptake of LDL cholesteryl esters in the arterial wall. *J Clin Invest.* 115, 2214-2222.

Shargorodsky, L., Veenman, L., Caballero, B., Pe'er, Y., Leschiner, S., Bode, J., Gavish, M. (2012). The nitric oxide donor sodium nitroprusside requires the 18 kDa Translocator Protein to induce cell death. *Apoptosis.* 17:647-65.

Sheng, H., Laskowitz, D.T., Bennett, E., Schmechel, D.E., Bart, R.D., Saunders, A.M., Pearlstein, R.D., Roses, A.D., & Warner, D.S. (1998). Apolipoprotein E isoform-specific differences in outcome from focal ischemia in transgenic mice. *J Cereb Blood Flow Metab.* 18:361-6.

Singh, V., Tiwari, R.L., Dikshit, M., & Barthwal, M.K. (2009). Models to Study Atherosclerosis: A Mechanistic Insight. *Curr Vasc Pharmacol.* 7, 75-109.

Stannard, A.K., Riddell, D.R., Sacre, S.M., Tagalakis, A.D., Langer, C., von Eckardstein, A., &

Steinberg, D., Parthasarathy, S., Carew, T.E., Khoo, J.C., & Witztum, J.L. (1989). Beyond cholesterol: modifications of low-density lipoprotein that increase its atherogenicity. *N Engl J Med.* 320:915-924

Steinberg, D. (2002). Atherogenesis in perspective: hypercholesterolemia and inflammation as partners in crime. *Nat Med* 8, 1211–1217.

Stephenson, D.T., Schober, D.A., Smalstig, E.B., Mincy, R.E., Gehlert, D.R., & Clemens, J.A. (1995). Peripheral benzodiazepine receptors are colocalized with activated microglia following transient global forebrain ischemia in the rat. *J Neurosci*. 15:5263-74.

Stocker, R & Keaney, JF Jr. (2004). Role of oxidative modifications in atherosclerosis. *Physiol Rev.* 84,1381–478.

Stocker, R & Keaney, J.F. Jr. (2005). New insights on oxidative stress in the artery wall. *J Thromb Haemost* 3, 1825-1834.

Stoebner, P.E., Carayon, P., Penarier, G., Fréchin, N., Barnéon, G., Casellas, P., Cano, J.P., Meynadier, J., & Meunier, L. (1999). The expression of peripheral benzodiazepine receptors in human skin: the relationship with epidermal cell differentiation. *Br J Dermatol.* 140:1010-6.

Stoebner, P.E., Carayon, P., Casellas, P., Portier, M, Lavabre-Bertrand, T., Cuq, P., Cano, J.P., Meynadier, J., & Meunier L. (2001). Transient protection by peripheral benzodiazepine receptors during the early events of ultraviolet light-induced apoptosis. *Cell Death Differ.* 8:747-53.

Strittmatter, W.J. & Bova Hill ,C. (2002). Molecular biology of apolipoprotein E. *Curr Opin Lipidol.* 13:119-23.

Taupin, V., Toulmond, S., Serrano, A., Benavides, J., & Zavala, F. (1993). Increase in IL-6, IL-1 and TNF levels in rat brain following traumatic lesion. Influence of pre- and post-traumatic treatment with Ro5 4864, a peripheral-type (p site) benzodiazepine ligand. *J Neuroimmunol.* 42:177-85.

Thoenen, H. (1987). Differential regulation of mRNA encoding nerve growth factor and its receptor in rat sciatic nerve during development, degeneration, and regeneration: role of macrophages. *Proc Natl Acad Sci* U S A. 84:8735-9.

Torres, S.R., Fröde, T.S., Nardi, G.M., Vita, N., Reeb, R., Ferrara, P., Ribeiro-do-Valle, R.M.,Farges, R.C. (2000). Anti-inflammatory effects of peripheral benzodiazepine receptor ligands in two mouse models of inflammation. *Eur J Pharmacol.* 408:199-211.

Truskey, G.A., Herrmann, R.A., Kait, J., & Barber, K.M. (1999). Focal increases in vascular cell adhesion molecule-1 and intimal macrophages at atherosclerosis-susceptible sites in the rabbit aorta after short-term cholesterol feeding. *Arterioscler Thromb Vasc Biol.* 19:393-401.

Veenman, L. & Gavish, M. (2000). Peripheral-type benzodiazepine receptors: Their implication in Brain Disease. *Drug Dev Res* 50:355-370

Veenman, L. & Gavish, M. (2006). The peripheral-type benzodiazepine receptor and the cardiovascular system. Implications for drug development. *Pharmacol Ther.*110, 503-24.

Veenman, L., Papadopoulos, V., & Gavish, M. (2007). Channel-like functions of the 18-kDa translocator protein (TSPO): regulation of apoptosis and steroidogenesis as part of the host-defence response. *Curr Pharm Des.* 13, 2385-405.

Veenman, L., Shandalov, Y., & Gavish, M. (2008). VDAC activation by the 18 kDa translocator protein (TSPO), implications for apoptosis. *J Bioenerg Biomembr.* 40(3):199-205.

Veenman, L., Gavish, M. (2012). The role of 18 kDa mitochondrial translocator protein (TSPO) in programmed cell death, and effects of steroids on TSPO expression. *Curr Mol Med.* 12(4): 398-412.

Veenman, L., Bode, J., Gaitner, M., Caballero, B., Pe'er, Y., Zeno, S., Kietz, S., Kugler, W., Lakomek, M., Gavish, M. (2012) Effects of 18-kDa translocator protein knockdown on gene expression of glutamate receptors, transporters, and metabolism, and on cell viability affected by glutamate. *Pharmacogenet Genomics.* 22:606-19.

Veiga, S., Azcoitia, I., Garcia-Segura, L.M. (2005). Ro5-4864, a peripheral benzodiazepine receptor ligand, reduces reactive gliosis and protects hippocampal hilar neurons from kainic acid excitotoxicity. *J Neurosci Res.* 80:129-3.

Vowinckel, E., Reutens, D., Becher, B., Verge, G., Evans, A., Owens, T., Antel, J.P.(1997). PK11195 binding to the peripheral benzodiazepine receptor as a marker of microglia activation in multiple sclerosis and experimental autoimmune encephalomyelitis. *J Neurosci Res.* 50:345-53.

Waterfield, J.D., McGeer, E.G., McGeer, P.L. (1999). The peripheral benzodiazepine receptor ligand PK 11195 inhibits arthritis in the MRL-lpr mouse model. Rheumatology (Oxford). 38:1068-73.

Weisgraber, K.H., Roses, A.D., Strittmatter, W.J.(1994). The role of apolipoprotein E in the nervous system. *Curr Opin Lipidol.* 5:110-6.

Whitman, S.C. (2004). A practical approach to using mice in atherosclerosis research. *Clin Biochem Rev.* 25(1), 81-93.

Wilms, H., Claasen, J., Röhl, C., Sievers, J., Deuschl, G., & Lucius, R. (2003). Involvement of benzodiazepine receptors in neuroinflammatory and neurodegenerative diseases: evidence from activated microglial cells in vitro. *Neurobiol Dis.* 14:417-24.

Wojta, J., Huber, K., & Valent, P. (2003). New aspects in thrombotic research: complement induced switch in mast cells from a profibrinolytic to a prothrombotic phenotype. *Pathophysiol Haemost Thromb.* 33:438-41.

Woods, A.A., Linton, S.M. & Davies, M.J. (2003). Detection of HOCl-mediated protein oxidation products in the extracellular matrix of human atherosclerotic plaques. *Biochem.* 370: 729-35.

Xu, P.T., Schmechel, D., Rothrock-Christian, T., Burkhart, D.S., Qiu, H.L., Popko, B., Sullivan, P., Maeda, N, Saunders, A.M., Roses, A.D., & Gilbert, J.R. (1996). Human apolipoprotein E2, E3, and E4 isoform-specific transgenic mice: human-like pattern of glial and neuronal immunoreactivity in central nervous system not observed in wild-type mice. *Neurobiol Dis.* 3:229-45.

Yang, H., Roberts, J.L., Shi, M.J., Zhou, C., Ballard, B.R., Richardson, A .& Guo, Z.M. (2004). Retardation of atherosclerosis by overexpression of catalase or both Cu/Zn-superoxide dismutase and catalase in mice lacking apoliporotein E. *Circ Res.* 95, 1075-1081.

Young, C.G., Knight, C., Vickers, K.C., Westbrook, D., Madamanchi, N.R., Runge, M.S., Ischiropoulos, H., & Ballinger, S.W. (2004). Differential effects of exercise on aortic mitochondria. *Am J Physol Heart Circ Physiol.* 288, H1683-H1689.

Zeno, S., Zaaroor, M., Leschiner, S., Veenman, L., & Gavish, M. (2009). CoCl(2) induces apoptosis via the 18kDa translocator protein in U118MG human glioblastoma cells. *Biochem.* 48, 4652-61.

Zeno, S., Veenman, L., Katz, Y., Bode, J., Gavish, M., & Zaaroor, M. (2012). The 18 kDa mitochondrial Translocator Protein (TSPO) prevents accumulation of protoporphyrin IX. Involvement of reactive oxygen species. *Curr Molecular Medicine.* 12(4): 494-501.

Zhao, Y., Kuge, Y., Zhao, S., Strauss, W.H., Blankenberg, F.G., & Tamaki, N. (2008). Prolonged high-fat feeding enhances aortic 18F-FDG and 99mTc-annexin A5 uptake in apolipoprotein E-deficient and wild type C57BL/6J mice. *J Nucl Med.* 49, 1707-1714.

Chapter 6

Metabolism of Plasma Membrane Lipids in Mycobacteria and Corynebacteria

Paul K. Crellin, Chu-Yuan Luo and Yasu S. Morita

Additional information is available at the end of the chapter

http://dx.doi.org/10.5772/52781

1. Introduction

Bacteria of the Corynebacterineae, a suborder of the Actinobacteria, comprise *Mycobacterium, Corynebacterium, Nocardia, Rhodococcus* and other genera. This suborder of high GC gram-positive bacteria includes a number of important human pathogens, such as *Mycobacterium tuberculosis, Mycobacterium leprae* and *Corynebacterium diphtheriae,* the causative agents of tuberculosis, leprosy and diphtheria, respectively. *M. tuberculosis* is the most medically significant species, a devastating human pathogen infecting around one-third of the entire human population and responsible for more than 1 million deaths annually. The Corynebacterineae also includes non-pathogenic species such as *Mycobacterium smegmatis,* a saprophytic species, and *Corynebacterium glutamicum,* an industrial workhorse for the production of amino acids and other useful compounds. These relatively fast-growing species serve as useful models to study metabolic processes essential to the growth and survival of the slow-growing pathogens.

All these bacteria share a common feature, a distinctive multilaminate cell wall composed of peptidoglycan, complex polysaccharides, and both covalently linked lipids and free lipids/lipoglycans (Fig. 1). Among them, mycolic acids are the hallmark of these species. These long chain α-branched, β-hydroxylated fatty acids are covalently linked to the arabinogalactan polysaccharide layer. This mycolic acid layer is complemented by a glycolipid layer to form an outer "mycomembrane" analogous to the outer membrane of Gram-negative bacteria. [1, 2]. The outer leaflet of the mycomembrane is composed of a variety of lipids including trehalose dimycolates (TDMs), glycopeptidolipids (GPLs), phthiocerol dimycocerosates (PDIMs), sulfolipids, phenolic glycolipids (PGLs), and lipooligosaccharides. Some of these lipids are widely distributed while others are restricted to particular species. For example, TDMs and their structural equivalents are found in both mycobacteria and corynebacteria, while PDIMs and PGLs are restricted to a subset of mycobacteria. The structure and hydrophobic properties of the cell wall make it a potent permeability barrier that is responsible for intrinsic resistance of mycobacteria to an array of host microbiocidal processes, many antibiotics and sterilization conditions [3, 4]. Many of the cell wall components of pathogenic mycobacterial species are essential for pathogenesis and *in vitro* growth, hampering efforts to characterize the function of individual proteins in their assembly. In contrast, some non-pathogenic species such as *C. glutamicum* can tolerate the loss of major cell wall components, making them useful model systems for delineating processes involved in the assembly of core cell wall structures.

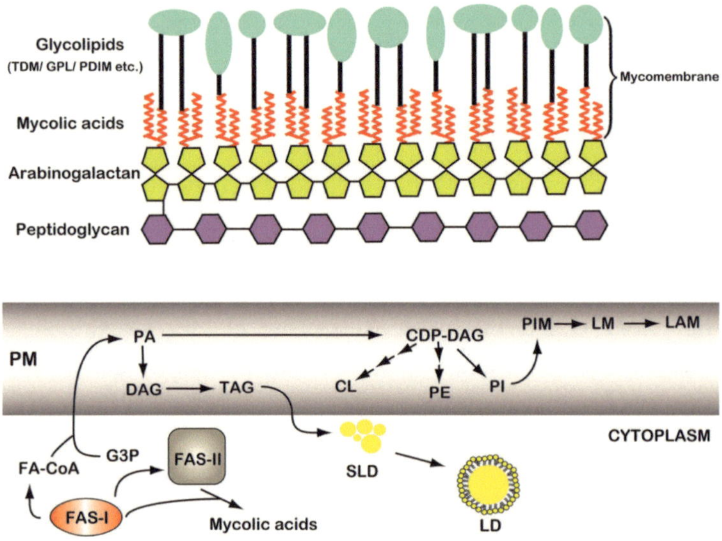

Figure 1. Mycobacterial plasma membrane and cell wall with flow of key metabolic pathways. Some of the metabolites are exported to the mycomembrane. SLD, small lipid droplet; LD, lipid droplet; FA-CoA, fatty acyl-CoA. See text for other abbreviations used in the figure.

Studies on mycobacteria and corynebacteria provide a unique opportunity to illustrate the complexity and diversity of lipid metabolic pathways in bacteria. They have a significantly higher lipid content than other bacteria with cell wall lipids comprising ~40% of the dry cell mass. *M. tuberculosis* produces a diversity of lipids unparalleled in bacteria, from simple fatty acids to highly complex long chain structures such as mycolic acids. It has devoted a significant proportion of its coding capacity to lipid metabolism and produces about 250 enzymes dedicated to fatty acid metabolism, which is around five times the number produced by *Escherichia coli* [5]. Lipid biosynthesis places a significant metabolic burden on the organism but is ultimately advantageous, allowing *M. tuberculosis* to survive and replicate in the inhospitable environment of host macrophages. While capable of *de novo* synthesis, these bacteria also scavenge and degrade host cell membrane lipids to acetyl-CoA, via broad families of β-oxidation and other catabolic enzymes, for incorporation into their own metabolic pathways and to fuel cellular processes.

The plasma membrane provides the platform for lipid metabolism. While some lipid metabolic reactions take place in the cytoplasm or cell wall, the plasma membrane is the pivotal site for the metabolism of lipids. At the same time, this membrane must perform many other functions associated with energy production, nutrient uptake, protein export, and various sensing/signaling reactions. Studies on how these metabolic and cellular processes might be organized within bacterial plasma membranes are in their infancy. Understanding the homeostasis of the plasma membrane is particularly important in Corynebacterineae organisms because this structure must support the high biosynthetic demands of sustaining such a lipid-rich cell wall. In this chapter, we focus our discussion on processes of lipid metabolism that are critical for the biogenesis and maintenance of the plasma membrane, and illustrate the recent progress on our understanding of plasma membrane biogenesis in mycobacteria and corynebacteria.

2. Functions of plasma membrane lipids in mycobacteria and corynebacteria

In this section we will describe the functions of plasma membrane lipids. First, we will describe the functions of major structural phospholipids. We will then describe quantitatively minor lipids, which have important metabolic/physiological functions. Lastly, we will discuss the functions of neutral lipids because their biosynthesis is closely linked to phospholipid metabolism and neutral lipid storage is a critical part of plasma membrane homeostasis.

2.1. Structural lipids

Major structural components of the mycobacterial plasma membrane are phospholipids such as cardiolipin (CL), phosphatidylethanolamine (PE), phosphatidylinositol (PI), and glycosylated PIs (*i.e.* phosphatidylinositol mannosides (PIM), lipomannans (LM) and lipoarabinomannans (LAM), see below). The ratio of these phospholipids may vary depending on the species and growth conditions [6-8]. For example, one study indicated that CL, PE, and PI/PIMs represent about 37, 32, and 28%, respectively, of the total phospholipids in the plasma membrane in *M. smegmatis* [9], while another reported the ratio in *Mycobacterium phlei* to be about 50, 10, and 40% [10]. Phosphatidylglycerol (PG), which is abundant in other bacteria, is a relatively minor species in mycobacteria. Deletion of the PI biosynthetic gene has been shown to be lethal in *M. smegmatis* [9], indicating that PI or glycosylated PIs are essential for mycobacterial viability. In *M. tuberculosis*, putative PI synthetase (*Rv2612c*) and PGP synthetase (*Rv2746c*, involved in CL synthesis) genes are predicted to be essential [11], while the PS synthetase gene (*Rv0436c*, involved in PE synthesis) is not [12]. In corynebacteria, major species of phospholipids are PI, PG, CL, and acylphosphatidylglycerol (APG) [13], and PE appears to be absent.

CL is widely found in both prokaryotes and eukaryotes. It forms aggregates within the membrane bilayer. Nonyl acridine orange (NAO) is a fluorescent dye which is proposed to bind the hydrophobic surface created by the CL cluster [14], allowing microscopic visualization of CL domains. Indeed, using NAO, CLs were found to be enriched in septa and poles of actively dividing *M. tuberculosis* and *M. smegmatis* cells [15, 16]. CL has a non-bilayer structure [17, 18], and carries a small partially immobilized head group that is more exposed to the aqueous environment than those of other glycerophospholipids [19]. Although the physiological function of CL is unclear, its physical properties may indicate that it provides a platform for membrane-protein interactions. Indeed, some mycobacterial enzymes require CL for activity [20-22], although the molecular basis for these observations has not been clarified. Recent fractionation studies in *C. glutamicum* revealed that CL (as well as other phospholipids) is enriched in the plasma membrane [23, 24]. However, a large proportion of CL is also found to be associated with the outer membrane [24], suggesting that some of these phospholipids are exported to the outer membrane in corynebacteria. Similarly, CL is released from *M. bovis* bacillus Calmette-Guerin residing in host phagosomes, and converted to lyso-CL by a host phospholipase A_2 [25]. It has been suggested that lyso-CL may influence host immune responses during infection.

PE is another major class of glycerophospholipids in mycobacteria. Although PE is generally found in all organisms, it is particularly abundant in bacterial plasma membranes [26]. Mycobacteria are no exception [20], but corynebacteria apparently lack the capacity to synthesize PE [27]. Indeed, PE biosynthetic enzymes, such as PS synthetase and PS decarboxylase, appear to be absent in corynebacterial genomes. *Corynebacterium aquaticum* has been reported to possess PE [28], but this species was later reclassified as *Leifsonia aquatica* [29], which belongs to the suborder Micrococcineae of the order Actinomycetales. The functions of PE remain elusive at the molecular level, but it appears to play important roles as a component of the plasma membrane. For example, TBsmr, a small multidrug resistance family protein from *M. tuberculosis*, shows enhanced catalytic activities when PE is supplemented in a reconstituted liposome [30].

PIs are an important class of phospholipids, and are known to be further modified by extensive glycosylation. The resultant lipoglycans, termed PIMs, LM, and LAM, are essential structural components of mycobacterial and corynebacterial cell walls. Furthermore, in pathogenic species, they have been suggested to perform additional roles in the modulation of host immune responses in favor of the pathogen through myriad effects on macrophages including cytokine production, inhibition of phagosome maturation and apoptosis [31-34]. PIMs are oligo-mannosylated PIs carrying up to 6 mannose residues while LM/LAM carry much longer mannose polymers with arabinan modifications. It remains controversial if these glycolipids are embedded in the plasma membrane or exported to the outer membrane. A recent study suggests that LM/LAM appear to be anchored to both the plasma membrane and outer membrane [35]. In *C. glutamicum*, the outer membrane and plasma membrane were fractionated on sucrose gradients upon cell lysis, and the analysis of these membrane sub-fractions demonstrated that PIMs, LM and LAM are all enriched in the plasma membrane fraction [23]. Another recent study also suggested that PI/PIMs are major components of the plasma membrane of *C. glutamicum* [24]. In the latter study, however, substantial amounts of PI/PIMs were detected in the outer membrane as well. The functional significance of these subcellular localizations, as well as the physiological roles of LM/LAM in each of these locations, remain important questions. The structural importance of PIMs remains unclear as well. For example, a *pimE*-deletion mutant that cannot produce mature

PIM6 species (see below) is viable, but shows severe plasma membrane abnormalities [36], suggesting that higher order PIMs may be involved in the maintenance of plasma membrane integrity.

It is notable that some unusual phospholipids have been identified in corynebacteria. APG is an acylated form of PG which is widespread in corynebacteria [37-40], and is a major phospholipid species in *Corynebacterium amycolatum*. Another interesting phospholipid from *C. amycolatum* is acyl-phosphatidylinositol (API), which was identified by electrospray ionization mass spectroscopy [41]. *C. amycolatum* lacks a mycolic acid-based outer membrane, and does not appear to have a fracture plane other than the plasma membrane [42]. Therefore, APG and API are likely to be components of the plasma membrane, and are suggested to play structural roles. Very little is known about their biosynthesis, and acyltransferases responsible for their synthesis remain to be identified for both lipid species.

2.2. Functional lipids

There are some examples of lipids that appear to play no structural roles in the plasma membrane. They often exist in low quantities but play important functional roles. Among these, polyprenol-phospho-sugars function as sugar donors. Two well-studied examples are polyprenol phosphomannose (PPM) and decaprenol phosphoarabinose (DPA). These molecules are the donors of mannose and arabinose, respectively, and their biosynthesis will be discussed in a later section.

PI 3-phosphate, recently identified in both *M. smegmatis* and *C. glutamicum* [43], may prove to be another interesting example of a functional lipid. It accumulates only transiently upon stimulation by high concentrations of salt, and behaves as if it is involved in a signaling cascade. However, whether PI 3-phosphate represents a mediator of stress responses remains to be addressed. More recently, lysinylated PG was identified as a minor phospholipid species in *M. tuberculosis* [44]. The synthesis of lysinylated PG is mediated by LysX and a *lysX* deletion mutant showed altered phospholipid metabolism and membrane integrity [16, 44], suggesting a regulatory role of lysinylated PG in plasma membrane homeostasis.

Carotenoids are photo-protective pigments and serve to scavenge free radicals or harvest light [45]. Several mycobacterial species are known to produce carotenoids with the notable exception of *M. tuberculosis*, despite the presence of a carotenoid oxidase in the human pathogen [46]. These hydrophobic pigments are thought to be present in the plasma membrane but whether they play structural roles in addition to a photo-protective role remains to be elucidated.

2.3. Lipid storage for energy and carbon

Neutral lipids are an important reservoir of stored energy and carbon, and their metabolism is closely linked to plasma membrane phospholipid metabolism. Unlike many other bacteria which use polyhydroxyalkanoates as a lipid storage material [47], Actinobacteria use triacylglycerides (TAGs) as a major form of lipid storage, and the presence of TAGs has been reported in *Mycobacterium, Streptomyces, Rhodococcus* and *Nocardia* [48-52]. Interestingly, corynebacteria seem to lack the capacity to synthesize TAG, indicating that some lineages of Actinobacteria have eliminated this capacity at some point in their evolution. Recent evidence suggests that *M. tuberculosis* accumulates TAG-based lipid droplets while residing in macrophages using fatty acids released from host TAGs, and this process is critical for acquiring a dormancy phenotype [53]. Nevertheless, a mutant defective in accumulating TAG remained viable under *in vitro* dormancy-inducing conditions [54]. These somewhat contradictory observations suggest that our understanding of TAG metabolism in mycobacteria is far from complete. As we illustrate later, there appear to be several redundant genes involved in the final step of TAG synthesis, suggesting that it is an important regulatory step of lipid metabolism in these bacteria.

Cholesterol has recently been suggested to be an alternative form of lipid storage in mycobacteria. Neither mycobacteria nor corynebacteria have the capacity to synthesize cholesterol. However, cholesterol is taken up by *M. tuberculosis* cells residing in the host, and components of the *mce4* operon have been shown to be involved in cholesterol import [55]. Cholesterol catabolism is critical in the chronic phase of animal infection, and a fully functional catabolic pathway is encoded by the *M. tuberculosis* genome [56]. Furthermore, cholesterol appears to accumulate in the mycobacterial cell envelope, and this might represent a potential form of lipid storage for *M. tuberculosis* during animal infection [57, 58]. Although the authors of this study suggested that cholesterol accumulates in the outer membrane, it remains possible that the plasma membrane is the true site of accumulation. Therefore, in addition to acting as a lipid storage molecule, cholesterol may play roles in plasma membrane structure and function, and these possibilities await further exploration.

Catabolism of cholesterol, amino acids and odd-chain-length/methyl branched fatty acids produces propionyl-coenzyme A (CoA). Propionate accumulation has been shown to be toxic in various organisms [59-61], and *M. tuberculosis* has multiple pathways to metabolize propionyl-CoA [62]. Metabolized propionyl-CoA is in part incorporated into TAG [63], and it has been suggested that TAG functions as a sink for reducing equivalents in addition to being a source of carbon and energy.

3. Structure and metabolism of plasma membrane lipids in mycobacteria and corynebacteria

In this section, we will describe the structure and metabolism of various lipids found in the plasma membrane of mycobacteria and corynebacteria in more detail. Lipids are categorized into the following four classes based on their key structural features.

3.1. Fatty acids

M. tuberculosis devotes a large proportion of its coding capacity to genes involved in fatty acid metabolism [5], highlighting the importance of lipids to the organism. Fatty acid metabolism is essential for intracellular survival of the pathogen since it forms the precursors of key membrane components such as plasma membrane phospholipids and outer membrane glycolipids. In particular, mycolic acids, which are very long chain α-alkyl β-hydroxy fatty acids, form the hydrophobic, protective mycomembrane described earlier. *M. tuberculosis* encodes two distinct enzyme systems for biosynthesis of fatty acids, designated FAS (fatty acid synthase) I and II (Fig. 2). Studies on fatty acid synthesis date back to the 1970s when *M. smegmatis* was shown to contain both type I fatty acid synthetase (FAS-I), involving a large multifunctional polypeptide, and type II fatty acid synthetase (FAS-II), consisting of a series of distinct enzymes [64]. The key elongation unit is malonyl-CoA, which is produced by acetyl-CoA carboxylase (ACCase) and the *M. tuberculosis* genome encodes several such enzymes (AccA1-3 and AccD1-6). The resultant malonyl-CoA is incorporated into fatty acids by the two FAS systems.

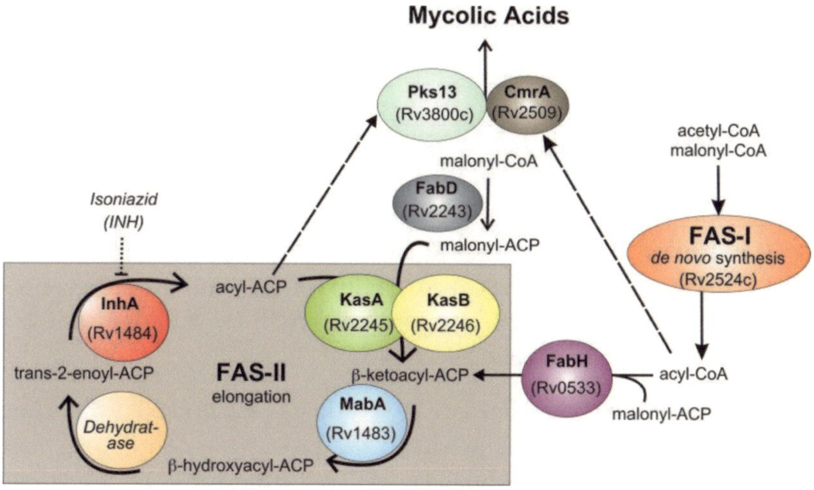

Figure 2. Fatty acid biosynthesis pathways in mycobacteria. Point of inhibition by the front-line tuberculosis drug isoniazid is indicated. Product profile of FAS-I is bimodal, and C_{16}-C_{18}-CoA and C_{24}-C_{26}-CoA are produced. Dashed lines indicate that some of the fatty acid products are further utilized for mycolic acid production.

3.1.1. *De novo synthesis by FAS-I*

Surprisingly, members of the Corynebacterineae use a eukaryote-like FAS-I system for *de novo* fatty acid synthesis. The single, essential [11], 9.2kb *fas* gene encodes a 326 kDa protein containing all seven domains necessary to perform the iterative series of reactions: acyl transferase, enoyl reductase, β-hydroxyacyl dehydratase, malonyl transferase, acyl carrier protein, β-ketoacyl reductase, and β-ketoacyl synthase [65, 66]. This very large protein elongates acetyl groups by 2-carbon (acetate) units using acetyl-CoA and malonyl-CoA. Early rounds of elongation yield C_{16} to C_{18}-CoA products that are used for synthesis of membrane phospholipids or to feed into the FAS-II system. More extensive elongation yields C_{24}-C_{26} products that ultimately form the α-branch of mycolic acids. Unlike *M. tuberculosis*, *C. glutamicum* encodes two *fas* genes (*fasA* and *fasB*) with FasA taking the dominant role [67]. The presence of two Fas proteins may compensate for the lack of a FAS-II system in this organism.

3.1.2. Elongation by FAS-II

The FAS-II system is commonly found in bacteria and plants and, unlike FAS-I, is composed of a series of separate enzymes, each performing one step in the pathway. FAS-II elongates medium chain fatty acids derived from FAS-I using malonyl-CoA, producing C_{18}-C_{30} fatty acids [68]. FAS-II has been extensively studied in *E. coli* [69] and orthologs of the *fab* genes have been identified in mycobacteria. AcpM is a mycobacterial acyl carrier protein (ACP) and plays a key role in transferring acyl groups between the various enzyme components [70]. The seven genes are located in two clusters on the *M. tuberculosis* chromosome [5], comprising *mtfabD-acpM-kasA-kasB-accD6* and *mabA-inhA*. Initially, the malonate group is transferred from malonyl-CoA to AcpM by the MtFabD protein. Then MtFabH performs a Claisen condensation of malonyl-ACP with acyl-CoA to form β–ketoacyl-ACP. A four-step cycle is then initiated [64] in which:

1. β–ketoacyl-ACP reductase MabA reduces the β–keto group with concomitant oxidation of NADPH
2. β-hydroxyacyl-ACP dehydratase dehydrates the β-hydroxyl to enoyl-ACP
3. enoyl-ACP reductase InhA, a target of the first-line anti-tuberculosis drug isoniazid (INH) [71], reduces enoyl-ACP to acyl-ACP with concomitant oxidation of NADPH
4. β-ketoacyl-ACP synthase KasA/B elongates acyl-ACP by 2 carbon units, forming β-ketoacyl-ACP, which can feed back into step 1.

In this way, the hydrocarbon chain increases by 2 carbons each cycle. Further elongation and processing of the products of FAS-II produces the precursors of the long meromycolate chains that are condensed with the α-branches derived from FAS-I by the large polyketide synthase Pks13 [72]. Reduction of the β–keto group by CmrA forms the mature C_{60}-C_{90} mycolic acid [73].

3.2. Glycerolipids

Glycerolipids include both nonpolar lipids and polar phospholipids. Their biosynthesis is overlapping and 1,2-diacyl-*sn*-glycerol 3-phosphate, commonly known as phosphatidic acid (PA), is an important intermediate at the branch point (Fig. 3) [74]. In this section, we focus our discussion on the biosynthesis of PA and its conversion to non-polar lipids. Non-polar lipids are generally divided into three different classes depending on the number of fatty acids attached to glycerol: monoacylglycerol (MAG), diacylglycerol (DAG) and TAG. TAG is a glycerol carrying three fatty acyl chains, and its biosynthesis diverges from phospholipid synthesis after the synthesis of PA. TAG is a major component of lipid droplets, which accumulate in the cytoplasm. How TAG is made in the plasma membrane and incorporated into lipid droplets remains largely unclear. Here, we provide an overview of the TAG metabolic pathway.

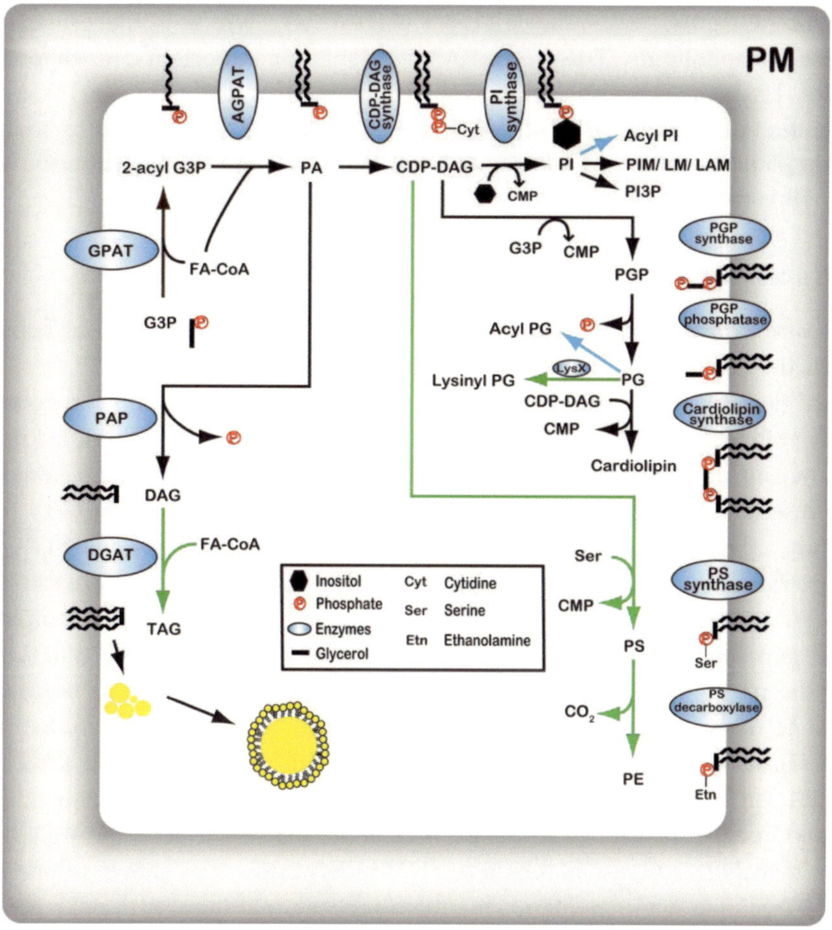

Figure 3. Glycerolipid/phospholipid biosynthesis pathways. Some pathways such as TAG and PE biosynthesis (shown as green arrows) do not occur in corynebacteria while some others (shown as blue arrows) are known to occur only in corynebacteria. PG is abundant in corynebacteria, but is a minor species in mycobacteria.

3.2.1. Biosynthesis of PA

The first step of PA biosynthesis is mediated by glycerol phosphate acyltransferase (GPAT) transferring an acyl chain from acyl-CoA to glycerol-3-phosphate, forming acyl-glycerol 3-phosphate. In general, this reaction produces 1-acyl-*sn*-glycerol 3-phosphate. However, mycobacteria are unusual in that 2-acyl-*sn*-glycerol 3-phosphate is used as the main intermediate for the production of PA [75]. Another unusual feature is that oleic acid, an unsaturated fatty acid often found at the *sn*-2 positions of glycerolipids, is found at the *sn*-1 position in mycobacteria. Instead, palmitic acid, a saturated fatty acid, is the preferred fatty acid attached to the *sn*-2 position in mycobacteria [75, 76]. In the second step, acylglycerol phosphate acyltransferase (AGPAT) further transfers a fatty acid from acyl-CoA to 2-acyl-*sn*-glycerol 3-phosphate, producing PA. PA can be diverted to TAG synthesis, or activated to form cytidine diphosphate-diacylglycerol (CDP-DAG), which is the precursor for the synthesis of phospholipids. Therefore, PA represents an important branch point for the synthesis of TAG and phospholipids [74]. An alternative pathway for PA synthesis is phosphorylation of DAG by DAG kinase, and Rv2252 has been suggested to be involved in this reaction [77]. Disruption of this enzyme results in altered PIM biosynthesis, but precise functions of this metabolic pathway remain unclear.

3.2.2. TAG Biosynthesis

TAG is *de novo* synthesized by two steps. First, PA is dephosphorylated to become DAG, and this reaction is mediated by phosphatidic acid phosphatase (PAP). PAP was discovered from animal tissues in 1957 by the group of Eugene Kennedy [78], and the gene encoding this activity was recently identified in *Saccharomyces cerevisiae* [79]. Nothing is known about this enzyme in mycobacteria or corynebacteria. In the second step, diacylglycerol acyltransferase (DGAT) catalyzes the addition of a fatty acyl-CoA to DAG to form TAG. Until recently, little was known about the genes involved in this final step of TAG synthesis in mycobacteria. Analysis of this final step is complicated because there are multiple genes encoding TAG synthetase in mycobacteria and corynebacteria. For example, the *M. tuberculosis* genome encodes 15 putative TAG synthetase genes [48, 80]. Despite the redundancies, recent studies reported that some of these *tgs* genes are critical for TAG synthesis in *M. tuberculosis* [48, 54]. Specifically, TAG synthetases encoded by *Rv3130c* (*tgs1*), *Rv3734c* (*tgs2*), *Rv3234c* (*tgs3*), and *Rv3088* (*tgs4*) have been shown to have TAG synthetase activities [53]. Furthermore, Tgs1 has been demonstrated to be the main contributor to TAG synthesis and lipid droplet formation in *M. tuberculosis* [53]. More recently, Ag85A, which is known as a mycolyltransferase involved in TDM biosynthesis, was shown to possess DGAT activity [81]. Ag85A is not homologous to other *tgs* genes, and may represent a novel class of TAG biosynthetic enzymes. TAG not only forms a lipid droplet in the cytoplasm, but also accumulates in the cell wall of mycobacteria [82]. Therefore, Ag85A located in the cell wall might be involved in the production of surface-exposed TAGs.

3.2.3. Utilization of TAG

Under starvation conditions where stored TAG needs to be mobilized for energy production, TAG is catabolized by lipases. In 1977, TAG lipase was purified from stationary phase *M. phlei* and predicted to have a molecular weight of about 40 kDa [83]. More recently, LipY, encoded by the *M. tuberculosis Rv3097c* gene, was identified as a TAG lipase [84]. LipY appears to play a critical role in TAG catabolism because a *M. tuberculosis lipY* deletion mutant cannot utilize accumulated TAG under starvation conditions. Another recent study demonstrated that LipY has a dual localization pattern [85]: while a fraction of LipY was found in the cytoplasm, consistent with its role in the catabolism of intracellular TAG, a significant fraction of LipY was also localized to the outer membrane of the cell wall, indicating that it may be involved in the breakdown of exogenously available TAGs. Indeed, it has been long known that *M. tuberculosis* depends on fatty acids as a preferred energy source during infection [86], and LipY may well be a critical enzyme for the utilization of host lipids during an *M. tuberculosis* infection. Another lipase encoded by *Rv0183* shows preference for MAG over DAG and TAG, and is localized to the cell wall [87], suggesting its involvement in subsequent reactions of TAG breakdown. However, whether it is involved in degradation of host-derived TAG or intracellular TAG remains to be determined.

3.2.4. Lipid droplet formation

In eukaryotes, lipid droplets form in between the two leaflets of the endoplasmic reticulum membrane [88]. In bacteria, a distinct mechanism of lipid body formation has been proposed. For example, in rhodococci, TAG is formed in the cytoplasmic surface of the plasma membrane. Small lipid droplets are then fused to each other, coated by a monolayer of phospholipids, and released from the surface of the plasma membrane into the cytoplasm as mature lipid droplets [89]. Although no endogenous proteins have been found to associate with lipid droplets in rhodococci or mycobacteria, heterologous expression of known lipid droplet-associated proteins resulted in correct targeting of these proteins to lipid droplets in both *R. opacus* and *M. smegmatis* [90, 91], allowing visualization of lipid droplets in these organisms.

3.3. Phospholipids

3.3.1. CDP-DAG

In both eukaryotic and prokaryotic cells, PA is activated by CTP to form CDP-DAG, and this reaction is mediated by CDP-DAG synthase [92]. The synthesis of CDP-DAG commits the pathway to phospholipid biosynthesis, and CDP-DAG is a common precursor for the biosynthesis of all glycerophospholipids in mycobacteria and corynebacteria. The activity of CDP-DAG synthetase is associated with plasma membrane in *M. smegmatis*, and is possibly encoded by the *cdsA* (*Rv2881c*) gene in *M. tuberculosis* H37Rv [93].

3.3.2. CL

CL is composed of four acyl chains, three glycerols and two phosphates, and is structured in a 1,3-diphosphatidylglycerol configuration [94]. It is a common phospholipid in bacteria, and is one of the abundant phospholipids in mycobacteria and corynebacteria. To initiate CL synthesis, PG phosphate synthase first produces PG phosphate (PGP) using CDP-DAG and glycerol 3-phosphate as substrates. An *M. smegmatis* strain engineered to overexpress *M. tuberculosis* PgsA3 (encoded by *Rv2746c*) was shown to overproduce PG, suggesting that PgsA3 is the PGP synthase [9]. PGP is then converted into PG via PGP phosphatase. Three phosphatases, PgpA, PgpB, and PgpC, have been identified as PGP phosphatases in *E. coli* [95-97]. Furthermore, Gep4 and PTPMT1 have been identified as PGP phosphatases in yeast and mammals, respectively [98, 99]. Some homologs exist in the genomes of mycobacteria and corynebacteria, but experimental verification of these genes remains to be performed.

Typically, the final step of CL synthesis in prokaryotes is mediated by a reaction that utilizes two PG molecules, producing one molecule of CL and one molecule of glycerol. However, in mycobacteria, the eukaryote-like reaction, which utilizes PG and CDP-DAG to produce CL, has been shown to occur [100], and Jackson and colleagues have suggested that PgsA2 might be the enzyme responsible for this reaction [9].

3.3.3. PE

The precise structure of PE was recently reported as 1-*O*-tuberculostearoyl-2-*O*-palmitoyl-*sn*-glycero-3-phosphoethanolamine in *M. tuberculosis* using tandem mass spectrometry [101]. In the initial step of PE synthesis, PS synthetase transfers serine to CDP-DAG and produces PS. In the second step, PE is produced by decarboxylation of PS mediated by PS decarboxylase. Genes encoding putative PS synthetase (*pssA, Rv0436c*) and PS decarboxylase (*psd, Rv0437c*) are found in tandem in the *M. tuberculosis* genome [9]. However, there is no experimental evidence demonstrating the identities of the genes. In *M. smegmatis*, PS synthetase and PS decarboxylase activities are enriched in different membrane fractions, which can be distinguished by sucrose gradient sedimentation [102]. However, the significance of differential membrane localization remains to be clarified.

3.3.4. PI

PI is a major phospholipid in both mycobacteria and corynebacteria and forms the anchor for the PIMs, which are substrates for heavy mannosylation to form LMs and additional arabinosylation to produce LAMs. PI is formed by the PI synthase PgsA (Rv2612c) from CDP-DAG and *myo*-inositol [9, 103]. Inositol is not a common metabolite in bacteria. It is therefore surprising that mycobacteria produce copious amounts of inositol through pathways shared with eukaryotes for incorporation into a range of metabolic pathways (recently reviewed in [104]). The enzyme D-*myo*-inositol 3-phosphate synthase (Ino1) converts glucose-6-phosphate to D-*myo*-inositol 3-phosphate, which is dephosphorylated by one of several inositol monophosphatases to produce *myo*-inositol [105].

3.3.5. PIMs

All Corynebacterineae synthesize PIMs that are important components of the cell envelope. Polar PIM species can also serve as membrane anchors for LM and LAM. Many of the steps of PIM/LM/LAM biosynthesis have now been elucidated [106]. Extensive genetic and biochemical studies have demonstrated that the synthesis of PIMs occurs linearly in mycobacteria with PI as the starting substrate (reviewed in [107]) (Fig. 4A). Early steps of the pathway occur on the cytoplasmic face of the plasma membrane. A PIM biosynthetic membrane, enriched in the early steps, has been purified by sucrose gradient fractionation as a membrane subdomain termed PMf, which is distinct from the bulk plasma membrane [102]. Mannosyltransferases performing the early steps utilize the water-soluble mannose donor, GDP-Man, which can be produced from exogenously acquired mannose or via *de novo* synthesis from the glycolytic pathway when fructose-6-phosphate is transformed by the enzymes ManA (Rv3255c), ManB (Rv3257c) and ManC (Rv3264c) [108-111], with a degree of redundancy reported at the ManC (NCgl0710) step in *C. glutamicum* [112]. The first step of PIM synthesis involves mannosylation of the C2-position of the inositol ring of PI by the enzyme PimA (Rv2610c) to form PIM1 [113, 114]. PimA is an essential enzyme in mycobacteria [11, 113] and absent in humans, making it a current target for drug development by several groups. The crystal structure of PimA from *M. smegmatis* has been solved in complex with GDP and GDP-Man at resolutions of 2.4Å and 2.6Å, respectively [115, 116]. PimA has a typical GT-B fold of glycosyltransferases consisting of two Rossmann-fold domains with a deep fissure at the interface, which contains the active site. Close to the GDP-Man binding site, the *N*-terminal domain displays a deep pocket containing highly conserved hydrophobic residues. This pocket is proposed to bind the acyl moieties of the acceptor substrate PI [116].

Next, *O*-6 mannosylation of the *myo*-inositol ring is performed by the cytoplasmic α-mannosyltransferase PimB' (Rv2188c) [117, 118] resulting in the formation of PIM2. While the mycobacterial enzyme Rv0557 was originally assigned this function [119], later studies showed that Rv2188c was the true PimB (designated PimB') [118], with Rv0557 being renamed MgtA and included in the LM-B pathway [120, 121] (see below). PimB' is an essential enzyme in mycobacteria [11, 117] and the crystal structure of the equivalent corynebacterial enzyme has been solved at high resolution complexed with nucleotide [122]. In corynebacteria, PIM2 is detected mainly in its mono-acylated form, but in mycobacteria PIM2 accumulates in the cell envelope as monoacyl (AcPIM2) and diacyl (Ac_2PIM2) forms, the former produced by the acyltransferase Rv2611c [123] which acts optimally on the product of the PimB' reaction [117].

The next enzyme in the pathway, PimC, has been identified in *M. tuberculosis* strain CDC1551 and could produce trimannosylated PIMs [124]. However, the absence of this enzyme in other strains indicates redundancy at this step and the enzymes involved remain to be identified, as does the putative "PimD" protein. Flipping of PIM intermediates from the cytoplasmic face of the membrane to the periplasm is thought to occur at this point of the pathway, but the precise intermediate and transporter involved are also undefined.

AcPIM4 species can be further mannosylated to form more polar PIMs in reactions thought to take place on the periplasmic side of the cytoplasmic membrane. These reactions are performed by glycosyltransferases that require a lipid sugar donor in the form of PPM, since these reactions are amphomycin-sensitive [36, 125-128]. In mycobacteria, AcPIM4 is proposed to be a branch point for synthesis of polar PIM end products and LM/LAM. PimE (Rv1159) has been shown to elongate AcPIM4 with one or more α1-2 linked mannoses to form AcPIM6 [36]. This polytopic membrane protein has sequence similarities with eukaryotic PIG-M mannosyltransferases and localizes to a cell wall-associated plasma membrane subdomain in *M. smegmatis*, termed PM-CW, to which enzymatic activities of AcPIM4-6 synthesis are enriched [102]. Its catalytic activity was successfully mapped to a conserved aspartate residue in the first outer loop of the protein. Whether PimE also forms AcPIM6 is unknown. Interestingly, no PimE orthologue is present in *C. glutamicum* and

Ac/Ac2PIM6 do not accumulate in this species, so the formation of Ac/Ac2PIM5/6 appears to be a mycobacterium-specific side-branch of the pathway.

Surprisingly, studies in *M. smegmatis* have revealed a role for a lipoprotein in PIM/LAM synthesis, since *lpqW* mutants produce reduced levels of LM/LAM [129]. As the only non-enzymatic component of the pathway identified to date, LpqW has been proposed to have a regulatory role at the bifurcation point of the pathways, as well as a functional connection with PimE, since mutations in the *pimE* gene can bypass the requirement for LpqW [130]. Very recent studies have implicated the corynebacterial ortholog of LpqW in the LM-B pathway as well (Rainczuk *et al*, submitted). Structural studies on the *M. smegmatis* LpqW revealed a scaffold similar to substrate binding proteins associated with ABC transporters, which has evolved to fulfill a new role in the regulation of PIM/LAM biosynthesis [131].

3.3.6. LM/LAM

A subpopulation of PIMs (AcPIM4 in mycobacteria [128, 129, 132] and AcPIM2 in corynebacteria [133]) can be extended with chains of α1-6 linked mannose to form LM that is further modified with a number of single α1-2 mannose side chains [134-136]. MptB is a PPM-dependent mannosyltransferase involved in extending AcPIM2 to form the proximal α1-6 mannan backbone of LM in *C. glutamicum* but is redundant in *M. smegmatis* [133], indicating additional complexity at this step in mycobacteria. Further elongation is performed by MptA (Rv2174) [135, 136], with MptC (Rv2181) required for addition of α1-2 linked Man side chains [106, 134, 137, 138]. Further additions of arabinose units by EmbC (Rv3793), AftC (Rv2673), AftD (Rv0236c) and at present unidentified α1-5 arabinofuranosyltransferases, result in the formation of mature LAM [139-142]. In *M. tuberculosis* and other pathogenic mycobacteria, additional mannose capping is present [143], synthesized by the enzymes MptC [137] and Rv1635c [144]. Alternatively, *M. smegmatis* LAM is capped with inositol phosphate [145].

While the general PI→PIM→LM→LAM pathway is conserved in corynebacteria, a second pathway of lipoglycan biosynthesis exists in which a sub-population of LM lipoglycans is assembled on a glucopyranosyluronic acid diacylglycerol (Gl-A, GlcADAG) glycolipid anchor [118, 121, 133]. In this pathway (Fig. 4B), Gl-A is first mannosylated by MgtA (NCgl0452 in *C. glutamicum* and previously termed PimB, see above) forming mannosyl-glucuronic acid diacylglycerol (Gl-X, ManGlcADAG), which is subjected to further α1-6 (backbone) and α1-2 (side unit) mannosylation resulting in LM [121]. This pathway shares some PPM-dependent enzymes with the PI-based LM pathway including MptB, since an *mptB* (*NCgl1505*) mutant of *C. glutamicum* fails to produce intermediates beyond Gl-X or AcPIM2 [133]. For clarity, the PI-based LM pool has been designated LM-A while this second pathway produces LM-B [121, 146], the major LM pool in *C. glutamicum* [118]. While *C. glutamicum* produces LAMs via LM-A using a similar pathway to mycobacteria, its LAMs are smaller and structurally distinct, with more extensive mannosylation and singular Ara*f* capping [147].

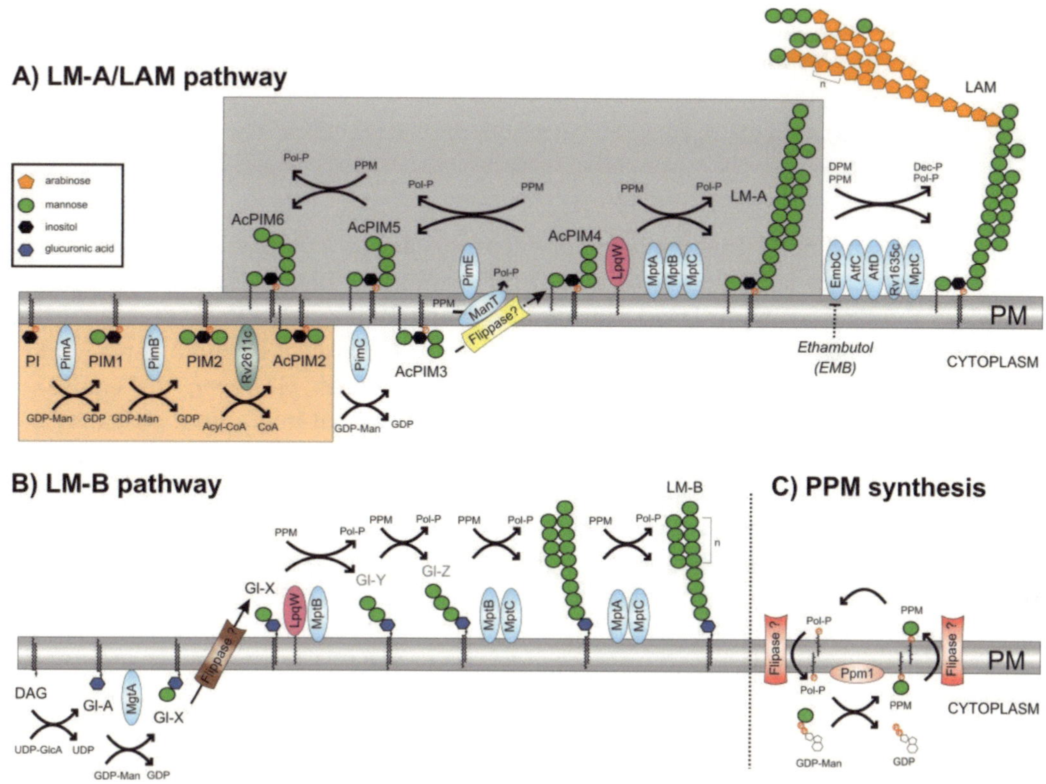

Figure 4. **Summary of Lipoglycan Biosynthesis Pathways in Corynebacterineae.** A) The mycobacterial pathway and structures for LM-A/LAM are shown, although several steps are inferred from studies in *C. glutamicum*. A progression from PIM1 to AcPIM2 via AcPIM1 can also occur but is sub-optimal in mycobacteria. AcPIM3 is shown as the substrate for the unidentified flippase but AcPIM2 may be the preferred substrate: AcPIM2 appears to be the flipped intermediate in *C. glutamicum*. Reactions associated with the PMf and PM-CW subfractions of *M. smegmatis* are shaded orange and grey, respectively. B) LM-B pathway in *C. glutamicum*. Its presence in mycobacteria remains to be determined. Intermediates representing Gl-Y and Gl-Z have been detected in very recent studies (Rainczuk et al, submitted). C) PPM serves as the lipid-linked donor of mannose for both pathways. The mechanism of flipping is undetermined. PM, plasma membrane. Other abbreviations are as defined in the text.

3.4. Prenol lipids

Polyprenol phosphate (Pol-P) is a key carrier lipid in synthesis of the core structures of the mycobacterial cell wall, including peptidoglycan and arabinogalactan. Unlike most bacteria, mycobacteria contain multiple types of Pol-P. For example, *M. smegmatis* produces decaprenol phosphate (C_{50}, Dec-P, [148]) and heptaprenol phosphate (C_{35}, Hep-P, [149]). Polyprenols are thought to be synthesized via the condensation of two C_5 lipids, isopentenyl diphosphate [150-152] and dimethylallyl diphosphate derived from the mevalonate-independent methylerythritol 4-phosphate (MEP) pathway. These reactions are catalyzed by prenol diphosphate synthases and two *M. tuberculosis* proteins, Rv2361c and Rv1086, acting sequentially, are thought to fulfill this role [148, 149, 153-155]. Finally, the C_{50} decaprenol diphosphate is dephosphorylated to produce Dec-P by an unknown phosphatase.

3.4.1. Polyprenol-phospho-sugars

3.4.1.1. PPM

PPM, a β-D-mannosyl-1-monophosphoryldecaprenol, is utilized by periplasmic mannosyltransferases for synthesis of polar PIM species and LMs [106]. C_{35}/C_{50}-P-Man*p* is formed by the PPM synthase Ppm1 (Rv2051c) from GDP-Man*p* and Pol-P [126, 127] (Fig. 4C). In *M. tuberculosis* Ppm1 consists of two domains: a C-terminal catalytic domain and a N-terminal membrane anchor with 6 transmembrane helices. However, the equivalent domains of the *M. smegmatis* PPM synthase are two distinct, but interacting, proteins [156]. The importance of PPM in cell wall synthesis has been highlighted by analysis of a *ppm1* mutant in *C. glutamicum* that failed to produce PPM, resulting in severe defects in lipoglycan biosynthesis. While the mutant could synthesize PIM2 species, all downstream products (LM, LAM) were absent, indicating their reliance on the PPM donor [127]. These findings were consistent with others showing that amphomycin, an antibiotic specific for PPM-dependent polymerases, blocked the PIM pathway at the PIM2 or PIM3 stage [125, 128]. The product of the *Rv3779* gene has also been implicated in PPM synthesis but its role remains unclear [157, 158].

3.4.1.2. DPA

DPA is the only known donor of arabinose (Ara) for mycobacterial cell wall synthesis, contributing Ara*f* units to arabinogalactan and LAM [106] with concomitant release of Pol-P. The Ara*f* portion is derived from the pentose-phosphate pathway [159-161]. 5-phosphoribose 1-diphosphate is transferred to Dec-P by the *Rv3806c* gene product [162] and the resultant Dec-P-β-D-5-phosphoribose is dephosphorylated to form Dec-P-β-D-ribose. Oxidation of the 2′ hydroxyl is followed by a reduction reaction to form DPA. This two-step epimerization reaction is catalyzed by the combined activities of DprE1 (Rv3790) and DprE2 (Rv3791) [163]. Since DPA is the sole donor of Ara*f* residues for mycobacterial cell wall synthesis, this pathway is of interest for drug development. Indeed, DprE1 is the target of dinitrobenzamide derivatives (DNBs) [164] and a set of nitro-compounds related to DNBs, the nitro-benzothiazinones (BTZ), a class of compounds with nanomolar anti-*M. tuberculosis* activities but minimal host-cell toxicity [165-167]. The essential nature of DprE1 in species beyond *M. tuberculosis* [168] reinforces it as a "magic" drug target [169]. The crystal structure of *M. tuberculosis* DprE1 complexed with BTZ inhibitors has been reported very recently, revealing the mode of inhibitor binding [170].

3.4.2. Carotenoids

Carotenoids are isoprenoid pigments widely distributed in biology and mostly based on C_{40}-polyene. Synthesis of these pigments has been poorly studied in mycobacteria but they have proven useful for taxonomic and identification purposes. Mycobacterial pigments are generally yellow or orange and most have been confirmed as carotenoids [171]. While carotenoid genetics has been best studied in plants, the key enzymes of the pathway have been identified in bacteria, including mycobacteria [172-174]. There are two classes of carotenoids in bacteria, carotenes and xanthophylls, the latter of which contain oxygen. Both classes are composed of eight isoprenoid units with a long central chain of double bonded carbons. A consensus pathway for carotenoid biosynthesis in bacteria has been elucidated with orthologues of key enzymes identified in several species of mycobacteria [175]. As described above for prenol lipids, the carotenoid pathway begins with isopentenyl diphosphate and dimethylallyl diphosphate derived from the MEP pathway [176]. Head-to-tail condensation of these terpenes produces geranylgeranyl pyrophosphate (GGPP) due to the activity of GGPP synthase (CrtE). Condensation of two GGPP molecules [177] is followed by desaturation to phytoene by phytoene synthase (CrtB). Phytoene desaturase (CrtI) converts phytoene to lycoprene followed by cyclization to β-carotene by lycoprene cyclase (CrtY) [178].

4. Concluding remarks

Lipid metabolism in mycobacteria and corynebacteria is a highly complex network of catabolic and anabolic reactions. While the metabolic pathways and many of the enzymes involved have been actively elucidated over the past decade, substantial efforts are still needed to draw a comprehensive map of lipid metabolism in these organisms. In particular, our understanding of regulatory mechanisms of lipid metabolism is currently at an early stage. In addition, there are very few studies describing the interactions between multiple metabolic pathways of lipid biosynthesis. One promising approach for the comprehensive understanding of lipid metabolism is lipidomics, which is the study of lipid biosynthetic and catabolic pathways at a global level [179]. In the past, metabolic pathways have generally been examined in isolation without consideration of how different pathways might interact with, and influence, one another. Since the plasma membrane is a shared platform for most lipid biosynthetic pathways, and some donors are shared between different pathways (see above), it seems unlikely that the various pathways are truly independent. Recent advances in mass spectrometry (*e.g.* MALDI-MS, ESI MS), nuclear magnetic resonance spectroscopy and associated computational methods have fuelled the development of this field [180]. Members of the Corynebacterineae, with their extensive lipid repertoires and complex metabolic pathways, would seem to be ideal targets to assess the true potential of lipidomics technologies. Recently, appropriate databases and methods for detection and identification of all major lipid classes of *M. tuberculosis* from a single crude extract have been developed [181, 182]. Very recently, a lipidomics profiling platform has been reported that uses high-performance liquid chromatography/mass spectrometry to resolve more than 12,000 molecules from *M. tuberculosis* [183]. These exciting advances provide a basis for future studies on the regulation of lipid metabolism and may allow, for the first time, a true appreciation of the interactive lipid networks of mycobacteria and corynebacteria.

Author details

Paul K. Crellin
Australian Research Council Centre of Excellence in Structural and Functional Microbial Genomics, Department of Microbiology, Monash University, Australia

Chu-Yuan Luo and Yasu S. Morita*
Department of Microbiology, University of Massachusetts, Amherst, USA

5. References

[1] 1. Hoffmann C, Leis A, Niederweis M, Plitzko JM, Engelhardt H. Disclosure of the mycobacterial outer membrane: cryo-electron tomography and vitreous sections reveal the lipid bilayer structure. Proc Natl Acad Sci U S A. 2008;105:3963-7.
[2] Zuber B, Chami M, Houssin C, Dubochet J, Griffiths G, Daffe M. Direct visualization of the outer membrane of mycobacteria and corynebacteria in their native state. J Bacteriol. 2008;190:5672-80.
[3] Barry CE, 3rd, Mdluli K. Drug sensitivity and environmental adaptation of mycobacterial cell wall components. Trends Microbiol. 1996;4:275-81.
[4] Daffe M, Draper P. The envelope layers of mycobacteria with reference to their pathogenicity. Adv Microb Physiol. 1998;39:131-203.
[5] Cole ST, Brosch R, Parkhill J, Garnier T, Churcher C, Harris D, et al. Deciphering the biology of *Mycobacterium tuberculosis* from the complete genome sequence. Nature. 1998;393:537-44.
[6] Nandedkar AK. Comparative study of the lipid composition of particular pathogenic and nonpathogenic species of *Mycobacterium*. J Natl Med Assoc. 1983;75:69-74.
[7] Subramoniam A, Subrahmanyam D. Light-induced changes in the phospholipid composition of *Mycobacterium smegmatis* ATCC 607. J Gen Microbiol. 1982;128:419-21.
[8] Khuller GK, Taneja R, Nath N. Effect of fatty acid supplementation on the lipid composition of *Mycobacterium smegmatis* ATCC 607, grown at 27 degrees and 37 degrees C. J Appl Bacteriol. 1983;54:63-8.
[9] Jackson M, Crick DC, Brennan PJ. Phosphatidylinositol is an essential phospholipid of mycobacteria. J Biol Chem. 2000;275:30092-9.
[10] Akamatsu Y, Nojima S. Separation and analyses of the individual phospholipids of mycobacteria. J Biochem. 1965;57:430-9.
[11] Sassetti CM, Boyd DH, Rubin EJ. Genes required for mycobacterial growth defined by high density mutagenesis. Mol Microbiol. 2003;48:77-84.
[12] Lamichhane G, Zignol M, Blades NJ, Geiman DE, Dougherty A, Grosset J, et al. A postgenomic method for predicting essential genes at subsaturation levels of mutagenesis: application to *Mycobacterium tuberculosis*. Proc Natl Acad Sci U S A. 2003;100:7213-8.

* Corresponding Author

[13] Yague G, Segovia M, Valero-Guillen PL. Phospholipid composition of several clinically relevant *Corynebacterium* species as determined by mass spectrometry: an unusual fatty acyl moiety is present in inositol-containing phospholipids of *Corynebacterium urealyticum*. Microbiology. 2003;149:1675-85.

[14] Mileykovskaya E, Dowhan W, Birke RL, Zheng D, Lutterodt L, Haines TH. Cardiolipin binds nonyl acridine orange by aggregating the dye at exposed hydrophobic domains on bilayer surfaces. FEBS Lett. 2001;507:187-90.

[15] Maloney E, Madiraju SC, Rajagopalan M, Madiraju M. Localization of acidic phospholipid cardiolipin and DnaA in mycobacteria. Tuberculosis (Edinb). 2011;91 Suppl 1:S150-5.

[16] Maloney E, Lun S, Stankowska D, Guo H, Rajagoapalan M, Bishai WR, et al. Alterations in phospholipid catabolism in *Mycobacterium tuberculosis* lysX mutant. Front Microbiol. 2011;2:19.

[17] Dahlberg M. Polymorphic phase behavior of cardiolipin derivatives studied by coarse-grained molecular dynamics. J Phys Chem B. 2007;111:7194-200.

[18] Powell GL, Marsh D. Polymorphic phase behavior of cardiolipin derivatives studied by 31P NMR and X-ray diffraction. Biochemistry. 1985;24:2902-8.

[19] Lewis RN, Zweytick D, Pabst G, Lohner K, McElhaney RN. Calorimetric, x-ray diffraction, and spectroscopic studies of the thermotropic phase behavior and organization of tetramyristoyl cardiolipin membranes. Biophys J. 2007;92:3166-77.

[20] Imai T, Kageyama Y, Tobari J. *Mycobacterium smegmatis* malate dehydrogenase: activation of the lipid-depleted enzyme by anionic phospholipids and phosphatidylethanolamine. Biochim Biophys Acta. 1995;1246:189-96.

[21] Kimura T, Tobari J. Participation of flavin-adenine dinucleotide in the activity of malate dehydrogenase from *Mycobacterium avium*. Biochim Biophys Acta. 1963;73:399-405.

[22] Tobari J. Requirement of flavin adenine dinucleotide and phospholipid for the activity of malate dehydrogenase from *Mycobacterium avium*. Biochem Biophys Res Commun. 1964;15:50-4.

[23] Marchand CH, Salmeron C, Bou Raad R, Meniche X, Chami M, Masi M, et al. Biochemical disclosure of the mycolate outer membrane of *Corynebacterium glutamicum*. J Bacteriol. 2012;194:587-97.

[24] Bansal-Mutalik R, Nikaido H. Quantitative lipid composition of cell envelopes of *Corynebacterium glutamicum* elucidated through reverse micelle extraction. Proc Natl Acad Sci U S A. 2011;108:15360-5.

[25] Fischer K, Chatterjee D, Torrelles J, Brennan PJ, Kaufmann SH, Schaible UE. Mycobacterial lysocardiolipin is exported from phagosomes upon cleavage of cardiolipin by a macrophage-derived lysosomal phospholipase A2. J Immunol. 2001;167:2187-92.

[26] Murzyn K, Rog T, Pasenkiewicz-Gierula M. Phosphatidylethanolamine-phosphatidylglycerol bilayer as a model of the inner bacterial membrane. Biophys J. 2005;88:1091-103.

[27] Brennan PJ, Lehane DP. The phospholipids of corynebacteria. Lipids. 1971;6:401-9.

[28] Khuller GK, Brennan PJ. Further studies on the lipids of corynebacteria. The mannolipids of *Corynebacterium aquaticum*. Biochem J. 1972;127:369-73.

[29] Suzuki KI, Suzuki M, Sasaki J, Park YH, Komagata KK. Leifsonia gen. nov., a genus for 2,4-diaminobutyric acid-containing actinomycetes to accommodate "*Corynebacterium aquaticum*" Leifson 1962 and Clavibacter xyli subsp. cynodontis Davis et al. 1984. J Gen Appl Microbiol. 1999;45:253-62.

[30] Charalambous K, Miller D, Curnow P, Booth PJ. Lipid bilayer composition influences small multidrug transporters. BMC Biochem. 2008;9:31.

[31] Chatterjee D, Khoo KH. Mycobacterial lipoarabinomannan: an extraordinary lipoheteroglycan with profound physiological effects. Glycobiology. 1998;8:113-20.

[32] Nigou J, Gilleron M, Rojas M, Garcia LF, Thurnher M, Puzo G. Mycobacterial lipoarabinomannans: modulators of dendritic cell function and the apoptotic response. Microbes Infect. 2002;4:945-53.

[33] Strohmeier GR, Fenton MJ. Roles of lipoarabinomannan in the pathogenesis of tuberculosis. Microbes Infect. 1999;1:709-17.

[34] Vercellone A, Nigou J, Puzo G. Relationships between the structure and the roles of lipoarabinomannans and related glycoconjugates in tuberculosis pathogenesis. Front Biosci. 1998;3:e149-63.

[35] Pitarque S, Larrouy-Maumus G, Payre B, Jackson M, Puzo G, Nigou J. The immunomodulatory lipoglycans, lipoarabinomannan and lipomannan, are exposed at the mycobacterial cell surface. Tuberculosis (Edinb). 2008;88:560-5.

[36] Morita YS, Sena CB, Waller RF, Kurokawa K, Sernee MF, Nakatani F, et al. PimE is a polyprenol-phosphate-mannose-dependent mannosyltransferase that transfers the fifth mannose of phosphatidylinositol mannoside in mycobacteria. J Biol Chem. 2006;281:25143-55.

[37] Lechevalier MP, Debievre C, Lechevalier H. Chemotaxonomy of aerobic actinomycetes - phospholipid composition. Biochem Syst Ecol. 1977;5:249-60.

[38] Yague G, Segovia M, Valero-Guillen PL. Acyl phosphatidylglycerol: a major phospholipid of *Corynebacterium amycolatum*. FEMS Microbiol Lett. 1997;151:125-30.

[39] Niepel T, Meyer H, Wray V, Abraham WR. Intraspecific variation of unusual phospholipids from *Corynebacterium* spp. containing a novel fatty acid. J Bacteriol. 1998;180:4650-7.

[40] Mazzella N, Molinet J, Syakti AD, Dodi A, Doumenq P, Artaud J, et al. Bacterial phospholipid molecular species analysis by ion-pair reversed-phase HPLC/ESI/MS. J Lipid Res. 2004;45:1355-63.

[41] Valero-Guillen PL, Yague G, Segovia M. Characterization of acyl-phosphatidylinositol from the opportunistic pathogen *Corynebacterium amycolatum*. Chem Phys Lipids. 2005;133:17-26.

[42] Puech V, Chami M, Lemassu A, Laneelle MA, Schiffler B, Gounon P, et al. Structure of the cell envelope of corynebacteria: importance of the non-covalently bound lipids in the formation of the cell wall permeability barrier and fracture plane. Microbiology. 2001;147:1365-82.

[43] Morita YS, Yamaryo-Botte Y, Miyanagi K, Callaghan JM, Patterson JH, Crellin PK, et al. Stress-induced synthesis of phosphatidylinositol 3-phosphate in mycobacteria. J Biol Chem. 2010;285:16643-50.
[44] Maloney E, Stankowska D, Zhang J, Fol M, Cheng QJ, Lun S, et al. The two-domain LysX protein of *Mycobacterium tuberculosis* is required for production of lysinylated phosphatidylglycerol and resistance to cationic antimicrobial peptides. PLoS Pathog. 2009;5:e1000534.
[45] Fraser PD, Bramley PM. The biosynthesis and nutritional uses of carotenoids. Prog Lipid Res. 2004;43:228-65.
[46] Scherzinger D, Scheffer E, Bar C, Ernst H, Al-Babili S. The *Mycobacterium tuberculosis* ORF *Rv0654* encodes a carotenoid oxygenase mediating central and excentric cleavage of conventional and aromatic carotenoids. FEBS J. 2010;277:4662-73.
[47] Steinbuchel A, Valentin HE. Diversity of bacterial polyhydroxyalkanoic acids. FEMS Microbiol Lett. 1995;128:219-28.
[48] Daniel J, Deb C, Dubey VS, Sirakova TD, Abomoelak B, Morbidoni HR, et al. Induction of a novel class of diacylglycerol acyltransferases and triacylglycerol accumulation in *Mycobacterium tuberculosis* as it goes into a dormancy-like state in culture. J Bacteriol. 2004;186:5017-30.
[49] Alvarez HM, Steinbuchel A. Triacylglycerols in prokaryotic microorganisms. Appl Microbiol Biotechnol. 2002;60:367-76.
[50] Alvarez HM, Kalscheuer R, Steinbuchel A. Accumulation and mobilization of storage lipids by *Rhodococcus opacus* PD630 and *Rhodococcus ruber* NCIMB 40126. Appl Microbiol Biotechnol. 2000;54:218-23.
[51] Alvarez HM, Luftmann H, Silva RA, Cesari AC, Viale A, Waltermann M, et al. Identification of phenyldecanoic acid as a constituent of triacylglycerols and wax ester produced by *Rhodococcus opacus* PD630. Microbiology. 2002;148:1407-12.
[52] Olukoshi ER, Packter NM. Importance of stored triacylglycerols in *Streptomyces*: possible carbon source for antibiotics. Microbiology. 1994;140 (Pt 4):931-43.
[53] Daniel J, Maamar H, Deb C, Sirakova TD, Kolattukudy PE. *Mycobacterium tuberculosis* uses host triacylglycerol to accumulate lipid droplets and acquires a dormancy-like phenotype in lipid-loaded macrophages. PLoS Pathog. 2011;7:e1002093.
[54] Sirakova TD, Dubey VS, Deb C, Daniel J, Korotkova TA, Abomoelak B, et al. Identification of a diacylglycerol acyltransferase gene involved in accumulation of triacylglycerol in *Mycobacterium tuberculosis* under stress. Microbiology. 2006;152:2717-25.
[55] Pandey AK, Sassetti CM. Mycobacterial persistence requires the utilization of host cholesterol. Proc Natl Acad Sci U S A. 2008;105:4376-80.
[56] Griffin JE, Gawronski JD, Dejesus MA, Ioerger TR, Akerley BJ, Sassetti CM. High-resolution phenotypic profiling defines genes essential for mycobacterial growth and cholesterol catabolism. PLoS Pathog. 2011;7:e1002251.
[57] Brzostek A, Pawelczyk J, Rumijowska-Galewicz A, Dziadek B, Dziadek J. *Mycobacterium tuberculosis* is able to accumulate and utilize cholesterol. J Bacteriol. 2009;191:6584-91.

[58] Av-Gay Y, Sobouti R. Cholesterol is accumulated by mycobacteria but its degradation is limited to non-pathogenic fast-growing mycobacteria. Can J Microbiol. 2000;46:826-31.

[59] Wright LD, Skeggs HR. Reversal of sodium propionate inhibition of *Escherichia coli* with beta-alanine. Arch Biochem. 1946;10:383-6.

[60] Brock M, Buckel W. On the mechanism of action of the antifungal agent propionate. Eur J Biochem. 2004;271:3227-41.

[61] Maruyama K, Kitamura H. Mechanisms of growth inhibition by propionate and restoration of the growth by sodium bicarbonate or acetate in *Rhodopseudomonas sphaeroides* S. J Biochem. 1985;98:819-24.

[62] Savvi S, Warner DF, Kana BD, McKinney JD, Mizrahi V, Dawes SS. Functional characterization of a vitamin B12-dependent methylmalonyl pathway in *Mycobacterium tuberculosis*: implications for propionate metabolism during growth on fatty acids. J Bacteriol. 2008;190:3886-95.

[63] Singh A, Crossman DK, Mai D, Guidry L, Voskuil MI, Renfrow MB, et al. *Mycobacterium tuberculosis* WhiB3 maintains redox homeostasis by regulating virulence lipid anabolism to modulate macrophage response. PLoS Pathog. 2009;5:e1000545.

[64] Bloch K. Control mechanisms for fatty acid synthesis in *Mycobacterium smegmatis*. Adv Enzymol Relat Areas Mol Biol. 1977;45:1-84.

[65] Fernandes ND, Kolattukudy PE. Cloning, sequencing and characterization of a fatty acid synthase-encoding gene from *Mycobacterium tuberculosis* var. bovis BCG. Gene. 1996;170:95-9.

[66] Bloch K, Vance D. Control mechanisms in the synthesis of saturated fatty acids. Annu Rev Biochem. 1977;46:263-98.

[67] Radmacher E, Alderwick LJ, Besra GS, Brown AK, Gibson KJ, Sahm H, et al. Two functional FAS-I type fatty acid synthases in *Corynebacterium glutamicum*. Microbiology. 2005;151:2421-7.

[68] Odriozola JM, Ramos JA, Bloch K. Fatty acid synthetase activity in *Mycobacterium smegmatis*. Characterization of the acyl carrier protein-dependent elongating system. Biochim Biophys Acta. 1977;488:207-17.

[69] Rock CO, Cronan JE. *Escherichia coli* as a model for the regulation of dissociable (type II) fatty acid biosynthesis. Biochim Biophys Acta. 1996;1302:1-16.

[70] Kremer L, Nampoothiri KM, Lesjean S, Dover LG, Graham S, Betts J, et al. Biochemical characterization of acyl carrier protein (AcpM) and malonyl-CoA:AcpM transacylase (mtFabD), two major components of *Mycobacterium tuberculosis* fatty acid synthase II. J Biol Chem. 2001;276:27967-74.

[71] Marrakchi H, Laneelle G, Quemard A. InhA, a target of the antituberculous drug isoniazid, is involved in a mycobacterial fatty acid elongation system, FAS-II. Microbiology. 2000;146:289-96.

[72] Portevin D, De Sousa-D'Auria C, Houssin C, Grimaldi C, Chami M, Daffe M, et al. A polyketide synthase catalyzes the last condensation step of mycolic acid biosynthesis in mycobacteria and related organisms. Proc Natl Acad Sci U S A. 2004;101:314-9.

[73] Lea-Smith DJ, Pyke JS, Tull D, McConville MJ, Coppel RL, Crellin PK. The reductase that catalyzes mycolic motif synthesis is required for efficient attachment of mycolic acids to arabinogalactan. J Biol Chem. 2007;282:11000-8.
[74] Athenstaedt K, Daum G. Phosphatidic acid, a key intermediate in lipid metabolism. Eur J Biochem. 1999;266:1-16.
[75] Okuyama H, Kameyama Y, Fujikawa M, Yamada K, Ikezawa H. Mechanism of diacylglycerophosphate synthesis in mycobacteria. J Biol Chem. 1977;252:6682-6.
[76] Okuyama H, Kankura T, Nojima S. Positional distribution of fatty acids in phospholipids from mycobacteria. J Biochem. 1967;61:732-7.
[77] Owens RM, Hsu FF, VanderVen BC, Purdy GE, Hesteande E, Giannakas P, et al. *M. tuberculosis Rv2252* encodes a diacylglycerol kinase involved in the biosynthesis of phosphatidylinositol mannosides (PIMs). Mol Microbiol. 2006;60:1152-63.
[78] Smith SW, Weiss SB, Kennedy EP. The enzymatic dephosphorylation of phosphatidic acids. J Biol Chem. 1957;228:915-22.
[79] Han GS, Wu WI, Carman GM. The *Saccharomyces cerevisiae* Lipin homolog is a Mg^{2+}-dependent phosphatidate phosphatase enzyme. J Biol Chem. 2006;281:9210-8.
[80] Kalscheuer R, Steinbuchel A. A novel bifunctional wax ester synthase/acyl-CoA:diacylglycerol acyltransferase mediates wax ester and triacylglycerol biosynthesis in *Acinetobacter calcoaceticus* ADP1. J Biol Chem. 2003;278:8075-82.
[81] Elamin AA, Stehr M, Spallek R, Rohde M, Singh M. The *Mycobacterium tuberculosis* Ag85A is a novel diacylglycerol acyltransferase involved in lipid body formation. Mol Microbiol. 2011;81:1577-92.
[82] Ortalo-Magne A, Lemassu A, Laneelle MA, Bardou F, Silve G, Gounon P, et al. Identification of the surface-exposed lipids on the cell envelopes of *Mycobacterium tuberculosis* and other mycobacterial species. J Bacteriol. 1996;178:456-61.
[83] Paznokas JL, Kaplan A. Purification and properties of a triacylglycerol lipase from *Mycobacterium phlei*. Biochim Biophys Acta. 1977;487:405-21.
[84] Deb C, Daniel J, Sirakova TD, Abomoelak B, Dubey VS, Kolattukudy PE. A novel lipase belonging to the hormone-sensitive lipase family induced under starvation to utilize stored triacylglycerol in *Mycobacterium tuberculosis*. J Biol Chem. 2006;281:3866-75.
[85] Mishra KC, de Chastellier C, Narayana Y, Bifani P, Brown AK, Besra GS, et al. Functional role of the PE domain and immunogenicity of the *Mycobacterium tuberculosis* triacylglycerol hydrolase LipY. Infect Immun. 2008;76:127-40.
[86] Munoz-Elias EJ, McKinney JD. Carbon metabolism of intracellular bacteria. Cell Microbiol. 2006;8:10-22.
[87] Cotes K, Dhouib R, Douchet I, Chahinian H, de Caro A, Carriere F, et al. Characterization of an exported monoglyceride lipase from *Mycobacterium tuberculosis* possibly involved in the metabolism of host cell membrane lipids. Biochem J. 2007;408:417-27.
[88] Waltermann M, Steinbuchel A. Neutral lipid bodies in prokaryotes: recent insights into structure, formation, and relationship to eukaryotic lipid depots. J Bacteriol. 2005;187:3607-19.

[89] Waltermann M, Hinz A, Robenek H, Troyer D, Reichelt R, Malkus U, et al. Mechanism of lipid-body formation in prokaryotes: how bacteria fatten up. Mol Microbiol. 2005;55:750-63.
[90] Hanisch J, Waltermann M, Robenek H, Steinbuchel A. Eukaryotic lipid body proteins in oleogenous actinomycetes and their targeting to intracellular triacylglycerol inclusions: Impact on models of lipid body biogenesis. Appl Environ Microbiol. 2006;72:6743-50.
[91] Hanisch J, Waltermann M, Robenek H, Steinbuchel A. The *Ralstonia eutropha* H16 phasin PhaP1 is targeted to intracellular triacylglycerol inclusions in *Rhodococcus opacus* PD630 and *Mycobacterium smegmatis* mc^{2}155, and provides an anchor to target other proteins. Microbiology. 2006;152:3271-80.
[92] Dowhan W. CDP-diacylglycerol synthase of microorganisms. Biochim Biophys Acta. 1997;1348:157-65.
[93] Nigou J, Besra GS. Cytidine diphosphate-diacylglycerol synthesis in *Mycobacterium smegmatis*. Biochem J. 2002;367:157-62.
[94] Lecocq J, Ballou CE. On the structure of cardiolipin. Biochemistry. 1964;3:976-80.
[95] Icho T, Raetz CR. Multiple genes for membrane-bound phosphatases in *Escherichia coli* and their action on phospholipid precursors. J Bacteriol. 1983;153:722-30.
[96] Funk CR, Zimniak L, Dowhan W. The pgpA and pgpB genes of *Escherichia coli* are not essential: evidence for a third phosphatidylglycerophosphate phosphatase. J Bacteriol. 1992;174:205-13.
[97] Lu YH, Guan Z, Zhao J, Raetz CR. Three phosphatidylglycerol-phosphate phosphatases in the inner membrane of *Escherichia coli*. J Biol Chem. 2011;286:5506-18.
[98] Osman C, Haag M, Wieland FT, Brugger B, Langer T. A mitochondrial phosphatase required for cardiolipin biosynthesis: the PGP phosphatase Gep4. EMBO J. 2010;29:1976-87.
[99] Zhang J, Guan Z, Murphy AN, Wiley SE, Perkins GA, Worby CA, et al. Mitochondrial phosphatase PTPMT1 is essential for cardiolipin biosynthesis. Cell Metab. 2011;13:690-700.
[100] Mathur AK, Murthy PS, Saharia GS, Venkitasubramanian TA. Studies on cardiolipin biosynthesis in *Mycobacterium smegmatis*. Can J Microbiol. 1976;22:354-8.
[101] Ter Horst B, Seshadri C, Sweet L, Young DC, Feringa BL, Moody DB, et al. Asymmetric synthesis and structure elucidation of a glycerophospholipid from *Mycobacterium tuberculosis*. J Lipid Res. 2010;51:1017-22.
[102] Morita YS, Velasquez R, Taig E, Waller RF, Patterson JH, Tull D, et al. Compartmentalization of lipid biosynthesis in mycobacteria. J Biol Chem. 2005;280:21645-52.
[103] Salman M, Lonsdale JT, Besra GS, Brennan PJ. Phosphatidylinositol synthesis in mycobacteria. Biochim Biophys Acta. 1999;1436:437-50.
[104] Morita YS, Fukuda T, Sena CB, Yamaryo-Botte Y, McConville MJ, Kinoshita T. Inositol lipid metabolism in mycobacteria: biosynthesis and regulatory mechanisms. Biochim Biophys Acta. 2011;1810:630-41.
[105] Nigou J, Besra GS. Characterization and regulation of inositol monophosphatase activity in *Mycobacterium smegmatis*. Biochem J. 2002;361:385-90.

[106] Mishra AK, Driessen NN, Appelmelk BJ, Besra GS. Lipoarabinomannan and related glycoconjugates: structure, biogenesis and role in *Mycobacterium tuberculosis* physiology and host-pathogen interaction. FEMS Microbiol Rev. 2011;35:1126-57.

[107] Guerin ME, Kordulakova J, Alzari PM, Brennan PJ, Jackson M. Molecular basis of phosphatidyl-*myo*-inositol mannoside biosynthesis and regulation in mycobacteria. J Biol Chem. 2010;285:33577-83.

[108] Ma Y, Stern RJ, Scherman MS, Vissa VD, Yan W, Jones VC, et al. Drug targeting *Mycobacterium tuberculosis* cell wall synthesis: genetics of dTDP-rhamnose synthetic enzymes and development of a microtiter plate-based screen for inhibitors of conversion of dTDP-glucose to dTDP-rhamnose. Antimicrob Agents Chemother. 2001;45:1407-16.

[109] McCarthy TR, Torrelles JB, MacFarlane AS, Katawczik M, Kutzbach B, Desjardin LE, et al. Overexpression of *Mycobacterium tuberculosis* manB, a phosphomannomutase that increases phosphatidylinositol mannoside biosynthesis in *Mycobacterium smegmatis* and mycobacterial association with human macrophages. Mol Microbiol. 2005;58:774-90.

[110] Ning B, Elbein AD. Purification and properties of mycobacterial GDP-mannose pyrophosphorylase. Arch Biochem Biophys. 1999;362:339-45.

[111] Patterson JH, Waller RF, Jeevarajah D, Billman-Jacobe H, McConville MJ. Mannose metabolism is required for mycobacterial growth. Biochem J. 2003;372:77-86.

[112] Mishra AK, Krumbach K, Rittmann D, Batt SM, Lee OY, De S, et al. Deletion of manC in *Corynebacterium glutamicum* results in a phospho-myo-inositol mannoside- and lipoglycan-deficient mutant. Microbiology. 2012;158:1908-17.

[113] Kordulakova J, Gilleron M, Mikusova K, Puzo G, Brennan PJ, Gicquel B, et al. Definition of the first mannosylation step in phosphatidylinositol mannoside synthesis. PimA is essential for growth of mycobacteria. J Biol Chem. 2002;277:31335-44.

[114] Gu X, Chen M, Wang Q, Zhang M, Wang B, Wang H. Expression and purification of a functionally active recombinant GDP-mannosyltransferase (PimA) from *Mycobacterium tuberculosis* H37Rv. Protein Expr Purif. 2005;42:47-53.

[115] Guerin ME, Buschiazzo A, Kordulakova J, Jackson M, Alzari PM. Crystallization and preliminary crystallographic analysis of PimA, an essential mannosyltransferase from *Mycobacterium smegmatis*. Acta Crystallograph Sect F Struct Biol Cryst Commun. 2005;61:518-20.

[116] Guerin ME, Kordulakova J, Schaeffer F, Svetlikova Z, Buschiazzo A, Giganti D, et al. Molecular recognition and interfacial catalysis by the essential phosphatidylinositol mannosyltransferase PimA from mycobacteria. J Biol Chem. 2007;282:20705-14.

[117] Guerin ME, Kaur D, Somashekar BS, Gibbs S, Gest P, Chatterjee D, et al. New insights into the early steps of phosphatidylinositol mannoside biosynthesis in mycobacteria: PimB' is an essential enzyme of *Mycobacterium smegmatis*. J Biol Chem. 2009;284:25687-96.

[118] Lea-Smith DJ, Martin KL, Pyke JS, Tull D, McConville MJ, Coppel RL, et al. Analysis of a new mannosyltransferase required for the synthesis of phosphatidylinositol

mannosides and lipoarabinomannan reveals two lipomannan pools in *Corynebacterineae*. J Biol Chem. 2008;283:6773-82.
[119] Schaeffer ML, Khoo KH, Besra GS, Chatterjee D, Brennan PJ, Belisle JT, et al. The *pimB* gene of *Mycobacterium tuberculosis* encodes a mannosyltransferase involved in lipoarabinomannan biosynthesis. J Biol Chem. 1999;274:31625-31.
[120] Mishra AK, Batt S, Krumbach K, Eggeling L, Besra GS. Characterization of the *Corynebacterium glutamicum* deltapimB' deltamgtA double deletion mutant and the role of *Mycobacterium tuberculosis* orthologues Rv2188c and Rv0557 in glycolipid biosynthesis. J Bacteriol. 2009;191:4465-72.
[121] Tatituri RV, Illarionov PA, Dover LG, Nigou J, Gilleron M, Hitchen P, et al. Inactivation of *Corynebacterium glutamicum NCgl0452* and the role of MgtA in the biosynthesis of a novel mannosylated glycolipid involved in lipomannan biosynthesis. J Biol Chem. 2007;282:4561-72.
[122] Batt SM, Jabeen T, Mishra AK, Veerapen N, Krumbach K, Eggeling L, et al. Acceptor substrate discrimination in phosphatidyl-myo-inositol mannoside synthesis: structural and mutational analysis of mannosyltransferase *Corynebacterium glutamicum* PimB'. J Biol Chem. 2010;285:37741-52.
[123] Kordulakova J, Gilleron M, Puzo G, Brennan PJ, Gicquel B, Mikusova K, et al. Identification of the required acyltransferase step in the biosynthesis of the phosphatidylinositol mannosides of *Mycobacterium* species. J Biol Chem. 2003;278:36285-95.
[124] Kremer L, Gurcha SS, Bifani P, Hitchen PG, Baulard A, Morris HR, et al. Characterization of a putative alpha-mannosyltransferase involved in phosphatidylinositol trimannoside biosynthesis in *Mycobacterium tuberculosis*. Biochem J. 2002;363:437-47.
[125] Besra GS, Morehouse CB, Rittner CM, Waechter CJ, Brennan PJ. Biosynthesis of mycobacterial lipoarabinomannan. J Biol Chem. 1997;272:18460-6.
[126] Gurcha SS, Baulard AR, Kremer L, Locht C, Moody DB, Muhlecker W, et al. Ppm1, a novel polyprenol monophosphomannose synthase from *Mycobacterium tuberculosis*. Biochem J. 2002;365:441-50.
[127] Gibson KJ, Eggeling L, Maughan WN, Krumbach K, Gurcha SS, Nigou J, et al. Disruption of Cg-Ppm1, a polyprenyl monophosphomannose synthase, and the generation of lipoglycan-less mutants in *Corynebacterium glutamicum*. J Biol Chem. 2003;278:40842-50.
[128] Morita YS, Patterson JH, Billman-Jacobe H, McConville MJ. Biosynthesis of mycobacterial phosphatidylinositol mannosides. Biochem J. 2004;378:589-97.
[129] Kovacevic S, Anderson D, Morita YS, Patterson J, Haites R, McMillan BN, et al. Identification of a novel protein with a role in lipoarabinomannan biosynthesis in mycobacteria. J Biol Chem. 2006;281:9011-7.
[130] Crellin PK, Kovacevic S, Martin KL, Brammananth R, Morita YS, Billman-Jacobe H, et al. Mutations in *pimE* restore lipoarabinomannan synthesis and growth in a *Mycobacterium smegmatis lpqW* mutant. J Bacteriol. 2008;190:3690-9.

[131] Marland Z, Beddoe T, Zaker-Tabrizi L, Lucet IS, Brammananth R, Whisstock JC, et al. Hijacking of a substrate-binding protein scaffold for use in mycobacterial cell wall biosynthesis. J Mol Biol. 2006;359:983-97.

[132] Besra GS, Brennan PJ. The mycobacterial cell wall: biosynthesis of arabinogalactan and lipoarabinomannan. Biochem Soc Trans. 1997;25:845-50.

[133] Mishra AK, Alderwick LJ, Rittmann D, Wang C, Bhatt A, Jacobs WR, Jr., et al. Identification of a novel alpha(1-->6) mannopyranosyltransferase MptB from *Corynebacterium glutamicum* by deletion of a conserved gene, *NCgl1505,* affords a lipomannan- and lipoarabinomannan-deficient mutant. Mol Microbiol. 2008;68:1595-613.

[134] Kaur D, Berg S, Dinadayala P, Gicquel B, Chatterjee D, McNeil MR, et al. Biosynthesis of mycobacterial lipoarabinomannan: role of a branching mannosyltransferase. Proc Natl Acad Sci U S A. 2006;103:13664-9.

[135] Kaur D, McNeil MR, Khoo KH, Chatterjee D, Crick DC, Jackson M, et al. New insights into the biosynthesis of mycobacterial lipomannan arising from deletion of a conserved gene. J Biol Chem. 2007;282:27133-40.

[136] Mishra AK, Alderwick LJ, Rittmann D, Tatituri RV, Nigou J, Gilleron M, et al. Identification of an alpha(1-->6) mannopyranosyltransferase (MptA), involved in *Corynebacterium glutamicum* lipomannan biosynthesis, and identification of its orthologue in *Mycobacterium tuberculosis*. Mol Microbiol. 2007;65:1503-17.

[137] Kaur D, Obregon-Henao A, Pham H, Chatterjee D, Brennan PJ, Jackson M. Lipoarabinomannan of *Mycobacterium*: mannose capping by a multifunctional terminal mannosyltransferase. Proc Natl Acad Sci U S A. 2008;105:17973-7.

[138] Sena CB, Fukuda T, Miyanagi K, Matsumoto S, Kobayashi K, Murakami Y, et al. Controlled expression of branch-forming mannosyltransferase is critical for mycobacterial lipoarabinomannan biosynthesis. J Biol Chem. 2010;285:13326-36.

[139] Birch HL, Alderwick LJ, Bhatt A, Rittmann D, Krumbach K, Singh A, et al. Biosynthesis of mycobacterial arabinogalactan: identification of a novel alpha(1-->3) arabinofuranosyltransferase. Mol Microbiol. 2008;69:1191-206.

[140] Alderwick LJ, Lloyd GS, Ghadbane H, May JW, Bhatt A, Eggeling L, et al. The C-terminal domain of the arabinosyltransferase *Mycobacterium tuberculosis* EmbC is a lectin-like carbohydrate binding module. PLoS Pathog. 2011;7:e1001299.

[141] Skovierova H, Larrouy-Maumus G, Zhang J, Kaur D, Barilone N, Kordulakova J, et al. AftD, a novel essential arabinofuranosyltransferase from mycobacteria. Glycobiology. 2009;19:1235-47.

[142] Zhang N, Torrelles JB, McNeil MR, Escuyer VE, Khoo KH, Brennan PJ, et al. The Emb proteins of mycobacteria direct arabinosylation of lipoarabinomannan and arabinogalactan via an N-terminal recognition region and a C-terminal synthetic region. Mol Microbiol. 2003;50:69-76.

[143] Chatterjee D, Hunter SW, McNeil M, Brennan PJ. Lipoarabinomannan. Multiglycosylated form of the mycobacterial mannosylphosphatidylinositols. J Biol Chem. 1992;267:6228-33.

[144] Appelmelk BJ, den Dunnen J, Driessen NN, Ummels R, Pak M, Nigou J, et al. The mannose cap of mycobacterial lipoarabinomannan does not dominate the *Mycobacterium*-host interaction. Cell Microbiol. 2008;10:930-44.

[145] Khoo KH, Dell A, Morris HR, Brennan PJ, Chatterjee D. Inositol phosphate capping of the nonreducing termini of lipoarabinomannan from rapidly growing strains of *Mycobacterium*. J Biol Chem. 1995;270:12380-9.

[146] Mishra AK, Klein C, Gurcha SS, Alderwick LJ, Babu P, Hitchen PG, et al. Structural characterization and functional properties of a novel lipomannan variant isolated from a *Corynebacterium glutamicum* pimB' mutant. Antonie Van Leeuwenhoek. 2008;94:277-87.

[147] Tatituri RV, Alderwick LJ, Mishra AK, Nigou J, Gilleron M, Krumbach K, et al. Structural characterization of a partially arabinosylated lipoarabinomannan variant isolated from a *Corynebacterium glutamicum* ubiA mutant. Microbiology. 2007;153:2621-9.

[148] Wolucka BA, McNeil MR, de Hoffmann E, Chojnacki T, Brennan PJ. Recognition of the lipid intermediate for arabinogalactan/arabinomannan biosynthesis and its relation to the mode of action of ethambutol on mycobacteria. J Biol Chem. 1994;269:23328-35.

[149] Takayama K, Schnoes HK, Semmler EJ. Characterization of the alkali-stable mannophospholipids of *Mycobacterium smegmatis*. Biochim Biophys Acta. 1973;316:212-21.

[150] Bailey AM, Mahapatra S, Brennan PJ, Crick DC. Identification, cloning, purification, and enzymatic characterization of *Mycobacterium tuberculosis* 1-deoxy-D-xylulose 5-phosphate synthase. Glycobiology. 2002;12:813-20.

[151] Dhiman RK, Schaeffer ML, Bailey AM, Testa CA, Scherman H, Crick DC. 1- Deoxy-D-xylulose 5-phosphate reductoisomerase (IspC) from *Mycobacterium tuberculosis*: towards understanding mycobacterial resistance to fosmidomycin. J Bacteriol. 2005;187:8395-402.

[152] Argyrou A, Blanchard JS. Kinetic and chemical mechanism of *Mycobacterium tuberculosis* 1-deoxy-deoxy-D-xylulose -5-phosphate isomeroreductase. Biochemistry. 2004;43:4375-84.

[153] Takayama K, Goldman DS. Enzymatic synthesis of mannosyl-1-phosphoryl-decaprenol by a cell-free system of *Mycobacterium tuberculosis*. J Biol Chem. 1970;245:6251-7.

[154] Wolucka BA, de Hoffmann E. The presence of beta-D-ribosyl-1-monophosphodecaprenol in mycobacteria. J Biol Chem. 1995;270:20151-5.

[155] Wolucka BA, de Hoffmann E. Isolation and characterization of the major form of polyprenyl-phospho-mannose from *Mycobacterium smegmatis*. Glycobiology. 1998;8:955-62.

[156] Baulard AR, Gurcha SS, Engohang-Ndong J, Gouffi K, Locht C, Besra GS. *In vivo* interaction between the polyprenol phosphate mannose synthase Ppm1 and the integral membrane protein Ppm2 from *Mycobacterium smegmatis* revealed by a bacterial two-hybrid system. J Biol Chem. 2003;278:2242-8.

[157] Scherman H, Kaur D, Pham H, Skovierova H, Jackson M, Brennan PJ. Identification of a polyprenylphosphomannosyl synthase involved in the synthesis of mycobacterial mannosides. J Bacteriol. 2009;191:6769-72.

[158] Skovierova H, Larrouy-Maumus G, Pham H, Belanova M, Barilone N, Dasgupta A, et al. Biosynthetic origin of the galactosamine substituent of arabinogalactan in *Mycobacterium tuberculosis*. J Biol Chem. 2010;285:41348-55.

[159] Klutts JS, Hatanaka K, Pan YT, Elbein AD. Biosynthesis of D-arabinose in *Mycobacterium smegmatis*: specific labeling from D-glucose. Arch Biochem Biophys. 2002;398:229-39.

[160] Scherman M, Weston A, Duncan K, Whittington A, Upton R, Deng L, et al. Biosynthetic origin of mycobacterial cell wall arabinosyl residues. J Bacteriol. 1995;177:7125-30.

[161] Scherman MS, Kalbe-Bournonville L, Bush D, Xin Y, Deng L, McNeil M. Polyprenylphosphate-pentoses in mycobacteria are synthesized from 5-phosphoribose pyrophosphate. J Biol Chem. 1996;271:29652-8.

[162] Huang H, Scherman MS, D'Haeze W, Vereecke D, Holsters M, Crick DC, et al. Identification and active expression of the *Mycobacterium tuberculosis* gene encoding 5-phospho-D-ribose-1-diphosphate: decaprenyl-phosphate 5-phosphoribosyltransferase, the first enzyme committed to decaprenylphosphoryl-d-arabinose synthesis. J Biol Chem. 2005;280:24539-43.

[163] Mikusova K, Huang H, Yagi T, Holsters M, Vereecke D, D'Haeze W, et al. Decaprenylphosphoryl arabinofuranose, the donor of the D-arabinofuranosyl residues of mycobacterial arabinan, is formed via a two-step epimerization of decaprenylphosphoryl ribose. J Bacteriol. 2005;187:8020-5.

[164] Christophe T, Jackson M, Jeon HK, Fenistein D, Contreras-Dominguez M, Kim J, et al. High content screening identifies decaprenyl-phosphoribose 2' epimerase as a target for intracellular antimycobacterial inhibitors. PLoS Pathog. 2009;5:e1000645.

[165] Makarov V, Manina G, Mikusova K, Mollmann U, Ryabova O, Saint-Joanis B, et al. Benzothiazinones kill *Mycobacterium tuberculosis* by blocking arabinan synthesis. Science. 2009;324:801-4.

[166] Makarov V, Riabova OB, Yuschenko A, Urlyapova N, Daudova A, Zipfel PF, et al. Synthesis and antileprosy activity of some dialkyldithiocarbamates. J Antimicrob Chemother. 2006;57:1134-8.

[167] Pasca MR, Degiacomi G, Ribeiro AL, Zara F, De Mori P, Heym B, et al. Clinical isolates of *Mycobacterium tuberculosis* in four European hospitals are uniformly susceptible to benzothiazinones. Antimicrob Agents Chemother. 2010;54:1616-8.

[168] Crellin PK, Brammananth R, Coppel RL. Decaprenylphosphoryl-beta- D-ribose 2'-epimerase, the target of benzothiazinones and dinitrobenzamides, is an essential enzyme in *Mycobacterium smegmatis*. PLoS One. 2011;6:e16869.

[169] Manina G, Pasca MR, Buroni S, De Rossi E, Riccardi G. Decaprenylphosphoryl-beta- D-ribose 2'-epimerase from *Mycobacterium tuberculosis* is a magic drug target. Curr Med Chem. 2010;17:3099-108.

[170] Batt SM, Jabeen T, Bhowruth V, Quill L, Lund PA, Eggeling L, et al. Structural basis of inhibition of *Mycobacterium tuberculosis* DprE1 by benzothiazinone inhibitors. Proc Natl Acad Sci U S A. 2012;109:11354-9.

[171] Tarnok I, Tarnok Z. Carotenes and xanthophylls in mycobacteria. II. Lycopene, alpha- and beta-carotene and xanthophyll in mycobacterial pigments. Tubercle. 1971;52:127-35.

[172] Houssaini-Iraqui M, Lazraq MH, Clavel-Seres S, Rastogi N, David HL. Cloning and expression of *Mycobacterium aurum* carotenogenesis genes in *Mycobacterium smegmatis*. FEMS Microbiol Lett. 1992;69:239-44.

[173] Ramakrishnan L, Tran HT, Federspiel NA, Falkow S. A crtB homolog essential for photochromogenicity in *Mycobacterium marinum*: isolation, characterization, and gene disruption via homologous recombination. J Bacteriol. 1997;179:5862-8.

[174] Viveiros M, Krubasik P, Sandmann G, Houssaini-Iraqui M. Structural and functional analysis of the gene cluster encoding carotenoid biosynthesis in *Mycobacterium aurum* A+. FEMS Microbiol Lett. 2000;187:95-101.

[175] Robledo JA, Murillo AM, Rouzaud F. Physiological role and potential clinical interest of mycobacterial pigments. IUBMB Life. 2011;63:71-8.

[176] Kim SW, Keasling JD. Metabolic engineering of the nonmevalonate isopentenyl diphosphate synthesis pathway in *Escherichia coli* enhances lycopene production. Biotechnol Bioeng. 2001;72:408-15.

[177] Ito M, Yamano Y, Tode C, Wada A. Carotenoid synthesis: retrospect and recent progress. Arch Biochem Biophys. 2009;483:224-8.

[178] Misawa N, Satomi Y, Kondo K, Yokoyama A, Kajiwara S, Saito T, et al. Structure and functional analysis of a marine bacterial carotenoid biosynthesis gene cluster and astaxanthin biosynthetic pathway proposed at the gene level. J Bacteriol. 1995;177:6575-84.

[179] Wenk MR. The emerging field of lipidomics. Nat Rev Drug Discov. 2005;4:594-610.

[180] Wenk MR. Lipidomics: new tools and applications. Cell. 2010;143:888-95.

[181] Layre E, Sweet L, Hong S, Madigan CA, Desjardins D, Young DC, et al. A comparative lipidomics platform for chemotaxonomic analysis of *Mycobacterium tuberculosis*. Chem Biol. 2011;18:1537-49.

[182] Sartain MJ, Dick DL, Rithner CD, Crick DC, Belisle JT. Lipidomic analyses of *Mycobacterium tuberculosis* based on accurate mass measurements and the novel "Mtb LipidDB". J Lipid Res. 2011;52:861-72.

[183] Madigan CA, Cheng TY, Layre E, Young DC, McConnell MJ, Debono CA, et al. Lipidomic discovery of deoxysiderophores reveals a revised mycobactin biosynthesis pathway in *Mycobacterium tuberculosis*. Proc Natl Acad Sci U S A. 2012;109:1257-62.

Chapter 7

Autophagy Regulates Lipid Droplet Formation and Adipogenesis

Yasuo Uchiyama and Eiki Kominami

Additional information is available at the end of the chapter

http://dx.doi.org/10.5772/51447

1. Introduction

Proteolysis in eukaryotic cells can be separated into two major pathways: one is mediated by the ubiquitin-proteasome system and by the autophagy-lysosome system. Substrates of lysosomes may be taken through heterophagocytosis, endocytosis, or autophagy into heterophagosomes, early endosomes, or autophagosomes, which receive lysosomal enzymes via transporting vesicles from the trans-Golgi network or lysosomes and become heterophagolysosomes, late endosomes, or autolysosomes [1-4]. Different from endocytosis and heterophagocytosis, substrates of autophagy are limited to intracellular constituents and include various membranous organelles together with a part of the cytoplasm [3]. Until recently, 18 autophagy-related proteins (Atgs) have been shown to be involved in autophagosome formation, although more than 30 Atgs have been uncovered to regulate autophagy [2, 5]. Such autophagy contributes to the maintenance of cellular homeostasis [6]. Impairment of autophagy, therefore, causes severe degenerative alterations in various tissue cells [1, 4, 7]. In addition to the maintenance of basal cellular metabolism, autophagy is induced in response to various stresses such as starvation and diseases [8-13].

Since one of the major sources in living organisms is lipid, the metabolism of lipid is finely regulated. Besides adipose tissues, neutral lipids, most of which are mainly triacylglycerol (TAG) and cholesterol ester (CE) in cells, are stored in a sort of inclusion body, called the lipid droplet or lipid body [14-16]. Under nutrient-rich situations, excess fatty acids may be converted to TAG through lipogenesis and stored in lipid droplets, whereas lipid droplets under starvation conditions may be a source to produce lipids by lipolysis for cell usage [16]. Under stress or starvation states, proteins are also degraded to produce an amino acid pool that is used in part for energy metabolism through glyconeogenesis, while free fatty acids (FFAs) from adipocytes are delivered to hepatocytes and cardiac myocytes where they are used as an energy source via β-oxidation [15, 16]. At the initial stage during fasting,

FFAs are also converted to triacylglycerol (TAG) and stored as lipid droplets (LDs) that are used for an energy source when starvation continues.

It has been shown that loss of Atg7 largely suppresses LD formations in hepatocytes and cardiac myocytes 24 hours after the start of starvation, although numerous LDs accumulate in normal hepatocytes and cardiac myocytes under the same conditions [11]. Moreover, a mouse model with a targeted deletion of *atg7* in adipose tissue has been generated; the mutant mice were slim and contained only 20% of the mass of white adipose tissue (WAT) found in wild-type mice [17]. These mutant mice exhibit a high sensitivity to insulin that reduces low fed plasma concentrations of FFAs, and also exhibit a marked decrease in plasma concentrations of leptin but not adiponectin, and lower plasma concentrations of TAG. LDs, initially considered inert lipid deposits, have gained the classification of cytosolic organelles during the last decade due to their defined composition and the multiplicity of specific cellular functions in which they are involved [18]. At present, it remains largely unknown how autophagy is involved in LD metabolism, although lipophagy may occur in cells.

One thing that we have found is that a lipidated form of LC3, representing the Atg8 family of proteins, is localized on the surface of LDs and also in LD fractions, in addition to ADRP and perilipin, representing the PAT family of proteins that cover the surface of LDs. In this review we will introduce the LC3 conjugation system that is involved in lipid metabolism via LD formation..

2. Microtubule-associated protein 1A/1B light chain 3 (LC3) localizes not only to autophagosomal membranes but also on the surface membrane of LDs in hepatic and cardiac tissues under starvation conditions

It is well known that hepatocytes are morphologically and functionally different between the periportal and perivenous regions; periportal hepatocytes are glycogenic and lipolytic, while perivenous hepatocytes are glycolytic and lipogenic [19]. Lysosomes in hepatocytes are also more abundant in the perivenous region than in the periportal region [19, 20].

Such a morphological difference is largely altered when mice are starved for 24 or 48 hours; numerous autophagosomes that contain part of the cytoplasm and possess the cisternal or double isolation membranes and autolysosomes appear near bile canaliculi in hepatocytes 24 hours after the commencement of starvation and those that in some cases contain mitochondria are seen 48 hours later [4, 9]. In addition to autophagosomes and autolysosomes, LDs accumulate abundantly in the cytoplasm of hepatocytes. When livers of conditional Atg7-deficient mice ($Atg7^{Flox/Flox}$: Albumin-Cre) at 22 days, or 6 or 8 weeks of age were examined, positive staining for LDs is sparsely detected in the hepatocytes under starvation conditions for 12 or 24 hours, although they are abundant in the cytoplasm of the hepatocytes of the control littermate mouse liver (Fig. 1). Size and amount of stained LDs were much smaller in hepatocytes deficient in Atg7 than in the control hepatocytes. When examined by electron microscopy, the diameter of LDs in the control hepatocytes is various and ranged up to 2.61 μm (the mean diameter (± SD)) is 1.12 ± 0.17 μm). Different from the control, mutant hepatocytes mainly possess smaller LDs whose diameter ranged up to 0.83 μm (the average diameter is 0.19 ± 0.17 μm). Moreover, small LD-like bodies were observed in the luminal space of rough surfaced endoplasmic reticulum (rER), Golgi cisternal ends, and vesicles near the Golgi apparatus of the cells, indicating that the lumenally-sorted LDs are normally produced in the rER of both mutant and control hepatocytes. Importantly, the total TAG amount in Atg7-deficient liver and control livers is half of that in the control liver. These data indicate that the conjugation system of LC3 by Atg7 is required for the formation of LDs.

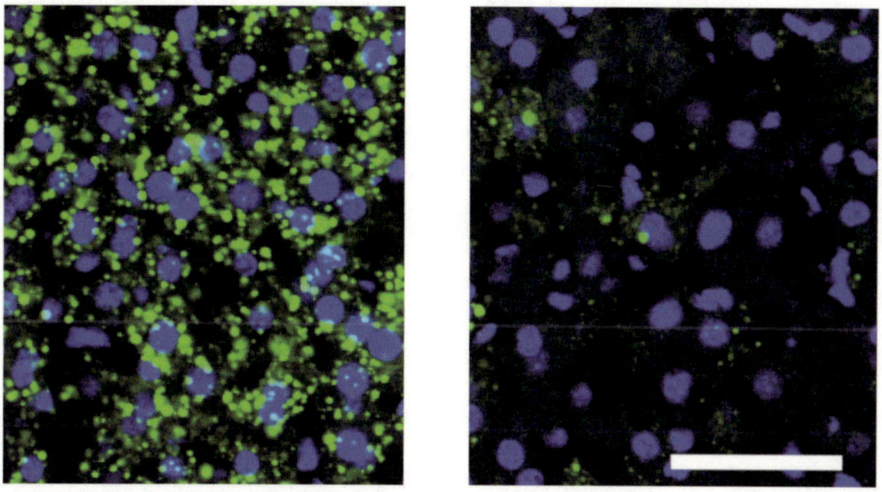

Figure 1. BODIPY staining (green) of hepatocytes obtained from control littermate (left) and Atg7-deficient (right) mice at the age of 6 weeks. Mice were housed under starvation conditions for 24 hours. BODIPY-positive LDs are abundant in hepatocytes from control littermate mouse, while positive LDs largely disappear from the Atg7-deficient hepatocytes. Bar= 50 μm

3. Inhibition of LD formation in hepatocytes deficient in Atg7 after deprivation

It has been shown that autophagy may play an important role in normal adipogenesis and that inhibition of autophagy by disrupting the *atg7* gene has a unique anti-obesity and insulin sensitization effect [17]. LDs are ubiquitous in eukaryotic cells, while excess free fatty acids and glucose in plasma are converted to TAG and stored as LDs (Fig. 1). However, the mechanism for the generation and growth of LDs in cells is largely unknown. As stated above, Atg7 that mediates LC3 lipidation and is essential for autophagy is involved in LD formation [4, 9]. LD formation accompanied by accumulation of TAG induced by starvation is largely suppressed in hepatocytes that cannot execute autophagy.

It is well known that LC3, microtubule-associated protein A/B light chain 3, is localized on the surface of the isolation membrane when starvation is induced [9]. Using GFP-LC3 transgenic mice, GFP-LC3 becomes dot-shaped, cap-shaped and ring-shaped in hepatocytes and cardiac myocytes under starvation conditions [21]. When immunostained for LC3 under starvation conditions, positive staining is, as shown by GFP-LC3 in TG mice, dot-shaped, cap-shaped, and ring-shaped in hepatocytes and cardiac myocytes (Figs. 2 and 3, Tables 1 and 2). Interestingly, positive staining of LC3 in cardiac myocytes is longitudinally arrayed in parallel to myofilaments. In both hepatocytes and cardiac myocytes, LDs are abundant 24 hours after the onset of starvation [9]. In particular, electron microscopic observations show that no clear-cut autophagosomes are detected in cardiac myocytes, although many large LDs are arranged longitudinally in parallel to the array of myofilaments together with mitochondria. This arrangement of LDs in cardiac myocytes is very similar to that of LC3-positive granules. To examine the relationship between staining patterns of LC3 and LDs in both hepatocytes and cardiac myocytes, double staining for perilipin with LC3 was performed. The results indicate that perilipin-positive LDs are also immunopositive for LC3 on the surface of LDs in both hepatocytes and cardiac myocytes [9]. In hepatocytes, there is also dotted staining of LC3 that is free of LD staining, whereas most LD-positive staining is co-localized with LC3 in cardiac myocytes (Figs. 2 and 3, Tables 1 and 2).

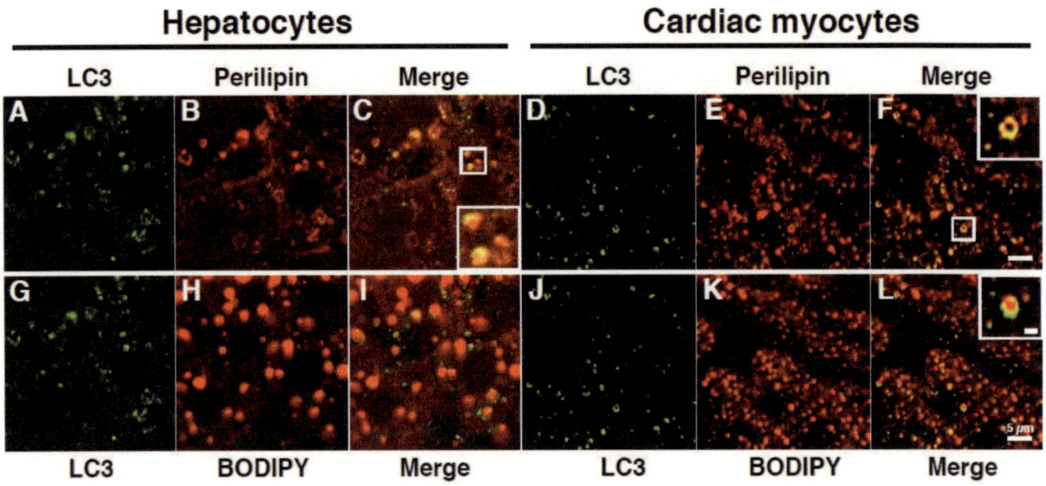

Figure 2. LC3 localizes not only to autophagosomes but also LDs in liver and heart tissues of mice under starvation conditions for 24 hours. (A-L) Double staining of LC3 (green) (A, D, G, J) and perilipin (B, E) or BODIPY (H, K) (red) in liver (A-C, G-I) and heart (D-F, J-L) tissues. Ring-shaped structures that were costained for LC3 and perilipin in boxed areas (C, F) are enlarged in insets. One of the ring-shaped structures that were costained for LC3 and BODIPY in a boxed area (L) was enlarged in an inset. Bar indicates 5 μm (1 μm in inset). This figure is referred from Biochemical and Biophysical Research Communications (Shibata et al., 382 (2009) 419–423).

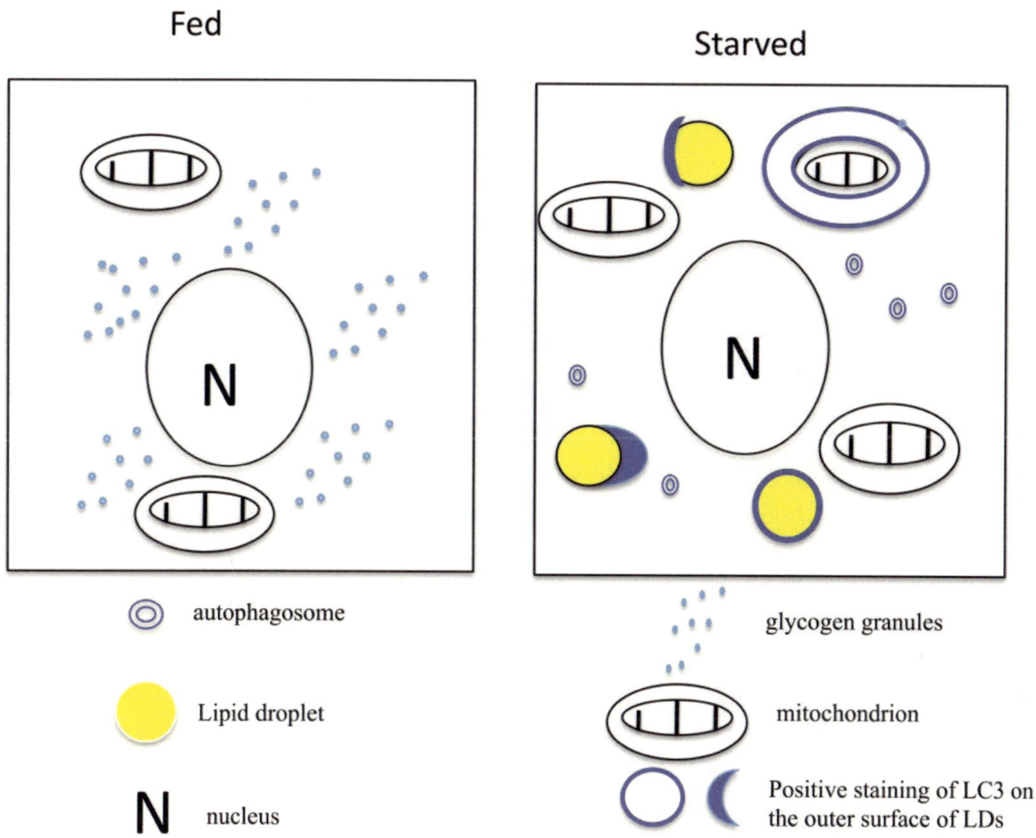

Figure 3. Schematic demonstrations of LC3 staining in cells from mice under fed (left panel) and starved (right panel) conditions. When mice are fed, cells start to produce and store glycogen granules, whereas under starved conditions, lipid droplets are increased and many autophagic granules with double membranes increase in the cytoplasm. In this situation, the lipidated form of LC3 is attached to the isolation membrane of autophagosomes (blue color) and the surface membrane of LDs (yellow). Starvation is further continued, and some mitochondria are enwrapped by the isolation membrane (mitophagy).

	hepatocytes				cardiac myocytes			
Starvation	Apg		LD		Apg		LD	
	24 h	48 h	24 h	48 h	24 h	48 h	24 h	48 h
	++	++	++	++	+/-	+/-	++	+
LC3 (ICH)	++	++	++	++	+/-	-	+	+/-
LC3-II (WB)	++	++	++	++	++	+/-	+	+/-
Mitophagy (EM)	+/-	+				not detected		

Apg, autophagosome; EM, electron microscopy; h, hours; ICH, immunocytochemistry; ++, highly positive; +, positive; +/-, rare; WB, Western blot

Table 1. Morphological changes detected in hepatocytes and cardiac myocytes after starvation

	Liver	heart
lipid fraction		
ADRP	++	++
LC3-II	+	+
Staining of LD in LD fraction from livers with anti-LC3	++	

++, highly positive; +, positive

Table 2. Proteins detected in lipid fractions

In fact, cytosolic LC3 is converted to membrane-bound LC3 (LC3-II) in both hepatocytes and cardiac myocytes 24 hours after the start of starvation. Electron microscopic morphometry reveals that the volume densities of autophagosomes/autolysosomes and LDs increase in hepatocytes 24 and 48 hours after the onset of starvation, whereas autophagosomes and autolysosomes are rarely found in cardiac myocytes and the volume density of LDs is only counted and significantly increased in them [9]. The amounts of TAG in hepatocytes and cardiac myocytes significantly increase after the onset of starvation, whereas the increase in TAG amount is much lower in cardiac myocytes than in hepatocytes and continues until 24 hours. Moreover, LC3 is localized on the surface of LDs and LC3-II (lipidated form) is fractionated into a perilipin and ADRP (LD marker)-positive lipid fraction from the starved liver and cardiac myocytes, respectively. In fact, the surface of such LDs obtained from the LD fraction is labeled by gold particles showing the antigenicity of LC3. Taken together, these results indicate that the LC3 conjugation system is critically involved in lipid metabolism via LD formation.

4. Generation of LDs is inhibited in various LC3 mRNA-knockdown cultured cells

The cytoplasmic LD is an organelle that has a neutral lipid core with a single phospholipid layer. LDs are believed to be generated between the two leaflets of the endoplasmic reticulum (ER) membrane and to play various roles, such as high efficiency energy storage [16]. However, it remains largely unknown how LDs are generated or grow in the cytoplasm. As has been shown previously, the Atg conjugation system that is essential for autophagosome formation is involved in LD formation in hepatocytes and cardiac myocytes. This tendency has also been confirmed in white adipose tissue of conditional Atg7-knockout mice that show less production fat bodies in the tissue [17].

It has been shown that LDs temporally accumulate in the cultured cell lines during proliferation [22]. We have confirmed that LDs are produced in cultured cells seeded at a density of 70% confluency [11]. Accordingly, it has been shown that LDs that are stained with BODIPY are significantly augmented in PC12 cells 12 hours after the start of cultures, while immunosignals for LC3 are colocalized with BODIPY-positive LDs [11]. By immunoelectron microscopy, gold particles indicating LC3 are found on the surface of LDs in PC12 cells. Moreover, by cell fractionation the membrane type of LC3 is demonstrated in the perilipin-positive LD fraction. It still remains unknown whether LC3 itself is involved in LD formation. Since LC3 is a substrate of Atg7, cultured cell lines such as HeLa cells, PC12 cells, HepG2 cells, and Cos-1 cells, were examined to check the relationship of LC3 and LD formation. Expression of LC3 was suppressed by the method of RNA interference (RNAi), and it was found that LD formation is largely inhibited in these cells. TAG, a major component of LDs, is synthesized and degraded in LC3 mRNA-knockdown cells as well as in control cells. Interestingly, the potential for bulk protein degradation in the knockdown-cells is also evident in the control cells.

3T3 L1 cells, a progenitor cell line of adipocytes, accumulate LDs 12 hours after the start of cultures and LD formation is suppressed in the cells when mRNA of LC3 is knocked down [11]. Differentiation of L1 cells into adipocytes is confirmed by the mRNA expression of sterol regulatory element binding factor 1 (SREBF1) and peroxisome proliferator activated receptor γ (PPARγ), adipose specific proteins. It takes 6days until the L1 cells differentiate, and as the cells differentiate, it is found that the amount of LC3 mRNA also increases. In this differentiated situations, the surface of LDs in L1 cells is covered with perilipin and LC3. In LC3 mRNA-knockdown L1 cells, however, BODIPY-positive LDs largely disappear.

These findings indicate that LC3 is involved in the LD formation regardless of the bulk degradation, and that LC3 has two pivotal roles in cellular homeostasis mediated by autophagy and lipid metabolism.

5. Connection between autophagy and lipid metabolism

Recent studies provide supporting evidence for a connection between autophagy and lipid metabolism, both lipid storage and lipolysis. The involvement of autophagy in lipolysis of LDs in hepatocytes has been reported by the groups of Czaja and Cuervo, who showed that loss of Atg7 ($Atg7^{Flox/Flox}$:albumin-Cre mice) results in accumulation of LDs in hepatocytes [18, 23-25]. Lipophagy, which is a form of autophagy that enwraps LDs by the isolation membrane has recently been considered important for the production of FFAs by degrading TAGs under acidic milieu and the FFAs produced fuel cellular rates of mitochondrial β-oxidation [18, 23-25]. This process, called lipophagy has recently been thought to function to regulate intracellular lipid stores, cellular levels of free lipids such as fatty acids and energy homeostasis [25]. On the contrary, as described in this chapter, it has been shown that loss of Atg7 (Atg7$^{Flox/Flox}$:albumin-Cre mice) largely suppresses LD formation in hepatocytes and cardiac myocytes 24 hours after the start of starvation, although numerous LDs accumulate in normal hepatocytes and cardiac myocytes under the same conditions [9] (Fig. 1).

Electron microscopic analysis of wild-type mice by the former group shows LD-containing autophagosomes (lipophagosomes) under starvation conditions, although the latter group indicates that it is hard to see the presence of LDs enwrapped by double membranes even under starvation conditions, and that different from lipophagy, mitophagy can easily be found in hepatocytes if the mice are starved for 48 hours.

Two groups used different experimental approaches in their studies, which may underlie different conclusions. One critical point is to consider that Atg7$^{Flox/Flox}$: albumin-Cre mice cause hepatomegaly and hepatitis with accumulation of abnormal organelles in hepatic cells [26].

Recently, metabolic contributions of amino acids released from liver by starvation-induced autophagy in adult animals using liver-specific Atg7-deficient mice have also been studied systematically [8]. That is, liver specific conditional Atg7-knockout mice (Atg7$^{Flox/Flox}$:Mx1 mice) are generated by the different method from Atg7$^{Flox/Flox}$:albumin-Cre mice [25]. To delete Atg7 from the liver, Cre expression in the liver was induced by intraperitoneal injection of polyinosinic acid-polycytidilic acid (pIpC), while complete deletion of the Atg7 protein in the liver was verified using immunoblotting analyses. Atg7-knockout mice are used 10 days after the injection of pIpC. No sign of hepatomegaly and hepatitis is observed within 2 weeks after the injection of pIpC. For synchronous induction of autophagy in the liver, mice previously fasted for 24 hours and preserve numerous LDs in hepatocytes, are fed by a pelleted laboratory diet for 2 hour (20:00–22:00) in the dark to suppress autophagic activity to a minimum [8]. The diet is then withdrawn and the mice are again starved. In separate experiments, it has been confirmed that the stomach and intestine are filled with a digested diet at the end of the 2 hour-feeding period. In this situation, hepatocytes become to change from the stage of lipogenesis and glycolysis to that of lipolysis and glycogenesis in hepatocytes. Electron microscopic examinations clearly show that in the control mice numerous LDs are continuously present in hepatocytes after 2 hour-feeding, and decrease during starvation [8]. Most LDs disappear in the liver after 24 hours of starvation, while glycogen granules increase in hepatocytes. In contrast, the number of autophagic vacuoles in the liver after 24 hour of starvation is increased dramatically. Such vacuoles and LDs are not observed in liver-specific Atg7-deficient mice [8].

These findings seem to indicate that LDs that accumulate in the liver during 24 hours fasting decrease in parallel with the following activation of autophagy after a 2 hour-feeding , but that loss of autophagy does not inhibit the disappearance of LDs in the liver. Thus another mechanism may operate in the removal of LDs from the liver that accumulated by starvation.

In adipose tissue, knock out of either Atg7 [9] or Atg5 [17] leads to reduced accumulation of lipid and impaired differentiation of adipocytes. The mutant white adipocytes are smaller with multiple LDs. It has been suggested that Atg5 deletion causes adipogenesis arrest at the later stages of mouse embryos. The possibility that a defect of Atg5-dependent Atg8 (LC3) lipidation and translocation to LDs of adipocytes may result in inefficient droplet fusion, which contributes to the defect of adipogenesis cannot be ruled out. The same authors observed reduced differentiation in Atg 5-deficient mouse embryonic fibroblasts (MEFs) model. An essential role of autophagy in lipid storage is also suggested in fat body cells of Drosophila. Knockdown of Atg1 or Atg6 led to small lipid droplets [27]. The paper has also indicated that Rab32 may regulate lipid storage by affecting autophagy [27]. Rab32 and several other Rabs have been found to affect the size of lipid droplets [27] and the mechanism of droplet fusion with atg8 (LC3) and Rab families awaits further studies. Thus, in adipocytes autophagy may contribute to LD formation and not significantly to lipolysis.

For hydrolysis of TAG in LDs of adipocytes, the molecular processes of lipolysis are becoming clear. Adipose tissue TAG lipase first acts on TAG to hydrolyze a fatty acyl chain [28]. Hormone sensitive lipase mediates the second step of lipolysis, diacylglycerol cleavage to monoacylglycerol. Finally monoacylglycerol lipase hydrolyzes the last side chain.

6. Concluding remarks

Lipid droplets (LDs) are key cellular organelles involved in lipid storage and mobilization. In non-adipocytes, LDs are small, mobile and interact with other cellular compartments. In contrast, adipocytes primarily contain very large, immotile LDs. The marked morphological differences between LDs in adipocytes and non-adipocytes suggest that key differences must exist in the manner in which LDs in different cell types interact with other organelles and undergo fusion and fission with other droplets. It has suggested that droplet fusion is dependent on microtubules, the motor protein dynein [29], Rab proteins [27] and the SNARE fusion machinery [31].

PAT proteins also target to the surface of LDs likely through different mechanisms. In adipocytes, TIP47 is found on smaller droplets and perilipin is found on larger LDs [31]. They may bind to different droplets associated proteins. Cleaved (and lipidated) LC3 demonstrated on isolated LDs from non-adipocytes [9] may be involved in LDs biology as well as PAT proteins (Figs. 2 and 3). Nakatogawa et al. [32] have shown that lipidated ATG8 (yeast homologue of LC3) mediates tethering between adjacent membranes of liposomes and stimulates membrane hemifusion, an event that may mimic expansion of the autophagosomal membrane during autophagy (Fig. 4). In LDs, homotropic interactions in adipocytes and non-adipocytes may involve a hemifusion type mechanism to facilitate lipid transfer (Fig.4). In adipocytes lipidated LC3 may also involved in growth of LDs (Fig. 4), as shown by morphological evidence that the mutant white adipocytes are smaller with multiple LDs [17].

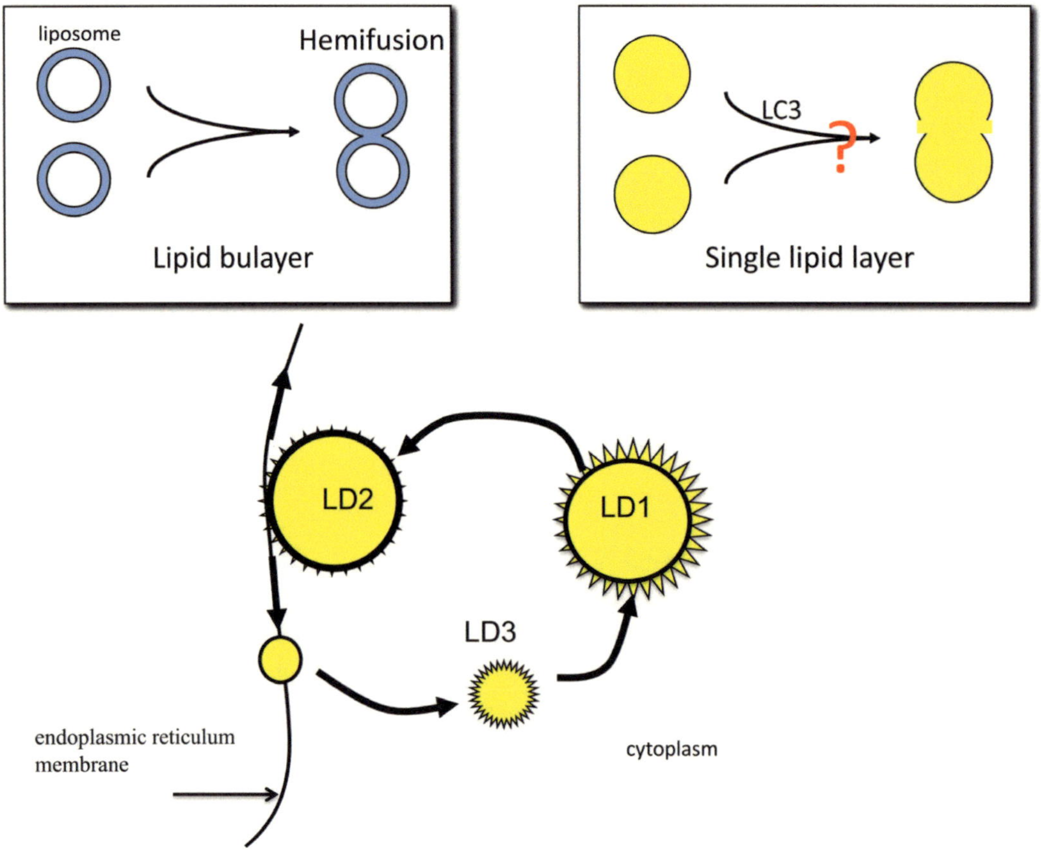

Figure 4. As shown by Murphy [16], a large LD3 that is attached to the endoplasmic reticulum may be degraded by ER-associated lipases and TAG may be re-synthesized. Newly formed LD1 would re-grow as LD2 in the cytoplasm. As has been shown by Nakatogawa et al. [32], bilayered liposomes with Atg8 undergo hemifusion (left upper), since Atg8 molecules are oligomerized with each other. If LC3 molecules are oligomelized on the surface of LDs (right upper), LDs would undergo fusion and grow in size.

It must be readdressed whether autophagy may affect lipid metabolism in a tissue- or cell-specific manner. If autophagy functions and regulates lipogenesis or lipolysis in a different way in non-adipocytes, it must be answered what molecular mechanisms work by which the autophagic machinery recognize LDs to enwrap for degradation or fuse with each other, and how they are regulated.

Author details

Yasuo Uchiyama and Eiki Kominami
Departments of Cell Biology and Neurosciences, and Biochemistry,
Juntendo University Graduate School of Medicine, Bunkyo-ku, Tokyo, Japan

Acknowledgement

This paper was supported by Grants-in-Aid for Scientific Research (B), (23390041) and partly for Scientific Research on Innovative Areas (23111004), and by MEXT-supported Program for the Strategic Research Foundation at Private Universities.

7. References

[1] Komatsu M, Waguri S, Chiba T, Murata S, Iwata J, Ueno Koike M, Uchiyama Y, Kominami E, Tanaka K. Loss of autophagy in the central nervous system causes neurodegeneration. Nature 2006 441: 880-884
[2] Komatsu M, Koike M, Ichimura Y, Uchiyama Y. Genetic mouse models for elucidation of autophagy-lysosomal systems in neurons under physiologic and pathologic conditions. In Ed. Zhenyu Yue, Charleen Chu: Autophagy of the nervous system – Cellular self-digestion in neurons and neurological diseases. World Scientific. (in press)
[3] Komatsu, M, Ueno, T, Waguri, S, Uchiyama, Y, Kominami, E, Tanaka, K. Constitutive autophagy: vital role in clearance of unfavorable proteins in neurons. Cell Death and Differentiation 2007 14:887-894
[4] Uchiyama Y, Shibata M, Koike M, Yoshimura K, Sasaki M. Autophagy - Physiology and Pathophysiology. Histochemistry and Cell Biology 2008 129: 407-420
[5] Mizushima M, Komatsu M. Autophagy: renovation of cells and tissues. Cell 2011 147:728-741
[6] Komatsu M, Waguri S, Koike M, Sou1 Y, Ueno T, Hara H, Mizushima N, Iwata J, Ezaki J, Murata S, Hamazaki J, Nishito Y, Iemura S, Natsume T, Yanagawa T, Uwayama J, Warabi E, Yoshida H, Ishii T, Kobayashi A, Yamamoto M, Yue Z, Uchiyama Y, Kominami E, Tanaka T. Homeostatic levels of p62 control cytoplasmic inclusion body formation in autophagy-deficient mice. Cell 2007 131: 1149-1163
[7] Mortimore GE, Pösö AR. Intracellular protein catabolism and its control during nutrient deprivation and supply. Annual Review of Nutrition 1987 7:539–564

[8] Ezaki J, Matsumoto N, Takeda-Ezaki M, Komatsu M, Takahashi K, Hiraoka Y, Taka H, Fujimura T, Takehana K, Yoshida M, Iwata J, Tanida I, Furuya N, Zheng DM, Tada N, Tanaka K, Kominami E, Ueno T. Liver autophagy contributes to the maintenance of blood glucose and amino acid levels. Autophagy 2011 7:727-736

[9] Shibata M, Yoshimura K, Furuya M, Koike M, Ueno T, Komatsu M, Arai H, Tanaka K, Kominami E, Uchiyama Y. The MAP1-LC3 conjugation system is involved in lipid droplet formation. Biochemical and Biophysical Research Communication 2009 382: 419-423

[10] Gotoh K, Lu Z, Morita M, Shibata M, Koike M, Waguri S, DonoK, DokiY, Kominami E, Sugioka A, Monden M, Uchiyama Y. Participation of autophagy in the initiation of graft dysfunction after rat liver transplantation. Autophagy 2009 5:351-360

[11] Shibata M, Yoshimura K, Tamura H, Ueno T, Nishimura T, Inoue T, Sasaki M, Koike M, Arai H, Kominami E, Uchiyama Y. LC3, a microtubule-associated protein1A/B light chain3, is involved in cytoplasmic lipid droplet formation. Biochemical and Biophysical Research Communication 2010 393:274-279

[12] Koike M, Shibata S, Tadakoshi T, Gotoh K, Komatsu M, Waguri S, Kawahara N, Kuida K, Nagata S, Kominami E, Tanaka K, Uchiyama Y. Inhibition of autophagy prevents hippocampal pyramidal neuron death after hypoxic-ischemic injury. American Journal of Pathology 2008 172: 454-469

[13] Koike M, Shibata M, Waguri S, Yoshimura K, Tanida I, Kominami E, Gotow G, Peters C, Figura Kv, Mizushima N, Saftig P and Uchiyama Y. Participation of autophagy in storage of lysosomes in neurons from mouse models of neuronal ceroid-lipofuscinoses (Batten disease). American Journal of Pathology 2005 167:1713-1728

[14] Martin S, Driessen K, Nixon SJ, Zerial M, Parton RG. Regulated localization of Rab18 to lipid droplets: effects of lipolytic stimulation and inhibition of lipid droplet catabolism. Journal of Biological Chemistry 2005 280:42325–42335

[15] Thiele C, Spandl J. Cell biology of lipid droplets. Current Opinion in Cell Biology 2008 20:378–385

[16] Murphy DJ. The biogenesis and functions of lipid bodies in animals, plants and microorganisms. Progress in Lipid Research 2001 40:325–438

[17] Zhang Y, Goldmana S, Baergaa R, Zhaoa Y, Komatsu M, Jin S. Adipose-specific deletion of autophagy-related gene 7 (atg7) in mice reveals a role in adipogenesis. Proceedings of the National Academy of Sciences of the United States of America 2009 106:19860–19865

[18] Singh R, Cuervo AM. Lipophagy: Connecting autophagy and lipid metabolism. International Journal of Cell Biology 2012 2012:1-12

[19] Uchiyama Y, Asari A. A morphometric study of the variations in subcellular structures of rat hepatocytes during 24 hours. Cell and Tissue Research 1984 236:305-315

[20] Waguri S, Kohmura M, Kanamori S, Watanabe T, Ohsawa Y, Koike M, Tomiyama Y, Wakasugi M, Kominami E, Uchiyama Y. Different distribution patterns of the two

mannose 6-phosphate receptors in rat liver. Journal of Histochemistry and Cytochemistry 2001 49: 1397-1405

[21] Mizushima N, Yamamoto A, Matsui M, Yoshimori T, Ohsumi Y. In vivo analysis of autophagy in response to nutrient starvation using transgenic mice expressing a fluorescent autophagosome marker. Molecular Biology of Cell 2004 15:1101–1111.

[22] Swinnen JV, Brusselmans K, Verhoeven G. Increased lipogenesis in cancer cells: new players, novel targets, Current Opinion in Clinical Nutrition and Metabolic Care 2006 9:358–365.

[23] Singh R, Kaushik S, Wang Y, Xiang Y, Novak I, Komatsu M, Tanaka K, Cuervo AM, Czaja MJ. Autophagy regulates lipid metabolism. Nature 2009 458:1131-1135

[24] Singh R, Xiang Y, Wang Y, Baikati K, Cuervo AM, Luu YK, Tang Y, Pessin JE, Schwartz GJ, Czaja MJ. Autophagy regulates adipose mass and differentiation in mice. Journal of Clinical Investigation 2009 119:3329-39

[25] Liu K, Czaja MJ. Regulation of lipid stores and metabolism by lipophagy. Cell Death and Differentiation 2012 doi:10.1038/cdd.2012.63

[26] Komatsu M, Waguri S, Ueno T, Iwata J, Murata S, Tanida I, Ezaki J, Mizushima N, Ohsumi Y, Uchiyama Y, Kominami E, Tanaka K, Chiba T. Impairment of starvation-induced and constitutive autophagy in Atg7-deficient mice. Journal of Cell Biology 2065 169: 425–434

[27] Wang C, Liu Z, Huang X. Rab32 Is Important for Autophagy and Lipid Storage in Drosophila. PLos ONE 2012 7e32086

[28] Zimmermann R, Strauss JG, Haemmerle G, Schoiswohl G, Birner-Gruenberger R, Riederer M, Lass A, Neuberger G, Eisenhaber F, Hermetter A, and Zechner R. Fat mobilization in adipose tissue is promoted by adipose triglyceride lipase. Science 2004 306;1383–1386

[29] Mendis-Handagama SMLC, Aten RF, Watkins PA, Scallen TJ, Berhman RH. Peroxisomes and sterol carrier protein-2 in luteal cell steroidogenesis: a possible role in cholesterol transport from lipid droplets to mitochondria. Tissue and Cell 1095 27+483-490

[30] Boström P, Rutberg M, Ericsson J, Holmdahl P, Andersson L, Frohman M, Borén J, Olofsson S. Cytosolic lipid droplets increase in size by microtubule-dependent complex formation. Arteriosclerosis, Thrombosis and Vascular Biology 2005 25:1945–1951.

[31] Boström P, Andersson Rutberg LM, Perman Lidberg JU, Johansson BR, Fernandez-Rodriguez J, Ericson j, Nilsson T, Boren j, Olofsson SO. SNARE proteins mediate fusion between cytosolic lipid droplets and are implicated in insulin sensitivity. Nature Cell Biology 2007 9:1286–1293

[32] Wolins N, Quaynor B, Skinner J, Schoenfish M, Tzekov A, Bickel P. S3-12, adipophilin, and TIP47 package lipid in adipocytes. Journal of Biological Chemistry 2005 280:19146–19155

[33] Nakatogawa H, Ichimura Y, Ohsumi Y. Atg8, a ubiquitin-like protein required for autophagosome formation, mediates membrane tethering and hemifusion. Cell 2007 130:165–178

Chapter 8

Metabolism of Short Chain Fatty Acids in the Colon and Faeces of Mice After a Supplementation of Diets with Agave Fructans

Alicia Huazano-García and Mercedes G. López

Additional information is available at the end of the chapter

http://dx.doi.org/10.5772/51248

1. Introduction

1.1. Fructans

Most plants store starch or sucrose as reserve carbohydrates, but approximately 12-15% of higher plants (representing more than 40,000 species) synthesizes fructans as their main source of carbohydrates [1]. Fructans are found naturally in plants as a heterogeneous mixture of different polymerization degrees, they are a polydisperse mixture. Among plants that store fructans, many are economically important, due to its content of fructans, as it is the case of chicory (*Cichorium intybus*), agave (*Agave spp.*), artichoke (*Cynara scolymus*), dahlia (*Dahlia variabilis*), garlic (*Allium sativum*) and wheat (*Triticum asetivum*) [2, 3]. Five different groups of fructans have been found in nature and distinguished according to the type of linkage between fructose units and the position of the glucose moiety within the structure. These groups consist of inulins, neoseries inulins, levans, neoseries levans and graminans. Inulins consist of a linear β(2-1) linked fructosyl chain; neoseries inulins are composed of two linear β(2-1) linked fructosyl chains, one bound to the fructosyl residue of the sucrose, the other bound to the glucosyl residue of the same sucrose molecule; levans consist a of linear β(2-6) linked fructosyl chain; neoseries levans are composed of two linear β(2-6) linked fructosyl chains, one bound to the fructosyl residue of the sucrose, the other bound to the glucosyl residue and graminans which present both linkages, β(2-1) and β(2-6) links to the fructose moiety of sucrose [4].

Currently, inulins are extracted from chicory roots, containing fructose chains having a degree of polymerization (DP) from 3 to 60 [2] (Figure 1a). The chemical or enzymatic (endoinulinases) hydrolysis of inulins produces inulins of shorter DP (DP<10), these are called fructooligosaccharides (FOS) [5, 6].

Mexico is considered the origin center of evolution and diversification of the *Agave genus*, since a large number of agave species are found in its territory. The *Agave genus* includes approximately 166 species and is the largest *genus* among the *Agavaceae* family that consists of 9 genera and approximately 293 species [7, 8]. The agave plants have the ability to grow in extremely dry-hot environments, where sometimes this plant is the predominant or exclusive flora in that type of a geo-climatic zone, however, they can also be found in diverse ecosystems, such as productive highlands and elevated humidity [9]. These plants present a crassulacean acid metabolism (CAM) and their principal photosynthetic products are fructans [10], fructans are synthesized and stored in the stems of agave plants. Agave is the most exploited genus and economically important as the raw materials are used on the production of alcoholic beverages such tequila (*A. tequilana*) and mezcal (*A. angustifolia, A. potatorum, A. cantala, A. duranguensis,* to mention some) in Mexico. *A. angustifolia* is an endemic plant that grows in different states of Mexico; however the main producing states are Oaxaca and Sonora. Fructans in *A. angustifolia* from Oaxaca represent more than 85% of total water soluble carbohydrates in the plant, with an estimated DP of 32 [11].

Agave fructans posses a molecular structure compose of a complex mixture containing highly branched molecules with β(2-1) and β(2-6) linkages, as well as internal and external glucose units, due to the existence of both types of glucose, agave fructans have been classified as graminans (external glucose) and agavins (internal glucose) [11] (Figure 1b).

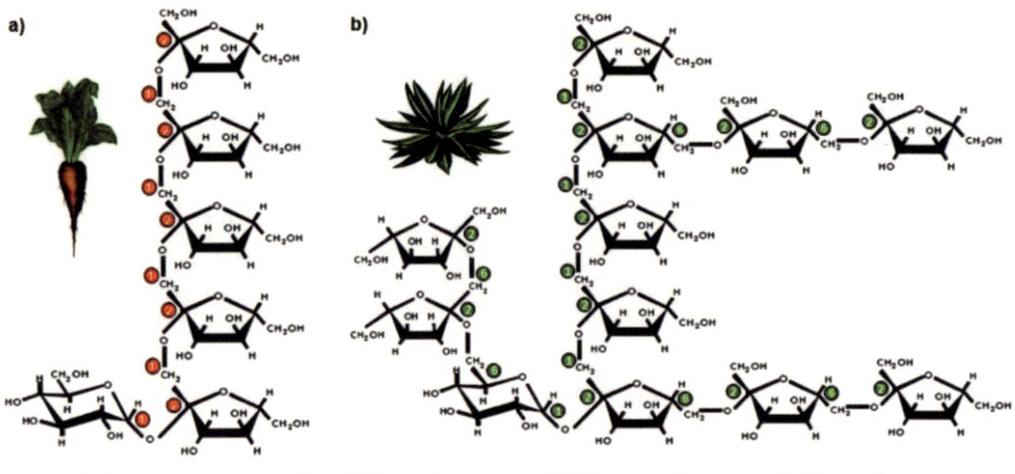

Figure 1. Schematic representation of the main structural differences between a) chicory fructans, "inulins" and b) agave fructans, "agavins".

All fructans are considered prebiotics molecules that serve as a substrate for the gut microbiota [6, 12-15]. A prebiotic is an ingredient selectively fermented by probiotics (*bifidobacteria* and *lactobacilli*) that induces specific changes on the composition and/or activity of the gastrointestinal microbiota, conferring benefits upon the host well-being and health in general [16, 17]. The fermentation of fructans in the colon generates short chain fatty acids (SCFAs). SCFAs formation is an important event since it favors the maintenance and the development of beneficial microbiota as well as the colonic epithelial cells [16].

1.2. Short chain fatty acids (SCFAs)

The gastrointestinal tract is an extremely complex ecosystem containing about 10^{11} CFU (colony forming units) of bacteria per gram of intestinal content. This large population of bacteria plays a key role in the nutrition and health of the host [18]. The colonic microbiota ferments organic material that cannot be digested otherwise by the host in the upper gut. These include resistant starch, non-digestible carbohydrates (fructans) as well as some proteins and amino acids [19]. The main products of fructans metabolism in the colon are linear SCFAs, mostly acetate ($C_{2:0}$), propionate ($C_{3:0}$) and butyrate ($C_{4:0}$) [19-21] (Figure 2). However, other fermentation products may be lactate, succinate as well as ethanol [6], which are sometimes only intermediates in the global process of carbohydrates fermentation by the microbiota, and are metabolized in varying degrees to SCFAs by interactions and/or collaboration of present bacteria in the ecosystem, so that generally do not accumulate to any significant extent in the colon [22]. Fructans fermentation also produces a few gases as CO_2, CH_4, H_2 and additionally heat [19, 23]. The presence of both, non-digestible carbohydrates and SCFAs in the colon can positively alter the colonic physiology drastically [24]. Various studies on microbial population have shown that SCFAs production is in the order of $C_{2:0} > C_{3:0} > C_{4:0}$ in a molar ratio of approximately 60:20:20 mainly in the proximal and distal colon [19, 25]. An increased in SCFAs synthesis also creates a more acidic environment in the gut, which is important *in vivo* in terms of colonization resistance against pathogens [18, 20]. The production of SCFAs is affected by many factors, including the source of substrate [26], in particular, the chemical composition of the fermentable substrate, the amount of substrate available, its physical form (e.g. particle size, solubility, association with undigestible complexes such as lignin) [27], the bacterial species composition of the microbiota [12], ecological factors (competitive and cooperative interactions between different groups of bacteria) and intestinal transit time [25]. The gut of mice comprises four sections: caecum, proximal, transverse (medial) and distal colon. The caecum and proximal colon are the main sites where fermentation is carried out, given the number of bacteria and the availability of substrate, because as it moves through the intestine toward the distal colon, there is a lower concentration of water as well as a depletion of carbohydrates and increased pH [22]. SCFAs are rapidly absorbed in the caecum and colon being excreted in the faeces only from 5% to 10% of them [24]. The major SCFAs ($C_{2:0}$, $C_{3:0}$ and $C_{4:0}$), are absorbed at comparable rates in different regions of the colon. Once absorbed, SCFAs are metabolized at three major sites in the body: 1) cells of the caecum-colonic epithelium that use $C_{4:0}$ as a major substrate for maintenance-energy; 2) liver cells that metabolize residual $C_{4:0}$ and $C_{3:0}$ used for gluconeogenesis and 50% to 70% of $C_{2:0}$ is also taken up by the liver; and 3) muscle cells that generate energy from the oxidation of residual $C_{2:0}$ [3].

1.2.1. Acetic ($C_{2:0}$), propionic ($C_{3:0}$) and butyric ($C_{4:0}$) acids

$C_{2:0}$ is the principal SCFA produced in the colon, this is readily absorbed and transported to the liver, and therefore is less metabolized in the colon [26]. The presence of acetyl-CoA synthetase in the cytosol of adipose and mammary glands allows the use of $C_{2:0}$ for lipogenesis once it enters the systemic circulation [24]. $C_{2:0}$ is the primary substrate for cholesterol synthesis. In the host, it may be absorbed and utilized by peripheral tissues also [29].

On the other hand, $C_{3:0}$ is produced via two main pathways: 1) by fixation of CO_2 to form succinate, which is subsequently decarboxylated (the "dicarboxylic acid pathway") and 2) forms lactate and acrylate (the "acrilate pathway") [30]. $C_{3:0}$ is also a substrate for hepatic gluconeogenesis and it has been reported that this acid inhibits cholesterol synthesis in hepatic tissue [31, 32]. The ratio of $C_{3:0}$ to $C_{2:0}$ in the colon is relevant since it lowers cholesterol synthesis coming from the $C_{2:0}$ pathway [32].

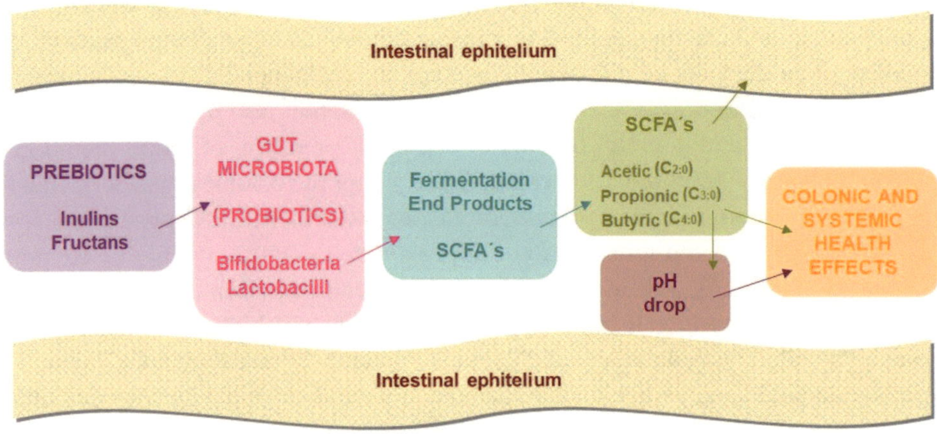

Figure 2. General events taken place in the large intestine. Prebiotics are the specific food for probiotics which ferment them to produce short chain fatty acids (SCFAs) to improve the host health.

Finally, $C_{4:0}$ is the preferred fuel by the colonic epithelial cells but also plays a major role in the regulation of cell proliferation and differentiation [19]. It is the most important SCFA in colonocytes metabolism, where 70% to 90% of $C_{4:0}$ is metabolized by the colonocytes. $C_{4:0}$ is used preferentially over $C_{3:0}$ and $C_{2:0}$ in a ratio of 90:30:50 [26]. Approximately 95% of the $C_{4:0}$ produced by colonic bacteria is transported across the epithelium, but concentrations in portal blood are usually undetectable as a result of a rapid utilization [33]. $C_{4:0}$ production might also occur through the use of other fermentation products such as $C_{2:0}$ or lactate that can act as precursors of $C_{4:0}$.

1.2.2. Production of SCFAs in vitro

In vitro SCFAs production can be measured using pure cultures of selected bacteria species of faecal slurry and some prebiotics (undigestible carbohydrates, for instance).

a. Inulins

Studies *in vitro* using faecal inocula incubation have shown that different substrates (prebiotics) yield various SCFAs patterns; Van de Wiele et al. [34] compared the fermentation of FOS and inulin *in vitro* with faecal inoculum, observing that FOS and inulin increased the production of SCFAs by about 30%. This increment in SCFAs production was attributed to an increase mainly in $C_{3:0}$ and $C_{4:0}$ acids. Where inulin showed a higher production of $C_{3:0}$ acid (almost 2-fold) than FOS. The authors concluded that these differences correlated well with the structural differences, FOS has a short DP and inulin a long DP. Stewart et al. [35] analyzed the fermentation of inulins with three different chain lengths (short, medium and long). These researchers found that short inulins were rapidly fermented and produced higher concentrations of $C_{4:0}$ compared with other inulins, hence, chain length is an important factor on the fermentation patterns of SCFAs (Table 1). Rycroft et al. [36] performed a comparative evaluation of different prebiotics *in vitro*, they observed that all the used substrates presented an increased concentration of $C_{2:0}$ acid. Inulins generated the highest concentrations of $C_{3:0}$ acid, but a mixture of FOS and inulin showed the highest production of $C_{4:0}$ acid than the other prebiotics by themselves. The differences in SCFAs patterns in these studies may be also attributed to differences in bacteria species present in the faecal inocula or fermentation process used.

Sample	DP (mean)	Time	$C_{2:0}$*		$C_{3:0}$*		$C_{4:0}$*	
			Mean	SEM	Mean	SEM	Mean	SEM
A	< 5	12 h	22.3^{a}	0.50	5.3^{a}	0.20	12.8^{a}	0.20
		24 h	16.9^{ab}	0.10	2.1	0.10	9.1^{a}	0.30
B	= 4.8	12 h	20.2^{ab}	1.50	4.1^{bc}	0.02	10.2^{b}	0.50
		24 h	15.1^{bd}	0.03	1.8	0.20	9.0^{a}	0.40
C	< 10	12 h	26.8^{a}	0.60	4.7^{ab}	0.20	12.8^{a}	0.30
		24 h	20.9^{c}	0.80	2.7	0.30	9.6^{a}	0.10
D	≈ 10	12 h	20.0^{ab}	0.10	2.1^{d}	0.10	9.3^{b}	0.20
		24 h	14.4^{d}	0.40	1.8	1.00	8.7^{a}	0.30
E	> 10	12 h	19.9^{ab}	1.30	3.6^{c}	0.10	9.2^{b}	0.02
		24 h	25.1^{a}	0.04	3.8	0.10	9.3^{a}	0.10
F	> 20	12 h	14.0^{b}	2.10	0.8^{e}	0.20	5.4^{c}	0.10
		24 h	18.7^{a}	0.20	2.4	0.10	6.8^{b}	0.10

*Concentration μmol/mL. Values with different letter within a time point are statistically different from each other ($P<0.05$). [35, with modifications].

Table 1. Concentration of acetic ($C_{2:0}$), propionic ($C_{3:0}$) and butyric ($C_{4:0}$) acids obtained after 12 and 24 h *in vitro* fermentation batch with inulins of different chain length.

b. Agave fructans

Urías-Silvas & López [37] analyzed the prebiotic potential of fructans extracted from five different species of *Agave* spp. grown in different regions of Mexico, *Dasylirion* sp. and commercial inulins, using strains of *bifidobacteria* and *lactobacilli*. These researchers found that branched fructans from *Dasylirion* (DSC) with a DP range from 3 to 20 and *A. tequilana* from the state of Guanajuato (ATG) with a DP between 3 and 22, stimulated better the growth of both bacteria genera in MRS medium (Figure 3). Moreover, the major SCFAs fermentation product, were acetic, formic and lactic acids, wherein the proportions of the acids varied depending on the prebiotic type used by the different bacteria. Figure 4 shows the fermentation products only for the two agave fructans (DSC and ATG) and commercial inulins (RSE and RNE) that better stimulated the growth of bacteria. In general, in figure 4 it can be observed that the branched fructans (agavins) were able to produce more acids than the linear fructans (inulins).

Santiago-García & López [38] studied the *in vitro* prebiotic effect of fructans from *A. angustifolia* of long-DP, short-DP and three combinations of them. The growth rate of *bifidobateria* and *lactobacilli* strains with *A. angustifolia* fructans was compared with commercial inulins (Raftiline and Raftilose). The authors observed that agave fructans stimulated the growth of *bifidobacteria* and *lactobacilli* more efficiently (2-fold) that commercial inulins, either long- or short-DP. They also reported that short-DP fructans in the mixtures highly influenced the rate of fermentation by probiotc bacteria. In this work, the main fermentation product in all treatments was $C_{2:0}$ acid. Moreover, Gomez et al. [39] compared the growth of *bifidobacteria* and *lactobacilli* on a complex faecal microbiota *in vitro* using fructans extracted from *A. tequilana Weber* var. azul and different commercial inulins. Their results indicated no significant differences among the growth of both bacteria genera with the different fructans used. With regard to the total SCFAs production by agave fructans and inulins was very similar. $C_{2:0}$ acid was the most prevalent SCFA in all treatments, only agave fructans and inulin of long-DP produced significantly higher amounts of $C_{3:0}$, however, there were no significant differences between the different fructans used.

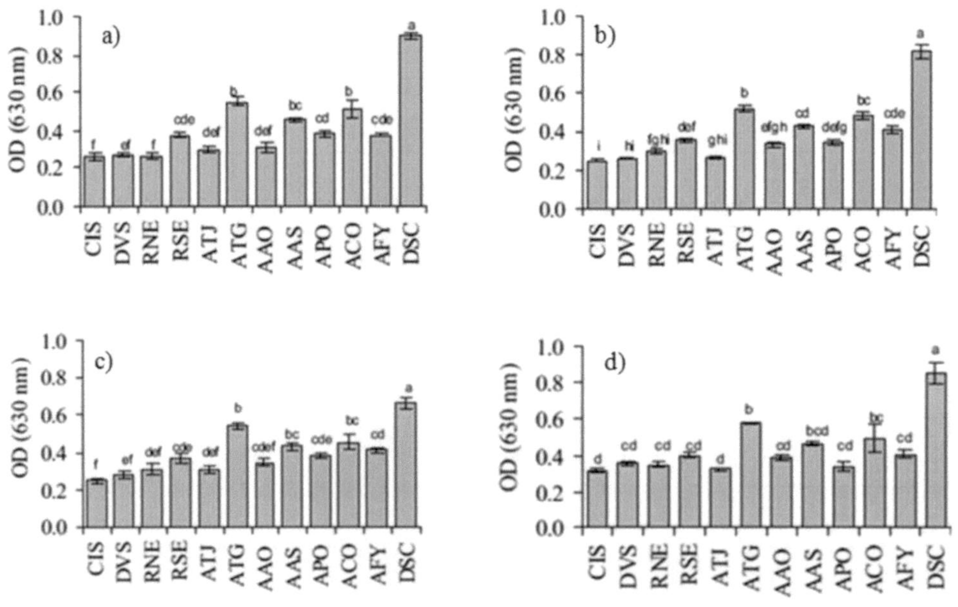

Figure 3. Effect of different fructans on the growth of **a)** *B. adolescentis;* **b)** *B. infantis;* **c)** *L. paracasei* and **d)** *L. rhamnosus* incubated anaerobically at 37°C in the presence of 10 g of fructan/L. OD, Optical density; CIS, *Cichorium intybus;* DVS, *Dahlia variabilis;* RNE, Raftiline; RSE, Raftilose; ATJ, *A. tequilana* Jalisco; ATG, *A. tequilana* Guanajuato; AAO, *A. angustifolia* Oaxaca; AAS, *A. angustifolia* Sonora; APO, *A. potatorum* Oaxaca; ACO, *A. cantala* Oaxaca; AFY, *A. fourcroydes* Yucatán; DSC, *Dasylirion* sp. Chihuahua.

1.2.3. *Production of SCFAs in vivo*

a. Inulins

Nilsson and Nyman [40] evaluated the formation of SCFAs in the hindgut of rats fed with lactulose, lactitol, FOS and inulins of different DP and solubility. The major acids formed were $C_{2:0}$, $C_{3:0}$ and $C_{4:0}$. The highest levels of $C_{3:0}$ acid were found in caecum and proximal and distal colon of rats fed with inulins, whereas the highest levels of $C_{4:0}$ acid were found in caecum and proximal and distal colon of rats fed with FOS. The authors concluded that the DP and solubility of the used prebiotics were of great importance on SCFAs production.

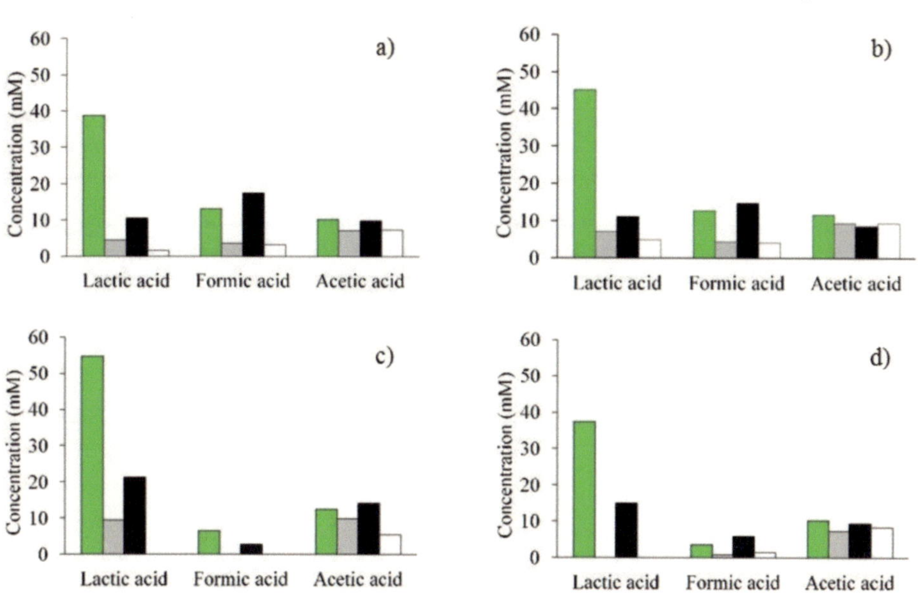

Figure 4. Concentration of short chain fatty acids generated by *bifidobacteria* and *lactobacilli* from the fermentation of *Dasylirion* sp. (DSC;■), Raftilose (RSE;■), *A. tequilana* GTO. (ATG;■) and Raftiline (RNE;□). **a)** *B. adolescentis;* **b)** *B. infantis;* **c)** *L. paracasei* and **d)** *L. rhamnosus.*

Similar results were obtained by Licht et al. [41] who fed rats with different dietary carbohydrates. These authors concluded that $C_{3:0}$ acid concentrations reached statistical significance in animals fed with inulins, whereas the concentration of $C_{4:0}$ acid was significantly higher in animals receiving FOS. Klessen et al. [42] also determined the production of SCFAs in the caecum and colon of germ-free rats associated with contents of human faecal, the rats were fed with inulins of different chain lengths (FOS, inulins and a mixture of FOS-inulins). They observed that FOS produced the greatest amount of $C_{2:0}$ acid in the colon of the rats whereas inulins increased the concentration of $C_{3:0}$ acid in the caecum of the animals that consumed this diet. Moreover, FOS, inulins and the mixture of FOS-inulins increased the amount of $C_{4:0}$ acid in the caecum and colon of the rats fed with the mixture regard to animals fed with standard diet. The authors concluded that the type of diet and the fermentation site in the colon affected the concentration of SCFAs (Table 2). In another work, Levrat et al. [43] fed rats with different percentages of inulins (5, 10 and 20%), finding that $C_{2:0}$ acid production was significantly lower in rats fed with 20% inulin diet. Moreover, all percentages of inulin increased the levels of $C_{3:0}$ acid in the caecum of the rats; the highest concentration was found in animals that consumed the 10% inulin diet whereas $C_{4:0}$ acid concentration was markedly enhanced in all supplemented diets in spite of the inulin percentage used. In another study, the same authors fed rats with 10% of inulin, they found a higher concentration of $C_{3:0}$ acid in the portal vein as well as a significant decrease in plasma cholesterol levels of the rats fed with this diet with regard to animals that consumed the standard diet [44]. On the other hand, a study carried out using obese rats that received a diet supplement with inulin, a two-fold greater $C_{3:0}$ concentration in the portal vein and a decrement on triglyceride accumulation in the liver of these animals was observed [45]. A similar result was seen in hamsters fed with different percentages of inulins (8, 12 and 16%). Plasma cholesterol and triglyceride concentrations were significantly lower with all the percentages of inulins studied with respect to hamsters fed with the standard diet [46].

Acid	**Segment**	**Diet**				**Pooled SEM**
		Standard	**FOS**	**Inulin**	**Mix (FOS-Inulin)²**	
	Caecum	49.8	55.4	45.9	51.2	1.3
$C_{2:0}$¹	Colon	41.1	50.8*	42.5	46.7	1.2
	Faeces	37.4	35.1	35.6	27.6*	1.3
	Caecum	21.1	22.8	32.5*	19.1	0.8
$C_{3:0}$¹	Colon	18.2	17.8	21.3	16.8	0.7
	Faeces	14.7	15.5	14.4	15.8	0.4
	Caecum	13.4	21.3*	25.4*	28.0*	1.3
$C_{4:0}$¹	Colon	9.3	18.6*	18.1*	22.3*	1.2
	Faeces	7.1	11.4	13.6*	15.7*	0.9

Mean values n=6; ¹Concentrations [μmol/g wet wt]; ²Mix FOS-Inulin (1:1 w/w). Mean values were significantly different from those of the standard diet group: *P<0.05. [42, with modifications].

Table 2. Production of short chain fatty acids in the caecum, colon and faeces in rats associated with human faecal contents and fed with inulins of different chain lengths.

b. Agave fructans

To date, there are no published reports on the production of SCFAs *in vivo* using agave fructans of any species. However, the physiological effects of fructans extracted from *A. tequilana* Gto. (ATG) and *Dasylirion* sp. (DSC) have shown that agave fructans positively impact some lipid metabolic molecules such triglycerides and cholesterol on serum of mice fed with diets supplemented with these types of fructans (Figure 5) they also affect glucose levels [47]. These effects were attributed to the production of $C_{3:0}$, which is largely produced through the fermentation of all fructans.

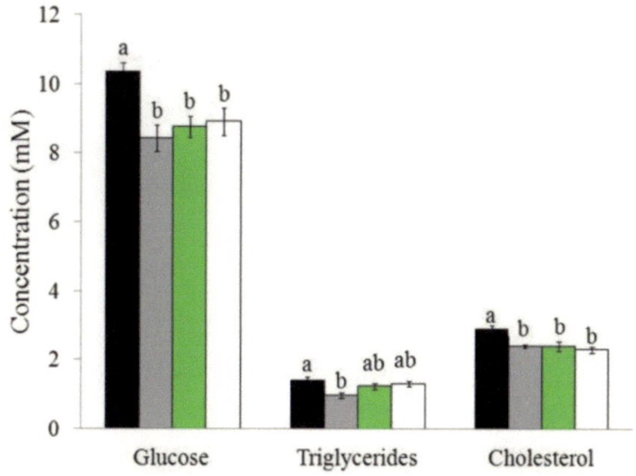

Figure 5. Concentration of glucose, triglycerides and cholesterol in mice after consumption of a standard diet (STD;■) or diet supplemented with fructans: chicory (RSE;□); *A. tequilana* Gto. (ATG;□) and *Dasylirion* sp. (DSC;□). Mean values n=8 with their standard errors of the mean for each parameter measured. Mean values with different letters were significantly different (P≤0.05).

In another study with fructans of *Dasylirion* sp. (DSC) and commercial inulin Raftilose (RSE), García-Pérez [48] reported that the diets supplemented with fructans had a beneficial effect on the concentration of glucose and cholesterol in blood of the portal vein of mice. Glucose concentrations were significantly lowered by 22 and 27% in mice fed DAS and RSE diets with respect to mice fed a standard diet. Cholesterol concentrations were also reduced by 20% in animals receiving DSC and 14% in mice fed RSE diet. However, levels of triglycerides were not significantly modified by any treatment. In this same study, SCFAs were determined only in faeces (Figure 6). In general, mice fed diets supplemented with DSC present higher amount of $C_{2:0}$, $C_{3:0}$ and $C_{4:0}$ acids in their faeces. Faecal concentrations of SCFAs are not of course the best way to measure the production rates since large proportion of SCFAs is taken up by the colonic mucosa. Nevertheless, faecal levels of SCFAs are a good marker or indicator of the differences on SCFAs taken place in the gut of mice that consumed fructans diets.

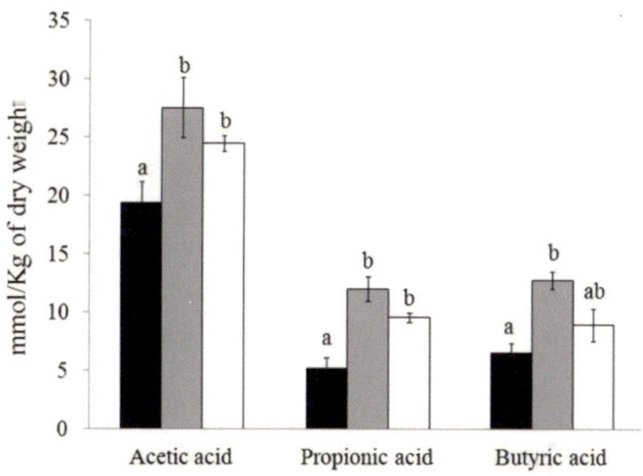

Figure 6. Concentration of SCFAs in faeces of mice fed with a standard diet (STD;■) or diet supplemented with Raftilose (RSE;□) or *Dasylirion* spp. (DSC;□). Mean values n=8 with their standard errors of the mean. Mean values with different letters were significantly different (P≤0.05).

With all the above, we decided to run an *in vivo* experiment feeding mice with *Agave angustifolia* fructans and evaluating the formation of SCFAs in caecum, colonic sections and faeces, as well as the pH drop in all these areas of the gut.

2. Materials and methods

2.1. Animals and diets

Twenty-four male C57BL/6J mice of 12 weeks old at the beginning of the experiment were obtained from the animal facilities of CINVESTAV-Zacatenco (Mexico). The mice were housed in a temperature and humidity controlled room with a 12 h light-dark cycle. They were divided into three groups (eight mice per group) according to diet. Mice were acclimated for 7 days, having free access to a pelleted 5053 standard diet (Laboratory Rodent Diet, USA) and water. During the experimental period (6 weeks), STD mice group were fed with 5053 standard diet, whereas inulins-RNE and agavins-AAO mice groups received a diet prepared by mixing 90 g of 5053 standard diet with 10 g of Raftiline or fructans from *A. angustifolia* (AAO). All diets were made by Laboratory Rodent Diet and were available *ad libitum* to mice.

2.2. Chemicals

Agavins were extracted in our laboratory as described by López et al. [10]. Briefly, one hundred grams of milled *Agave angustifolia* stems were extracted twice with 100 ml of 80% v/v ethanol with continuous shaking for 1 h at 55 °C. The sample was filtered and the plant material re-extracted with 100 ml of water for 30 min at 55 °C. The supernatants were mixed; chloroform was used to eliminate the organic fraction. The aqueous phase was concentrated by rotary evaporation under reduced pressure. The sample was dried using a spray dryer and stored in a humidity-free container. RNE were from Beneo Orafti. The average degree polymerization for agavins is 32[11] and for RNE >23.

2.3. Faeces and blood samples

Faeces collection was performed once a week during the experimental period to evaluate the SCFAs. On day 45, mice were anaesthetized by intra-peritoneal injection of sodium pentobarbital solution. Portal vein blood samples were collected in EDTA tubes; after centrifugation for 10 minutes at 2500 r.p.m., plasma was stored at -80 °C. The concentration of serum triglycerides, cholesterol and glucose was measured using kits coupling enzymatic reaction and spectrophotometric detection of reaction end-products (BioVision).

2.4. pH and SCFAs

Segments of the caecum and proximal, medial and distal colon were immediately excised. Caecal and colonic contents of each section were collected in tubes and frozen at -80 °C. The pH measurements were made using a microelectrode (PHR-146, Lazar Research

Laboratories, Inc.). Analysis of SCFAs was carried out by gas chromatography and flame ionization detection as described by Pietro Femia et al. [49] with some modifications. Briefly, 0.05 g of caecal and faecal contents were acidified with 0.05 ml of sulfuric acid and SCFAs were extracted by shaking with 0.6 ml of diethyl ether and subsequent centrifugation at 14000 r.p.m. for 30 s. One microliter of the organic phase was injected immediately into the capillary column (Nukol) of the gas chromatograph coupled to a flame ionization detector. The initial temperature was 80 °C and the final temperature was 200 °C. Nitrogen was used as carrier gas and the quantification of the samples was carried out using calibration curves for $C_{2:0}$, $C_{3:0}$ and $C_{4:0}$ acids. A standard curve for each acid was done for their quantitation in the samples.

2.5. Statistical analysis

Results are expressed as mean values with their standard errors of the mean. Statistical differences between groups were evaluated using one-way ANOVA followed by a Tukey test using GraphPad Prism version 5 for Windows. $P<0.05$ was regarded as statistically significant.

3. Results

3.1. Feed intake and body weight

The intake of all mice independently of the diet fed ranged between 3.3 and 4.2 g/d with an average of 3.7 g/d, it is worth to mention that the intake fluctuated weekly throughout the study. The feed intake was 9% lower for the AAO group compared to the STD and RNE diets. Mice fed with the diet supplemented with RNE ate 10% more food than even the STD group. Initial body weights ranged from 21.4 to 24.4 g with final body weights ranging between 24.3 and 25.9 g. No significant differences among all groups were noted in body weight even though mice fed AAO reduced their intake.

3.2. Production of SCFAs and pH drop

The total production of SCFAs was greater for the group of mice fed with AAO in the caecum and proximal and medial colon. However in the distal colon, the production of SCFAs were not significantly different among supplemented diets but it did with the STD diet (Table 3).

$C_{2:0}$ was the most abundant acid formed in the caecum and colon of all mice followed by $C_{3:0}$ and $C_{4:0}$ acid. The concentrations of $C_{2:0}$ acid were significantly higher in the caecum and the first two sections of the colon (proximal and medial) in mice fed with AAO diet compared to RNE or STD groups. However, in the distal colon there were no significant differences on the production of $C_{2:0}$ acid between groups of mice fed fructans (Figure 7a). The higher concentration of $C_{3:0}$ acid was found in the caecum of mice fed with AAO diet. This increment was significant with regard to RNE but not for the STD diet. In the proximal and medial colon $C_{3:0}$ acid production was greater for mice fed AAO, but these enhancements were not significant. Interestingly, in the distal colon of mice fed fructans (AAO and RNE) the enhancement was significantly for the production of $C_{3:0}$ acid (Figure 7b). The concentration of $C_{4:0}$ acid increased approximately 24% in the caecum of mice fed with RNE diet. This enhanced was significant with regard to AAO but not for the STD diet. Finally, an increment of $C_{4:0}$ acid was observed in the medial and distal colon, this change was significant in mice fed with AAO and RNE diets compared to mice fed with the STD diet (Figure 7c).

SCFAs changes were confirmed when the pH was measured in all the same samples. The mice fed AAO diet showed a pronounced pH drop in the caecum and all sections of the colon. The group of mice fed RNE showed significant pH drop only in the medial and distal colon and the pH of the mice fed a STD diet did not change significantly in any sections of the gut (Figure 8). The pH drop changes positively correlated with the total production of SCFAs (Table 3).

Section	STD*		RNE*		AAO*	
	Mean	SEM	Mean	SEM	Mean	SEM
Caecum	73.93^{a}	1.98	70.90^{a}	2.08	83.48^{b}	1.54
Proximal colon	71.98^{a}	2.11	76.93^{a}	2.62	106.92^{b}	4.61
Medial colon	51.44^{a}	1.25	64.26^{b}	2.59	107.25^{b}	2.41
Distal colon	28.58^{a}	0.86	49.65^{b}	2.91	66.84^{b}	2.97

*[mmol/Kg of fresh weight]. Mean values n=8 with their standard errors of the mean. ^{a,b} Mean values with unlike superscript letters were significantly different ($P \leq 0.05$).

Table 3. Concentration of total short chain fatty acids production in the caecum and the three sections of the colon in mice fed a standard (STD) diet or diet supplemented with Raftiline (RNE-inulin) or *Agave angustifolia* Oax. (AAO-agavins).

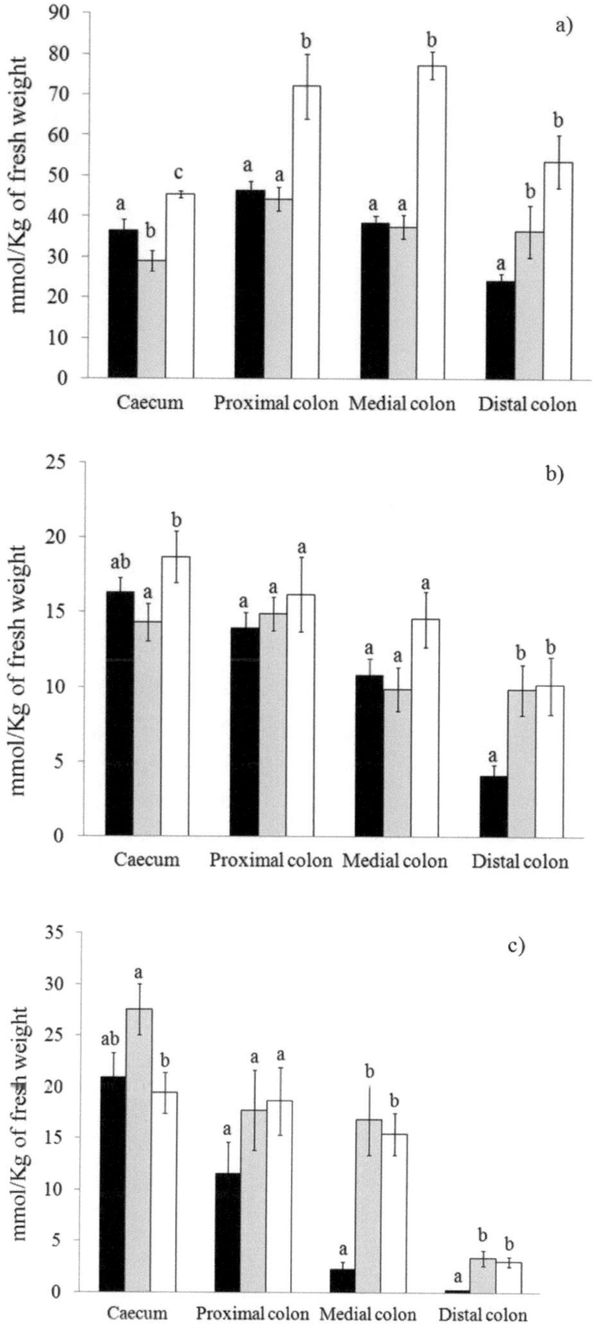

Figure 7. Concentrations of SCFAs in the caecum and the three sections of the colon of mice fed with a standard diet (STD; ■) and supplemented diets containing Raftiline (RNE; ■) and *A. angustifolia* Oax. (AAO; □). A) Acetic acid ($C_{2:0}$); B) Propionic acid ($C_{3:0}$); and C) Butyric acid ($C_{4:0}$). Mean values n=8 with their standard errors of the mean for each parameter measured. Mean values with different letters were significantly different ($P \leq 0.05$).

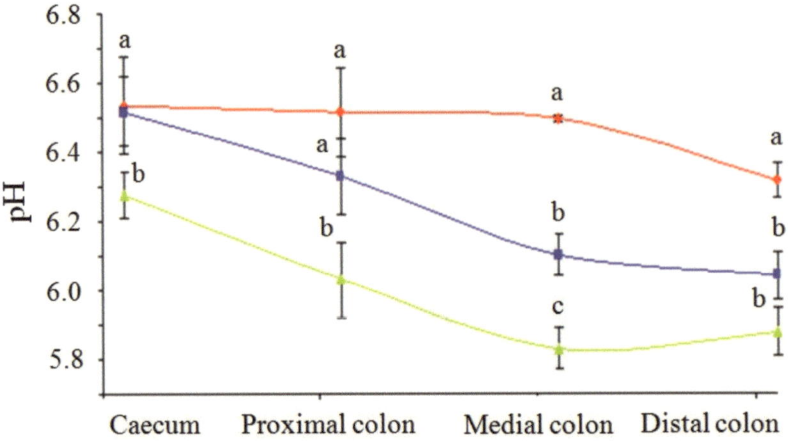

Figure 8. pH values in the caecum and the three sections of the colon of mice fed a standard diet (STD; ■) or diet supplemented with Raftiline (RNE;■) or *A. angustifolia* Oax. (AAO;■). Mean values n=8 with their standard errors of the mean. Mean values with different letters were significantly different ($P \leq 0.05$).

3.3. SCFAs in the faeces

The analyses of SCFAs in the collected faeces showed that $C_{2:0}$ acid was again the most abundant acid in the faeces of all mice followed by $C_{3:0}$ and $C_{4:0}$ acids. However, the amounts of $C_{2:0}$ and $C_{3:0}$ acids excreted in the faeces were not affected significantly by any dietary treatment. Surprisingly, only the mice fed with agavins (AAO) or inulin (RNE) diets, showed a significant increment on the amount of $C_{4:0}$ acid compared with the STD diet (Figure 9).

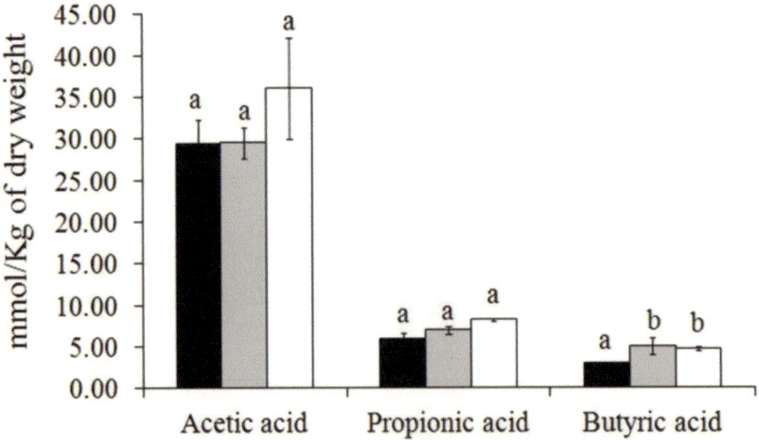

Figure 9. Concentration of acetic ($C_{2:0}$), propionic ($C_{3:0}$) and butyric ($C_{4:0}$) acids excreted in the faeces of mice fed a standard diet (STD;■) or diet supplemented with Raftiline (RNE;□) or *A. angustifolia* Oax. (AAO;□). Mean values n=8 with their standard errors of the mean. Mean values with different letters were significantly different ($P \leq 0.05$).

3.4. Plasma glucose, triglyceride and cholesterol

Besides SCFAs some other physiological parameters were determined in the plasma of all mice groups, among them glucose, triglycerides and cholesterol. Glucose concentrations of mice fed AAO and RNE diets were significantly lowered by 12% and 17% respectively when compared to the STD diet. On the other hand, triglycerides concentrations of the supplemented groups compared with the STD were reduced by 37% and 38 % in mice fed AAO and RNE diets, respectively. A reduction of cholesterol concentrations by 36 % and 38 % in animals receiving AAO and RNE diets was also observed *vs* STD diet (Table 4).

Diet	Glucose (mM)		Triglyceride (mM)		Cholesterol (mM)	
	Mean	SEM	Mean	SEM	Mean	SEM
STD	6.690^{a}	0.25	3.070^{a}	0.09	3.087^{a}	0.10
RNE	5.932^{b}	0.27	2.233^{b}	0.27	1.876^{b}	0.14
AAO	5.857^{b}	0.31	2.378^{b}	0.18	1.756^{b}	0.09

(Mean values n=8 with their standard errors of the mean for each parameter measured) ^{a,b}Mean values with unlike superscript letters were significantly different (P≤0.05).

Table 4. Glucose, triglycerides and cholesterol levels in plasma of mice fed with a standard (STD) diet or diet supplemented with Raftiline (RNE) and *A. angustifolia* Oax. (AAO).

4. Discussion

The determination of the production of $C_{2:0}$, $C_{3:0}$ and $C_{4:0}$ acids in the caecum, proximal, medial and distal colon of mice fed with different diets, was performed with the aids to evaluate the profiles of these acids throughout the caecum, large intestine and faeces of mice, and also to be able to establish the main sites of fermentation of inulins such Raftiline (RNE) and fructans extracted from *A. Angustifolia* (AAO) supplemented in the diets. These objectives basically arise from the knowledge on the structural differences between the two fructans types. Raftiline is an inulin type fructan with an average DP of 25 and it is know that its structure is completely linear, therefore containing a terminal glucose molecule. On the other hand, *A. angustifolia* fructans have an average DP of 32, with molecular structures very complex, they are highly branched and present a terminal glucose molecule (graminans) or internal glucose (agavins) [11]. Many reports have established that the structure of undigested carbohydrates and the microbiota present in an ecosystem are determining factors that control fermentation in the gut [50]. It is also know that the profiles of the production and distribution of SCFAs in the gut are influenced not only by the type of consumed carbohydrates, but also by the place where fermentation of those carbohydrates takes place, essentially in the caecum in mice and in the upper colon in humans, but the type of substrate may also affect the site of fermentation [51]. Previous reports mentioned that high DP fructans are fermented more slowly in the caecum and proximal colon, thus reaching the distal colon almost unchanged [6, 34], but bacteria present in this section produce mainly $C_{4:0}$ acid as the end product of such fermentation [51]. In the present work, inulins were fermented poorly in the caecum and proximal colon but an increment was observed on the concentration of $C_{4:0}$ acid in the distal colon, which agrees well with previous reports. However, mice fed with agave fructans (AAO) produced greater amounts of SCFAs in the caecum and proximal and medial colon than those mice fed with inulins (RNE), suggesting that AAO fructans were easily fermentable, independently of the their high DP, therefore, the difference might be due to the presence of branches in the agave fructans, which could make the molecule more accessible to enzymes (fructosyltransferases), in other words, there are more terminal fructose available for the fructosyltransferases of bacteria. According to the production of SCFAs, proximal and medial colon, were the main sites where fermentation of *A. angustifolia* fructans was carried out. In general, an increment was observed in the production of $C_{3:0}$ and $C_{4:0}$ acids in the distal colon of mice that received diets supplemented with fructans. On the other hand, total SCFAs and individual SCFAs concentrations in the different sections of the colon are very important since they have been associated with many diseases of the colon, especially with colon cancer and gastrointestinal disorders. Therefore, increased SCFAs production and a greater delivery of them distally, especially $C_{4:0}$ acid, may have an important role in preventing some of these diseases and other metabolic problems. Moreover, $C_{3:0}$ acid has been reported to have a positive metabolic effect, through the inhibition of hepatic cholesterol synthesis from $C_{2:0}$ acid [32]. Interestingly, a significant decrease in plasma triglycerides and cholesterol levels of animals fed with fructans was observed in this work. Finally, the mice that consumed agave fructans showed the more pronounced drop on pH in the caecum and the three sections of the colon, which creates a more acid environment which is highly beneficial for the grow of bacteria such as *bifidobacteria* and/or *lactobacilli* but is detrimental for the growth of potentially pathogenic species [17,18].

As a general conclusion, we can mention that the supplementation of diets with inulins or agavins altered the large intestine environment by increasing the amounts of SCFAs and lowering the pH in the colon, consequently reducing few health risks. Finally, we would like to close this work saying that these SCFAs had a positive effect on the host lipid metabolism, since they decreased the levels of triglycerides, cholesterol and glucose in blood of mice fed with supplemented diets.

Based on all the previous data, agave fructans may offer a good prebiotic potential, opening new and excited alternatives as food supplements. Even do, further research is definitely needed on specific health problems and should be performed using supplemented diets with agavins of different structures as well as different mixtures and concentrations, because more knowledge is needed on health issues such obesity, diabetes, colon cancer and in general, gut associated risks that might be improved with this type of ingredients.

Author details

Alicia Huazano-García and Mercedes G. López
Departamento de Biotecnología y Bioquímica,
Centro de Investigación y de Estudios Avanzados del IPN, México

Acknowledgement

Alicia Huazano-García thanks the Consejo Nacional de Ciencia y Tecnología (CONACYT) for her scholarship and also thanks M.S. Patricia Santiago for the agave fructans sample.

5. References

[1] Cairns A., Pollock C., Gallagher J., Harrison J. Fructans: Synthesis and Regulation. Leegood R., Sharkey T., Caemmerer S. von (eds) Photosynthesis: Physiology and Metabolism. Kluwer Academic Publishers; 2000. p 301-320.

[2] Niness K. Inulin and Oligofructose: What are They? The Journal of Nutrition 1999; 129(7) 1402S-1406.

[3] Van Loo J., Coussement P., De Leenheer L., Hoebregs H., Smits G. On the Presence of Inulin and Oligofructose as Natural Ingredients in the Western Diet. Critical Reviews in Food Science and Nutrition 1995; 35(6) 525-552.

[4] Ritsema T., Smeekens S. Engineering Fructan Metabolism in Plants. Journal of Plant Physiology 2003; 160(7) 811-820.

[5] Roberfroid M. Prebiotics: The Concept Revisited. The Journal of Nutrition 2007; 137(3) 830S-837.

[6] Roberfroid M., Van Loo J., Gibson G. The Bifidogenic Nature of Chicory Inulin and its Hydrolysis Products. The Journal of Nutrition 1998; 128(1) 11-19.

[7] Good-Avila S., Souza V., Gaut B., Eguiarte L. Timing and Rate of Speciation in Agave (*Agavaceae*). Proceedings of the National Academy of Sciences of the United States of America 2006;103(24) 9124-9129.

[8] Eguiarte L., Souza V., Silva-Montellano A. Evolución de la Familia *Agavaceae*: Filogenia, Biología Reproductiva y Genética de Poblaciones. Bolletin de la Sociedad Botánica de México 2000; 66 131-150.

[9] Gentry H. Agaves of continental North America. The University of Arizona Press; 1998.

[10] López M., Mancilla-Margalli N., Mendoza-Díaz G. Molecular Structures of Fructans from *Agave tequilana* Weber var. azul. Journal of Agricultural and Food Chemistry 2003; 51(27) 7835-7840.

[11] Mancilla Margalli N., López G. Water soluble Carbohydrates and Fructan Structure Patterns from Agave and Dasylirion Species. Journal of Agricultural and Food Chemistry 2006; 54(20) 7832-7839.

[12] Roberfroid M. Introducing Inulin Type Fructans. British Journal of Nutrition 2005;93(1) 13S-25.

[13] Roberfroid M. Prebiotics and Probiotics: Are they Functional Foods? The American Journal of Clinical Nutrition 2000; 71(1) 1682S-1687.

[14] Kolida S., Gibson G. Prebiotic Capacity of Inulin-type Fructans. The Journal of Nutrition 2007; 137(11) 2503S-2506.

[15] López M., Urías-Silvas J. Agave Fructans as Prebiotics. Norio S., Noureddine B., Shuichi O. (eds) Recent Advances in Fructooligosaccharides Research. Research Signpost; 2007. p 1-14.

[16] Gibson G., Probert H., Van Loo J., Rastall R., Roberfroid M. Dietary Modulation of the Human Colonic Microbiota: Updating the Concept of Prebiotics. Nutrition Research Reviews 2004; 17(2) 259-275.
[17] Gibson G., Roberfroid M. Dietary modulation of the human colonic microbiota: introducing the concept of prebiotics. The Journal of Nutrition 1995; 125(6) 1401-1412.
[18] Roberfroid M. Fructo-oligosaccharide Malabsorption: Benefit for Gastrointestinal Functions. Current Opinion in Gastroenterology 2000; 16(2) 173-177.
[19] Topping D., Clifton P. Short-chain Fatty Acids and Human Colonic Function: Roles of Resistant Starch and Nonstarch Polysaccharides. Physiological Reviews 2001; 81(3) 1031-1063.
[20] Gibson G. Dietary Modulation of the Human Gut Microflora Using the Prebiotics Oligofructose and Inulin. The Journal of Nutrition 1999; 129(7) 1438S-1441.
[21] Cummings J., Macfarlane G. The Control and Consequences of Bacterial Fermentation in the Human Colon. Journal of Applied Bacteriology 1991; 70(6) 443-459.
[22] Bernalier A., Dore J., Durand M. Biochemistry of fermentation. Gibson G., Roberfroid M. (eds) Colonic Microbiota, Nutrition and Health. Dordrecht:Kluwer Academic Publishers; 1999. p 37-53.
[23] Flamm G., Glinsmann W., Kritchevsky D., Prosky L., Roberfroid M. Inulin and Oligofructose as Dietary Fiber: A Review of Evidence. Critical Reviews in Food Science and Nutrition 2001; 41(5) 353;362.
[24] Wong J., De Souza R., Kendall C., Emam A., Jenkins D. Colonic Health: Fermentation and Short Chain Fatty Acids. Journal of Clinical Gastroenterology 2006; 40(3) 235-243.
[25] Cummings J., Roberfroid M., Andersson H., Barth C., Ferro-Luzzi A., Ghoos Y., Gibney M., Hermonsen K., James W., Korver O. A New Look at Dietary Carbohydrate: Chemistry, Physiology and Health. European Journal of Clinical Nutrition 1997; 51(7) 417-423.
[26] Cook S., Sellin J. Short Chain Fatty Acids in Health and Disease. Alimentary Pharmacology and Therapeutics 1998; 12(6) 499-507.
[27] Macfarlane G., Macfarlane S. Models for Intestinal Fermentation: Association between Food Components, Delivery Systems, Bioavailability and Functional Interactions in the Gut. Current Opinion in Biotechnology 2007; 18(2) 156-162.
[28] Zeng J., Tan Z. Metabolic Homeostasis and Colonic Health: The Critical Role of Short Chain Fatty Acids. Current Nutrition and Food Science 2010; 6(3) 209-222.
[29] Pomare E., Branch W., Cummings J. Carbohydrate Fermentation in the Human Colon and its Relation to Acetate Concentrations in Venous Blood. The Journal of Clinical Investigation 1985; 75(5) 1448-1454.
[30] Cummings J. Short Chain Fatty Acids in the Human Colon. GUT 1981; 22(9) 763-779.
[31] Venter C., Vorster H., Cummings J. Effects of Dietary Propionate on Carbohydrate and Lipid Metabolism in healthy volunteers. The American Journal of Gastroenterology 1990; 85(5) 549-553.
[32] Cheng H., Lai M. Fermentation of resistant rice starch produces propionate reducing serum and hepatic Cholesterol in Rats. The Journal of Nutrition 2000; 130(8) 1991-1995.

[33] Pryde S., Duncan S., Hold G., Stewart C., Flint H. The Microbiology of Butyrate Formation in the Human Colon. FEMS Microbiology Letters 2002; 217(2) 133-139.

[34] Van de Wiele T., Boon N., Possemiers S., Jacobs H., Verstraete W. Inulin-type Fructans of Longer Degree of Polymerization Exert More Pronounced *in vitro* Prebiotic Effects. Journal of Applied Microbiology 2007; 102(2) 452-460.

[35] Stewart M., Timm D., Slavin J. Fructooligosaccharides Exhibit More Rapid Fermentation than Long-chain Inulin *in* an *vitro* fermentation system. Nutrition Research 2008; 28(5) 329-334.

[36] Rycroft C., Jones M., Gibson G., Rastall R. A Comparative *in vitro* Evaluation of the Fermentation Properties of Prebiotic Oligosaccharides. Journal of Applied Microbiology 2001; 91(5) 878-887.

[37] Urías-Silvas J., López M. *Agave* spp. and *Dasylirion* sp. Fructans as a Potential Novel Source of Prebiotics. Dynamic Biochemistry, Process Biotechnology and Molecular Biology 2009; 3(1) 59-64.

[38] Santiago-García P., López M. Prebiotic Effect of Agave Fructans and Mixtures of Different Degrees of Polymerization from *Agave angustifolia* Haw. Dynamic Biochemistry, Process Biotechnology and Molecular Biology 2009; 3(1) 52-58.

[39] Gomez E., Tuohy K., Gibson G., Klinder A., Costabile A. *In vitro* Evaluation of the Fermentation Properties and Potential Prebiotic Activity of Agave Fructans. Journal of Applied Microbiology 2010; 108(6) 1859-2228.

[40] Nilsson U., Nyman M. Short-chain Fatty Acid Formation in the Hindgut of Rats Fed Oligosaccharides Varying in Monomeric Composition, Degree of Polymerization and Solubility. British Journal of Nutrition 2005; 94(5) 705-713.

[41] Licht T., Hansen M., Poulsen M.,Dragsted L. Dietary Carbohydrate Source Influences Molecular Fingerprints of the Rat Faecal Microbiota. BMC Microbiology 2006; 6(1) 98-107.

[42] Klessen B., Hartmann L., Blaut M. Oligofructose and Long-chain Inulin: Influence on the Gut Microbial Ecology of Rats Associated with a Human Faecal Flora. British Journal of Nutrition 2001; 86(2) 291-300.

[43] Levrat M., Remesy C., Demigne C. High Propionic Acid Fermentations and Mineral Accumulation in the Cecum of Rats Adapted to Different Levels of Inulin. The Journal of Nutrition 1991; 121(11) 1730-1737.

[44] Levrat M., Favier M., Moundras C., Remesy C., Demigne C., Morand C. Role of Dietary Propionic Acid and Bile Acid Excretion in the Hypocholesterolemic Effects of Oligosaccharides in Rats. The Journal of Nutrition 1994; 124(4) 531-538

[45] Daubioul C., Rousseau N., Demeure R., Gallez B., Taper H., Declerck B., Delzenne N. Dietary Fructans, but not Cellulose, Decrease Triglyceride Accumulation in the Liver of Obese Zucker *fa/fa* Rats. The Journal of Nutrition 2002; 132(5) 967-973.

[46] Trautwein E., Rieckhoff D., Erbersdobler H. Dietary Inulin Lower Plasma Cholesterol and Triacylglycerol and Alters Biliary Bile Acid Profile in Hamsters. The Journal of Nutrition 1998; 128(11) 1937-1943.

[47] Urías-Silvas J., Cani P., Delmee E., Neyrinck A., López M., Delzenne N. Physiological Effects of Dietary Fructans Extracted from *Agave tequilana* Gto. and *Dasylirion* spp. British Journal of Nutrition 2008; 99(2) 254-261.

[48] García-Pérez M. Efecto de los Fructanos de *Dasylirion* sp. en la Secreción de Grelina y GLP-1 en Ratones. MS thesis. CINVESTAV-Irapuato; 2008.

[49] Pietro F., Luceri C., Dolara P., Giannini A., Biggeri A., Salvadori M., Clune Y., Collins K., Paglierani M., Cademi G. Antitumorigenic Activity of the Inulin Enriched with Oligofructose in Combination with the Probiotics *Lactobacillus rhamnosus* and *Bifidobacterium lactis* on Azoximethane-induced Colon Carcinogenesis in Rats. Carcinogenesis 2002; 23(11) 1953-1960.

[50] Henningsson A., Björck I., Nyman G. Combinations of Indigestible Carbohydrates Affect Short-chain Fatty Acid Formation in the Hindgut of Rats. The Journal of Nutrition 2002; 132(10) 3098-3104.

[51] Hughes R., Rowland I. Stimulation of Apoptosis by Two Prebiotic Chicory Fructans in the Rat Colon. Carcinogenesis 2000; 22(1) 43-47.

Section 3

Lipid Metabolism in Health and Disease

Chapter 9

Lipid Metabolism, Metabolic Syndrome, and Cancer

Fang Hu, Yingtong Zhang and Yuanda Song

Additional information is available at the end of the chapter

http://dx.doi.org/10.5772/51821

1. Introduction

Metabolism is the process of making energy and cellular molecules from breaking down the food that made up of proteins, carbohydrates and fats etc. A metabolic disorder occurs when abnormal chemical reactions disrupt this process. When this happens, our body might have too much of some substances or too little of other ones that we need to stay healthy. Metabolic syndrome, a combination of several metabolic risk factors including abdominal obesity, insulin resistance, hypertension, and atherogenic dyslipidemia, is one of the most common health problems in the modern society. Increasingly accumulated evidence from epidemiologic and basic research data, as well as translational, clinical, and intervention studies suggested that metabolic syndrome may be an important etiologic factor for the onset of cancer. In fact cancer has long been indicated as a metabolic disease due to aberrant energy metabolism caused by mitochondrial damage.

In living cells, processes of carbohydrate metabolism, lipid metabolism and energy metabolism are closely related. Metabolic syndrome (MS), such as diabetes, obesity, hyperlipidimia, and hypertension, is, more or less, associated with abnormal lipid metabolism. As a metabolic disease, cancer is caused by impaired energy metabolism due to impaired mitochondrial function, which is linked with abnormal mitochondrial membrane lipids, especially cardiolipin content [1]. Recent studies have indicated that abnormalities in cellular lipid metabolism are involved in both pathogenesis of metabolic syndrome and various cancers [2, 3].

As the major component of membranes and energy resources, cellular lipids, including phospholipids and neutral lipids (mainly triacylglycerols and sterol esters), play a crucial role for both cellular and physiological energy homeostasis. As cellular membrane structure components, phospholipids are important for cellular membrane remodeling and cellular proliferation. Disruption of phospholipid homeostasis may lead to carcinogenesis and MS [4, 5]. Triacylglycerol, as an important energy storage form, is closely related to glucose homeostasis and its disregulation is associated with onset of MS such as diabetes, obesity, and cardiovascular diseases [6].

In this chapter, we focused on the metabolism of phospholipid and triacylglycerol (including fatty acids) and discussed the association of lipid metabolism disorders with pathogenesis of MS and cancer as shown in Figure1. We also discussed the emerging role of omega-3 polyunsaturated fatty acids in preventing lipid disorder associated MS and cancer.

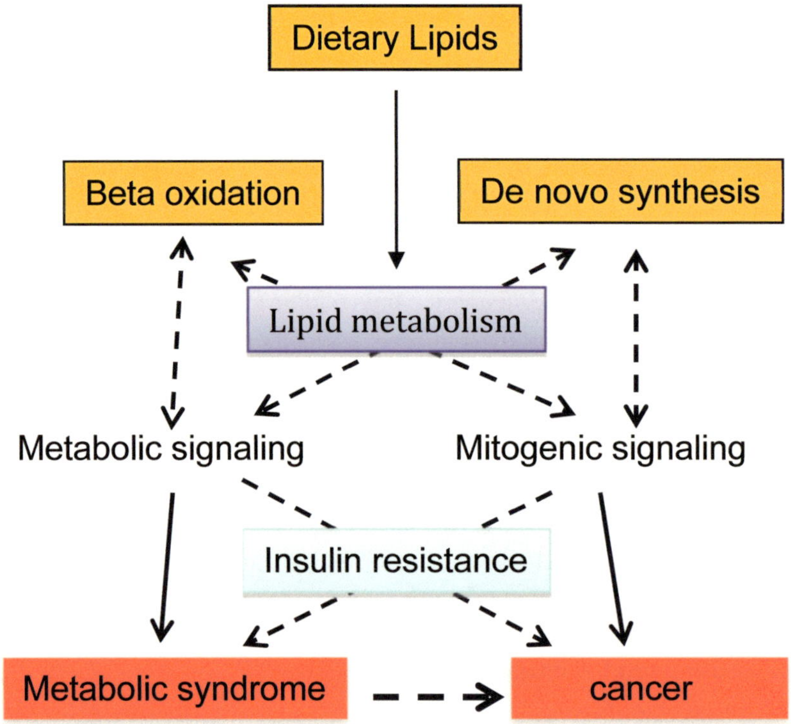

Figure 1. Inter-relationship between lipid metabolism, metabolic syndrome and cancer

2. Dietary lipids and metabolic diseases

2.1. Dietary lipids and metabolic syndrome

MS, also known as syndrome X, or the insulin resistance syndrome, is a combination of medical disorders comprising an array of metabolic risk factors including central obesity, dyslipidemia, hypertension, glucose intolerance, and insulin resistance[7]. The worldwide prevalence of MS causes lots of health problems not only in the developed countries, but also in the developing countries as well. Individuals with MS are at high risk for diabetes and cardiovascular disease. Increasingly accumulated evidence shows that aberrations in lipid metabolism are the central to the etiology of MS.

As one of the most abundant lipid species and major components of very-low-density lipoprotein (VLDL) and chylomicrons, triacylglycerols (TAG) play an important role in metabolism as energy sources. It can be acquired from de novo synthesis in liver or dietary lipids. Depending on the oil source, TAGs are either the main constituents of vegetable oils (typically more unsaturated) or animal fats (typically more saturated). Animal fat comprises about 40% of the energy intake in the human diet in Western countries, and a high proportion of this is TAG. Fat tissue, liver and intestine are the major places where TAG is synthesized and stored. There is also some intracellular storage of TAG e.g. in the muscle and brain cells. The storage of TAG can be replenished from dietary fat, or by endogenous synthesis of fat from carbohydrates or proteins, which mainly takes place in the liver.

The overabundance of nutrients such as lipids in obesity and caloric surplus leads to aberrant lipid management and ectopic fat accumulation (i.e., ''lipotoxicity''), which is a fundamental component of metabolic disease and insulin resistance [8, 9].

2.1.1. Fatty acids and insulin resistance

Insulin resistance is the center underlying the different metabolic abnormalities in the metabolic syndrome, in which pathophysiological conditions insulin becomes less effective in lowering blood glucose. Insulin resistance can be induced by various environmental factors, including dietary habits. Muscle, liver and fat are the three major tissues for maintaining blood glucose levels. In the presence of insulin, fat and muscle cells absorb glucose, and the liver regulates glucose levels by reducing its secretion and increasing its storage in the form of glycogen. However, in the condition of insulin resistance, glucose uptake by muscle and fat cells is disrupted, and glycogen synthesis and storage are also reduced in liver cells, resulting in failure of suppressing glucose production and releasing into the blood. Impaired glucose metabolism is associated with molecular alterations of insulin signaling, which is particularly well characterized in muscle [10].

Insulin also facilitates the uptake and storage of amino acids and fatty acids by converting them to protein and lipid, respectively. Besides the diminished glucose- lowering effects, insulin resistance also causes reduced actions of insulin on lipids and results in decreased uptake of circulating lipids and increased hydrolysis of stored triglycerides and, as a consequence, elevates free fatty acids in the blood plasma. Elevated levels of free fatty acids and triglycerides in the blood and tissues have been reported to contribute to impaired insulin sensitivity in many studies [11, 12]. Increased contents of fatty acids and their metabolites cause phosphorylation of insulin receptor substrate 1 (IRS-1) at serine, which blocks IRS-1 tyrosine phosphorylation and the associated activation of phosphatidylinositol-3' kinase (PI3K) activity, and results in a decreased translocation of the glucose transporter GLUT4 to membrane of muscle and liver cells [13, 14].

The conversion of fatty acids to acetyl-CoA, the process known as β-oxidation, mainly occurs in the mitochondria. Defects in mitochondrial fatty acid oxidation and in adipocyte fat metabolism may increase fatty acid content in muscle and liver, which, in turn, cause impaired transport of glucose and defective glycogen synthesis in muscle, and sustained output of glucose from the liver, which finally lead to hyperinsulinemia and insulin resistance. In addition, oxidative stress and cytokine induction in liver may lead to the development of nonalcoholic fatty liver (NAFLD). Considerable experimental evidence suggests that increased hepatic fat synthesis contributes to nonalcoholic steatohepatitis and associated insulin resistance [15].

Dietary fat composition is the major sources of free fatty acids in the blood and tissue. Consumption of high fat diets is strongly and positively associated with overweight that, in turn, deteriorates insulin sensitivity, particularly when the excess of body fat is located in abdominal region. Epidemiological evidence and experimental animal studies clearly show that saturated fat significantly worsen insulin resistance, while monounsaturated (MUFA) and polyunsaturated fatty acids (PUFA) improve it through modifications in the composition of cell membranes, and an elevated ratio of saturated fats to unsaturated fats is a risk factor for MS [16, 17].

A multicenter study has shown that shifting from a diet rich in saturated fatty acids (SFAs) to one rich in monounsaturated fat improves insulin sensitivity in healthy people [18]. Substitution of unsaturated fat for saturated fat reduces both LDL cholesterol and plasma triglycerides in insulin resistant individuals [16]. Several early cross- sectional studies have found a positive association between saturated fat intake and hyperinsulinaemia, and insulin resistance [19, 20], while polyunsaturated fat intake was inversely associated with plasma insulin levels whereas linoleic acid intake was positively associated with fasting plasma insulin concentrations, and increased unsaturated fat intake is associated with improved insulin sensitivity [16, 21].

In addition, numerous observations in rodent and cell culture models as well as obese and diabetic humans have shown that chronic lipid exposure is associated with insulin resistance [22-24], and fatty acid composition in body tissues is related to the incidence of diabetes [25]. Particular, intramuscular or hepatic content of TAG, diacylglycerol (DAG), or ceramide is negatively correlated with insulin sensitivity [26-28], which may be caused by disrupted insulin-stimulated translocation of the GLUT4 by ectopic accumulation of TAG and other lipid molecules in liver and muscle.

More and more evidence suggests that ceramide, composition of sphingosine and fatty acid and found in high concentrations within the cell membrane, plays a critical role in insulin resistance [29]. Both *in vitro* and *in vivo* studies have produced a large body of data implicating that accumulation of ceramide and its metabolites is associated with nutrient-induced pathogenesis of insulin resistance and metabolic diseases, including diabetes, cardiomyopathy, and atherosclerosis [28-30]. In cultured cells, ceramide inhibits insulin-stimulated glucose uptake by blocking translocation of the glucose transporter GLUT4, and glycogen synthesis [31, 32]. These effects are due to the ability of ceramide to block activation of Akt/PKB, a serine/threonine kinase that is activated by insulin and growth-factors. It is also found that accumulation of ceramide may impair mitochondrial function by altering mitochondrial membrane permeability, inhibiting electron transport chain intermediates, and promoting oxidative stress [33].

In rodents, inhibition of ceramide de novo synthesis pathway by serine palmitoyltransferase inhibitor myriocin improves insulin sensitivity and prevents insulin resistance associated metabolic diseases [30, 34-36]. In humans, it is well documented the association of ceramides accumulation in peripheral tissues, including muscle and fat, of obese subjects with insulin resistance [37-40].

2.1.2. *Fatty acids and cardiovascular diseases*

Since the 1950s, it has long been believed that consumption of foods containing high amounts of SFAs, including meat fats, milk fat, butter, lard, coconut oil, etc, is not only a risk factor for dyslipidemia and insulin resistance, but also a risk factor for cardiovascular diseases. However, recent evidence from systematic reviews, meta-analyses and prospective cohort studies indicates that SFAs alone maybe not associated with an increased risk of cardiovascular disease. A randomized controlled dietary intervention trial that compared a carbohydrate restricted diet to a low fat diet over a 12-week period in overweight subjects with atherogenic dyslipidemia found that carbohydrate restriction, rather than a low fat diet may improve features of MS and cardiovascular risk [41]. In a recent cross-sectional study conducted in Japanese to exam the relationship between dietary ratio of PUFA to SFA with cardiovascular risk factors and MS, the data showed that dietary polyunsaturated to saturated fatty acid ratio was significantly and inversely related to serum total and LDL cholesterol, but did not significantly relate to single metabolic risk factors or the prevalence of MS [42].

However, on the other hand, some SFAs such as stearic acid and fatty acids found in milk and milk products appear to be beneficial and may diminish the risk for cardiovascular disease. In a systematic review, after comparing with those of trans, other saturated, and unsaturated fatty acids (USFAs), Hunter et al [43] found that stearic acid raised LDL cholesterol, and compared with USFA, stearic acid lowered HDL cholesterol and increased the total cholesterol/HDL cholesterol ratio [43].

Palmitoleic acid (cis-16:1, n-7) has been linked to both beneficial metabolic effects. It has been reported that adipose-produced cis-palmitoleate directly improved hepatic and skeletal muscle insulin resistance and related metabolic abnormalities, and suppressed hepatic fat synthesis as well [44]. A prospective cohort study showed that circulating trans-palmitoleate (trans-16:1, n-7) is associated with lower insulin resistance, decreased presence of atherogenic dyslipidemia, and incidence of diabetes incidence [45] suggesting metabolic benefits of dairy consumption. There is also strong evidence collected by systematic review and meta-analysis of randomized controlled trials showing that consumption of polyunsaturated fat as a replacement for saturated fat alleviates coronary heart disease risk [46]. While many studies have found that replacement of saturated fats with polyunsaturated fats in the diet produces more beneficial outcomes on cardiovascular health [47, 48], the effects of substituting monounsaturated fats or carbohydrates are still unclear.

2.1.3. *Omega-3 PUFAs and metabolic syndrome*

Omega-3 PUFAs (also called ω–3 fatty acids or n–3 fatty acids are commonly found in marine and plant oils, which contain a double bond at the third carbon atom from the methyl-end of the carbon chain. These PUFAs, including α-linolenic acid (ALA, 18:3, n-3), eicosapentaenoic acid (EPA, 20:5, n–3) and docosahexaenoic acid (DHA, 22:6, n–3), are considered as essential fatty acids because they can not be de novo synthesized by the human body. In human diets, ALA is usually derived from botanical sources such as perilla, flaxseed, canola, rapeseed, soybean, linseed and walnut. EPA and DHA are found in fish and some other sea foods [49]. Recent researches have shown that, while diets rich in saturated fatty acids (SFAs) are associated with an increased prevalence of obesity and type 2 diabetes, supplement of omega-3 PUFAs rich in eicosapentaenoic acid (EPA) and docosahexaenoic acid (DHA) has anti-inflammatory and anti-obesity effects and protect against metabolic abnormalities [50].

Earlier epidemiologic observations showed the beneficial properties of n-3 PUFAs in populations consuming large amounts of fatty fish and marine mammal oils [51]. Later studies showed that a 3-wk supplement with fish oil rich in n-3 PUFA in healthy humans resulted in improved sensitivity to insulin, higher fat oxidation, and increased glycogen storage [52]. Most subsequent studies confirmed these effects and observed that supplementation with n-3 PUFAs, either EPA or DHA alone, or with their combination in fish oil, has favorably effects on many adverse serum and tissue lipid alterations related to the metabolic syndrome by reducing levels of fasting and postprandial serum triacylglycerols and free fatty acids [53, 54]. Some of the effects of n-3 PUFAs on lipid and lipoprotein metabolism could remain in subjects who become overtly diabetic.

In addition, other recognized benefits of n-3 PUFAs include a reduction in inflammatory status, decreased platelet activation, mild reduction in blood pressure, improved endothelial function, and increased cellular antioxidant defense, all of which may prove particularly favorable in overweight, hypertensive patients [55]. Furthermore, supplementation with fish oil also blunted the sympathetic activity elicited by mental stress in healthy volunteers [56]. However, the beneficiary effects of n-3 PUFA supplementation on cardiovascular risk prevention are association with other components of lifestyle, ie, weight control, regular physical activity, and consumption of other dietary ingredients contributing to risk reduction [57].

The mechanisms underlying beneficiary effects of use n-3 PUFAs/fish oils or a combination of EPA and DHA have been extensively analyzed. Studies in animal and humans have demonstrated that, in addition to be used as fuels and structural components of the cell, the dietary intake of marine fish oil is also effective in lowering both triglyceride (Tg) and VLDL-Tg concentration in experimental animals and normal and hyper- triglyceridemic men [58, 59], which might be related to decreased mRNA encoding several proteins involved in hepatic lipogenesis including SREBP1, and enhanced fatty acid oxidation throughout a peroxisome proliferator- activated receptors (PPARs)—stimulated process [60, 61]. Moreover, n-3 PUFAs elevate the fatty acid composition of membrane phospholipids that modify membrane-mediated processes such as insulin transduction signals, activities of lipases and biosynthesis of eicosanoids [62].

Furthermore, dietary fish oil consumption normalizes the function of many tissues or cells involved in insulin sensitivity in the sucrose-rich diet (SRD) fed rats. It reverses dyslipidemia and improves insulin action and adiposity by reducing adipocytes cell size, increasing insulin sensitive and decreasing the release of fatty acids. Both oxidative and non-oxidative glucose pathways are improved in muscle. In isolated beta cells, lipid contents and glucose oxidation return to normal [63]. All these effects lead to the improvement of glucose- stimulated insulin secretion and muscle insulin insensitivity.

Adipose tissue plays a key role in the development of MetS and improvement of adipose tissue function is specifically linked to the beneficial effects of n-3 PUFA [64]. In accordance with the general anti-inflammatory action, n-3 PUFA supplementation induces production and secretion of adiponectin [65], the major adipokine exerting an insulin-sensitizing effect, and prevents adipose tissue hyperplasia and hypertrophy, and induces mitochondrial biogenesis in adipocytes [66], which effects maybe mediated by n-3 PUFA induced AMP-activated protein kinase (AMPK), a metabolic sensor controlling intracellular metabolic fluxes [64].

2.2. Dietary lipids and cancer

Case–control and cohort studies have found positive associations between several cancers such as prostate cancer[67], ovarian cancer[68], breast cancer[69], colon cancer[70] etc, and an intake of foods with high levels of saturated fats, such as red meat, eggs, and dairy products. However, controversial results have also been reported about the role of high fat diet in carcinogenicity [71, 72]. This is largely due to the complexity of the diet, not only the fat components such as SFA, MUFA, and PUFA may vary among people in different regions, but also other non-fat nutrients may also alter the function of fat. Therefore only preclinical animal studies with clearly-defined fat composition may help elucidate the causal relationship between dietary fat and cancer. Up to now, it is generally accepted that cis-MUFA and omega-3 PUFAs are inversely associated with the increased risk of cancer, while SFA and omega-6 PUFAs are associated with the development of cancer [73]. However, physiologically, the metabolism of fatty acids are connected, any results based on a single fatty acids may be incomprehensive, therefore a fat containing diet with elevated MUFA and low ratio of omega-6/omega-3 fatty acid is suggested to be associated with cancer prevention and protection [74]. Interested readers are advised to read recent review articles about the association of dietary lipids with prostate [75] and breast cancer [76], and potential mechanisms for the association of dietary lipids with cancer [77-79].

2.2.1. Saturated fatty acids

Recent studies have shown that high fat diet with saturated animal fat as major fat in the diet is associated with several cancer such as prostate cancer [67], colon cancer [80], ovarian cancer [68] and breast cancer [81] etc, whereas high fat diet with plant oils is not associated with cancer risk, however this may not be true, plant oils high in omega-6 fatty acids may be risk factors for cancer, which will be discussed in the polyunsaturated fatty acid section.

2.2.2. Monounsaturated fatty acids

It has been found that cancer incidence in the Mediterranean countries, where the main source of fat is olive oil, is lower than in other areas of the world. Such effects may be due to the main MUFA in olive oil, oleic acid, and to certain minor compounds such as squalene and phenolic compounds [82]. Recent studies have also shown that canola oil, with high MUFA, oleic acid, can decrease colon and breast cancer incidence significantly [83, 84]. Although the authors suggested that such effect may be caused by omega-3 fatty acids, ALA, as high as 10% in canola oil, however, the role of oleic acid, as high as 61% in canola oil, cannot be excluded. So far, no epidemiological studies or animal studies can clearly demonstrate the preventive effect of MUFA on cancer, However, *in vivo* analysis of the fatty acid composition of the adipose tissue of breast cancer and healthy women showed that elevated adipose MUFA, oleic acid, are associated with reduced odds of breast cancer [85]. Although the mechanism underling the protective function of oleic acid on cancer is, so far, not clear, it has been found that oleic acid, when complexed with the molten globule form of alpha-lactalbumin (α-LA), acquires tumoricidal activity [86]. Carrillo et al found that oleic acid can inhibit store-operated Ca(2+) entry (SOCE), a Ca(2+) influx pathway, involved in the control of multiple cellular and physiological processes including cell proliferation, thus regulating the growth of colon carcinoma cells [87].

2.2.3. Polyunsaturated fatty acids

Increasing evidences from animal and in vitro studies indicate that populations who ingest high amounts of omega-3 fatty acids in their diets have lower incidences of breast, colon, and, perhaps, prostate cancers. Paola et al. [88] used MTT viability test and expression of apoptotic markers to evaluate the effect of PUFAs on cancer growth, and their results indicated that EPA and DHA might induce modifications of tumor cell membrane structure leading to an obviously decreased induction rate of breast cancer. Menéndez et al. [89] also reported that omega-3 PUFAs ALA suppresses the overexpression of HER2, which plays an important role in aetiology, progression and chemosensitivity of various types of human cancers, suggesting that ALA is a potential anticancer agent. However, the clinical roles of omega-3 PUFAs may rely not only on the absolute content but also on the proportion of omega-3 PUFAs to omega-6 PUFAs in the cells due to the inverse biological functions of these two series of PUFAs. A higher omega-6/omega-3 PUFAs ratio contributes to many diseases including cancer, cardiovascular and inflammation. Reducing the omega-6/omega-3 PUFAs ratio can help lower the risk of initiation and development of cancer. Berquin et al. established a prostate-specific phosphatase and tension homolog (PTEN) knockout mouse model, and the result demonstrated that a dietary ratio of omega-6/omega-3 PUFA lower than 5 was effective in suppressing tumor growth, and extending animal lifespan [90] The recent research suggested that a balanced ratio of omega-6/omega-3 PUFAs (1:1) exerts a beneficial effects on cell function and physiology [91].

2.2.4. Potential mechanisms of the association of dietary lipids with cancer

Although it has been generally accepted that dietary lipids are associated with carcinogenesis and the development of cancer, the detailed mechanism is still far from clear. When lipids are digested and absorbed by small intestine mucosa cells, they can be transported to adipocytes for storage, or used for energy production by peripheral cells through fatty acid β-oxidation. They can also be used for membrane lipid biosynthesis. Upon environmental stimulus, these lipids may be hydrolyzed and free fatty acids are released. Omega-6 PUFAs such as ARA released from membrane lipids will be converted to normal eicosanoids, and regulate cellular physiology; however elevated levels of these eicosanoids may accelerate cell proliferation and lead to inflammation and carcinogenesis, etc [92]. Whereas omega-3 PUFAs such as EPA, when released from membrane lipids, may be converted to eicosanoids with opposite activity to the product of omega-6 fatty acids, which inhibit cell proliferation and COX-2 activity, thus providing cancer preventive function [93]. Another mechanism of regulation of cancer initiation and development may be elucidated by fatty acid signaling pathway through its receptors. In particular, two transcription factors, sterol regulatory element binding protein-1c (SREBP-1c) and peroxisome proliferator activated receptor alpha (PPAR alpha), have emerged as key mediators of gene regulation by FA [94, 95]. SREBP-1c induces a set of lipogenic enzymes in liver. PUFA, but not SFA or MUFA, suppressES the induction of lipogenic genes by inhibiting the expression and processing of SREBP-1c. Thus inhibits the de novo lipogenesis of fatty acids, which is of particular importance for cancer cells [96].

PPAR alpha plays an essential role in metabolic adaptation to fasting by inducing the genes for mitochondrial and peroxisomal FA oxidation as well as those for ketogenesis in mitochondria. FAs released from adipose tissue during fasting are considered as ligands of PPAR alpha. Dietary PUFA, except for 18:2 n-6, are likely to induce FA oxidation enzymes via PPAR alpha as a "feed-forward " mechanism. PPAR alpha is also required for regulating the synthesis of highly unsaturated FA, indicating pleiotropic functions of PPAR alpha in the regulation of lipid metabolic pathways. Thus, in addition to its inhibition of fatty acid biosynthesis through SREBP, omega-3 fatty acids induce fatty acid degradation through PPAR alpha, in so doing, they regulate fatty acid metabolism and metabolic diseases. Multiple mechanisms of omega-3 fatty acids mediated inhibition of cancer may include suppression of neoplastic transformation and cell growth, and enhanced apoptosis and antiangiogenicity etc [97].

3. De novo lipogenesis in metabolic disease

3.1. De novo lipogenesis in metabolic syndrome

De novo fatty acid biosynthesis occurs in essentially all cells, but adipose tissue and liver are the major sites. The first committed step in fatty acid synthesis is catalyzed by fatty acid synthase (FAS), a multifunctional cytosolic protein that primarily synthesizes palmitate. Variations in FAS expression and enzyme activity have been implicated in insulin resistance and obesity in humans [98]. A circulating form of FAS has been reported as a biomarker of metabolic stress and insulin sensitivity. In humans it changes with weight loss and may reflect improved insulin sensitivity [99].

Fatty acid elongation is catalyzed by Elovl (elongation of very long-chain fatty acid) proteins. Elovl6 is thought to be involved in de novo lipogenesis and is regulated by dietary, hormonal and developmental factors. Mice with Elov6 deficiency are obese but protected from insulin resistance [100, 101].

Citrate produced by the tricarboxylic acid cycle in mitochondria is converted by ATP-citrate lyase (ACL) to acetyl-CoA, which is next converted to malonyl-CoA by acetyl CoA carboxylase (ACC). Malonyl-CoA is a potent inhibitor of carnitine- palmitoyl transferase 1 (CPT1), which transports FAs into the mitochondria for oxidation, thus plays a key role in the regulation of both mitochondrial fatty acid oxidation and fat synthesis. ACC catalyzes a key rate-controlling step in both de novo lipogenesis and fatty acid oxidation. The absence of ACC decreases the cellular concentration of malonyl-CoA, removes the inhibition of CPT1 and maintains FA oxidation. In rats with NAFLD, suppression or knockdown of ACC isoforms significantly reduced hepatic malonyl-CoA levels, lowered hepatic lipids including long-chain acyl-CoAs, DAG, and triglycerides, and improved hepatic insulin sensitivity [102].

Lipogenesis and FA oxidation are highly integrated processes. Studies in genetically modified mice have demonstrated that inhibition of FA synthesis and storage is associated with upregulation of FA oxidation [103]. For examples, knockout the diacylglycerol acyltransferase (DGAT), an enzyme that catalyses the final acylation step of TAG synthesis, reduced fat deposition and protected mice against diet- induced obesity and, in the meanwhile, elevated mice energy expenditure and increased activity, suggesting a correlation of disrupted FA storage and increased FA oxidation [104, 105]. Similarly, deletion of acetyl-CoA carboxylase 2 (ACC2), an isoform of ACC and key enzyme for de novo FA synthesis, leads to a lean mouse with increased FA oxidation [106].

As a major component of the metabolic syndrome, NAFLD characterizes with the accumulation of TAGs in hepatocytes, and development of steatohepatitis, cirrhosis, and hepatocellular carcinoma. FAs stored in adipose tissue and newly made through liver de novo lipogenesis are the major sources of TAGs in the liver [107].

Lipogenesis is also an insulin- and glucose-dependent process that is under the control of specific transcription factors. SREBP1 is such a transcription factor and activates most genes involved in FA synthesis. It occurs in two isoforms, SREBP1a and 1c, through alternative splicing. SREBP-1c is highly expressed in the WAT, liver, adrenal gland, brain, and muscle and regulates the expression of many of the genes involved in de novo FA and TAG synthesis including ACC and FAS [108, 109]. Insulin increases lipogenesis through activating SREBP-1c that is dependent on the mammalian target of rapamycin (mTOR) complex 1 (mTORC1) [110]. SREBP1 gene expression is decreased in adipose tissue of obese subjects and the aberrant activation of SREBPs may contribute to obesity-related pathophysiology in various organs, including cardiac arrhythmogenesis and hepatic insulin resistance.

Lipogenesis is also regulated by glucose activated carbohydrate response element-binding protein (ChREBP), which induces gene expression of liver-type pyruvate kinase, a key regulatory enzyme in glycolysis; this enzyme in turn provides the precursors for lipogenesis [111]. ChREBP also stimulates expression of genes involved in lipogenesis [112] including SREBP-1c, which in turn activates glycolytic gene expression, promoting glucose metabolism, and lipogenic genes in conjunction with ChREBP [113]. ChREBP knockout mice show decreased liver triglyceride but increased liver glycogen content indicating that ChREBP may regulate metabolic gene expression to convert excess carbohydrate into triglyceride rather than glycogen [114]. In addition, complete inhibition of ChREBP in ob/ob mice reduces the effects of the MS such as obesity, fatty liver, and glucose intolerance, indicating it as a potential target for treatment of MS [115].

3.2. De novo lipogenesis in cancer

Enhanced flux of glucose derivatives through glycolysis, which sustain the redirection of mitochondrial ATP to glucose phosphorylation, and de novo FA synthesis is a hallmark of aggressive cancers. Although most normal cells use FA from dietary lipids, tumor cells de novo synthesize more than 95% of lipids required for cell proliferation despite having enough nutritional supply of lipids. Lipogenic enzymes such as, FAS, ACC, and ACL involved in FA biosynthesis, glycerol-3-phosphate dehydrogenase involved in lipid biosynthesiss, and SREBP1, the master regulator of lipogenic gene expression, are found to be overexpressed in a number of cancer or cancer cells, such as prostate cancer [116], ovarian cancer [117], breast cancer [118], lung cancer [119], colon cancer [120], and etc. Some research has been carried out to provide insights into the molecular mechanism of the association of lipogenesis and cancer. In this chapter we focused on three main lipogenic genes: FAS, ACC, and ACL.

3.2.1. Fatty acid synthase

High levels of FAS expression have been found in many human cancers, including prostate cancer [121], ovarian cancer [117, 122], breast cancer [123], bladder cancer [124], colon cancer [125] mantle cell lymphoma [126], and etc. However, the cellular mechanism by which FAS is up-regulated in cancer cells is not fully understood. Nevertheless a few studies suggested that steroid hormones and human epidermal growth factor receptor (HER) family ligands, especially HER2 could increase FAS expression via the PI3K/Akt or mitogen-activated protein kinases (MAPK) pathways[117]. Recently Mukherjee et al [117] demonstrated that bioactive lipid lysophosphatidic acid (LPA) induces FAS expression and lipogenesis through LPA2-G12/13-Rho-SREBP signaling pathway in ovarian cancer cells. Moreover over-expression of FAS in non-cancerous epithelial cells is sufficient to induce a cancer-like phenotype through the induction of HER1/HER2 [127], therefore FAS over-expression may play a role in carcinogenesis. Furthermore FAS overexpression is found to be associated with the advanced stage of colorectal cancer and liver metastasis, thus it may also play a role in the progression of cancer [128]. So far abundant evidences have shown that FAS contributes to both tumorigenesis and metastasis, and it becomes an ideal target for cancer therapy. In deed inhibition of FAS activity by FAS specific inhibitors or siRNA can significantly inhibit cancer or cancer cell growth, induce cancer cell apoptosis, and reduce the metastasis of several cancers[124, 129]. Both synthetic chemicals and natural products of

FAS inhibitors have been developed [123[130], and the recent progress in developing FAS inhibitors as cancer drugs has been reviewed by Pandey et al [131].

3.2.2. ATP-Citrate lyase and acetyl CoA carboxylase

Apart from FAS, other key lipogenic enzymes for de novo FA biosynthesis include ACL and ACC. While ACL produce the substrate acetyl-CoA from glycolytic product citrate, ACC activates the substrate to generate malanyl-CoA, the building block for fatty acid synthesis. Both ACC and ACL have been found to be over-expressed in many cancers such as breast, liver, lung, ovarian, prostate and leukemia cancers [132, 133]. Inhibition of either ACL or ACC induces growth arrest and apoptosis in several cancer cell lines [134-136]. The potential mechanism of ACL overexpression in tumorigenesis is through PI3K/AKT and MAPK signaling pathway [135, 137]. Yoon et al [138] found that the major mechanism of HER2-mediated induction of ACC alpha in breast cancer cells is translational regulated primarily through mTOR signaling pathway. While Mukherjee et al [117] found that LPA induced induction of ACC in ovarian cancer cells is through LPA2-Gq-PLC-AMPK signaling pathway. Many small molecule inhibitors for ACL and ACC have been developed as potential therapeutic agents for cancer [133, 139].

4. Phospholipids metabolism in metabolic diseases

Phospholipids are polar lipids as major component of membrane structure and some intracellular complex such as lipoproteins. Enzymes involved in the metabolism of phospholipids include phospholipase A_2 (PLA_2), phospholipase C (PLC), phospholipase D (PLD), and lysophospholipase D (autotoxin), and alterations of these enzymes have been found to be linked with metabolic diseases, such as MS and cancer. In addition, the intermediates or end products of phospholipid metabolism such as phosphatidic acid (PA), DAG, LPA, sphingosine-1-phoshate (S-1-P), and free fatty acid arichidonic acid (ARA), are also involved in the pathogenesis of metabolic diseases.

4.1. Phospholipid metabolism in metabolic syndrome

Phosphatidylcholine (PC) is the most abundant phospholipids in animal cells. Blocking S-adenosylmethionine (SAMe) or PC synthesis in C. elegans, mouse liver, and human cells have been found to cause elevated SREBP-1-dependent transcription and lipid droplet accumulation [4], suggesting nutritional or genetic conditions limiting SAMe or PC production may activate SREBP-1, and contribute to human metabolic disorders.

Phosphatidylethanolamine (PE) is another abundant phospholipid in mammals. PE and its downstream signaling events play an important role in the heart function, and alteration in the asymmetrical transbilayer distribution of PE in sarcolemmal membranes during ischemia causes sarcolemmal disruption [140]. Moreover, abnormalities in the molecular species profile of PE may contribute to membrane dysfunction and defective contractility of the diabetic heart [141, 142].

SREBPs may play critical roles in phospholipid homeostasis and lipotoxic cardiomyopathy. Dysregulated phospholipid signaling that alters SREBP activity has been reported to contribute to the progression of impaired heart function in flies and also act as a potential link to lipotoxic cardiac diseases in humans [143]. Thus the role of SREBPs in modulating heart function and its associated phospholipid signaling maybe a candidate target for future therapies for obesity- and diabetes- related cardiac dysfunction.

4.2. Phospholipid metabolism in cancer

An aberrant choline phospholipid metabolism is another major hallmark of cancer cells. In deed alterations of choline phospholipid metabolism have been reported in ovarian cancer and also in breast cancer [144, 145]. Altered choline phospholipid metabolism in ovarian cancer has been found to be linked with the regulation of FAS. Because the drop in the level of PC (59%) was significantly correlated with a drop in *de novo* synthesized FA levels, PC was identified as a potential noninvasive magnetic resonance spectroscopy–detectable biomarker of FAS inhibition *in vivo* [146]. Phospholipids and their metabolism have been found to be involved in ovarian cancer in several forms, including LPA, PLA_2, PLD, and autotoxin (ATX). Although aberrant phospholipid metabolism has been found in other cancers, the most detailed research work has been carried out using ovarian cancer as a model, so in this section we summarized the recent advances in the research of phospholipid metabolism and ovarian cancer.

4.2.1. Lysophosphatidic acid

The LPAs, with their various FA side chains, are the constituents of a growth-stimulating factor—ovarian cancer activating factor—that has been identified from ascites in patients with ovarian cancer [147]. As a bioactive compound, LPA works to induce cell proliferation or differentiation, prevents apoptosis induced by environmental stress or stimuli, induce platelet aggregation and smooth muscle contraction, and stimulate morphological changes, adhesion and migration of cells. It thus is involved in a broad range of biologic processes in a variety of cellular systems [148, 149]. As an established mitogen, LPA also promotes the invasiveness of hepatoma cells into monolayers of mesothelial cells, and stimulates proliferation of ovarian and breast cancer cell lines even in the absence of other growth promoters such as serum. Furthermore, LPA stimulates rapid neurite retraction and rounding of the cell body in serum-deprived neuroblastoma cells [150], and plays a critical role in regulation of gene expression in normal and neoplastic cells. It is a potent modulator of the expression of genes involved in inflammation, angiogenesis, and carcinogenesis such as interleukin [151-154], vascular endothelial growth factor (VEGF) [155], urokinase plasminogen activator [156], and cyclooxygenase-2 [157]. Thus LPA may contribute to cancer progression by triggering expression of those target genes, resulting in a more invasive and metastatic microenvironment for tumor cells [152, 158]. A significant increase in the expression of LPA receptors (LPA2 and LPA3) with VEGF was found by Fujita *et al.* [159], who suggested that LPA receptors might be involved in VEGF expression mediated by LPA signals in human ovarian oncogenesis. The recent identification of metabolizing enzymes that mediate the degradation and production of LPA and the development of receptor selective-analogs has opened a potential new approach to the treatment of ovarian cancer [160]. LPA also stimulates VEGF expression independent of hypoxia-inducible factor 1 (H1F1) and promotes tumor angiogenesis by activation of c-Myc and Sp-1 transcription factors [161]. A very recent study shows that LPA induces de novo lipogenesis through LPA2-G12/13-SREBP-FAS, and LPA2-G(q)-AMPK-ACC signaling pathway.

4.2.2. Phospholipase A_2

The PLA_2 enzyme has been implicated in the activation of cell migration and the production of LPA in ovarian carcinoma cells [162]. Autonomous replication and growth-factor-stimulated proliferation of ovarian cancer cells are highly sensitive to inhibition of calcium-independent PLA_2 ($iPLA_2$), but are refractory to inhibition of cytosolic PLA_2 [162]. Activation of $iPLA_2$ plays a critical role in cell migration, which is involved in many important biologic processes such as development, the immunologic and inflammatory responses, and tumor biology [162]. When ovarian cancer cells were grown under growth-factor-independent conditions, suppression of $iPLA_2$ activity led to an accumulation of cell populations in both the S and the G2/M-phases [163]. Supplementation with exogenous growth factors such as LPA and epidermal growth factor in culture released the S-phase arrest, but did not affect the G2/M arrest associated with inhibition of $iPLA_2$. In addition to the prominent effect on the cell cycle, inhibition of $iPLA_2$ also induced weak-to-modest increases in apoptosis [163]. Downregulation of $iPLA_2$ ◎with lentivirus-mediated RNA interference targeting $iPLA_2$ ◎expression inhibited cell proliferation in culture and decreased tumorigenicity of ovarian cancer cell lines in athymic nude mice [163]. Recently $iPLA_2$ has been found to play a role in breast cancer metastasis as $iPLA_2$ deficiency protects breast cancer from metastasis to the lung [164].

4.2.3. Phospholipase D

PLD, a family of signaling enzymes that most commonly responsible to generate most lipid second messenger phosphatidic acid (PA), is found in diverse organisms from bacteria to humans and functions in multiple cellular pathways. It has been increasingly recognized as a critical regulator of cell proliferation and tumorigenesis and the expression and activity of PLD are elevated in many different types of human cancers.

In ovarian cancer cells, PLD is involved in the formation of PA, which may be further converted to LPA by PLA_2. It was suggested that PLD is also involved in cancer progression and metastasis and elevated PLD expression has been reported in various cancer tissues [165]. Moreover, PLD was found to stimulate cell protrusions in v-Src–transformed cells [166]. Furthermore, PLD activity was elevated by the integrin receptor signaling pathway in OVCAR-3 cells, and PLD blocking was found to inhibit integrin-mediated Rac translocation in, and the spreading and migration of, OVCAR-3 cells [167]. Thus, the PLD-PA-Rac pathway plays an important role in the metastasis of cancer cells, and might provide a connection for integrin and PLD-mediated cancer metastasis [167]. A new mechanism has also been suggested for PLD and PA mediated carcinogenesis through Wnt/β-catenin signaling network [168].

4.2.4. Autotaxin

The ATX protein is a member of the ectonucleotide pyrophosphatase and phosphodiesterase family of enzymes, but unlike other members of this group, ATX possesses lysophospholipase D activity. This enzyme hydrolyzes lysophosphatidylcholine (LPC) to generate bioactive lipid LPA, which is an important signaling molecule regulates a variety of biological process through its receptors. ATX is essential for normal development and is implicated in various physiological processes. It also acts as a potent tumor growth factor and mitogen that is, associated with pathological conditions such as cancer, pain and fibrosis. Exogenous addition of VEGF-A to cultured cells induces ATX expression and secretion, resulting in increased extracellular LPA production [169]. This elevated LPA, acting through LPA4, modulates VEGF responsiveness by inducing VEGF receptor 2 expression. Downregulation of ATX secretion in SKOV3 cells significantly attenuates cell motility responses to VEGF, ATX, LPA, LPC [169]. Through their respective G protein–coupled receptors, LPC and LPA have both been reported to stimulate migration [170]. LPC was unable to stimulate the cellular migration by itself, ATX had to be present. Knocking down ATX secretion, or inhibiting its catalytic activity, blocked cellular migration by preventing LPA production and the subsequent activation of LPA receptors [170].

5. Summary

As a combination of central obesity, dyslipidemia, and insulin resistance, MS is the central of world–wide prevalence of Type 2 Diabetes Mellitus (T2DM), cardiovascular diseases and inflammation. Current animal and clinical evidence strongly suggest that abnormal lipid metabolism is closely associated with onset of insulin resistance and cancer. Importantly, more and more evidence show that most of the components of the MS are linked in some way to the development of various cancers [171-173], although epidemiological studies linking the MS to cancer are highly required. Obesity and diabetes have been reported to be associated with breast, endometrial, colorectal, pancreatic, hepatic or renal cancer [174, 175]. The molecular links between MS and cancer are still unclear, but insulin/insulin-like growth factor (IGF) systems and associated intracellular signaling cascades may play an important role in mediating MS related cancers [173]. However, the mechanisms by which actually promote tumor cell growth in patients with MS need further investigation. Since lipids and their metabolites and metabolism pathways are related to metabolic diseases and cancer cell growth, we propose that lipids may link to MS and cancers and exploring the related molecules and understanding the underlying mechanisms will be helpful in developing potential therapies for both MS and cancer. Based on the discoveries of current research results, a diet with high amount of oleic acid and balanced ratio of omega-3/omega-6 PUFAs would be helpful for health and prevention of both MS and cancer.

Author details

Fang Hu
Center for Food Biotechnology, School of Food Science and Technology,
State Key Laboratory of Food Science and Technology, Jiangnan University, Jiangsu, China

Metabolic Syndrome Research Center, the Second Xiangya Hospital, Central South University, Changsha, China

Yingtong Zhang and Yuanda Song
Center for Food Biotechnology, School of Food Science and Technology,
State Key Laboratory of Food Science and Technology, Jiangnan University, Jiangsu, China

Acknowledgement

Fang Hu is supported by National Key Basic Research Program of China (973 Program) 2012CB524900, National Science Foundation of China (NSFC) grant 31071921, and NSFC grant 81170783. Yuanda Song is supported by NSFC grant 81071685, Open Project Program of State Key Laboratory of Food Science and Technology, Jiangnan University (SKLF-TS-201101), and starting grant from Jiangnan University.

6. References

[1] Kiebish M A, et al. (2008) Cardiolipin and electron transport chain abnormalities in mouse brain tumor mitochondria: lipidomic evidence supporting the Warburg theory of cancer. J Lipid Res. 49: 2545-56.

[2] Swinnen J V and G Verhoeven (1998) Androgens and the control of lipid metabolism in human prostate cancer cells. J Steroid Biochem Mol Biol. 65: 191-8.

[3] Lee C H, P Olson, and R M Evans (2003) Minireview: lipid metabolism, metabolic diseases, and peroxisome proliferator-activated receptors. Endocrinology. 144: 2201-7.

[4] Walker A K, et al. (2011) A conserved SREBP-1/phosphatidylcholine feedback circuit regulates lipogenesis in metazoans. Cell. 147: 840-52.

[5] Podo F, et al. (2011) MR evaluation of response to targeted treatment in cancer cells. NMR Biomed. 24: 648-72.

[6] Pegorier J P, et al. (1985) Effect of intragastric triglyceride administration on glucose homeostasis in newborn pigs. Am J Physiol. 249: E268-75.

[7] Eckel R H, S M Grundy, and P Z Zimmet (2005) The metabolic syndrome. Lancet. 365: 1415-28.

[8] Unger R H (2002) Lipotoxic diseases. Annu Rev Med. 53: 319-36.

[9] Unger R H and P E Scherer (2010) Gluttony, sloth and the metabolic syndrome: a roadmap to lipotoxicity. Trends Endocrinol Metab. 21: 345-52.

[10] Hotamisligil GS P P, Budavari A, Ellis R, White MF, Spiegelman BM. (1996) IRS-1-mediated inhibition of insulin receptor tyrosine kinase activity in TNF-alpha- and obesity-induced insulin resistance. Science. 271(5249): 665-8.

[11] Schinner S, et al. (2005) Molecular mechanisms of insulin resistance. Diabet Med. 22: 674-82.

[12] Storlien LH J A, Chisholm DP, Pascoe WS, Kraegen EW. (1991) Influence of dietary fat composition on development of insulin resistance in rats: relationship to muscle triglyceride and omega-3 fatty acids in muscle phospholipids. Diabetes. 40: 280-9.

[13] Shulman G I (2000) Cellular mechanisms of insulin resistance. J Clin Invest. 106: 171-6.

[14] Shulman G I (2004) Unraveling the cellular mechanism of insulin resistance in humans: new insights from magnetic resonance spectroscopy. Physiology (Bethesda). 19: 183-90.

[15] Postic C and J Girard (2008) Contribution of de novo fatty acid synthesis to hepatic steatosis and insulin resistance: lessons from genetically engineered mice. J Clin Invest. 118: 829-38.

[16] Riccardi G, R Giacco, and A A Rivellese (2004) Dietary fat, insulin sensitivity and the metabolic syndrome. Clin Nutr. 23: 447-56.

[17] Parillo M and G Riccardi (2004) Diet composition and the risk of type 2 diabetes: epidemiological and clinical evidence. Br J Nutr. 92: 7-19.

[18] Vessby B, et al. (2001) Substituting dietary saturated for monounsaturated fat impairs insulin sensitivity in healthy men and women: The KANWU Study. Diabetologia. 44: 312-9.

[19] Mayer E J, et al. (1993) Usual dietary fat intake and insulin concentrations in healthy women twins. Diabetes Care. 16: 1459-69.

[20] Parker D R, et al. (1993) Relationship of dietary saturated fatty acids and body habitus to serum insulin concentrations: the Normative Aging Study. Am J Clin Nutr. 58: 129-36.

[21] Feskens EJ L J, Kromhout D. (1994) Diet and physical activity as determinants of hyperinsulinemia: the Zutphen Elderly Study. Am J Epidemiol. Am J Epidemiol. 140(4): 350-60.

[22] An J, et al. (2004) Hepatic expression of malonyl-CoA decarboxylase reverses muscle, liver and whole-animal insulin resistance. Nat Med. 10: 268-74.

[23] Hulver M W, et al. (2003) Skeletal muscle lipid metabolism with obesity. Am J Physiol Endocrinol Metab. 284: E741-7.

[24] Nagle C A, E L Klett, and R A Coleman (2009) Hepatic triacylglycerol accumulation and insulin resistance. J Lipid Res. 50 Suppl: S74-9.

[25] Vessby B A A, Skarfos E, Berglund L, Salminen I, Lithell H. (1994) The risk to develop NIDDM is related to the fatty acid composition of the serum cholesterol esters. Diabetes. 43: 1353-7.

[26] Erion D M and G I Shulman (2010) Diacylglycerol-mediated insulin resistance. Nat Med. 16: 400-2.

[27] Goodpaster B H and D E Kelley (2002) Skeletal muscle triglyceride: marker or mediator of obesity-induced insulin resistance in type 2 diabetes mellitus? Curr Diab Rep. 2: 216-22.

[28] Holland W L and S A Summers (2008) Sphingolipids, insulin resistance, and metabolic disease: new insights from in vivo manipulation of sphingolipid metabolism. Endocr Rev. 29: 381-402.
[29] Chavez J A and S A Summers (2012) A ceramide-centric view of insulin resistance. Cell Metab. 15: 585-94.
[30] Holland W L, et al. (2007) Inhibition of ceramide synthesis ameliorates glucocorticoid-, saturated-fat-, and obesity-induced insulin resistance. Cell Metab. 5: 167-79.
[31] Wang C-N O B, L., Brindley, D.N (1998) Effects of cell-permeable ceramides and tumor necrosis factor-a on insulin signaling and glucose uptake in 3T3-L1 adipocytes. Diabetes. 47: 24–31.
[32] Hajduch E, et al. (2001) Ceramide impairs the insulin-dependent membrane recruitment of protein kinase B leading to a loss in downstream signalling in L6 skeletal muscle cells. Diabetologia. 44: 173-83.
[33] Bikman BT S S (2011) Ceramides as modulators of cellular and whole-body metabolism. J Clin Invest. 121(11): 4222-30.
[34] Glaros E N, et al. (2008) Myriocin slows the progression of established atherosclerotic lesions in apolipoprotein E gene knockout mice. J Lipid Res. 49: 324-31.
[35] Park TS H Y, Noh HL, Drosatos K, Okajima K, Buchanan J, et al. (2008) Ceramide is a cardiotoxin in lipotoxic cardiomyopathy. J Lipid Res. 49(10): 2101-12.
[36] Ussher J R, et al. (2010) Inhibition of de novo ceramide synthesis reverses diet-induced insulin resistance and enhances whole-body oxygen consumption. Diabetes. 59: 2453-64.
[37] Adams J M, et al. (2004) Ceramide content is increased in skeletal muscle from obese insulin-resistant humans. Diabetes. 53: 25-31.
[38] Schenk S and J F Horowitz (2007) Acute exercise increases triglyceride synthesis in skeletal muscle and prevents fatty acid-induced insulin resistance. J Clin Invest. 117: 1690-8.
[39] Straczkowski M, et al. (2007) Increased skeletal muscle ceramide level in men at risk of developing type 2 diabetes. Diabetologia. 50: 2366-2373.
[40] Dube J J, et al. (2011) Effects of weight loss and exercise on insulin resistance, and intramyocellular triacylglycerol, diacylglycerol and ceramide. Diabetologia. 54: 1147-1156.
[41] Volek J S, et al. (2009) Carbohydrate Restriction has a More Favorable Impact on the Metabolic Syndrome than a Low Fat Diet. Lipids. 44: 297-309.
[42] Guo Z, et al. (2010) Relationship of the polyunsaturated to saturated fatty acid ratio to cardiovascular risk factors and metabolic syndrome in Japanese: the INTERLIPID study. J Atheroscler Thromb. 17: 777-84.
[43] Hunter J E, J Zhang, and P M Kris-Etherton (2010) Cardiovascular disease risk of dietary stearic acid compared with trans, other saturated, and unsaturated fatty acids: a systematic review. Am J Clin Nutr. 91: 46-63.
[44] Cao H, et al. (2008) Identification of a lipokine, a lipid hormone linking adipose tissue to systemic metabolism. Cell. 134: 933-44.

[45] Mozaffarian D, et al. (2010) Trans-palmitoleic acid, metabolic risk factors, and new-onset diabetes in U.S. adults: a cohort study. Ann Intern Med. 153: 790-9.

[46] Mozaffarian D, R Micha, and S Wallace (2010) Effects on coronary heart disease of increasing polyunsaturated fat in place of saturated fat: a systematic review and meta-analysis of randomized controlled trials. PLoS Med. 7: e1000252.

[47] Jebb S A, et al. (2010) Effect of changing the amount and type of fat and carbohydrate on insulin sensitivity and cardiovascular risk: the RISCK (Reading, Imperial, Surrey, Cambridge, and Kings) trial. Am J Clin Nutr. 92: 748-58.

[48] Astrup A, et al. (2011) The role of reducing intakes of saturated fat in the prevention of cardiovascular disease: where does the evidence stand in 2010? American Journal of Clinical Nutrition. 93: 684-688.

[49] Lee J H, et al. (2009) Omega-3 fatty acids: cardiovascular benefits, sources and sustainability. Nature Reviews Cardiology. 6: 753-758.

[50] Carpentier Y A, L Portois, and W J Malaisse (2006) n-3 fatty acids and the metabolic syndrome. Am J Clin Nutr. 83: 1499S-1504S.

[51] Bang H O, J Dyerberg, and A B Nielsen (1971) Plasma lipid and lipoprotein pattern in Greenlandic West-coast Eskimos. Lancet. 1: 1143-5.

[52] Delarue J, et al. (1996) Effects of fish oil on metabolic responses to oral fructose and glucose loads in healthy humans. Am J Physiol. 270: E353-62.

[53] Weintraub M S, et al. (1988) Dietary polyunsaturated fats of the W-6 and W-3 series reduce postprandial lipoprotein levels. Chronic and acute effects of fat saturation on postprandial lipoprotein metabolism. J Clin Invest. 82: 1884-93.

[54] Woodman R J, et al. (2002) Effects of purified eicosapentaenoic and docosahexaenoic acids on glycemic control, blood pressure, and serum lipids in type 2 diabetic patients with treated hypertension. Am J Clin Nutr. 76: 1007-15.

[55] Mori T A and R J Woodman (2006) The independent effects of eicosapentaenoic acid and docosahexaenoic acid on cardiovascular risk factors in humans. Curr Opin Clin Nutr Metab Care. 9: 95-104.

[56] Delarue J, et al. (2003) Fish oil prevents the adrenal activation elicited by mental stress in healthy men. Diabetes Metab. 29: 289-95.

[57] Hu F B, et al. (2002) Fish and omega-3 fatty acid intake and risk of coronary heart disease in women. JAMA. 287: 1815-21.

[58] Connor W E (2000) Importance of n-3 fatty acids in health and disease. Am J Clin Nutr. 71: 171S-5S.

[59] Lombardo Y B and A G Chicco (2006) Effects of dietary polyunsaturated n-3 fatty acids on dyslipidemia and insulin resistance in rodents and humans. A review. J Nutr Biochem. 17: 1-13.

[60] Clarke S D (2001) Polyunsaturated fatty acid regulation of gene transcription: a molecular mechanism to improve the metabolic syndrome. J Nutr. 131: 1129-32.

[61] Jump D B, et al. (2005) Fatty acid regulation of hepatic gene transcription. J Nutr. 135: 2503-6.

[62] Clamp A G, et al. (1997) The influence of dietary lipids on the composition and membrane fluidity of rat hepatocyte plasma membrane. Lipids. 32: 179-84.
[63] Lombardo Y B, G Hein, and A Chicco (2007) Metabolic syndrome: effects of n-3 PUFAs on a model of dyslipidemia, insulin resistance and adiposity. Lipids. 42: 427-37.
[64] Kopecky J, et al. (2009) n-3 PUFA: bioavailability and modulation of adipose tissue function. Proc Nutr Soc. 68: 361-9.
[65] Neschen S, et al. (2006) Fish oil regulates adiponectin secretion by a peroxisome proliferator-activated receptor-gamma-dependent mechanism in mice. Diabetes. 55: 924-8.
[66] Flachs P, et al. (2005) Polyunsaturated fatty acids of marine origin upregulate mitochondrial biogenesis and induce beta-oxidation in white fat. Diabetologia. 48: 2365-75.
[67] Huang M, et al. (2012) A high-fat diet enhances proliferation of prostate cancer cells and activates MCP-1/CCR2 signaling. Prostate.
[68] Blank M M, et al. (2012) Dietary fat intake and risk of ovarian cancer in the NIH-AARP Diet and Health Study. Br J Cancer. 106: 596-602.
[69] Rockenbach G, et al. (2011) Dietary intake and oxidative stress in breast cancer: before and after treatments. Nutricion Hospitalaria. 26: 737-744.
[70] Perse M, et al. (2012) High fat mixed lipid diet modifies protective effects of exercise on 1,2 dimethylhydrazine induced colon cancer in rats. Technol Cancer Res Treat. 11: 289-99.
[71] Freedland S J, et al. (2008) Carbohydrate restriction, prostate cancer growth, and the insulin-like growth factor axis. Prostate. 68: 11-9.
[72] Lloyd J C, et al. (2010) Effect of isocaloric low fat diet on prostate cancer xenograft progression in a hormone deprivation model. J Urol. 183: 1619-24.
[73] Othman R (2007) Dietary lipids and cancer. Libyan J Med. 2: 180-4.
[74] Bougnoux P, B Giraudeau, and C Couet (2006) Diet, cancer, and the lipidome. Cancer Epidemiol Biomarkers Prev. 15: 416-21.
[75] Suburu J and Y Q Chen (2012) Lipids and prostate cancer. Prostaglandins Other Lipid Mediat. 98: 1-10.
[76] Escrich E, et al. (2011) Modulatory effects and molecular mechanisms of olive oil and other dietary lipids in breast cancer. Curr Pharm Des. 17: 813-30.
[77] Djuric Z (2011) The Mediterranean diet: effects on proteins that mediate fatty acid metabolism in the colon. Nutr Rev. 69: 730-44.
[78] Rose D P and J M Connolly (2000) Regulation of tumor angiogenesis by dietary fatty acids and eicosanoids. Nutr Cancer. 37: 119-27.
[79] Lee J Y, L Zhao, and D H Hwang (2010) Modulation of pattern recognition receptor-mediated inflammation and risk of chronic diseases by dietary fatty acids. Nutr Rev. 68: 38-61.
[80] Park H, et al. (2011) A high-fat diet increases angiogenesis, solid tumor growth, and lung metastasis of CT26 colon cancer cells in obesity-resistant BALB/c mice. Mol Carcinog.

[81] Thiebaut A C, et al. (2007) Dietary fat and postmenopausal invasive breast cancer in the National Institutes of Health-AARP Diet and Health Study cohort. J Natl Cancer Inst. 99: 451-62.
[82] Escrich E, et al. (2007) Molecular mechanisms of the effects of olive oil and other dietary lipids on cancer. Mol Nutr Food Res. 51: 1279-92.
[83] Bhatia E, et al. (2011) Chemopreventive effects of dietary canola oil on colon cancer development. Nutr Cancer. 63: 242-7.
[84] Cho K, et al. (2010) Canola oil inhibits breast cancer cell growth in cultures and in vivo and acts synergistically with chemotherapeutic drugs. Lipids. 45: 777-84.
[85] Mamalakis G, et al. (2009) Adipose tissue fatty acids in breast cancer patients versus healthy control women from Crete. Ann Nutr Metab. 54: 275-82.
[86] Mercer N, et al. (2011) Applications of site-specific labeling to study HAMLET, a tumoricidal complex of alpha-lactalbumin and oleic acid. PLoS One. 6: e26093.
[87] Carrillo C, M D Cavia, and S R Alonso-Torre (2011) Oleic acid inhibits store-operated calcium entry in human colorectal adenocarcinoma cells. Eur J Nutr.
[88] Corsetto P A, et al. (2011) Effects of n-3 PUFAs on breast cancer cells through their incorporation in plasma membrane. Lipids Health Dis. 10.
[89] Menendez J A, et al. (2006) HER2 (erbB-2)-targeted effects of the omega-3 polyunsaturated fatty acid, alpha-linolenic acid (ALA; 18:3n-3), in breast cancer cells: the "fat features" of the "Mediterranean diet" as an "anti-HER2 cocktail". Clin Transl Oncol. 8: 812-20.
[90] Berquin I M, et al. (2007) Modulation of prostate cancer genetic risk by omega-3 and omega-6 fatty acids. J Clin Invest. 117: 1866-75.
[91] Doughman S D, S Krupanidhi, and C B Sanjeevi (2007) Omega-3 fatty acids for nutrition and medicine: considering microalgae oil as a vegetarian source of EPA and DHA. Curr Diabetes Rev. 3: 198-203.
[92] Wang D and R N Dubois (2010) Eicosanoids and cancer. Nat Rev Cancer. 10: 181-93.
[93] Larsson S C, et al. (2004) Dietary long-chain n-3 fatty acids for the prevention of cancer: a review of potential mechanisms. Am J Clin Nutr. 79: 935-45.
[94] Nakamura M T, et al. (2004) Mechanisms of regulation of gene expression by fatty acids. Lipids. 39: 1077-83.
[95] Georgiadi A and S Kersten (2012) Mechanisms of gene regulation by fatty acids. Adv Nutr. 3: 127-34.
[96] Swinnen J V, K Brusselmans, and G Verhoeven (2006) Increased lipogenesis in cancer cells: new players, novel targets. Curr Opin Clin Nutr Metab Care. 9: 358-65.
[97] Baracos V E, V C Mazurak, and D W L Ma (2004) n-3 Polyunsaturated fatty acids throughout the cancer trajectory: influence on disease incidence, progression, response to therapy and cancer-associated cachexia. Nutrition Research Reviews. 17: 177-192.
[98] Roberts R, et al. (2009) Markers of de novo lipogenesis in adipose tissue: associations with small adipocytes and insulin sensitivity in humans. Diabetologia. 52: 882-90.
[99] Fernandez-Real J M, et al. (2010) Extracellular fatty acid synthase: a possible surrogate biomarker of insulin resistance. Diabetes. 59: 1506-11.

[100] Matsuzaka T, et al. (2007) Crucial role of a long-chain fatty acid elongase, Elovl6, in obesity-induced insulin resistance. Nat Med. 13: 1193-202.

[101] Lodhi I J, X C Wei, and C F Semenkovich (2011) Lipoexpediency: de novo lipogenesis as a metabolic signal transmitter. Trends in Endocrinology and Metabolism. 22: 1-8.

[102] Savage D B, et al. (2006) Reversal of diet-induced hepatic steatosis and hepatic insulin resistance by antisense oligonucleotide inhibitors of acetyl-CoA carboxylases 1 and 2. J Clin Invest. 116: 817-24.

[103] Lelliott C and A J Vidal-Puig (2004) Lipotoxicity, an imbalance between lipogenesis de novo and fatty acid oxidation. International Journal of Obesity. 28: S22-S28.

[104] Cases S, et al. (1998) Identification of a gene encoding an acyl CoA:diacylglycerol acyltransferase, a key enzyme in triacylglycerol synthesis. Proc Natl Acad Sci U S A. 95: 13018-23.

[105] Smith S J, et al. (2000) Obesity resistance and multiple mechanisms of triglyceride synthesis in mice lacking Dgat. Nat Genet. 25: 87-90.

[106] Abu-Elheiga L, et al. (2001) Continuous fatty acid oxidation and reduced fat storage in mice lacking acetyl-CoA carboxylase 2. Science. 291: 2613-6.

[107] Donnelly K L, et al. (2005) Sources of fatty acids stored in liver and secreted via lipoproteins in patients with nonalcoholic fatty liver disease. Journal of Clinical Investigation. 115: 1343-1351.

[108] Shimomura I, et al. (1997) Differential expression of exons 1a and 1c in mRNAs for sterol regulatory element binding protein-1 in human and mouse organs and cultured cells. J Clin Invest. 99: 838-45.

[109] Shimano H, et al. (1997) Isoform 1c of sterol regulatory element binding protein is less active than isoform 1a in livers of transgenic mice and in cultured cells. J Clin Invest. 99: 846-54.

[110] Yecies J L, et al. (2011) Akt Stimulates Hepatic SREBP1c and Lipogenesis through Parallel mTORC1-Dependent and Independent Pathways (vol 14, pg 21, 2011). Cell Metab. 14: 280-280.

[111] Yamashita H, et al. (2001) A glucose-responsive transcription factor that regulates carbohydrate metabolism in the liver. Proc Natl Acad Sci U S A. 98: 9116-9121.

[112] Iizuka K, et al. (2004) Deficiency of carbohydrate response element-binding protein (ChREBP) reduces lipogenesis as well as glycolysis. Proc Natl Acad Sci U S A. 101: 7281-7286.

[113] Ferre P and F Foufelle (2010) Hepatic steatosis: a role for de novo lipogenesis and the transcription factor SREBP-1c. Diabetes Obesity & Metabolism. 12: 83-92.

[114] Iizuka K and Y Horikawa (2008) ChREBP: A glucose-activated transcription factor involved in the development of metabolic syndrome. Endocr J. 55: 617-624.

[115] Dentin R, et al. (2006) Liver-specific inhibition of ChREBP improves hepatic steatosis and insulin resistance in ob/ob mice. Diabetes. 55: 2159-2170.

[116] Verhoeven G (2002) [Androgens and increased lipogenesis in prostate cancer. Cell biologic and clinical perspectives]. Verh K Acad Geneeskd Belg. 64: 189-95; discussion 195-6.

[117] Mukherjee A, et al. (2012) Lysophosphatidic acid activates lipogenic pathways and de novo lipid synthesis in ovarian cancer cells. J Biol Chem.

[118] Wang G, et al. (2012) Endoplasmic Reticulum Factor ERLIN2 Regulates Cytosolic Lipid Content in Cancer Cells. Biochem J.

[119] Migita T, et al. (2008) ATP citrate lyase: activation and therapeutic implications in non-small cell lung cancer. Cancer Res. 68: 8547-54.

[120] Martel P M, et al. (2006) S14 protein in breast cancer cells: direct evidence of regulation by SREBP-1c, superinduction with progestin, and effects on cell growth. Exp Cell Res. 312: 278-88.

[121] Lin V C, et al. (2012) Activation of AMPK by Pterostilbene Suppresses Lipogenesis and Cell-Cycle Progression in p53 Positive and Negative Human Prostate Cancer Cells. J Agric Food Chem. 60: 6399-407.

[122] Rahman M T, et al. (2012) Fatty acid synthase expression associated with NAC1 is a potential therapeutic target in ovarian clear cell carcinomas. Br J Cancer. 107: 300-7.

[123] Turrado C, et al. (2012) New synthetic inhibitors of Fatty Acid synthase with anticancer activity. J Med Chem. 55: 5013-23.

[124] Jiang B, et al. (2012) Inhibition of Fatty-acid Synthase Suppresses P-AKT and Induces Apoptosis in Bladder Cancer. Urology.

[125] Kuchiba A, et al. (2012) Body mass index and risk of colorectal cancer according to fatty acid synthase expression in the nurses' health study. J Natl Cancer Inst. 104: 415-20.

[126] Gelebart P, et al. (2012) Blockade of fatty acid synthase triggers significant apoptosis in mantle cell lymphoma. PLoS One. 7: e33738.

[127] Vazquez-Martin A, et al. (2008) Overexpression of fatty acid synthase gene activates HER1/HER2 tyrosine kinase receptors in human breast epithelial cells. Cell Prolif. 41: 59-85.

[128] Zaytseva Y Y, et al. (2012) Inhibition of fatty acid synthase attenuates CD44-associated signaling and reduces metastasis in colorectal cancer. Cancer Res. 72: 1504-17.

[129] Chen H W, et al. (2012) Targeted therapy with fatty acid synthase inhibitors in a human prostate carcinoma LNCaP/tk-luc-bearing animal model. Prostate Cancer Prostatic Dis.

[130] Yang T P, et al. (2012) Mulberry Leaf Polyphenol Extract Induced Apoptosis Involving Regulation of Adenosine Monophosphate-Activated Protein Kinase/Fatty Acid Synthase in a p53-Negative Hepatocellular Carcinoma Cell. J Agric Food Chem.

[131] Pandey P R, et al. (2012) Anti-cancer drugs targeting fatty acid synthase (FAS). Recent Pat Anticancer Drug Discov. 7: 185-97.

[132] Wang C R S, Watabe K, Liao DF, Cao D. (2010) Acetyl-CoA carboxylase-a as a novel target for cancer therapy. Front Biosci. 2: 515-26.

[133] Zu X Y, et al. (2012) ATP citrate lyase inhibitors as novel cancer therapeutic agents. Recent Pat Anticancer Drug Discov. 7: 154-67.

[134] Zaidi N, et al. (2012) ATP-citrate lyase (ACLY)-knockdown induces growth arrest and apoptosis through different cell- and environment-dependent mechanisms. Mol Cancer Ther.

[135] Hanai J, et al. (2012) Inhibition of lung cancer growth: ATP citrate lyase knockdown and statin treatment leads to dual blockade of mitogen-activated protein kinase (MAPK) and phosphatidylinositol-3-kinase (PI3K)/AKT pathways. J Cell Physiol. 227: 1709-20.

[136] Wang C, et al. (2009) Acetyl-CoA carboxylase-alpha inhibitor TOFA induces human cancer cell apoptosis. Biochem Biophys Res Commun. 385: 302-6.

[137] Bauer D E, et al. (2005) ATP citrate lyase is an important component of cell growth and transformation. Oncogene. 24: 6314-22.

[138] Yoon S, et al. (2007) Up-regulation of acetyl-CoA carboxylase alpha and fatty acid synthase by human epidermal growth factor receptor 2 at the translational level in breast cancer cells. J Biol Chem. 282: 26122-31.

[139] Luo D X, et al. (2012) Targeting acetyl-CoA carboxylases: small molecular inhibitors and their therapeutic potential. Recent Pat Anticancer Drug Discov. 7: 168-84.

[140] Post J A, J J Bijvelt, and A J Verkleij (1995) Phosphatidylethanolamine and sarcolemmal damage during ischemia or metabolic inhibition of heart myocytes. Am J Physiol. 268: H773-80.

[141] Leonardi R, et al. (2009) Elimination of the CDP-ethanolamine pathway disrupts hepatic lipid homeostasis. J Biol Chem. 284: 27077-89.

[142] Vecchini A, et al. (2000) Molecular defects in sarcolemmal glycerophospholipid subclasses in diabetic cardiomyopathy. J Mol Cell Cardiol. 32: 1061-74.

[143] Lim H Y, et al. (2011) Phospholipid homeostasis regulates lipid metabolism and cardiac function through SREBP signaling in Drosophila. Genes & Development. 25: 189-200.

[144] Glunde K, C Jie, and Z M Bhujwalla (2004) Molecular causes of the aberrant choline phospholipid metabolism in breast cancer. Cancer Res. 64: 4270-6.

[145] Iorio E, et al. (2005) Alterations of choline phospholipid metabolism in ovarian tumor progression. Cancer Res. 65: 9369-76.

[146] Ross J, et al. (2008) Fatty acid synthase inhibition results in a magnetic resonance-detectable drop in phosphocholine. Mol Cancer Ther. 7: 2556-65.

[147] Lu J, et al. (2002) Role of ether-linked lysophosphatidic acids in ovarian cancer cells. J Lipid Res. 43: 463-76.

[148] Moolenaar W H (1999) Bioactive lysophospholipids and their G protein-coupled receptors. Exp Cell Res. 253: 230-8.

[149] Liscovitch M and L C Cantley (1994) Lipid second messengers. Cell. 77: 329-34.

[150] Westermann A M, et al. (1998) Malignant effusions contain lysophosphatidic acid (LPA)-like activity. Ann Oncol. 9: 437-42.

[151] Freeman M R and K R Solomon (2004) Cholesterol and prostate cancer. J Cell Biochem. 91: 54-69.

[152] Fang X, et al. (2004) Mechanisms for lysophosphatidic acid-induced cytokine production in ovarian cancer cells. J Biol Chem. 279: 9653-61.
[153] Li H Y, et al. (2003) Cholesterol-modulating agents kill acute myeloid leukemia cells and sensitize them to therapeutics by blocking adaptive cholesterol responses. Blood. 101: 3628-34.
[154] Sivashanmugam P, L Tang, and Y Daaka (2004) Interleukin 6 mediates the lysophosphatidic acid-regulated cross-talk between stromal and epithelial prostate cancer cells. J Biol Chem. 279: 21154-9.
[155] Hu Y L, et al. (2001) Lysophosphatidic acid induction of vascular endothelial growth factor expression in human ovarian cancer cells. J Natl Cancer Inst. 93: 762-8.
[156] Pustilnik T B, et al. (1999) Lysophosphatidic acid induces urokinase secretion by ovarian cancer cells. Clin Cancer Res. 5: 3704-10.
[157] Symowicz J, et al. (2005) Cyclooxygenase-2 functions as a downstream mediator of lysophosphatidic acid to promote aggressive behavior in ovarian carcinoma cells. Cancer Res. 65: 2234-42.
[158] Oyesanya R A, et al. (2008) Transcriptional and post-transcriptional mechanisms for lysophosphatidic acid-induced cyclooxygenase-2 expression in ovarian cancer cells. FASEB J. 22: 2639-51.
[159] Fujita T, et al. (2003) Expression of lysophosphatidic acid receptors and vascular endothelial growth factor mediating lysophosphatidic acid in the development of human ovarian cancer. Cancer Lett. 192: 161-9.
[160] Tanyi J and J Rigo, Jr. (2009) [Lysophosphatidic acid as a potential target for treatment and molecular diagnosis of epithelial ovarian cancers]. Orv Hetil. 150: 1109-18.
[161] Song Y, et al. (2009) Sp-1 and c-Myc mediate lysophosphatidic acid-induced expression of vascular endothelial growth factor in ovarian cancer cells via a hypoxia-inducible factor-1-independent mechanism. Clin Cancer Res. 15: 492-501.
[162] Zhao X, et al. (2006) Caspase-3-dependent activation of calcium-independent phospholipase A2 enhances cell migration in non-apoptotic ovarian cancer cells. J Biol Chem. 281: 29357-68.
[163] Song Y, et al. (2007) Inhibition of calcium-independent phospholipase A2 suppresses proliferation and tumorigenicity of ovarian carcinoma cells. Biochem J. 406. 427-36.
[164] McHowat J, et al. (2011) Platelet-activating factor and metastasis: calcium-independent phospholipase A2beta deficiency protects against breast cancer metastasis to the lung. Am J Physiol Cell Physiol. 300: C825-32.
[165] Eder A M, et al. (2000) Constitutive and lysophosphatidic acid (LPA)-induced LPA production: role of phospholipase D and phospholipase A2. Clin Cancer Res. 6: 2482-91.
[166] Shen Y, Y Zheng, and D A Foster (2002) Phospholipase D2 stimulates cell protrusion in v-Src-transformed cells. Biochem Biophys Res Commun. 293: 201-6.
[167] Chae Y C, et al. (2008) Phospholipase D activity regulates integrin-mediated cell spreading and migration by inducing GTP-Rac translocation to the plasma membrane. Mol Biol Cell. 19: 3111-23.

[168] Kang D W, K Y Choi, and S Min do (2011) Phospholipase D meets Wnt signaling: a new target for cancer therapy. Cancer Res. 71: 293-7.
[169] Ptaszynska M M, et al. (2008) Positive feedback between vascular endothelial growth factor-A and autotaxin in ovarian cancer cells. Mol Cancer Res. 6: 352-63.
[170] Gaetano C G, et al. (2009) Inhibition of autotaxin production or activity blocks lysophosphatidylcholine-induced migration of human breast cancer and melanoma cells. Mol Carcinog. 48: 801-9.
[171] Cowey S and R W Hardy (2006) The metabolic syndrome: A high-risk state for cancer? Am J Pathol. 169: 1505-22.
[172] Pothiwala P, S K Jain, and S Yaturu (2009) Metabolic syndrome and cancer. Metab Syndr Relat Disord. 7: 279-88.
[173] Braun S, K Bitton-Worms, and D LeRoith (2011) The link between the metabolic syndrome and cancer. Int J Biol Sci. 7: 1003-15.
[174] Calle E E, et al. (2003) Overweight, obesity, and mortality from cancer in a prospectively studied cohort of U.S. adults. N Engl J Med. 348: 1625-38.
[175] Emily Jane Gallagher R N, Shoshana Yakar , Derek LeRoith (2010) The Increased Risk of Cancer in Obesity and Type 2 Diabetes: Potential Mechanisms. Principles of Diabetes Mellitus. 579-99.

Chapter 10

Impacts of Nutrition and Environmental Stressors on Lipid Metabolism

Heather M. White, Brian T. Richert and Mickey A. Latour

Additional information is available at the end of the chapter

http://dx.doi.org/10.5772/51204

1. Introduction

Mediation of nutrition and environmental stressors through hormonal and physiological responses alters growth performance and lipid metabolism in nonruminants, resulting in substantial impacts on carcass lipid quality. Understanding and managing the factors that control carcass fat quality is a challenge for the swine industry yet provides opportunities to improve final carcass quality and profitability of pork production. Three major contributors to lipid quality in swine are regulation of *de novo* lipogenesis, dietary lipid composition, and environmental stressors. This chapter will evaluate these contributors and their effects on lipid deposition and quality, as well as nutritional and managerial interventions.

2. De novo lipogenesis

In general, the fatty acid profiles of swine carcass lipids are reflective of dietary fatty acid composition and *de novo* lipogenesis. The level of unsaturation in dietary fat sources is mimicked in the carcass fatty acid profile, altering the lipid firmness by increasing the degree of unsaturation. Stress has also been shown to impact growth performance, and can have an impact on the swine industry both by altering growth performance and carcass lipid firmness. Fatty acids synthesized *de novo* are products of pathways tightly regulated by rate-limiting enzymes. Nutritional and hormonal regulators of the enzymes which regulate these pathways can alter rates in lipid synthesis, oxidation, and desaturation.

The first step in *de novo* lipogenesis is the generation of the main fatty acid subunit, malonyl-CoA. The production of malonyl-CoA from acetyl-CoA is catalyzed by acetyl-CoA carboxylase (ACC; EC 6.4.1.2) [1]. Acetyl-CoA is a single polypeptide chain which contains a biotin carboxyl carrier protein, biotin carboxylase, and carboxyl transferase domains [2, 3]. Acetyl-CoA is present as ACCα (~265 kDa) in liver and adipose tissue and catalyzes fatty acid synthesis [2, 3, 4]. In liver, heart, and muscle tissues ACCβ (~280 kDa) controls fatty acid oxidation [2, 3, 4]. The ACC reaction is a two-step reaction in which the biotin molecule, covalently attached by holo-carboxylase synthetase to the ε-amino group of a lysine residue, acts as the carboxyl carrier [5]. The first step results in the formation of carboxy-biotinyl-ACC at the biotin carboxylase active site and is ATP-dependent. During the second step, the carboxyl group is transferred from biotin to acetyl-CoA forming the malonyl-CoA product [5].

The fatty acid synthase (FAS; EC 2.3.1.85) pathway is responsible for *de novo* lipogenesis which stores excess energy as fatty acids in liver and adipose tissue [1,6]. This pathway occurs within the cytosol and is a sequence of seven steps which are NADPH-dependent and utilize one acetyl-CoA and seven malonyl-CoAs as the base molecules to produce palmitate [1]. The NADPH required for each reaction is derived from activity of malic enzyme and the pentose phosphate shunt [7]. Though palmitate is the main product, stearic, mysristic and shorter fatty acids may also be produced [7]. Fatty acids produced from *de novo* lipogenesis are primarily saturated or monounsaturated and may be used in phospholipid and triacylglycerol synthesis [7].

Fatty acid synthase is a multifunctional enzyme composed of two identical monomers, each ~270 kDa [3]. Each monomer contains six functional domains which are β-ketoacyl synthase (KS), acetyl/malonyl transacylase (AT/MT), β-hydroxyacyl dehydratase (DH), enoyl reductase (ER), β-ketoacyl reductase (KR), acyl carrier protein (ACP) and thioesterase (TE) in order from the N-terminus [3]. The condensation of seven C_2 moieties to the acetyl unit involves specific functions of the monomer components [3]. The reaction begins when the two substrates, acetyl-CoA and malonyl-CoA, are transferred to the KS and ACP, respectively, which is catalyzed by acetyl and malonyl transacylases. The condensation of these two substrates is catalyzed by KS and thus acetoacetyl-ACP is formed and CO_2 is released. Acetoacetyl is reduced to a β-hydroxyacyl chain by KR and the product is then dehydrated and reduced a second time by DH and ER, respectively. The resulting product is a four-carbon fatty acid which is attached to ACP and transferred, by KS, from the ACP to a Cys-SH group on the KS. The ACP is then free to accept another malonyl unit. The addition of two carbon units from malonyl-CoA to the growing acyl chain leads to the synthesis of palmitate which is released after being hydrolyzed by TE [3].

2.1. Regulation of de novo lipogenesis

Regulation of ACC and FAS are important as they are the rate limiting steps of lipogenesis. Transcriptional regulation of ACC-α and -β is controlled by three promoters, PI, II, and III [5]. These promoters respond to glucose, insulin, thyroid hormone, catabolic hormones, and leptin [5]. Additional regulation occurs by sterol-regulatory-element-binding protein 1c (SREBP1c) and peroxisome-proliferator-activated receptors (PPAR) [5]. Fasting inhibits ACC expression though re-feeding returns expression to normal levels. Insulin exposure activates ACC, while catecholamines or glucagon exposure will inhibit ACC [5]. Activation and inhibition by insulin, catecholamines and glucagon, respectively, occur within minutes of exposure [5].

Acetyl-CoA carboxylase is also allosterically regulated, resulting in active and inactive protein conformations [1,5]. Phosphorylation of four or more serine residues on ACC results in inactivation [5, 8]. Phosphorylation of ACCα is by AMP-activated protein kinase (AMPK) while phosphorylation of ACCβ is by protein kinase A (PKA) [5, 8]. In liver and heart cells, insulin activates ACCα by dephosphorylating the AMPK site although this mechanism has not been observed in fat or liver cells [5].

Transcriptional regulation is the primary means of controlling FAS [1, 7]. The FAS promoter has been studied in the rat, human, and chicken and the sequence is highly conserved among species [7]. The 5′ flanking region of the promoter is 2.1 kb long and has transcription factor binding sites which determine tissue specificity of expression [7]. Promoter activity and FAS expression have been shown to increase in transgenic mice when high carbohydrate diets are fed, after fasting, and with increased insulin and glucocorticoid levels. Dietary polyunsaturated fatty acids (PUFA) decrease hepatic and adipose FAS mRNA levels and is a part of the mechanism of dietary fats to reduce *de novo* fatty acid synthesis [7]. Another mode of FAS regulation is stability of FAS mRNA [7]. In diabetic rats, thyroid hormone regulates FAS mRNA stability and in fetal rat lung, glucocorticoids stabilize FAS mRNA [7].

2.2. Desaturation of fatty acids

Stearoyl-CoA desaturase (SCD; EC 1.14.19.1), also known as Δ^9 desaturase, is an endoplasmic reticulum associated enzyme that catalyzes the conversion of saturated fatty acids to monounsaturated fatty acids (MUFA) [9, 10]. Palmitoyl-CoA and stearoyl-CoA are the primary substrates of the desaturation reaction and are converted to palmitoleoyl-CoA and oleoyl-CoA, respectively [10, 11]. In liver, SCD is also required for synthesis of cholesteryl esters [9]. There are four isomers of SCD: SCD-1, found in adipose and liver tissue; SCD-2 and -3, found in the brain and harderian gland; and SCD-4, found in the heart [9]. The action of SCD to add a double bond to the Δ^9 position of a saturated fatty acid starts the desaturation process. More double bonds can then be added by the elongation pathways discussed below [11]. Desaturation of 12 to 19 carbon fatty acyl-CoAs catalyzed by SCD-1, -2, -3, and -4 results in the addition of a *cis*-double bond between carbons nine and 10 and this reaction requires NADH, oxygen, NADH-cytochrome *b*5 reductase and cytochrome *b*5 [9].

Control of SCD-1, -2, -3, and -4 is mainly by transcriptional regulation [9]. Dietary omega-3 and -6 PUFAs, thyroid hormone, glucagon, thiazolidinediones, and leptin suppress SCD-1 expression, while cholesterol, vitamin A, PPARα, SREBP-1c, and high carbohydrate feeding induce expression [9, 12]. Increased SCD-1 activity thus increases the conversion of saturated fatty acids to unsaturated fatty acids and changes the ratio of carcass fatty acids.

2.3. β-oxidation

β-oxidation is the catabolic process, occurring primarily in the mitochondria of the cell, that breaks down fatty acids into acyl-CoA molecules. These two carbon molecules can then enter the tricarboxylic acid cycle for energy production. β-oxidation involves three key components: activation of fatty acids in the cytosol of the cell, transport of activated fatty acids into the cell mitochondria, and oxidation.

The mechanism of the carnitine pathway is an ordered reaction where the binding of acyl-CoA begins the transport action [13]. Long chain fatty acids are converted to acyl-CoAs by acyl-CoA synthetase [14]. Acyl-CoAs are converted to acyl-carnitine molecules and transferred across the outer mitochondrial membrane by carnitine palmitoyltransferase-I (CPT; EC 2.3.1.21) [14]. Carnitine palmitoyltransferase-II is located on the inner mitochondrial membrane and liberates the carnitine from the acylcarnitine after transfer across the inner mitochondrial membrane [15]. After liberation, the acyl-CoA units are available for β-oxidation within the mitochondrial matrix [14]. Because CPT-II is not regulated [1] it is not pertinent to this discussion.

Carnitine palmitoyltransferase-I is located on the outer mitochondrial membrane and limits the rate of fatty acid oxidation by controlling the transportion of fatty acyl-CoA to the mitochondrial matrix where β-oxidation occurs [13, 1]. Two transmembrane domains anchor CPT-I to the outer mitochondrial membrane [13]. There are three isoforms of CPT-I [1]. In liver, kidney, lung, and heart tissue, CPT-Ia is present; CPT-Ib is present in skeletal muscle, heart, and adipose tissue; and CPT-Ic is brain tissue specific [1].

Regulation of β-oxidation occurs during the initial transport step. The main route of CPT-I regulation is by malonyl-CoA, the first product of lipogenesis, which inhibits CPT-I and aids to prevent simultaneous oxidation and synthesis [1, 16]. Regulation of CPT-I allows β-oxidation to be regulated by controlling the availability of acyl-CoA in the mitochondrial matrix [1, 14]. Though the sensivitiy of the CTP-Ia and CPT-Ib to malonyl-CoA are different, they both contain binding sites on the same side of the membrane as the active site [13]. The N-terminus of the enzyme, which is not required for catalytic activity, controls the response to malonyl-CoA [13]. The kinetics of inhibition by malonyl-CoA are responsive to temperature, pH, and lipids [13, 14].

Fasting and glucagon increases CPT-I gene expression while hypothyroidism decreases expression by regulating the transcription level [13]. The insulin growth factor I receptor also controls CPT-I expression by mediating the inhibitory effects of insulin [13, 14]. Expression of CPT-I is also transcriptionally upregulated by PPARα [13]. Long chain fatty acids increase CPT-Ia mRNA expression in liver tissue by both increasing transcription levels as well as improving CPT-I mRNA stability [14].

2.4. Regulation of lipid metabolism by transcription factors

Sterol regulatory element binding proteins (SREBP) are helix loop helix proteins that are within the leucine zipper family of transcription factors [9]. The SREBPs are present as two isoforms, SREBP-1 (a and c subforms) and SREBP-2 [9]. While SREBP-2 is primarily involved in activation of cholesterol synthesis and metabolism, SREBP-1c is involved solely in regulation of fatty acid synthesis and SREBP-1a is capable of inducing both synthesis of cholesterol and fatty acids [9]. In the liver, SREBP-1c increases expression of SCD, ACC, FAS and acetyl CoA synthase [9].

Long-chain fatty acids are oxidized in the peroxisome by catalase, producing acetyl-CoA and hydrogen peroxide [15]. The catalase enzyme is induced by high-fat diets and proliferation of the peroxisomes is controlled by the peroxisome proliferator activated receptor (PPAR), which is part of the nuclear receptor family [9, 15]. The PPARα form is involved in regulation of β-oxidation and lipolysis in hepatocytes while PPARγ is involved in regulation of fatty acid synthesis in adipocytes [17, 18, 19]. The PPAR binding site contains both a hydrophobic ligand-binding pocket and a DNA-binding domain [9]. Stimulation of fatty acid oxidation by PPARα is by induction of CPT-I. Peroxisome proliferators also stimulate SCD-1 transcription levels [9].

Intracellular fatty acids contribute to the overall regulation of synthesis and oxidative pathways. Fatty acids enter cells through diffusion or transporters, specifically fatty acid transport protein (FATP) or fatty acid transporter CD36 (FAT). Fatty acyl CoA synthetases or FATP then convert fatty acids into fatty acyl CoA (FACoA). Fatty acid binding proteins (FABP) then bind to and transport FACoA into intracellular compartments where they influence transcription through regulation of PPARα, γ and SREBP-1 [17, 20]. Intracellular PUFA inhibit SREBP-1 by downregulating enzymes involved in fatty acid synthesis [17, 18]. Intracellular PUFA activate PPAR to upregulate the transcription of the corresponding enzymes [17].

3. Dietary lipid composition

Dietary triacylglycerol composition plays a major role in determining adipose tissue composition. Monogastric animals incorporate dietary fatty acids directly into tissue lipid deposits [21, 22] and, therefore, to manipulate carcass lipid quality, it is important to understand the interactions of dietary lipids with carcass lipid. Carcass fatty acid profiles closely mimic dietary fatty acid profile [21, 23], and therefore, potential exists to modify carcass lipid properties (i.e., firmness, fatty acid profile, etc.) by altering dietary lipid composition.

One of the strongest determinants of carcass fat quality in pigs is the level and composition of lipids in the diet [24]. Because the utilization efficiency of dietary fat is 90% in pigs fed above maintenance [24] and the transfer coefficient of dietary fat to carcass lipid is as high as 31-40% [25] the carcass lipid composition is a reflection of dietary fat. The impact of dietary lipids on carcass lipid may differ depending on the timing of feeding relative to growth and finishing, levels included in the diet, and interactions with other stressors.

3.1. Dietary fat

Dietary triacylglycerols alter carcass lipid composition at the level of the fatty acid profile [21]. Saturated fatty acids lack double bonds and have melting temperatures above 40ºC. Mono-, di- and poly-unsaturated fatty acids have one, two, or many double bonds, respectively and as the level of unsaturation increases, the melting point decreases [21]. The ratio of saturated to unsaturated fatty acids is a way of describing the relative saturation of a fatty acid profile [21]. Iodine value, a measure of double bonds in a lipid, is a method used to composite characteristics of lipids in regard to fluidity [21, 26]. Saturated to unsaturated ratios and iodine values can be utilized to describe the composition of lipids in both feedstuffs, total rations, and animal tissue.

Fat is commonly added in swine diets from 0.5% up to 7% of the ration and increases growth rate, reduces feed intake, and improves feed efficiency [21]. Because of the previously mentioned utilization efficiency and transfer coefficients, the level of saturation and iodine value of the feed lipid source will be strongly reflected in the carcass fatty acid profile and therefore, sources of dietary fats play a critical role in final carcass lipid quality. Vegetable oils are typically high in linoleic acid, have an unsaturated to saturated fatty acid ratio of 12:1 [22] and an iodine value greater than 100 [21]. Diets high in these unsaturated vegetable oils will result in oily, soft carcass fat [21]. Conversely, tallow, which is high in palmitate and stearate, has a saturated to unsaturated fatty acid ratio of 1:1 [22], an iodine value between 40 and 45 [21] and will result in firmer carcass fat when fed in the diet. Greater saturated:unsaturated fatty acid ratio in fat contained in pig carcasses results in fewer difficulties during processing [27] due to increased firmness at typical processing temperatures (2 to 4°C). Due to differences in calculation of these indices, some variations in fatty acid profile are captured with one ration but not the other, as seen in Figure 1. For this reason, it is best to utilize both the IV and saturated:unsaturated indices when characterizing fat quality, in order to identify all variations in fatty acid profile.

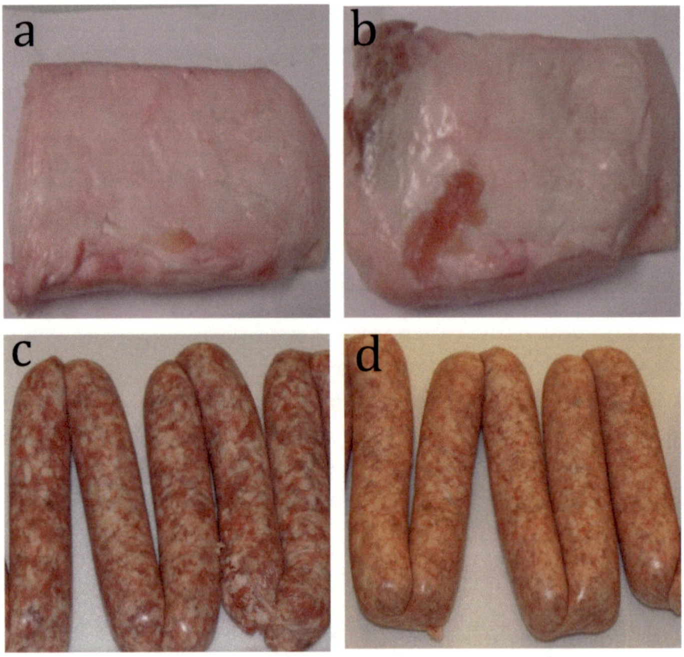

Figure 1. Differences in carcass lipid quality alter final product characteristics. Higher iodine values (IV) are associated with fat that is softer, resulting in increased difficulty slicing and processing. Panel *a* is backfat with an IV of 69 which represents fat that is firm and maintains shape and structure, while panel *b* is backfat with an IV of 79 which represents fat that will lack the firmness required for processing. Saturated to unsaturated fatty acid ratios are also used to characterize fatty acid profiles. While sausages (bottom panels) made from different animals have the same IV (59), the differences in saturated:unsaturated fatty acids results in a higher quality, firmer product in panel *c* (0.62) that has less smearing compared with panel *d* (0.59).

3.2. Dried Distillers Grains with Solubles

Dried distillers grains with solubles (DDGS) is the by-product of yeast fermentation of grains such as corn for ethanol production [28]. During fermentation, corn starch is converted into alcohol and the remaining grain components, protein, fat, fiber, minerals, and vitamins are concentrated in the fermentative co-product approximately 3-times that of corn [28]. The nutritional value of corn DDGS is variable and a function of DDGS processing [28, 29, 30].

There are two processes by which ethanol can be extracted from corn, wet milling and dry grinding. Dry grinding is more commonly used and accounts for 70% of ethanol production processes [31]. Dry grinding yields the maximum ethanol from corn while wet milling yields other products including corn oil and corn gluten meal [31, 32]. The dry grind process begins by grinding the corn and mixing it with water (Figure 2). The resulting mash is then heated with enzymes to convert the starches to sugars which can be fermented by yeast. The product contains particulates and solubles which are distilled and dehydrated, producing ethanol and wet distiller's grains. The distiller's grains are then dried in order to increase shelf life [31, 32].

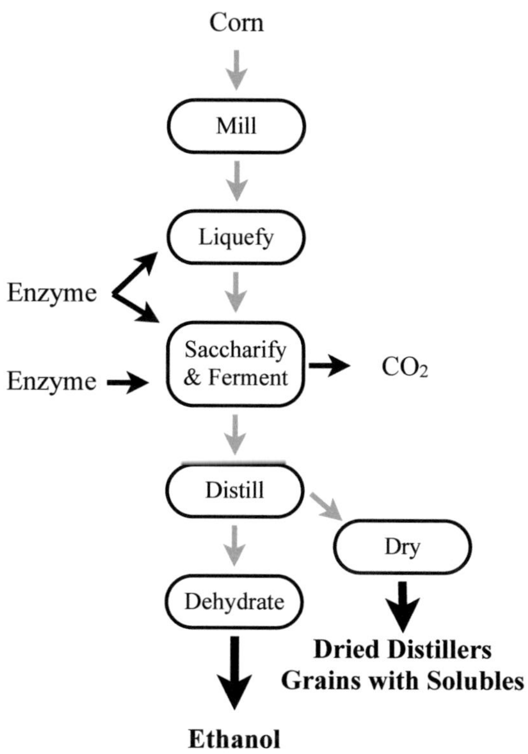

Figure 2. Dry grind processing of corn to produce ethanol. Progression of processing steps are shown in ovals and gray arrows, with inputs and outputs indicated by black arrows. The major byproduct of ethanol production is dried distillers grains with solubles.

The nutritional value of DDGS for pigs is influenced by the processing procedure and production plant equipment and techniques [33, 34]. The nutrient profile of DDGS remains highly variable even within the same production site [30, 35]. The NRC published content for DDGS is 93% dry matter, 2.82 Mcal/kg metabolizable energy, 27.7% crude protein, 8.4% crude fat and 34.6% neutral detergent fiber [36], however there is significant plant to plant variation, as noted above.

Two limiting factors for including DDGS in swine diets are the high level of unsaturation in the dietary fatty acid profile and the high fiber content [28, 31]. As discussed above, the composition of these fat sources is important when considering the carcass fat firmness [21]. Dietary fiber has also shown beneficial effects in swine diets including reduction of gastric ulceration and restriction of pathogenic bacteria in the intestinal tract; however, when fiber content of the diet exceeds 7%, growth is inhibited [37]. The high level of fat and fiber in DDGS have been shown to result in both decreased feed intake and increased unsaturated content of adipose tissue. In a trial utilizing 0, 10, 20, and 30% DDGS in grow-finish diets, pigs fed 20 or 30% DDGS had decreased growth performance and increased IV when compared to control fed pigs [38]. Incorporation of 0, 20, or 40% DDGS in diets during the final 30 days of the finishing phase resulted in reduced percent lean in bacon and decreased carcass firmness (based on IV and saturation); however, no effect on growth performance was observed [39].

The future direction of DDGS as a feed ingredient will likely be defined by the final use in global energy needs and not how it might be valued as a feed ingredient; that is, DDGS still contains a considerable amount of oil, a highly valued potential energy source. Today, DDGS is well suited for non-ruminants in terms of energy and protein content, price, and availability; however, the high linoleic acid content known to alter fat quality must be considered when determining dietary inclusions. As refiners investigate new approaches to removing the oil and protein, which may be of more value extracted, the future product could resemble a more fiber-like product, which would have wide range implications on non-ruminant animals and likely reduce it's future use in swine diets.

3.3. Omega-3 and -6 fatty acids

The levels of omega-3 and omega-6 fatty acids in the human diet are important for optimal health. Animals, including humans, lack the enzymes required to add double bonds between the methyl group and ninth carbon and therefore cannot synthesize omega-3 and -6 fatty acids, making these fatty acids essential in the diet [22]. Fatty acids in the omega-6 family, linoleic (LA; 18:2n-6) and arachidonic (AA; 20:4n-6), and those in the omega-3 family, α-linolenic (ALA; 18:3n-3) and subsequently eicosapentaenoic acid (EPA; 20:5n-3) and docosahexaenoic acid (DHA; 22:6n-3), must be supplied in animal diets [16, 21, 22). The synthesis pathways of omega-3 and -6 fatty acids and the parallel omega-9 pathways are shown in Figure 3. The omega-3 and -6 pathways compete for the Δ^5 and Δ^6 desaturases though both enzymes preferentially catalyze the reactions of the omega-3 pathway [40, 41].

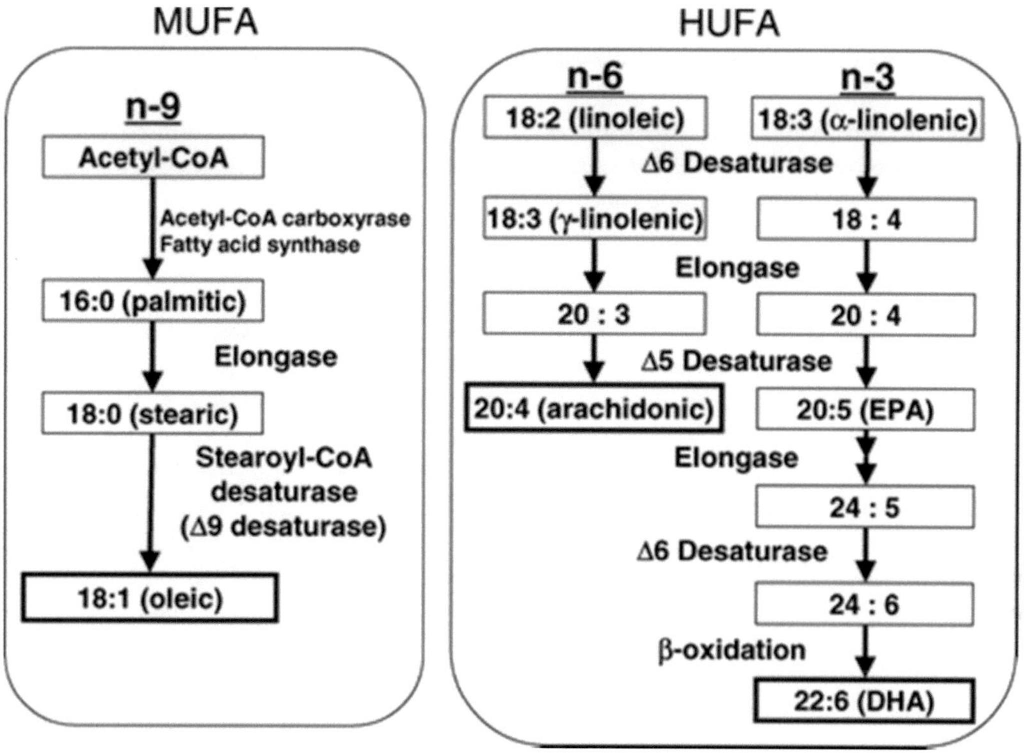

Figure 3. Synthesis pathways for omega-3, -6, and -9 fatty acids in mammals. MUFA, monounsaturated fatty acid; HUFA, highly unsaturated fatty acid; EPA, eicosapentaenoic acid; DHA, docosahexaenoic acid [9].

The ideal ratio of omega-6 to omega-3 fatty acids in human diets is between 4 to 6:1, although the average American diet is between 10 to 30:1 [42]. The change in this ratio is due to the increase in omega-6 intake relative to the level of omega-3 fatty acids [41]. The need to increase dietary intake of omega-3 fatty acids, specifically EPA and DHA, has increased demand for products with a ratio of omega-6 to -3 fatty acids more closely related to American Heart Association (AHA) recommendations.

The many health benefits of omega-3 fatty acids, such as lowering serum cholesterol and triacylglycerol concentrations, reduce platelet aggregation, reduction of blood pressure, and decreasing very-low-density and low-density lipoproteins, make dietary inclusion important [40]. The overall anti-inflammatory effects of omega-3 fatty acids have shown beneficial effects for arthritis and joint health in rats and humans [40]. Though it has not been directly studied in swine, omega-3 fatty acids could decrease the prevalence of lameness in sows if they result in the same joint and anti-inflammatory benefits noted in humans and rats. In Canada, 8-11% of sows culled were due to lameness [43] and in the United States lameness accounts for about 10% of culled sows during parity zero, one, and two or more, respectively [44]. Lameness results in the removal of sows at a younger age than other culling reasons, thus decreasing breeding herd productivity [44].

Omega-6 fatty acids are the precursors of eicosanoids which include prostaglandins, thromboxanes and leukotrienes. These metabolites of n-6 fatty acids exhibit inflammatory effects [45]. Omega-3 fatty acids inhibit eicosanoid synthesis by decreasing the available arachidonic acid available for eicosanoid production [18, 45]. In addition to decreasing eicosanoid production, omega-3 fatty acids also decrease other inflammatory cytokines such as interleukin-1 and -6, and tumour necrosis factor [18, 45].

3.4. Conjugated linoleic acid

Conjugated linoleic acids (CLA) are a group of polyunsaturated fatty acids that are positional and geometric isomers of linoleic acid (C18:2). Because CLA and its precursor, *trans* vaccenic acid, are naturally produced during bacterial fermentation in the rumen of ruminant animals, the main sources of CLA in human nutrition are ruminant milk and meats [46, 47]. The main isomers of CLA are *cis*-9, *trans*-11(c9t11) and *trans*-10, *cis*-12 (t10c12; Figure 4). Though the main isomer produced by ruminants is c9t11, commercially available products commonly contain equal proportions of c9t11 and t10c12 [46, 47]. Research in rodents, pigs, and humans has been conducted on the effects of CLA and has shown beneficial effects of CLA against obesity, cancer, atherosclerosis, and diabetes, some of which are isomer specific [46, 47, 48].

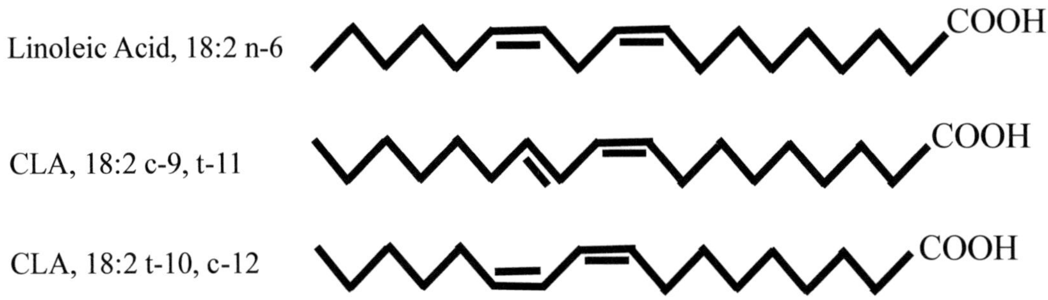

Figure 4. Structure of linoleic acid compared with *cis*-9, *trans*-11 and *trans*-10, *cis*-12 conjugated linoleic acid (CLA).

Many studies have shown CLA mixtures are able to reduce adipose tissue depots in rodents, pigs, and humans and that this effect is specific to the t10c12 isomer or a mixture containing greater than 50% t10c12 [46, 48]. Postweanling mice fed 1% CLA for 28-30 d had a 50% reduction in total adipose tissue compared to control mice [49]. In pigs, CLA inclusion in feed has resulted in decreased backfat thickness at finishing [50, 51]. Overweight or obese humans supplemented with CLA for 12 weeks also demonstrated reduced body fat mass, although their body mass index remained unchanged [52].

Another noted effect of CLA is the inhibition of cancer, specifically, mammary, prostate, skin, colon, and stomach cancers [48]. The anti-carcinogenic effects of CLA have been mainly attributed to the c9t11 isomer [46]. In studies of mammary and prostate cancer cell lines, feeding 1% CLA significantly reduced growth of the cancerous cells. Other studies of the same cell lines have not demonstrated these effects of CLA [48].

Atherosclerotic plaque formation is reduced by CLA [48]. Inclusion of 0.5 g/day in hypercholesterolemic diets fed to rabbits for 12 weeks resulted in significantly reduced serum triacylglycerols, low density lipoprotein (LDL) cholesterol levels and atherosclerotic plaque formation in the aorta [53]. The reduction of plaque deposits by CLA was proposed to be due to changes in LDL oxidative susceptibility [48].

Effects of CLA on the onset of diabetes and insulin resistance are inconsistant. Rats fed CLA have shown significantly reduced fasting glucose, insulinemia, triglyceridemia, free fatty acids, and leptinemia [48]. Butter enriched with c9t11 CLA failed to reduce glucose tolerance, lower adipose tissue or enhance glucose uptake leading to the conclusion that perhaps it is the t10c12 isomer which is responsible for the antidiabetogenic responses [48]. Insulin tolerance testing on CLA-fed mice showed marked insulin resistance without changes to blood glucose concentrations after oral glucose tolerance testing [54]. Other studies have examined the reduction of plasma leptin by CLA and the concomitant changes in blood glucose level due to regulation by leptin [46]. Feeding male mice high-fat diets with 1% CLA has resulted in reduced plasma leptin levels in one study [55] while resulting in no change in plasma leptin or glucose levels in another [56].

3.4.1. Feeding CLA to pigs

The effects of feeding CLA to pigs have been evaluated in regard to fat quality [57]. Gilts fed 1% CLA for seven weeks had firmer bellies, higher levels of saturated fatty acids, lower levels of unsaturated fatty acids and decreased IV when compared to controls [58]. Barrows fed CLA had improved feed efficiency, decreased backfat, and improved loin marbling and firmness when CLA was included at 0.75% of grow-finish diets [51]. When CLA was fed to genetically lean gilts for eight weeks, an increase in average daily gain and gain:feed was observed [59]. The same study also noted an increase in saturated fatty acids, decrease in unsaturated fatty acids, and an increased level of saturation of the belly tissue [59]. Several studies have shown that CLA feeding increases fatty acid saturation, and firmness in back fat and belly fat [60, 61, 62]. Additionally, use of CLA when feeding by-products may alleviate some or all of the negative impact on carcass quality. When feeding 0, 20, or 40% DDGS during the final 30 days of the finishing period, the addition of 0.6% CLA minimized the negative impact of 20% DDGS inclusion on carcass lipid quality but was unable to overcome the negative effects of feeding 40% DDGS [63].

3.4.2. Mechanism of CLA to alter lipid metabolism

Dietary CLA in several species alters the activity of SCD-1, FAS, and ACC in adipose and liver. Conjugated linoleic acids decrease mRNA for FAS and ACC to significantly inhibit the capacity for *de novo* lipogenesis [47, 60]. In barrows and gilts fed 0.25 or 0.5% CLA for the finishing diet from 97 to 172 kg, ACC activity was significantly reduced compared to control pigs [64]. Alleviation of negative impacts of nutritional stress of lipid quality, such as during DDGS feeding, is likely through altered lipid metabolism as adipose mRNA expression of ACC was decreased with CLA supplementation with all inclusion levels of DDGS [39].

Reductions in SCD-1 expression were observed with CLA feeding in both mouse liver and cultured preadipocytes [48]. Previous studies indicate that CLA tends to decrease both SCD-1 [65] and decreases the Δ^9 desaturase index in pigs [65, 66]. Decreasing SCD-1 mRNA expression, and thereby decreasing the amount of saturated fatty acids being converted to unsaturated fatty acids, may be responsible for the increased levels of saturated fatty acids observed after feeding CLA [65, 66].

The c10 t12 isomer of CLA decreases the expression of PPARγ in adipose tissue and increases the expression of PPARα in liver tissue [67, 68, 69]. By acting as a PPARγ modulator, CLA is able to prevent lipid accumulation as shown in cultured adipocytes [70]. Conjugated linoleic acid also acts as a PPARα activator and induces accumulation of PPAR-responsive mRNAs in hepatic cells [67] serving to upregulate PPAR-responsive pathways.

4. Environmental stressors

Environmental stressors on pigs can impact lipid metabolism and overall carcass quality. Impacts of environmental stressors, including thermal stress and housing density, are through both direct effects of decreased growth efficiency and indirect effects of altered regulation of *de novo* lipogenesis. Managerial and nutritional strategies during critical growth periods may alleviate the impact of these environmental stressors. Additionally, the regulation of *de novo* lipogenesis is influenced by the health status of the animal. Insults to health through disease or constant stress decrease feed intake and reduce *de novo* lipid synthesis. This decrease in *de novo* synthesis shifts the ratios of fatty acids in the adipose tissue to more unsaturated FA, further reducing lipid quality.

4.1. Spatial allocation, growth, and carcass composition

Decreasing space allocation reduces growth performance and the minimal spatial requirements for grow-finish pigs have been examined [36, 71]. Housing densities between 0.76 and 0.93 m^2/pig have been reported as the threshold for grow-finish swine, below which ADG and ADFI are reduced [71].

Stress from spatial allocation is not a simple reflection of floor space, it is also reflective of pen dimensions, size, location of feeders and waters, and size of the pigs. One allometric calculation for spatial allocation is $f = k \times BW^{.667}$ (f = floor allowance, m^2; k = coefficient of housing area; BW = body weight, kg) which accounts for the relationship between body weight and surface area [71]. In a study using this approach, housing densities of 0.578, 0.761 and 0.942 m^2/pig corresponding to housing area coefficients of 0.030, 0.039 and 0.048, respectively; resulted in decreased ADG and ADFI in pigs housed at floor area allowances with coefficients between 0.030 and 0.039 [71]. These results were within in the range of other reported housing threshold values [71].

4.2. Heat stress, pork quality and animal growth

The thermal neutral zone of a mammal is the range of ambient temperatures within which the animal can control its core body temperature without elevating its metabolic rate [72].

Within the thermoneutral zone of mammals, core body temperature is maintained without expending additional energy to warm or cool basal body temperature [72, 73]. If the environmental conditions are below this zone, additional energy of metabolism is devoted to generating heat to maintain the desired core temperature [72]. Conversely, at temperatures above this zone, the animal must dissipate energy to maintain core body temperature through additional heat loss mechanisms such as evaporative heat loss, convection, and conduction [72]. When environmental temperature rises above the point where heat production and heat loss are balanced, the animal is in a state of heat stress [74]. In swine, evaporative heat loss is limited due to their inability to sweat; therefore, heat loss is primarily by respiration, evaporation, and exposure to cool air and wet surfaces for convection and conduction, respectively [72, 73, 75]. As an adaptive mechanism to further cool the body and maintain a homeothermic temperature, the animal decreases feed intake in order to decrease the thermal effect of feeding [74].

The optimum temperature for a finishing pig between 54.5 and 118.2 kg of body weight is 18.3°C, with a desirable temperature range between 10°C to 23.9°C [76]. The heat stress index (HSI; Figure 5), published by Iowa State University [77], is a practical guideline outlining temperature and humidity ranges for growing pigs. The HSI classifies environmental temperature and humidity conditions into three zones: alert, danger, and emergency. Within the alert range, producers are advised to monitor animal behavior, increase ventilation, and ensure that water is readily available. The danger range requires additional cooling by spraying or misting with water and increasing air flow. Under emergency conditions, producers are advised to avoid transporting animals, withdraw feed during the hottest part of the day, and reduce light levels. For example, when relative humidity is between 45 and 60%, 25.6°C is the alert threshold, 27.2°C is the danger threshold and 30°C is the emergency threshold.

For grow-finish swine, housing temperatures above 23.9°C decrease voluntary feed intake and growth rate compared to optimum housing temperatures [76, 78]. Voluntary decreases in feed intake decrease metabolic heat production to help maintain homeothermy [79]. Pigs challenged with heat-stress will have decreased feed consumption and average daily gain; however, feed efficiency is maintained when compared to control animals [80].

Nienaber et al. [81] noted that elevated temperature decreased daily feed consumption in both cattle and swine, through decreases in meal size and frequency. Feed intake was reduced by 55 g per degree of temperature increase above 22ºC [82]. A similar decrease in feed intake observed by Collin et al. [75] was coupled to reductions in thermic effect of feeding and heat production.

Humidity is also influential in the animal's ability to dissipate heat by evaporative heat loss [74]. In a study comparing 50, 65, and 80% humidity levels, respiration rate and rectal temperatures were increased at lower temperatures and 80% humidity compared to when humidity was 50 and 65% [74]. Increasing environmental humidity decreases the efficiency of evaporative cooling, resulting in symptoms of heat-stress occurring at lower temperatures.

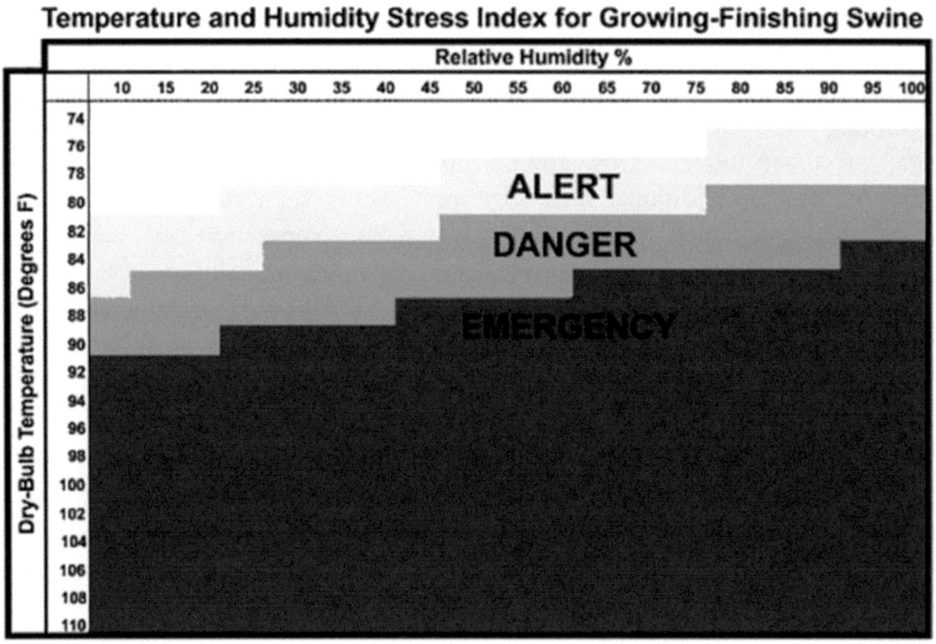

Figure 5. Heat Stress Index for Swine published by Iowa State University [77].

Physiological response to stressors, such as heat, results in the activation of the stress-activated sympathetic nervous system and the release of catecholamines and glucocorticoids [83]. When animals are exposed to a stressor, the hypothalamus releases corticotrophin-releasing hormone which stimulates adrenocorticotropin hormone (ACTH) from the pituitary gland [84]. The release of ACTH stimulates the adrenal cortex to release cortisol [84]. Cortisol regulates growth, immunity, and intermediary metabolism including gluconeogenesis, glycogen synthesis, and lipogenesis [7, 85]. The regulation of these processes by stress-activated hormones is one source of altered metabolism during periods of stress that may contribute to changes in feed intake, weight gain, and carcass lipid quality.

Decreases in acetyl-CoA-carboxylase and stearoyl-CoA-desaturase in adipose and liver tissues have been noted in heat-stressed pigs [79]. Kouba et al. [79] noted a decrease in acetyl-CoA-carboxylase activity in heat-stressed pigs and a decrease in *de novo* fatty acid synthesis. Acetyl-CoA-carboxylase and stearoyl-CoA-desaturase catalyze the first step of the synthesis of fatty acids and the synthesis of monounsaturated fatty acids from saturated fatty acids, respectively, and therefore would be key points of potential change in lipid metabolism.

Kouba et al. [86] noted 20-35 kg pigs maintained at 31°C compared to 20°C had slightly thicker backfat with a greater lipid content and an increase in lipoprotein lipase expression in backfat and an increase in VLDL-lipid concentration in heat-stressed pigs. The increase in fat thickness of heat-stressed pigs was thus attributed to increases in lipid metabolism in the liver, and in adipose tissue, noted through increased VLDL production and LPL activity, respectively. Increased lipid circulation between liver and adipose tissue is also part of the adaptation of pigs to high environmental temperatures [86].

Interactions between environmental stressors can amplify or alleviate the impact of an individual stressor. Pigs challenged with increased temperature and decreased spatial allocation demonstrated that both temperature and spatial allocation affected growth performance and carcass quality [63]. Temperature stress decreased ADG, ADFI, and G:F ratios. Pigs housed at minimum required spatial allocation of 0.66 m^2/pig [36] and high environmental temperatures (32.2°C) had a 50% reduction in ADFI and an 85% reduction in ADG when compared with pigs housed in their thermal neutral zone; when pigs were housed at increased spatial allocation (0.93 m^2/pig) and a temperature above 23.9°C, there was a 29% reduction of ADFI and a 36% reduction in ADG. Additionally, the level of saturation in adipose tissue was decreased in heat stressed pigs; however, increasing the spatial allocation in the 32.2°C environment ameliorated these effects and increased the fatty acid saturation to match the 23.9°C-housed pigs. The effects of spatial allocation on carcass quality demonstrate that challenging pigs with elevated temperature and reduced spatial allocation decreased feed intake, as demonstrated in the literature [87], and also decreased carcass lipid firmness. These relationships demonstrate that almost 50% of the negative growth performance effects of temperature can be ameliorated by a 28% increase in spatial allocation. In addition, an increase in housing allocation during heat stress may ameliorate the negative effects of temperature on belly weight, carcass quality, and growth performance.

5. Carcass quality

5.1. Bacon quality

The belly is the most expensive cut of the carcass, thus, the quality of bacon produced from the belly is linked to overall carcass value. Bacon is scored according to lean content and slice thickness to identify premium quality slices [88]. Premium slices have greater than 50% lean content and are wider than 1.9 cm at all points [88]. Accordingly, bacon slices are graded as either number one slices, number two slices, or as ends and pieces [88]. Pork bellies that are classified below standard based on these characteristics represent a decrease in carcass value.

The swine industry has shifted to genetically lean lines with decreased backfat and thus, bellies of have become thinner, leaner, and softer [89, 90]. Thinner bellies are generally softer, produce fewer grade one slices, and present more problems with processing and storage [89, 90]. Providing saturated fat in the diet of pigs increases belly thickness and improves belly firmness [90]. Likewise, feeding CLA improves belly firmness in finishing pigs [59, 90].

5.2. Carcass lipid quality

Many processors utilize IV as numerical evaluation of carcass fat quality and thus have target IV values. An IV greater than 65, for some processors may be unacceptably high [58], while an IV greater than 75 may be the threshold for other processors. Increased IV [29] and decreased saturated to unsaturated fatty acid ratios [21] indicate decreases in carcass quality due to decreased fat firmness. High levels of unsaturated fatty acids result in rapid oxidation which decreases shelf life [91]. Furthermore, high levels of unsaturated fatty acids in the diets also produce bacon which is smeary, separates and causes processing difficulties

[88]. As discussed above, dietary fatty acid composition contributes to the carcass fatty acid composition; therefore, feeding more saturated dietary lipid sources will result in firmer carcass lipids with decreased IV [21].

5.3. Shelf-life of meat products

Shelf-life is defined as the period of time between packaging of a product and its end use when product properties remain acceptable to the consumer [92]. Shelf-life properties may include appearance, texture, flavor, color, and nutritive value [93]. One of the major factors affecting the shelf-life of meat products is rancidity or lipid oxidation, which occurs when fatty acids react to oxygen sources in the environment [94]. Oxidation produces low molecular weight aldehydes, acids, and ketones that cause the meat to exhibit distinct odors and flavors, typically unacceptable to consumers [94]. The level of unsaturation greatly affects the susceptibility of fat to oxidation with high degrees of unsaturation resulting in rapid oxidation and subsequently decreased shelf-life [95].

6. Summary

The fatty acid profiles of swine carcass lipids are reflective of dietary fatty acid composition and *de novo* lipogensis [21]. The level of unsaturation in dietary fat sources is mimicked in the carcass fatty acid profile, altering the lipid firmness by increasing the degree of unsaturation [21, 22]. Feed alternatives such as DDGS, which are high in PUFA, decrease carcass lipid firmness and bacon lean when fed to grow-finish pigs [38]. Conversely, feeding CLA positively impacts growth performance and carcass fat quality [57, 58]. Stress has also been shown to impact growth performance, and low spatial allocation and heat stress have an impact on the swine industry both by altering growth performance and carcass lipid firmness [36, 76]. Fatty acids synthesized *de novo* are products of pathways tightly regulated by rate-limiting enzymes. Nutritional and hormonal regulators of the enzymes, which regulate these pathways, can alter rates in lipid synthesis, oxidation, and desaturation [5, 7, 13].

Environmental and nutritional stressors on pigs can impact lipid metabolism and carcass quality and thus alter final product quality and profitability. While the interactions of these stressors can additively worsen the impact on growth or lipid quality, understanding these interactions can also be used as a basis for managerial or nutritional interventions to alleviate the negative impact of unavoidable stressors.

Author details

Heather M. White
Department of Animal Science, University of Connecticut, USA

Brian T. Richert
Department of Animal Science, Purdue University, Brian, USA

Mickey A. Latour
Department of Animal Science, Southern Illinois University, Carbondale, USA

7. References

[1] Ronnett, G. V., A. M. Kleman, E. K. Kim, L. E. Landree, and Y. Tu. 2006. Fatty acid metabolism, the central nervous system, and feeding. *Obesity.* 14Suppl:201-207.

[2] Munday, M. R. 2002. Regulation of mammalian acetyl-CoA carboxylase. *Biochem Soc Trans.* 30:1059-1064.

[3] Chirala, S. S., and S. J. Wakil. 2004. Structure and function of animal fatty acid synthase. *Lipids.* 39(11):1045-1053.

[4] Tong, L. 2005. Acetyl-coenzyme A carboxylase: crucial metabolic enzyme and attractive target for drug discovery. *Cell Mol Life Sci.* 62:1784-1803.

[5] Brownsey, R. W., A. N. Boone, J. E. Kulpa, and W. M. Lee. 2006. Regulation of acetyl-CoA carboxylase. *Biochem Soc Trans.* 34:223-227.

[6] Ronnett, G. V., A. K. Kim, L. E. Landree, and Y. Tu. 2005. Fatty acid metabolism as a target for obesity treatment. *Phsyiol Behav.* 85:25-35.

[7] Semenkovich, C. F. 1997. Regulation of fatty acid synthase (FAS). *Prog Lipid Res.* 36(1):43-53.

[8] Boone, A. N., A. Chan, J. E. Kulpa, and R. W. Brownsey. 2000. Bimodal activation of acetyl-CoA carboxylase by glutamate. *J Biol Chem.* 275(15):10819-10825.

[9] Nakamura, M. T., and T. Y. Nara. 2004. Structure, function and dietary regulation of Δ6, Δ5, and Δ9 desaturases. *Annu Rev Nutr.* 24:345-376.

[10] Dobrzyn, A., and J. M. Ntambi. 2005. The role of stearoyl-CoA desaturase in the control of metabolism *Prostaglandins Leukot Essent Fatty Acids.* 73(1):35-41.

[11] Mayes, P. A., and K. M. Botham. 2003a. Metabolism of unsaturated fatty acids & Eicosanoids. Pg. 190 in Harper's Illustrated Biochemistry. R.K. Murray, D.K. Granner, P.A. Mayes and V.W. Rodwell, ed. McGraw-Hill, New York.

[12] Ntambi, J. M., M. Miyazaki, and A. Dobrzyn. 2004. Regulation of stearoyl-CoA desaturase expression. *Lipids.* 39(11):1061-1065.

[13] Ramsay, R. R., R. D. Gandour, and F. R. van der Leij. 2001. Molecular enzymology of carnitine transfer and transport. *Biochim Biophys Acta.* 1546:21-43.

[14] Louet, J. F., C. L. May, J. P. Pegorier, J. F. Decaux, and J. Girard. 2001. Regulation of liver carnitine palmitoyltransferase I gene expression by hormones and fatty acids. *Biochem Soc Trans.* 29:310-316.

[15] Mayes, P. A., and K. M. Botham. 2003b. Oxidation of fatty acids: ketogenesis. Pg. 180 in Harper's Illustrated Biochemistry. R.K. Murray, D.K. Granner, P.A. Mayes and V.W. Rodwell, ed. McGraw-Hill, New York.

[16] Drackley, J. K. 2000. Lipid Metabolism. Page 97 in Farm Animal Metabolism and Nutrition. J.P.F. D'Mello, ed. CABI Publishing, Oxon, UK.

[17] Jump, D. B., and S. D. Clarke. 1999. Regulation of gene expression by dietary fat. *Annu Rev Nutr.* 19:63-90.

[18] Jump, D. B. 2002. The biochemistry of n-3 polyunsaturated fatty acids. *J Biol Chem.* 277(11):8755-8758.

[19] Sampath, H., and J. M. Ntambi. 2005. Polyunsaturated fatty acid regulation of genes of lipid metabolism. *Ann Rev Nutr.* 25:317-340.

[20] Jump, D. B., D. Botolin, Y. Wang, J. Xu, B. Christian, and O. Demeure. 2005. Fatty acid regulation of hepatic gene transcription. *J Nutr.* 135:2503-2506.
[21] Azain, M. J. 2001. Fat in swine nutrition. Pg 95 in Swine Nutrition 2nd Ed. A.J. Lewis and L.L. Southern, ed. CRC Press, Boca Raton.
[22] Wiseman, J. 2006. Value of fats and oils in pig diets. Page 368 in Whittemore's Science and Practice of Pig Production. 3rd ed. I. Kyriazakis and C.T. Whittemore, ed. Blackwell Publishing, Oxford, UK.
[23] Allen, C. E., D. C. Beitz, B. A. Cramer, and R. G. Kauggman. 1976. Biology of fat in meat animals. Research Division, College of Agricultural and Life Sciences, University of Wisconsin-Madison.
[24] Freeman, C. P. 1983. Fat supplementation in animal production -- monogastric animals. *Proc Nutr Soc.* 42:351-359.
[25] Kloareg, M., J. Noblet, and J. van Milgen. 2007. Deposition of dietary fatty acids, *de novo* synthesis and anatomical partitioning of fatty acids in finishing pigs. *Brit J Nutr*. 97:35-44.
[26] Madsen, A., K. Jakoben, and H. P. Mortensen. 1992. Influence of dietary fat on carcass fat quality in pigs. A review. *Acta Agric Scand, Sect. A., Animal Sci.* 42:220-225.
[27] Teye, G. A., J. D. Wood, F. M. Whittington, A. Stewart, and P. R. Sheard. 2006. Influence of dietary oils and protein level on pork quality. 2. Effects on properties of fat and processing characteristics of bacon and frankfurter-style sausages. *Meat Science*. 73: 166-177.
[28] Newland, H. W., and D. C. Mahan. 1990. Distillers By-Products. Page 161 in Nontraditional Feed Sources for Use in Swine Production. P.A. Thacker and R.N. Kirkwood, ed. Butterworths, Stoneham, MA.
[29] Cromwell, G. L., K. L. Herkelman, and T. S. Stahly. 1993. Physical, chemical, and nutritional characteristics of distillers dried grains with solubles from chicks and pigs. *J Anim Sci*. 71:679-686.
[30] Pahm, A.A., C. Pedersen, D. Hoehler, and H.H. Stein. 2008. Factors affecting the variability in ileal amino acid digestibility in corn distillers dried grains with solubles fed to growing pigs. *J. Anim. Sci.* 86:2180-2189.
[31] Rausch, K. D., and R. L. Belyea. 2006. The future of coproducts from corn processing. *Appl Biochem Biotechnol.* 128:47-86.
[32] Bothast, R. J., and M. A. Schlicher. 2005. Biotechnological processes for conversion of corn into ethanol. *App Microbiol Biotechnol.* 67:19-25.
[33] Spiehs, M. J., M. H. Whitney, and G. C. Shurson. 2002. Nutrient database for distiller's dried grains with solubles produced from new ethanol plants in Minnesota and South Dakota. *J Anim Sci*. 80:2639-2645.
[34] Belyea, R. L., K. D. Rausch, and M. E. Tumbleson. 2004. Composition of corn and distillers dried grains with solubles from dry grind ethanol processing. *Bioresour Technol.* 94:293-298.
[35] Shurson, G., M. Spiehs, and M. Whitney. 2004. The use of maize distiller's dried grains with solubles in pig diets. *Pig news and information*. 25(2):75N-83N.

[36] NRC. 1998. Nutrient Requirements of Swine. 10th rev. ed. Natl. Acad. Press, Washington, DC.
[37] Varel, V. H. and J. T. Yen. 1997. Microbial perpective on fiber utilization by swine. *J Anim Sci.* 75:2715-2722.
[38] Whitney, M. H., G. C. Shurson, L. J. Johnston, D. M. Wulf, and B. C. Shanks. 2006. Growth performance and carcass characteristics of grower-finisher pigs fed high-quality corn distillers dried grain with solubles origninating from a modern Midwestern ethanol plant. *J Anim Sci.* 84:3356-3363.
[39] White, H. M., B. T. Richert, J. S. Radcliffe, A. P. Schinckel, J. R. Burgess, S. L. Koser, S. S. Donkin, and M. A. Latour. 2009. Feeding CLA partially recovers carcass quality in pigs fed dried distillers grains with solubles. *J. Anim. Sci.* 87:157-66.
[40] Simopoulos, A. P. 1991. Omega-3 fatty acids in health and disease and in growth and development. *Am J Clin Nutr.* 54:438-463.
[41] Kris-Etherton, P. M., W. S. Harris, and L. J. Appel. 2002. Fish consumption, fish oil, omega-3 fatty acids, and cardiovascular disease. *Circulation.* 106:2747-2757.
[42] Leskanich, C. O., K. R. Matthews, C. C. Warkup, R. C. Noble, and M. Hazzledine. 1997. The effect of dietary oil containing (n-3) fatty acids on the fatty acid, physicochemical, and organoleptic characteristics of pig meat and fat. *J Anim Sci.* 75(3):673-683.
[43] Dewey, C. E., R. M. Friendship, and M. R. Wilson. 1992. Lameness in breeding age swine – a case study. *Can Vet J.* 33:747-748.
[44] Anil, S. S., L. Anil, and J. Deen. 2005. Elavulation of patterns of removal and associations among culling because of lameness and sow productivity traits in swine breeding herds. *JAVMA.* 226(6):956-961.
[45] Calder, P. C. 2006. Polyunsaturated fatty acids and inflammation. *Prostaglandins Leukot Essent Fatty Acids.* 75:197-202.
[46] Wang, Y. W. and P. J. H. Jones. 2004. Conjugated linoleic acid and obesity control: efficacy and mechanisms. *Int J Obes.* 28:941-955.
[47] House, R. L., J. P. Cassady, E. J. Eisen, M. K. McIntosh, and J. Odle. 2005. Conjugated linoleic acid evokes de-lipidation through the regulation of genes controlling lipid metabolism in adipose and liver tissue. *Obes Rev.* 6:247-258.
[48] Belury, M. A. 2002. Dietary Conjugated Linoleic Acid in Health: Physiological Effects and Mechanisms of Action. *Annu Rev Nutr.* 22:505-531.
[49] Park Y., K. J. Albright, J. M. Storkson, W. Liu, M.E. Cook, and M. W. Pariza. 2001. Changes in body composition in mice during feeding and withdrawl of conjugated linoleic acid. *Lipids.* 34:243-248.
[50] Tischendorf, F., F. Schone, U. Kirchheim, and G. Jahreis. 2002. Influence of a conjugated linoleic acid mixture on growth, organ weights, carcass traits and meat quality in growing pigs. *J Anim Physiol Anim Nutr (Berl).* 86:117-128.
[51] Wiegand, B. R., F. C. Parrish, Jr., J. E. Swan, S. T. Larsen, and T. J. Baas. 2001. Conjugated linoleic acid improves feed efficiency, decreases subcutaneous fat, and improves certain aspects of meat quality in Stress-Genotype pigs. *J Anim Sci.* 79:2187-2195.

[52] Blankson, H., J. A. Stakkestad, H. Fagertun, E. Thom, J. Wadstein, and O. Gudmundsen. 2000. Conjugated linoleic acid reduces body fat mass in overweight and obese humans. *J Nutr.* 130:2943-2948.

[53] Lee, K. N, D. Kritchevsky and M. W. Pariza. 1994. Conjugated linoleic acid and atherosclerosis in rabbits. *Atherosclerosis.* 108:19-25.

[54] Tsuboyama-Kasaoka, N., M. Takahashi, K. Tanemura, H. J. Kim, T. Tange, H. Okuyama, M. Kasai, S. Ikemoto, and O. Ezaki. 2000. Conjugated linoleic acid supplementation reduces adipose tissue by apoptosis and evelops lipodystrophy in mice. *Diabetes.* 49:1534-1542.

[55] DeLany, J. P., F. Blohm, A. A. Truett, J. A. Scimeca, and D. B. West. 1999. Conjugated linoleic acid rapidly reduces body fat content in mice without affecting energy intake. *Am J Physiol.* 276:R1172-R1179.

[56] West, D. B., F. Y. Blohm, A. A. Truett, and J. P. DeLany. 2000. Conjugated linoleic acid persistently increases total energy expenditure in AKR/J mice without increasing uncoupling protein gene expression. *J Nutr.* 130:2471-2477.

[57] Cox, A. D. 2005. Added dietary fat effects on market pigs and sows. M.S. Thesis, Purdue University, West Lafayette.

[58] Eggert, J. M., M. A. Belury, A. Kempa-Steczko, S. E. Mills, and A. P. Schinckel. 2001. Effects of conjugated linoleic acid on the belly firmness and fatty acid composition of genetically lean pigs. *J Anim Sci.* 79:2866-2872.

[59] Weber, T. E., B. T. Richert, M. A. Belury, Y. Gu, K. Enright, and A. P. Schinckel. 2006. Evaluation of the effects of dietary fat, conjugated linoleic acid, and ractopamine on growth performance, pork quality, and fatty acid profiles in genetically lean gilts. *J Anim Sci.* 84:720-732.

[60] Ostrowska, E., M. Muralitharan, R. F. Cross, D. E. Bauman, and F. R. Dunshea. 1999. Dietary conjugated linoleic acids increase lean tissue and decrease fat deposition in growing pigs. *J Nutr.* 129:2037-2042.

[61] Aalhus, J. L., and M. E. R. Dugan. 2001. Improving meat quality through nutrition. *Advances in Pork Production.* 12:145.

[62] Dugan, M. E. R., J. L. Aalhus, and B. Uttaro. 2004. Nutritional manipulation of pork quality: current opportunities. *Advances in Pork Production.* 15:237.

[63] White, H. M., J. R. Burgess, A. P. Schinckel, S. S. Donkin, and M. A. Latour. 2008. Effects of temperature stress on growth performance and bacon quality in grow-finish pigs housed at two densities. *J. Anim. Sci.* 86:1789-98.

[64] Corino, C., S. Magni, G. Pastorelli, R. Rossi, and J. Mourot. 2003. Effect of conjugated linoleic acid on meat quality, lipid metabolism, and sensory characteristics of dry-cured hams from heavy pigs. *J Anim Sci.* 81:2219-2229.

[65] Smith, S. B., T. S. Hively, G. M. Cortese, J. J. Han, K. Y. Chung, P. Castenada, C. D. Gilbert, V. L. Adams, and H. J. Mersmann. 2002. Conjugated linoleic acid depresses the delta9 desaturase index and stearoyl coenzyme A desaturase enzyme activity in porcine subcutaneous adipose tissue. *J Anim Sci.* 80:2110-2115.

[66] Demaree, S. R., C. D. Gilbert, H. J. Mersmann, and S. B. Smith. 2002. Conjugated Linoleic Acid Differentially Modifies Fatty Acid Composition in Subcellular Fractions of

Muscle and Adipose Tissue but Not Adiposity of Postweanling Pigs. *J Nutr.* 132:3272-3279.

[67] Moya-Camarena, S. Y., J. P. Vanden Heuvel, S. G. Blanchard, L. A. Leesnitzer, and M. A. Belury. 1999. Conjugated linoleic acid is a potent naturally occurring ligand and activator of PPARα. *J Lipid Res.* 40:1426-1433.

[68] Evans, M. E., J. M. Brown, and M. K. McIntosh. 2002. Isomer-specific effects of conjugated linoleic acid (CLA) on adiposity and lipid metabolism. *J Nutr Biochem.* 13:508-516.

[69] Kang, K., W. Liu, K. J. Albright, Y. Park, and M. W. Pariza. 2003. *trans*-10, *cis*-12 CLA inhibits differentiation of 3T3-L1 adipocytes and decreases PPARγ expression. *Biochem Biophys Res Commun.* 303:795-799.

[70] Granlund, L., L. K. Juvet, J. I. Pedersen, and H. I. Nebb. 2003. *Trans*10, *cis*12-conjugated linoleic acid prevents triacylglycerol accumulation in adipocytes by acting as a PPARγ modulator. *J Lipid Res.* 44:1441-1452.

[71] Gonyou, H. W. and W. R. Stricklin. 1998. Effects of floor area allowance and group size on the productivity of growing/finishing pigs. *J Anim Sci.* 76:1326-1330.

[72] Mount, L. E. 1976. Heat loss in relation to plane of nutrition and thermal environment. *Proc Nutr Soc.* 35:81-86.

[73] Noblet, J., J. L. Dividich, and J. Van Milgen. 2001. Thermal environment and swine nutrition. Page 519 in Swine Nutrition 2nd Ed. A.J. Lewis and L.L. Southern, ed. CRC Press, Boca Raton.

[74] Huynh, T. T. T., A. J. A. Aarnink, M. W. A. Verstegen, W. J. J. Gerrits, M. J. W. Heetkamp, B. Kemp, and T. T. Canh. 2005. Effects of increasing temperatures on physiological changes in pigs at different relative humidities. *J Anim Sci.* 83:1385-1396.

[75] Collin, A., J. van Milgen, S. Dubois, and J. Noblet. 2001. Effect of high temperature on feeding behavior and heat production in group-housed young pigs. *Br J Nutr.* 86:63-70.

[76] Myer, R., and R. Bucklin. 2001. Influence of hot-humid environment on growth performance and reproduction of swine. University of Florida, IFAS Extension. Available: http://edis.ifas.ufl.edu/AN107. Accessed May 30, 2007.

[77] Iowa State University. 2002. Heat stress index chart for swine producers. Available: http://www.thepigsite.com/articles/5/housing-and-environment/669/heat-stress-index-chart-for-swine-producers. Accessed May 30, 2007.

[78] Verstegen, M. W. A., W. H. Close, I. B. Start, and L. E. Mount. 1973. The effects of environmental temperature and plane of nutrition on heat loss, energy retention and deposition of protein and fat in groups of growing pigs. *Br J Nutr.* 30:21-35.

[79] Kouba, M., D. Hermier, and J. Le Dividich. 1999. Influence of a high ambient temperature on stearoyl-CoA desaturase activity in the growing pig. *Comp Biochem Physiol.* 124B:7-13.

[80] Lopez, J., G. W. Jesse, B. A. Becker, and M. R. Ellersieck. 1991. Effects of temperature on the performance of finishing swine: I. Effects of a hot, diurnal temperature on average daily gain, feed intake, and feed efficiency. *J Anim Sci.* 69:1843-1849.

[81] Nienaber, J. A., G. L. Hahn, and R. A. Eigenberg. 1999. Quantifying livestock responses for heat-stress management: a review. *Int J Biometeorol.* 42:183-188.

[82] Le Bellego, L., J. van Milgen, and J. Noblet. 2002. Effect of high temperature and low-protein diets on the performance of growing-finishing pigs. *J Anim Sci.* 80:691-701.86. Kouba, M., D. Hermier, and J. Le Dividich. 2001. Influence of a high ambient temperature on lipid metabolism in the growing pig. *J Anim Sci.* 79:81-87.

[83] Breinekova, K., M. Svoboda, M. Smutna, L. Vorlova. 2006. Markers of acute stress in pigs. *Physiological Research Pre-Press Article.*

[84] Becker, B. A., J. A. Nienaber, R. K. Christenson, R. C. Manak, J. A. DeShazer, and G. L. Hahn. 1985. Peripheral concentrations of cortisol as an indicator of stress in the pig. *Am J Vet Res.* 46(5):1034-1038.

[85] Chrousos, G. P. 2007. Adrenocorticosteroids & Adrenocortical Antagonists. Ch 39 in Basic & Clinical Pharmacology, 10th Ed. B.G. Katzung, ed. McGraw-Hill, New York, NY.

[86] Missing Reference

[87] Kerr, C. A., L. R. Giles, M. R. Jones, and A. Reverter. 2005. Effects of grouping unfamiliar cohorts, high ambient temperature and stocking density on live performance of growing pigs. *J Anim Sci.* 83:908-915.

[88] Person, R. C., D. R. McKenna, D. B. Griffin, F. K. McKeith, J. A. Scanga, K. E. Belk, G. C. Smith, and J. W. Savell. 2005. Benchmarking value in the pork supply chain: Processing characteristics and consumer evaluations of pork bellies of different thicknesses when manufactured into bacon. *Meat Science.* 70:121-131.

[89] Morgan, J. B., G. C. Smith, J. Cannon, F. McKeith, and J. Heavner. 1994. Pork distribution channel audit report. In: Pork Chain Quality Audit-Progress Repork. D. Meeker and S. Sonka, ed. NCCP, Des Moines, IA.

[90] Gatlin, L. A., M. T. See, J. A. Hansen, D. Sutton, and J. Odle. 2002. The effects of dietary fat sources, levels, and feeding intervals on pork fatty acid composition. *J Anim Sci.* 80:1606-1615.

[91] Wood, J. D., R. I. Richardson, G. R. Nute, A. V. Fisher, M. M. Campo, E. Kasapidou, P. R. Sheard, and M. Enser. 2003. Effects of fatty acids on meat quality: a review. *Meat Science.* 66:21-32.

[92] Delmore, R. J. (2009). Beef Shelf-life. Cattlemen's Beef Board and National Cattlemen's Beef Association.

[93] Singh, R. K., & Singh, N. (2005). Quality of packaged foods. In J. H. Han (Ed.), Innovations in Food Packaging, (pp. 22-24). Amsterdam: Elsevier Academic Press.

[94] Gerrard, D. E. and A. L. Grant. 2003. Principles of Animal Growth and Development (1st ed.). Dubuque, IA: Kendall/Hunt Publishing Co.

[95] Wood, J. D., R. I. Richardson, G. R. Nute, A. V. Fisher, M. M. Campo, E. Kasapidou, P. R. Sheard, and M. Enser. 2004. Effects of fatty acids on meat quality: a review. Meat Science, 66:21-32.

Chapter 11

Polydextrose in Lipid Metabolism

Heli Putaala

Additional information is available at the end of the chapter

http://dx.doi.org/10.5772/51791

1. Introduction

Dietary fiber include fibers from natural sources (such as fruits, vegetables, and wholegrain cereals), fibers that are extracted or obtained by other means from food material, and synthetic carbohydrate polymers, that have been shown to possess physiological health benefits [1, 2]. Dietary fiber can be classified analytically as soluble and insoluble based on their solubility in water, but can also be characterized as viscous or non-viscous and fermentable or non-fermentable depending upon the physiological characteristics the fiber might have [2]. Insoluble dietary fiber includes cellulose, part of hemicellulose, and lignin, whereas soluble fibers include components such as pectin, some hemicelluloses, lignin, gums and mucilage [2, 3]. Whilst there have been difficulties in achieving a global definition for dietary fiber, it is now generally accepted that dietary fiber can be defined as carbohydrate polymers with a degree of polymerization of 3 or more monomeric units which are not hydrolysed in the small intestine by the endogenous enzymes [4]. As fiber is resistant to digestion and absorption in the human small intestine, it enters the colon where it can be partially or completely fermented [5].

Polydextrose is a polysaccharide produced by the random polymerization of glucose in the presence of sorbitol and a suitable acid catalyst, at a high temperature and under partial vacuum [6]. Polydextrose is composed of a mixture of glucose oligomers, with an average degree of polymerization ~12, but ranging from residual monomer to dp >100 [6, 7]. It is a branched molecule, and contains all different combinations of α- and β-linked $1\rightarrow2$, $1\rightarrow3$, $1\rightarrow4$ and $1\rightarrow6$ glycosidic linkages (Figure 1) [7, 8]. As polydextrose is only partially digested during gastrointestinal transit, it acts as a substrate for saccharolytic fermentation throughout the colon, even to the distal parts [9-12]. Polydextrose has a low caloric value: about 1 kcal/g, and it is widely used as a bulking agent and to replace the structure and texture of sucrose in low-calorie products by the food industry in confectionery applications, in pastry and bread, in dairy products, meat products, pasta and noodles, and in beverages [7, 13]. Polydextrose is widely accepted as a soluble fiber and has scientifically substantiated fiber characteristics, including increase in stool weight, decreased transit time, improved stool consistency and ease of defecation, and reduced fecal pH [7]. It is safe to use, and well tolerated, with a mean laxative threshold of 90 g/day, or 50 g as a single bolus dose [14-16].

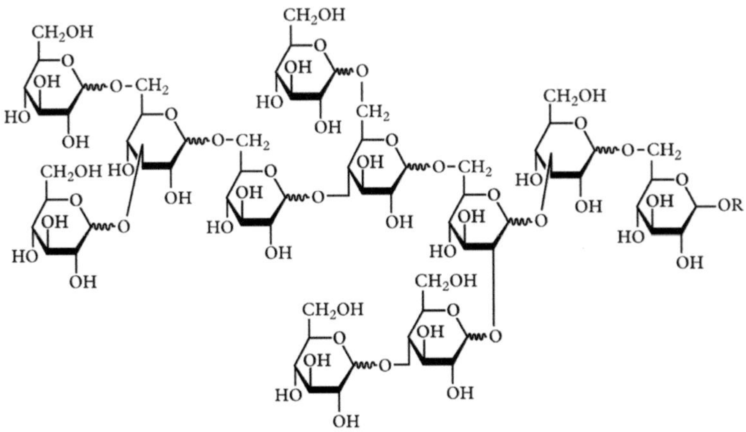

Figure 1. Structure for the polydextrose. The letter R can be either hydrogen (H), sorbitol, sorbitol bridge, of more polydextrose. Polydextrose has highly branched complex three-dimensional structure with all different combinations of α- and β-linked 1→2, 1→3, 1→4 and 1→6 glycosidic linkages.

Several beneficial effects have been linked to the consumption of polydextrose. Consumption of polydextrose promotes the growth of beneficial bifidobacteria and lactobacilli while preventing the growth of harmful ones, such as clostridia [17, 18]. It has been suggested to possess anti-inflammatory actions and to improve the signs of osteoarthritis in canines [19], to increase IgA amount in the rat cecum [20], to reduce cyclo-oxygenase 2 expression in pigs distal colon, and to reduce lesions in rat colitis model [21]. Furthermore, it has been suggested to improve the absorption of magnesium, calcium [22-25] and iron [26].

Soluble fiber, both viscous (e.g. gums, pectin and β-glucan) and non-viscous (e.g. polydextrose, resistant maltodextrin and inulin), has been suggested to have beneficial metabolic advantages. These include increasing satiety and reduction of body weight, control of postprandial glycemic and insulin responses, and hypocholesterolemic effects on serum lipid parameters [5, 27]. The inverse relationship of higher HDL to coronary artery disease risk has been recognized and is evident across numerous populations, and the increment of its relative amount over LDL has been generally accepted as a hallmark of better cardiovascular health [28]. Soluble fiber has been associated inversely with serum total and LDL cholesterol, while HDL cholesterol concentration has been reported to either slightly decrease or remain unchanged [29, 30]. This effect has been attributed as an effect of soluble viscous fibers, as insoluble fibers do not appear to affect serum cholesterol concentrations [31, 32]. The ability of soluble fibers to reduce serum triglyceride levels is also controversial, as in some studies an inverse association has been suggested, while in many studies no effect has been observed [29, 33]. Soluble viscous fibers have a characteristic of being hypocholesterolemic, reducing serum cholesterol by about 5-10 % for a 5-10 g dose in subjects with hypercholesterolemia, whereas insoluble fibers have not shown this effect [34].

2. Polydextrose studies in animals, human and *in vitro*: Contribution of polydextrose in lipid metabolism

Polydextrose is a fermentable non-viscous fiber, and has been shown to exhibit lipid metabolism regulating effects [5]. Typically these effects have been associated with two physiochemical properties of soluble fibers: viscosity and fermentability. Viscous soluble fibers may work by slowing down gastric emptying and prevention of bile salt re-absorption which would increase the secretion of bile acids and neutral sterols into feces and interruption of the enterohepatic circulation of bile acids [35, 36]. Soluble fiber can also decrease intestinal cholesterol absorption by affecting micelle formation and mobility [37, 38], and reduce glycemic response leading to lower insulin stimulation and hepatic cholesterol synthesis [39]. Fibers can also promote satiety [40]. Additionally, colonic fermentation products of these fibers, short chain fatty acids (SCFAs), mainly propionate, have been shown to inhibit hepatic fatty acid synthesis [41]. Polydextrose has been reported to confer lipid modulating effects in human clinical intervention studies, as well as in animal studies. However, some of the characteristics of polydextrose are different to other soluble fibers, such as low viscosity, and sustained fermentation throughout the colon [11].

2.1. Polydextrose studies in animals

The ability of polydextrose to modulate triglycerides, total, LDL, and HDL cholesterol has been studied in animals both in normal diets without additional lipid load or in diets in which lipids have been included as part of the normal diet. There is a clear difference between the types of studies, as the two studies without lipid load have not shown any effect on the blood lipid values. In a 6-week feeding study in normal rats with 5 % (w/w) inclusion of polydextrose no change in plasma triglycerides, total cholesterol, and HDL cholesterol or liver cholesterol, triglycerides and phospholipids was observed [42]. Another, 15-day feeding trial with rats, did not show differences in serum total and free cholesterol, triacylglycerols, and phospholipids even though 3 % polydextrose was administered together with 3 % pectin or 3 % cellulose [43].

However, in two other rat feeding studies in which polydextrose was accompanied with a lipid load, reduced lipid levels were reported. In one study rats were given two different dosages of corn oil, 10 % and 20 %, to represent a moderate or high fat diet, for 8 weeks, with or without 5 % polydextrose [44]. Rats in the polydextrose group showed decreased serum triglycerides as compared to a guar gum control in the high-fat diet, and increased levels of serum HDL cholesterol both in the moderate fat and high fat diet [44]. Serum total lipids and cholesterol remained at the level of the control [44]. One study has been done with gerbils: in the 4-week study the gerbils were fed with 0.15 % cholesterol with 30 % of the energy coming from fat and with inclusion of 6 % polydextrose [45]. Both liver and plasma total cholesterol as well as free and esterified cholesterol from liver decreased in the polydextrose group [45]. The effect was presumed by the authors to be related to the reduction of VLDL and LDL, since no change in HDL was observed [45]. In the same gerbil study, it was additionally investigated whether polydextrose can remove cholesterol from

Table 1. Polydextrose studies in relation to lipid metabolism done in animals.

Study design					Cholesterol				
Ref	Animals	Dose	Time	Lipid load	Total	LDL	HDL	TG	Remarks
[42]	Sprague-Dawley rats	5 %	6 w	No load	N.C.	n.a.	N.C.	N.C.	Lipids measured both from plasma and liver
[43]	Sprague-Dawley rats	3 %	15 d	No load	N.C.	n.a.	n.a.	N.C.	Together with pectin or cellulosa
[44]	Sprague-Dawley rats	5 %	8 w	10 % and 20 % from corn oil	N.C.	n.a.	↑	↓	Compared to guar gum group
[45]	Gerbils	6 %	4 w	30 % energy from fat, 0.15 % from cholesterol	↓	↓ (or VLDL)[a]	N.C.	N.C.	Liver total ↓, free ↓, esterified cholesterol ↓ Total to HDL ratio trend ↓ in plasma
[45]	Gerbils	6 %	3 w	0.4 % choleterol preload[b]	↓	n.a.	↓	N.C.	Liver total ↓, Esterified cholesterol ↓
[46]	Wistar rats	28 % as 3 ml/200 g body weight	Acute	Fats as in chocolate	n.a.	n.a.	n.a.	↓	Together with 25.7 % lactitol

n.a. not available; d days; w weeks; m months; a ↓reduced; ↑increased; Trend ↓or Trend ↑only a tendency for reduced or increased values were observed; N.C. no change

[a] Indirect evidence, LDL and VLDL were not directly measured but authors concluded that as total cholesterol decreased and there was no change in HDL, then preferential target is then VLDL and/or LDL.

[b] 0.4 % cholesterol administered to the gerbils 2 weeks prior the feeding with polydextrose in order to expand the endogenous cholesterol pools.

[c] 0.4 % cholesterol administered to the gerbils 2 weeks prior the feeding with polydextrose in order to expand the endogenous cholesterol pools.

endogenous pools by first artificially expanding the endogenous cholesterol pools of the gerbils with a preload of 0.4 % cholesterol for two weeks before 6 % polydextrose was fed for an additional three weeks. Polydextrose was shown to hasten the endogenous clearance of cholesterol pools, and to reduce liver and plasma total cholesterol, esterified cholesterol from liver and plasma HDL cholesterol [45].

The acute response of polydextrose on serum lipid values has also been studied in rats, but together with lactitol [46]. Polydextrose was administered as a 28 % solution in a dose of 3 ml/200 g of body weight in a solution also containing 26 % lactitol and a fat emulsion which was comparable to one in chocolate. The rats showed reduced serum triglyceride levels, and an increase in luminal triglyceride levels in the cecum after 150 minutes of ingestion of polydextrose, which would indicate that the combination of polydextrose and lactitol reduced either the level of fat absorption in the earlier part of small intestine or promoted the transit time of fat through the intestine [46]. No change in total, HDL, or LDL cholesterol were found in that study.

These studies are summarised in Table 1. There is an indication from these studies that polydextrose can lower total cholesterol and has a tendency to lower LDL cholesterol and tendency to increase HDL cholesterol.

2.2. Polydextrose lipid metabolism studies in clinical intervention studies

Clinical intervention studies with polydextrose have been conducted either with healthy adults, with individuals having hypercholesterolemia or with individuals with impaired glucose tolerance.

In a human study with normal healthy adults with no reported hypercholesterolemia a reduction in the amount of total HDL by administration of 15 g of polydextrose for two months with concomitant decrease in apolipoprotein A-I, which is the main component of the HDL cholesterol, has been observed [47]. Apolipoprotein B levels, found in all atherogenic apolipoprotein particles, and the LDL cholesterol levels itself had also a tendency to be reduced after the 2-month and 1-month intervention period, respectively [47]. In another study with healthy adults, administration of 10 g of polydextrose for 18 days was shown to decrease LDL cholesterol and total cholesterol values with no effect on HDL cholesterol or triglycerides [48]. There are also contradictory results with healthy humans, as administration of polydextrose in an amount from 4 to 12 g per day for 29 days did not affect triacylglycerol, or cholesterol [49]. However, in that study no data was shown, and in addition to which the cholesterol type measured was not specified.

In hypercholesterolomic individuals, the effect of polydextrose has been studied in a 4-week study with administration of 15 g and 30 g polydextrose daily [45]. The study was quite small, with only 12 subjects participating, and each individual subject serving as a control for him/herself. In this study it was noted that 5 of the 6 individuals ingesting 30 g of polydextrose were in a separate responder group, and in this group the LDL cholesterol values declined significantly, and there was a tendency for reduced total cholesterol, but no change in HDL cholesterol. However, when all 6 individuals were studied together, no change compared to control was observed.

In diabetic patients, diets containing high amounts of fiber have improved plasma lipid control [50, 51]. The effect of polydextrose on lipid values has been of interest in two studies with individuals showing abnormal glucose metabolism or type 2 diabetes. In subjects with impaired glucose metabolism, polydextrose administered for 12 weeks at 16 g/day has been observed to lower LDL cholesterol, increase HDL cholesterol and cause no change in triglycerides [52]. In this study, LDL cholesterol decreased also in the control group probably because of simultaneous nutrition consultation by a nutritionist [52]. In a combination study with 7 g polydextrose and 3 g oligofructose administered daily for 6 weeks in adults with type 2 diabetes, a decrease in total cholesterol, triglycerides, VLDL cholesterol, and ratios of total cholesterol to HDL cholesterol, and LDL cholesterol to HDL cholesterol was observed, while HDL cholesterol increased [53].

The acute effect of polydextrose has been studied in humans too, together with lactitol, in the triglyceride levels after consumption of 46 g of chocolate supplemented with 15.1 % of the weight with polydextrose. The intervention group had reduced serum triglycerides in comparison to control chocolate during the 150 minutes the triglycerides were measured from the blood [46]. During intense exercise, polydextrose has been shown to reduce the amount of free fatty acids in plasma [54]. In addition, an abstract has been published about ingestion of 12.5 g polydextrose during a hamburger meal observing a reduction in total postprandial hypertriglyceridemia by 25 % [55].

2.2.1. *Effect of polydextrose on different HDL subfractions*

HDL is highly heterogeneous, and subfractions of it can be identified on the basis of density, size, charge, and protein composition [56]. Different fractions of HDL can be identified by ultracentrifugation, gradient gel electrophoresis, and nuclear magnetic resonance (NMR) spectroscopy, and these different fractions could play diverse roles in protective function [56, 57]. It is thought that certain fractions of HDL cholesterol could be better predictors of cardiovascular diseases and its risk. However, controversy about the role of the different forms still exists, as in [58] and in [59] increased HDL2 and apoA-I levels were associated as protective against coronary heart disease. In other studies, in turn, such as in [60], and [61], the HDL3 has had a stronger inverse association with coronary heart disease. The early studies, however, more strongly indicate that reduced levels of HDL2 over HDL3 is associated more strongly to CVD risk [62].

The different subfractions of HDL and the impact of ingestion of polydextrose on their distribution has been investigated in one study [47], and in this study HDL3 was increased during the 2-month intervention period and one month after finishing the study. At the same time, a reduced level of HDL2, apoA-I and LCAT activity was observed. In other studies with soluble fibers, such as with guar gum, no changes in HDL2 and HDL3 subfractions or their ratio were observed [63, 64]. No difference between serum HDL2 and HDL3 cholesterol subfractions could be observed between high-fiber, consisting partially of soluble fiber from psyllium, and low-fiber diets [65] or with beta-glucan as an oat fiber extract [66]. In addition, lack of standardization among the analytical methods that are used to measure size distribution of different HDL2 and HDL3 subfractions may cause approximation of HDL subclass levels [67, 68].

Study design					Cholesterol				
Ref		Dose	Time	Lipid load	Total	LDL	HDL	TG	Remarks
[47]	Healthy	15 g/day	2 m		N.C.	N.C.[a]	HDL2↓ HDL3↑	N.C.[a]	ApoA-I ↓ ApoA-II ↓
[69]	Healthy	15 g/day	4 w		Trend↓[b]	Trend↓[b]	N.C.	N.C.	ApoB ↓
[48]	Healthy	10 g/day	18 d		↓	↓	N.C.	N.C.	
[49]	Healthy	4, 8, or 12 g/day	28 d		N.C.	N.C.	N.C.	N.C.	Measured lipid values were not specific
[46]	Healthy	15.1 % in 46 g of chololate	Acute	Lipids from chocolate	n.a.	n.a.	n.a.	↓	Together with 19.4 % lactitol
[45]	With hypercholesterolemia	15 or 30 g/day	4 w		Trend ↓[c]	↓[c]	N.C.[d]	N.C.[d]	
[52]	With impaired glucose metabolism	16 g/day	12 w		N.C.	↓	↑	N.C.	Total to HDL ratio ↓
[53]	With type 2 diabetes	1[illegible].2 g/day	6 w		↓	↓	↑	↓	With 6.8 g oligofructose/day. Total/HDL cholesterol ↓, VLDL cholesterol ↓

n.a. not available; d days; w weeks; m months; ↓reduced; ↑increased; Trend ↓or Trend ↑only tendency for reduced or increased values were observed; N.C. no change

[a] had a tendency to be reduced 1 month after intervention

[b] Total cholesterol and LDL cholesterol were reduced by 6 % but not significantly

[c] When studied form a group that responded to the 30 daily dose of polydextrose

[d] Both in the responder group that ingested 30g/day polydextrose and in a group in which in addition to responders, a non-responder was included.

Table 2. Polydextrose clinical intervention studies in which lipid values have been measured.

Table 2 summarizes the different human clinical intervention studies done with polydextrose in relation to HDL, LDL, total cholesterol and triglycerides. From these studies it can be concluded that polydextrose in the diet can lower serum total and LDL cholesterol and triglycerides. There are two studies in which definite increases in HDL have been observed.

3. Mechanisms for polydextrose action on lipid values

3.1. Role of polydextrose in enterohepatic bile circulation and in cholesterol absorption

One of the mechanisms by which soluble viscous fibers induce hypocholesterolemic responses is the disruption of enterohepatic bile acid circulation, which reduces absorption of intestinal bile acids. The major route by which cholesterol in the liver is eliminated is through the de novo synthesis of primary bile acids from cholesterol [70]. The bile is released into the small intestine, where bile salt micelles help in the solubilisation of lipophilic components, such as cholesterol, fat soluble vitamins, and other lipids [70]. The diffusion of the micelles with solubilised components as well as the biliary and dietary cholesterol across the unstirred water layer, covering the luminal side of the enterocytes facilitate the uptake of cholesterol and other lipophilic components by the enterocytes [71]. When the bile salt micelles have accomplished their role they transit the remainder of small and large intestine where they are progressively absorbed into the enterohepatic circulation by the hepatic portal vein [70]. The bile salts that escape the intestinal absorption are transformed through colonic bacterial enzymatic activity to form secondary bile salts, from which deoxycholic acid is absorbed passively through colonic epithelium into the enterohepatic circulation, while lithocholic acid is secreted into the feces [72]. The amount of bile salts, both primary and secondary, is maintained in a rather constant level, and the daily bile salt losses are compensated by de novo hepatic biosynthesis [73]. The enterohepatic circulation is very efficient, as 95 % of the bile salts released into the intestine is absorbed back to the liver [70].

The presence of viscous soluble fiber has been shown to prevent bile salt reabsorption, which leads to enhanced excretion of bile salts into feces [35, 36]. This depletes the bile acids from liver and leads to rapid catabolisation of cholesterol through activation of 7alpha-hydroxylase. At the same time cholesteryl esters are metabolised, and in order to replace these production of LDL surface membrane receptors and concomitant LDL cholesterol uptake from blood stream are increased. This leads to lowering of the blood cholesterol concentration [74]. The fibers presumably interact with bile acids directly at the molecular level or entrap bile salt micelles in the gelatinous network formed by the polymeric fiber [35, 75]. The fiber can also form a barrier which can prevent the formation of bile acid micelles, and increase the unstirred water layer lining the intestinal mucosal surface [76].

Polydextrose is a non-viscous fiber and its capacity to bind bile salts has been studied in one clinical intervention study [77]. In this study, administration of polydextrose in healthy adults at 8 g/day for three weeks was not found to increase fecal excretion of total bile acids and secondary bile acids, but rather decreased values were observed during the intervention period compared to the run-in period before [77]. A similar observation was made in normal rats, in which administration of 5 % polydextrose for 6 weeks did not increase the fecal output of bile acids [42]. The low ability of polydextrose to bind bile acids is not, however, surprising. In order for a fiber to bind bile acids, it is required to be viscous in nature, and polydextrose is lower in viscosity for instance in comparison to pectin and guar gum which have high water binding capacity with higher viscosity and thus increased capability to bind bile acids [42, 78]. Polydextrose has a high capacity to bind water, and it can for instance relieve constipation presumably due to this characteristic, but there is no gel formation by polydextrose in water and little viscosity [43, 79, 80].

Even though no clear effect on bile acid binding can be detected, the fact that cholesterol and triglyceride absorption can still be modulated, are indications that polydextrose can retard the transportation of lipids from the intestinal lumen to the lymph. When polydextrose was infused as 5 % and 10 % to duodenum together with cholesterol and triglyceride on mesenteric lymph-fistulated rats, the amount of cholesterol and triglycerides in the lymph decreased dose-dependently, and concomitantly the amount of the unabsorbed lipids increased in the lumen of the intestine [81]. It was concluded that since most of the luminal triglyceride and cholesterol was detected in the proximal part of the small intestine, the absorption of the lipids was inhibited. There was a tendency to have increased amount of cholesterol and a significant increase of triglycerides remaining in the colon which could indicate that some of the lipids were not absorbed [81]. However, polydextrose did not seem to increase secretion of cholesterol into feces in rats even though some tendency was observed in another study [82].

In an acute response study of polydextrose in combination with lactitol in rats with lipid load similar to the composition of chocolate an increase in luminal triglyceride in the cecum was observed with concomitant decrease in serum triglycerides [46]. This would indicate that the combination of polydextrose and lactitol reduced either the level of fat absorption in the earlier part of small intestine or promoted the transit time of fat through the intestine [46].

Cholesterol that escapes absorption is partially degraded to coprostanol and coprostanone by colon microbes [83]. A decrease of the degradation products coprostanol, coprostanon and cholestanol has been observed [77] which would indicate that the amount of cholesterol entering the colon is less in humans receiving polydextrose.

3.2. Role of polydextrose on intestinal microbiota and its impact on cholesterol metabolism

When soluble fiber enters the large intestine, it is fermented by the residual microbes forming short-chain fatty acids (SCFAs), butyrate, acetate, and propionate, end-products of bacterial carbohydrate fermentation. The SCFAs have been indicated to possess different physiological functions. Butyrate has been implicated to be the most important SCFA for colonic and immune cells due to its ability to serve as energy source for colonic epithelium as well as regulate cell growth and differentiation [84, 85]. It is a preferred energy source by colonocytes over glucose, glutamine, or other SCFA, and 70 to 90 % of butyrate is metabolized by colonocytes [86]. It has been implicated to inhibit intestinal cholesterol biosynthesis [87]. Acetate, as a direct substrate for acetyl-CoA synthetase, an enzyme that converts acetate to acetyl-CoA for entering to the cholesterol and fatty acid synthesis cycle, has been implicated to increase liver cholesterol, and fatty acid levels [41, 88]. Acetate has been shown to associate negatively with visceral adipose tissues and insulin levels in obese people [89]. Propionate has been shown to possess antilipogenic and cholesterol-lowering effects. While acetate is a substrate for sterol and fatty acid synthesis, propionate counteracts this by inhibiting acetate incorporation to serum lipids [41]. Propionate has been shown to to reduce the rate of cholesterol synthesis [87, 90], to inhibit fatty acid synthesis [91], to decrease liver lipogenesis [92], and to decrease hepatic and plasma and serum cholesterol levels [93, 94]. Propionate supplementation has been shown increase serum HDL cholesterol and triglyceride levels without effect on total cholesterol [92, 95]. However, contradictory results about its efficacy on cholesterol metabolism has been also observed [96-98].

The production of short-chain fatty acids during polydextrose fermentation has been studied with batch fermentations, colon simulators as well as from feces in animal and human studies. The differences in the results reflect individual variation, sampling, and differences in the methods used. Fecal SCFA concentration measurements are not the best indicators of SCFA produced as the majority of fecal SCFA is absorbed rapidly by the colonic epithelial cells [99]. Polydextrose has been observed to increase the production of butyrate, acetate and propionate in vitro [18, 100-102], in rats [20], pigs [11], in dogs [103] and in humans [17, 49]. When compared to other fibers, polydextrose produced similar quantities of SCFAs, and the molecular ratio of acetate/propionate/butyrate produced was found to be similar to that of fructo-oligosaccharides and xylo-oligosaccharides and other carbohydrates, such as inulin, pectin, and arabinose [104, 105] while in other studies polydextrose produced less total SCFAs compared to FOS, inulin and GOS [102, 106, 107]. The lower production of SCFAs by polydextrose can be explained by the lower digestability of polydextrose and its more sustained fermentation throughout the gut due to its branched complex structure. Furthermore, polydextrose fermentation has been shown to reduce putrefactive microbial metabolites, or branched-chain fatty acids and biogenic amines produced from protein fermentation [11, 20, 49, 100, 101, 107-109] but the decrease of these in relation to lipid metabolism and absorption is unknown. Figure 2 shows an example of how fermentation of polydextrose increases the amount short chain fatty acids in an in vitro colon simulation both when the amount of polydextrose is increased, and when the simulation proceeds from vessel V1 representing proximal part of the colon towards the vessels representing more distal parts of the colon [108].

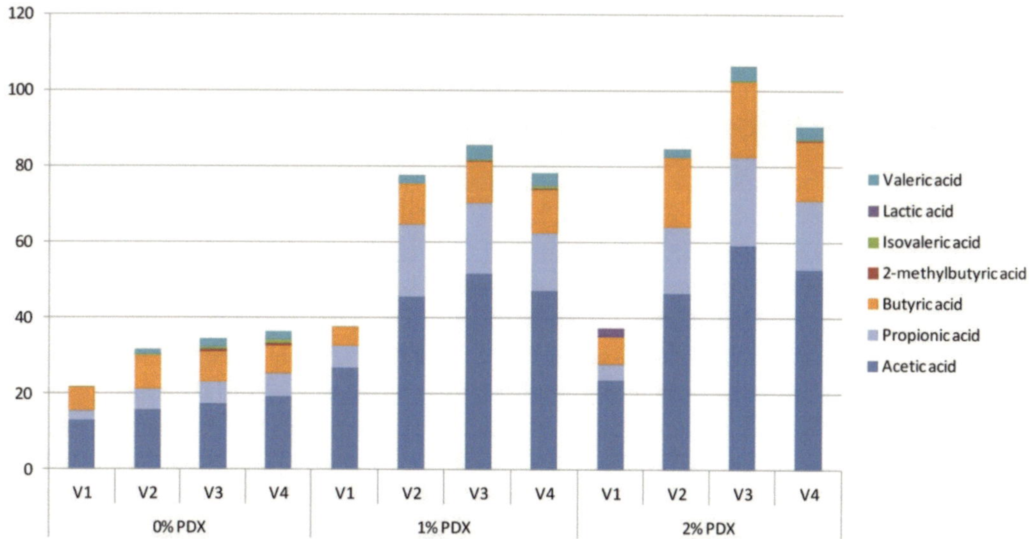

Figure 2. Concentration (mM) of short chain fatty acids (SCFAs) in the different vessels V1, V2, V3, and V4 after 48h in vitro colon fermentation simulation. An increase in the concentration of SCFAs can be observed both dose-dependently as well as from vessels representing proximal colon V1 towards vessels representing more distal parts of the colon, V3 and V4.

When polydextrose enters the colon, it is fermented by the indigenous microbiota, thus serving as an energy-source to promote their growth and survival. In germ-free mice, the transplantation of the colonic microbiota from normal mice resulted in a 60 % increase in body fat in an unchanged diet [110] and there are an increasing number of reports that the gut microbiota may play an important role in cholesterol and lipid homeostasis, in obesity and metabolic syndrome [111-113].

Bacterial DNA of fecal samples from 20 individuals consuming 21 g of polydextrose in 3 doses per day were pyrosequenced, and the amount of Clostridiaceae, and Veillonea increased while Lachnospiraeae and Eubacteriaceae decreased compared to the control group without additional supplemental fiber [114]. Well-known butyrate-producers were increased in number, such as Faecalibacterium, and especially Faecalibacterium prausnitzii, whereas other SCFA producers, such as Lachnospiraceae, and Eubacteriaceae were reduced in number by administration of polydextrose [114]. Polydextrose also decreased the number of Coriobacteriaceae, which have been shown to have a positive association to non-HDL cholesterol [111, 114]. Interestingly, bifidobacteria have shown a positive correlation with HDL-cholesterol [111], but the bifidobacterial counts were decreased by polydextrose when studied with pyrosequencing [114]. In other studies polydextrose administration has been shown to increase the amount of bifidobacteria and lactobacilli [17, 18, 49, 106, 107, 115] while in some studies this effect has not been noted [103] or that there was no effect on the growth of lactobacilli [102]. This kind of inconsistency in the response could reflect the interindividual differences in indigenous microbiota to begin with. These kind of fluctuations in the indigenous microbiota, however, might explain why there are differencies in the studies with polydextrose and its effect on cholesterol values, for instance in [45] in which a responder group with a decrease in LDL was observed.

3.3. Polydextrose effect on glycemic control and insulin response

Fibers can affect blood glucose levels by decreasing the glycemic load of a meal or by affecting glucose absorption or release of glucose [5], and especially soluble fiber has been shown to attenuate the absorption of glucose [27]. Soluble dietary fibers may affect total and LDL cholesterol levels through effects on postprandial glycemia, as reduction in the glucose absorption, which would lower the insulin level and its production in the pancreas, would then lead to a decrease in cholesterol synthesis [116]. When soluble dietary fibers are being digested they delay the emptying of digested food from the stomach to the small intestine, slow down the transportation and mixing of digestive enzymes in the chyme and increase the resistance of the unstirred water layer lining the mucosa [117, 118]. This leads to reduction in the absorption of glucose and macronutrients, and lowered level of postprandial glucose is accompanied with lowered insulin level which would possibly lead to lowered hepatic cholesterol synthesis. [39]. There has been studies describing inverse relationship between glycemic load and HDL cholesterol [119, 120], and an indirect regulation of intestinal lipid uptake by dietary glucose has been presumed. Short-term incubation with intestinal epithelial cells, Caco-2 cells, with glucose on the apical side induces a significant uptake of cholesterol in a dose-dependent manner [121], and in addition cholesterol synthesis seems to dependent on glucose intake [122].

The effect of polydextrose ingestion on glucose and postprandial insulin response has been investigated in several studies. Polydextrose has a very low glycemic index (4 to 7) with glycemic load of 1 compared to the reference glucose (100) [7, 123]. Polydextrose has been reported to attenuate the blood glucose raising potential of glucose, as the glycemic index of glucose was reduced from 100 to 88 when 12 grams of polydextrose was ingested together with glucose by healthy adults [49]. Similar results were observed in a study with healthy adults when 14 g was ingested together with 50 g of glucose or 106 g of bread [124]. Plasma glucose levels were decreased by 28 % and 35 %, compared to glucose and bread without polydextrose, respectively, with significantly reduced serum insulin levels in the glucose plus polydextrose group [124]. These observations indicate that polydextrose could reduce the absorption of glucose. When the effect of polydextrose was studied with human subjects with impaired glucose tolerance or impaired fasting glucose, no change in plasma glucose or insulin has been observed [52]. However, this study [52] had a moderately high fructose intake which could have affected the results as fructose does not induce endogenous secretion of insulin [125]. Diurnally polydextrose did not seem to change plasma sugar levels, but a decrease in insulin after meals was noted [69]. In dogs, polydextrose showed an attenuated postprandial glycemic and lower relative insulin responses than the control sugar maltitol [126].

Polydextrose has been also studied in trials in which the reference group received a normal meal/snack with glucose, and the intervention group the same but with the glucose partially replaced with polydextrose. In volunteers with type 2 diabetes, cranberries with 10g of polydextrose showed attenuated plasma glucose and insulin response compared to cranberries with glucose [127]. In one study with healthy adults, significantly lower postprandial glucose levels were observed after ingestion of strawberry jam with 40 % polydextrose than after ingestion of strawberry jam sweetened with sugar, corn syrup, or apple juice, but this study did not measure insulin [128].

These above results indicate that polydextrose might have a role in postprandial glucose absorption and insulin response. One good candidate to modify insulin response is again the SCFAs, especially propionate, which have been shown to improve insulin sensitivity during glucose tolerance tests [95]. Polydextrose also might interfere the release and absorption of the glucose in the small intestine which would lead to slower and lower blood sugar rise [5]. In some of these studies the response is observed because polydextrose was used as sugar substitute to lower the caloric content of the snack/product [127, 128]. In [127] the beneficial insulin reduction was observed not to be in 1:1 ratio with caloric reduction so there might be additional beneficial effect apart from lowering the overall calorie content.

3.4. Polydextrose as a satiety increasing agent

Meals dense in fiber have also been demonstrated to be able to control the sense of hunger, satiety, inhibit the desire for another meal, or induce satiation, limit the size of the meal, possibly by lowering caloric density or slowing down gastric emptying [40, 129] This would further decrease the sugar load of the individual, since high-fiber diets usually have a lower glycemic load.

Polydextrose has been observed to significantly reduce the feeling of hunger in subjects with impaired glucose metabolism [52], and to have tendency towards reduced snacking [10]. It has been shown to increase satiety and to reduce food intake when combined with yoghurt preloads [130]. However, evidence has been conflicting - in one study when 25 g polydextrose was preloaded in two servings before lunch, no difference in the desire to eat, sense of hunger and fullness was observed beween polydextrose and the other fibers tested [131]. In this study polydextrose did not decrease the energy consumed in lunch. In another study when polydextrose was consumed as 9.5 g in a muffin no difference in the feeling of hungriness or food intake was observed between polydextrose and the other fibers studied [132]. In the two most recent studies, polydextrose intake of 12 g in a fruit smoothie, consumed as a single dose preload, significantly reduced the intake of energy in a buffet lunch 1 hour after the consumption of the smoothie [133]. Similar observations with a single dose of 6.25 g or 12.5 g of polydextrose before a test lunch were also made in another study [134, 135].

Both butyrate and propionate have been shown to induce gut hormones and reduce food intake [136]. Propionate has been shown to act as a satiety-inducing agent, with strong effects on energy intake and feeding behaviour with significantly greater feeling of fullness and lower desire to eat [137, 138]. This could be introduced by the modulation of the colonic mucosa secreted peptide hormones that regulate appetite, such as glucagon like peptide -1

(GLP-1), peptide YY (PYY), oxyntomodulin, or SCFA receptors, GPR43 or GPR41, which have been localized in intestinal enteroendocrine L cells, that are responsible for the production of the appetite regulating hormones [139, 140] but whether polydextrose ingestion causes changes in these peptide hormones remains to be investigated.

3.5. Modulation of genes regulating energy metabolism by polydextrose fermentation in colon

Microbial metabolites have been shown to modulate gene expression, for instance butyrate acts as a histone deacetylase (HDAC) inhibitor, and affects gene transciption [141]. Polydextrose has been shown to increase expression of PPARγ in the colon of mice [142]. This has been attributed to be mediated at least by butyrate, which can not only up regulate gene expression of PPARγ, but also activate it [143]. When intestinal epithelial cells were treated with polydextrose fermentation metabolites, a gene expression signature was induced that approached the response of butyrate [144]. In the study [144] 1 or 2 % polydextrose was fermented in a four-stage semicontinuous colon simulation model, in which each vessel in sequence represents different parts of the colon. Caco-2 cells were treated with the polydextrose fermentation metabolites from each vessel, and the idea was to analyse gene expression pattern of the Caco-2 cells treated with fermentation metabolome representing the whole colon. The weakness of this study was that the cells were not differentiated, but were used as a cancer cell model, and that fermentation metabolites originated from a fecal sample only from one individual. In the gene ontology analysis of this study, enrichment of class "lipid metabolism" by the polydextrose fermentation metabolites was noted, which indicated that genes involved in energy metabolism were regulated. Indeed, induction of PPARα, PGC-1α, and Lipin 1which are major regulators of the metabolism, were observed. Additionally, some PPARα responsive genes were observed to be up regulated, such as SORBS1, LPIN1, NPC1, FATP1, HMOX1, and ACSL1 [144].

In the intestine, activation of PPARα results in the specific induction of genes involved in fatty acid uptake, binding, transport, and catabolism. In addition, genes involved in triacylglycerol and glycerolipid metabolism have been suggested to function as fatty acid sensors, and in nutrient absorption [145, 146]. PGC-1α participates to the regulation of both carbohydrate and lipid metabolism, and it has been involved in the adaptation of and maintenance of energy homeostais in caloric restriction [147]. Drosophila PGC-1α homolog increases mitochondrial gene expression and activity and protects against age-related loss of intestinal homeostasis and integrity, and is suggested to extend life span [148]. Lipin 1 is induced by PGC-1α in liver and acts to amplify PGC-1α and to activate many of the genes of mitochondrial fatty acid oxidative metabolism [149]. Lipin 1 has been associated with insulin sensitivity in adipose tissue and liver which indicates that it has a profound role in maintaining systemic metabolic homeostasis [150, 151].

One of the genes regulated by polydextrose fermentation metabolites was Niemann Pick C1 (NPC1), a significant contributor to plasma HDL cholesterol formation [152]. NPC1 facilitates the movement of cholesterol to ABCA1, a cholesterol transporter that is located in the basolateral membrane of enterocytes, that is involved in the efflux process of cholesterol to circulating HDL particles [153]. Approximately 30 % of the steady-state HDL was contributed by the intestinal ABCA1 in mice [154]. In NPC1 deficient cells the HDL cholesterol formation is reduced [155].

4. Conclusions

Based on the current research there is clear evidence that polydextrose has the ability to attenuate glucose absorption, reduce insulin response and lower blood LDL, total cholesterol and triglyceride levels. HDL cholesterol shows a tendency to be increased, but this has not been consistently demonstrated in all studies. This kind of ability to increase HDL would be quite unique among soluble fermentable fibers. Animal studies also indicate that polydextrose could interfere with cholesterol and triglyceride absorption.

Figure 3 summarises the possible mechanisms of how polydextrose could affect cholesterol and lipid metabolism. Polydextrose is used as a bulking agent, and increases the bulk of the material that transits along the colon. This can provide a sense of fullness and satiety. The effect of polydextrose on bile acid secretion cannot be definitely concluded at this point but is unlikely due to its non-viscous characteristic. It seems, that polydextrose attenuates the blood glucose raising potential of glucose itself, and the insulin response. Glucose and insulin are linked to hepatic de novo cholesterol synthesis, cholesterol absorption and HDL formation. The mechanism of the lipid metabolism modulating effect of polydextrose might be indirect, through its fermentation by the indigenous microbiota either the luminal or mucosal, that at the same time increase SCFA production. The microbiota can affect cholesterol degradation, but could also for instance affect chylomicron formation and cholesterol absorption. The absorbed SCFAs, propionate and butyrate, are linked to diminishing de novo cholesterol synthesis in the liver. Acetate, in contrast, has an opposite effect. Whether SCFAs are the molecules exerting the effect of the polydextrose is not known. During the fermentation of soluble fibers other metabolites apart from SCFAs are formed [156]. The complex structure of polydextrose facilitates its fermentation throughout colon. This differentiates it from other fibers which are fermented early in the colon, and it serves as an energy source for bacteria throughout the colon, and changes in the composition of the microbiota are observed with an increase in butyrate-producing bacteria [114]. It is possible that due to its fermentation characteristics the long-term effect on microbiota composition might be different to other soluble fibers. The mechanism of polydextrose might also be direct, through modulation of surface receptors, but currently there is no evidence for this.

The microarray study has given ideas of how polydextrose fermentation metabolites might affect the intestinal tissue. The evidence is, however, at the transcriptional level only, and is speculative. Additional studies in the possible regulation of PPARα, PGC1α, Lipin1, NPC1, and others by polydextrose is thus needed. In vitro studies could be used for instance to study the role of polydextrose fermentation in HDL formation using a differentiated Caco-2 cell model which has shown to be good model to study de novo ApoA-I production [157].

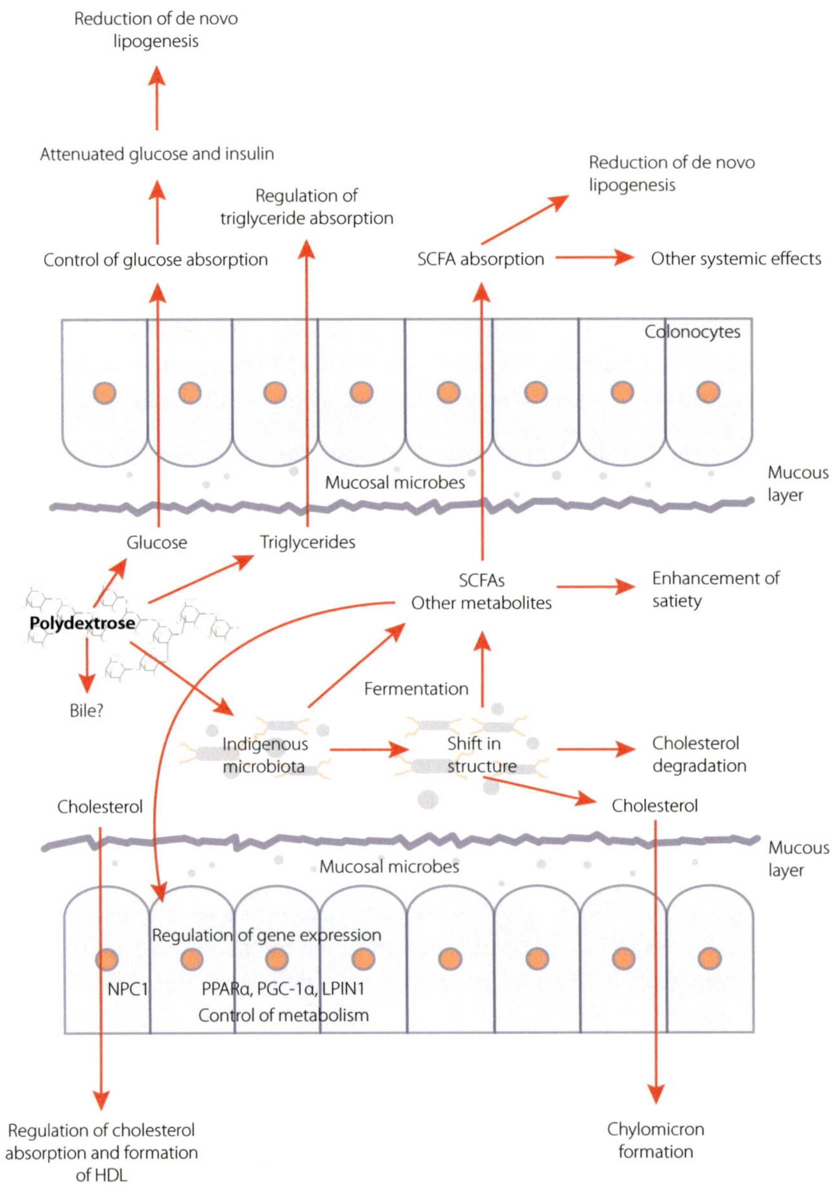

Figure 3. Summary of the polydextrose function in lipid metabolism.

It could be worthwhile to investigate to what extent polydextrose fermentation metabolites cause systemic effects for instance in liver, and its de novo cholesterol synthesis, not forgetting the role of the intestine. When lipidemic conditions are normal, the liver is the most important site of cholesterol biosynthesis, followed by the intestine. Biosynthesis in the liver and intestine account for about 15 and 10 %, respectively, in the total amount of cholesterol biosynthesis each day [158] [159]. In hypercholesterolemia, when cholesterol biosynthesis is supressed in most organs by fasting, the intestine becomes the major site of cholesterol biosynthesis, and its contribution can increase up to 50 %[160, 161]. Mixtures of short chain fatty acids have been show to suppress cholesterol synthesis in the rat liver and intestine [162], and whether fermentation metabolites from polydextrose can inhibit cholesterol biosynthesis in the intestine, or even in the liver, is an open question.

Author details

Heli Putaala
DuPont Nutrition and Health, Active Nutrition, Kantvik, Finland

Acknowledgement

Michael Bond, Stuart Craig, and Kirsti Tiihonen (DuPont Nutrition and Health) are thanked for their valuable contribution on the manuscript.

5. References

[1] Phillips GO, Cui SW. An Introduction: Evolution and Finalisation of the Regulatory Definition of Dietary Fibre. Food Hydrocolloids 2011;25 (2) 139-143.
[2] DeVries JW, Camire ME, Cho S, Craig S, Gordon D, Jones JM, Li B, Lineback D, Prosky L, Tungland BC. The Definition of Dietary Fiber. Cereal Foods World 2001;46 (3) 112-129.
[3] Roberfroid M, Gibson GR, Hoyles L, McCartney AL, Rastall R, Rowland I, Wolvers D, Watzl B, Szajewska H, Stahl B, Guarner F, Respondek F, Whelan K, Coxam V, Davicco MJ, Leotoing L, Wittrant Y, Delzenne NM, Cani PD, Neyrinck AM, Meheust A. Prebiotic Effects: Metabolic and Health Benefits. British Journal of Nutrition 2010;104 (S2) S1-S63.
[4] Howlett JF, Betteridge VA, Champ M, Craig SAS, Meheust A, Jones JM. The Definition of Dietary Fiber - Discussions at the Ninth Vahouny Fiber Symposium: Building Scientific Agreement. Food and Nutrition Research 2010;54 (1)
[5] Raninen K, Lappi J, Mykkänen H, Poutanen K. Dietary Fiber Type Reflects Physiological Functionality: Comparison of Grain Fiber, Inulin, and Polydextrose. Nutrition Reviews 2011;69 (1) 9-21.
[6] Craig SAS, Holden JF, Troup JP, Auerbach MH, Frier HI. Polydextrose as Soluble Fiber: Physiological and Analytical Aspects. Cereal Foods World 1998;43 (5) 370-376.
[7] Stowell JD. Polydextrose. In: Sungsoo S, Samuel P (ed.) Fiber Ingredients, Food Applications and Health Benefits, Boca Raton: CRC Press; 2009. p173-201.
[8] Stumm I, Baltes W. Analysis of the Linkage Positions in Polydextrose by the Reductive Cleavage Method. Food Chemistry 1997;59 (2) 291-297.
[9] Achour L, Flourie B, Briet F, Pellier P, Marteau P, Rambaud JC. Gastrointestinal Effects and Energy Value of Polydextrose in Healthy Nonobese Men. American Journal of Clinical Nutrition 1994;59 (6) 1362-1368.

[10] Costabile A, Fava F, Röytiö H, Forssten SD, Olli K, Klievink J, Rowland IR, Ouwehand AC, Rastall RA, Gibson GR, Walton GE. Impact of Polydextrose on the Faecal Microbiota: A Double-Blind, Crossover, Placebo-Controlled Feeding Study in Healthy Human Subjects. British Journal of Nutrition 2011;1-11.

[11] Fava F, Makivuokko H, Siljander-Rasi H, Putaala H, Tiihonen K, Stowell J, Tuohy K, Gibson G, Rautonen N. Effect of Polydextrose on Intestinal Microbes and Immune Functions in Pigs. British Journal of Nutrition 2007;98 (1) 123-133.

[12] Lahtinen SJ, Knoblock K, Drakoularakou A, Jacob M, Stowell J, Gibson GR, Ouwehand AC. Effect of Molecule Branching and Glycosidic Linkage on the Degradation of Polydextrose by Gut Microbiota. Bioscience Biotechnology and Biochemistry 2010;74 (10) 2016-2021.

[13] Auerbach MH, Craig SAS, Howlett JF, Hayes KC. Caloric Availability of Polydextrose. Nutrition Reviews 2007;65 (12) 544-549.

[14] Flood MT, Auerbach MH, Craig SAS. A Review of the Clinical Toleration Studies of Polydextrose in Food. Food and Chemical Toxicology 2004;42 (9) 1531-1542.

[15] Burdock GA, Flamm WG. A Review of the Studies of the Safety of Polydextrose in Food. Food and Chemical Toxicology 1999;37 (2-3) 233-264.

[16] Herfel TM, Jacobi SK, Lin X, Walker DC, Jouni ZE, Odle J. Safety Evaluation of Polydextrose in Infant Formula Using a Suckling Piglet Model. Food and Chemical Toxicology 2009;47 (7) 1530-1537.

[17] Beards E, Tuohy K, Gibson G. A Human Volunteer Study to Assess the Impact of Confectionery Sweeteners on the Gut Microbiota Composition. British Journal of Nutrition 2010;104 (5) 701-708.

[18] Beards E, Tuohy K, Gibson G. Bacterial, Scfa and Gas Profiles of a Range of Food Ingredients Following in Vitro Fermentation by Human Colonic Microbiota. Anaerobe 2010;16 (4) 420-425.

[19] Beynen AC, Saris DHJ, de Jong L, Staats M, Einerhand AWC. Impact of Dietary Polydextrose on Clinical Signs of Canine Osteoarthritis. American Journal of Animal and Veterinary Sciences 2011;6 (3) 93-99.

[20] Peuranen S, Tiihonen K, Apajalahti J, Kettunen A, Saarinen M, Rautonen N. Combination of Polydextrose and Lactitol Affects Microbial Ecosystem and Immune Responses in Rat Gastrointestinal Tract. British Journal of Nutrition 2004;91 (6) 905-914.

[21] Witaicenis A, Fruet AC, Salem L, Di Stasi LC. Dietary Polydextrose Prevents Inflammatory Bowel Disease in Trinitrobenzenesulfonic Acid Model of Rat Colitis. Journal of Medicinal Food 2010;13 (6) 1391-1396.

[22] Legette LL, Lee W, Martin BR, Story JA, Campbell JK, Weaver CM. Prebiotics Enhance Magnesium Absorption and Inulin-Based Fibers Exert Chronic Effects on Calcium Utilization in a Postmenopausal Rodent Model. J Food Sci 2012;77 (4) H88-94.

[23] dos Santos EF, Tsuboi KH, Araújo MR, Ouwehand AC, Andreollo NA, Miyasaka CK. Dietary Polydextrose Increases Calcium Absorption in Normal Rats. ABCD. Arquivos Brasileiros de Cirurgia Digestiva (São Paulo) 2009;22 201-205.

[24] Mineo H, Hara H, Kikuchi H, Sakurai H, Tomita F. Various Indigestible Saccharides Enhance Net Calcium Transport from the Epithelium of the Small and Large Intestine of Rats in Vitro. Journal of Nutrition 2001;131 (12) 3243-3246.

[25] Weaver CM, Martin BR, Story JA, Hutchinson I, Sanders L. Novel Fibers Increase Bone Calcium Content and Strength Beyond Efficiency of Large Intestine Fermentation. Journal of Agricultural and Food Chemistry 2010;58 (16) 8952-8957.

[26] dos Santos EF, Tsuboi KH, Araújo MR, Falconi MA, Ouwehand AC, Andreollo NA, Miyasaka CK. Ingestion of Polydextrose Increase the Iron Absorption in Rats Submitted to Partial Gastrectomy. Acta Cirurgica Brasileira 2010;25 518-524.

[27] Dikeman CL, Fahey Jr GC. Viscosity as Related to Dietary Fiber: A Review. Critical Reviews in Food Science and Nutrition 2006;46 (8) 649-663.

[28] Kapur NK, Ashen D, Blumenthal RS. High Density Lipoprotein Cholesterol: An Evolving Target of Therapy in the Management of Cardiovascular Disease. Vascular Health and Risk Management 2008;4 (1) 39-57.

[29] Brown L, Rosner B, Willett WW, Sacks FM. Cholesterol-Lowering Effects of Dietary Fiber: A Meta-Analysis. American Journal of Clinical Nutrition 1999;69 (1) 30-42.

[30] Hunninghake DB, Miller VT, LaRosa JC, Kinosian B, Jacobson T, Brown V, Howard WJ, Edelman DA, O'Connor RR. Long-Term Treatment of Hypercholesterolemia with Dietary Fiber. American Journal of Medicine 1994;97 (6) 504-508.

[31] Jenkins DJA, Kendall CWC, Vuksan V, Augustin LSA, Mehling C, Parker T, Vidgen E, Lee B, Faulkner D, Seyler H, Josse R, Leiter LA, Connelly PW, Fulgoni Iii V. Effect of Wheat Bran on Serum Lipids: Influence of Particle Size and Wheat Protein. Journal of the American College of Nutrition 1999;18 (2) 159-165.

[32] Jenkins DJA, Vuksan V, Kendall CWC, Würsch P, Jeffcoat R, Waring S, Mehling CC, Vidgen E, Augustin LSA, Wong E. Physiological Effects of Resistant Starches on Fecal Bulk, Short Chain Fatty Acids, Blood Lipids and Glycemic Index. Journal of the American College of Nutrition 1998;17 (6) 609-616.

[33] Truswell AS. Dietary Fibre and Plasma Lipids. European Journal of Clinical Nutrition 1995;49 (SUPPL. 3) S105-S109.

[34] Jenkins DJA, Kendall CWC, Axelsen M, Augustin LSA, Vuksan V. Viscous and Nonviscous Fibres, Nonabsorbable and Low Glycaemic Index Carbohydrates, Blood Lipids and Coronary Heart Disease. Current Opinion in Lipidology 2000;11 (1) 49-56.

[35] Ellegård L, Andersson H. Oat Bran Rapidly Increases Bile Acid Excretion and Bile Acid Synthesis: An Ileostomy Study. European Journal of Clinical Nutrition 2007;61 (8) 938-945.

[36] Marlett JA, Fischer MH. A Poorly Fermented Gel from Psyllium Seed Husk Increases Excreta Moisture and Bile Acid Excretion in Rats. Journal of Nutrition 2002;132 (9) 2638-2643.

[37] Gunness P, Flanagan BM, Gidley MJ. Molecular Interactions between Cereal Soluble Dietary Fibre Polymers and a Model Bile Salt Deduced from 13c Nmr Titration. Journal of Cereal Science 2010;52 (3) 444-449.

[38] Shelat KJ, Vilaplana F, Nicholson TM, Gidley MJ, Gilbert RG. Diffusion and Rheology Characteristics of Barley Mixed Linkage B-Glucan and Possible Implications for Digestion. Carbohydrate Polymers 2011;86 (4) 1732-1738.

[39] Potter JG, Coffman KP, Reid RL. Effect of Test Meals of Varying Dietary Fiber Content on Plasma Insulin and Glucose Response. American Journal of Clinical Nutrition 1981;34 (3) 328-334.

[40] Burton-Freeman B. Dietary Fiber and Energy Regulation. Journal of Nutrition 2000;130 (2 SUPPL.) 272S-275S.

[41] Wolever TMS, Spadafora PJ, Cunnane SC, Pencharz PB. Propionate Inhibits Incorporation of Colonic [1,2-13c]Acetate into Plasma Lipids in Humans. American Journal of Clinical Nutrition 1995;61 (6) 1241-1247.

[42] Choi YS, Cho SH, Kim HJ, Lee HJ. Effects of Soluble Dietary Fibers on Lipid Metabolism and Activities of Intestinal Disaccharidases in Rats. Journal of Nutritional Science and Vitaminology 1998;44 (5) 591-600.

[43] Oku T, Fujii Y, Okamatsu H. Polydextrose as Dietary Fiber - Hydrolysis by Digestive Enzyme and Its Effect on Gastrointestinal Transit-Time in Rats. Journal of Clinical Biochemistry and Nutrition 1991;11 (1) 31-40.

[44] Choe M, Kim JD, Ju JS. Effects of Polydextrose and Hydrolysed Guar Gum on Lipid Metabolism of Normal Rats with Different Levels of Dietary Fat. Korean Journal of Nutrition 1992;25 (3) 211-220.

[45] Pronczuk A, Hayes KC. Hypocholesterolemic Effect of Dietary Polydextrose in Gerbils and Humans. Nutrition Research 2006;26 (1) 27-31.

[46] Shimomura Y, Maeda K, Nagasaki M, Matsuo Y, Murakami T, Bajotto G, Sato J, Selno T, Kamiwaki T, Suzuki M. Attenuated Response of the Serum Triglyceride Concentration to Ingestion of a Chocolate Containing Polydextrose and Lactitol in Place of Sugar. Bioscience Biotechnology and Biochemistry 2005;69 (10) 1819-1823.

[47] Saku K, Yoshinaga K, Okura Y, Ying H, Harada R, Arakawa K. Effects of Polydextrose on Serum-Lipids, Lipoproteins, and Apolipoproteins in Health Subjects. Clinical Therapeutics 1991;13 (2) 254-258.

[48] Liu S, Tsai CE. Effects of Biotechnically Synthesized Oligosaccharides and Polydextrose on Serum Lipids in the Human. Journal of the Chinese Nutrition Society 1995;20 (1) 1-12.

[49] Jie Z, Bang-Yao L, Ming-Jie X, Hai-Wei L, Zu-Kang Z, Ting-Song W, Craig SA. Studies on the Effects of Polydextrose Intake on Physiologic Functions in Chinese People. American Journal of Clinical Nutrition 2000;72 (6) 1503-1509.

[50] Riccardi G, Rivellese A, Pacioni D. Separate Influence of Dietary Carbohydrate and Fibre on the Metabolic Control in Diabetes. Diabtologia 1984;26 (2) 116-121.

[51] Rivellese A, Riccardi G, Giacco A. Effect of Dietary Fibre on Glucose Control and Serum Lipoproteins in Diabetic Patients. Lancet 1980;2 (8192) 447-449.

[52] Schwab U, Louheranta A, Torronen A, Uusitupa M. Impact of Sugar Beet Pectin and Polydextrose on Fasting and Postprandial Glycemia and Fasting Concentrations of Serum Total and Lipoprotein Lipids in Middle-Aged Subjects with Abnormal Glucose Metabolism. European Journal of Clinical Nutrition 2006;60 (9) 1073-1080.

[53] Cicek B, Arslan P, Kelestimur F. The Effects of Oligofructose and Polydextrose on Metabolic Control Parameters in Type-2 Diabetes. Pakistan Journal of Medical Sciences 2009;25 (4) 573-578.

[54] Chinevere TD, Sawyer RD, Creer AR, Conlee RK, Parcell AC. Effects of L-Tyrosine and Carbohydrate Ingestion on Endurance Exercise Performance. Journal of Applied Physiology 2002;93 (5) 1590-1597.

[55] Vasankari TJ, Ahotupa M. Supplementation of Polydextrose Reduced a Hamburger Meal Induced Postprandial Hypertriglyceridemia. Circulation 2005;112 (17) 3849.

[56] Movva R, Rader DJ. Laboratory Assessment of Hdl Heterogeneity and Function. Clinical Chemistry 2008;54 (5) 788-800.

[57] Kwiterovich PO, Jr. Lipoprotein Heterogeneity: Diagnostic and Therapeutic Implications. American Journal of Cardiology 2002;90 (8, Supplement 1) 1-10.

[58] Salonen JT, Salonen R, Seppanen K, Rauramaa R, Tuomilehto J. Hdl, Hdl2, and Hdl3 Subfractions, and the Risk of Acute Myocardial Infarction. A Prospective Population Study in Eastern Finnish Men. Circulation 1991;84 (1) 129-139.

[59] Lamarche B, Moorjani S, Cantin B, Dagenais GR, Lupien PJ, Despres JP. Associations of Hdl2 and Hdl3 Subfractions with Ischemic Heart Disease in Men. Prospective Results from the Quebec Cardiovascular Study. Arteriosclerosis, Thrombosis, and Vascular Biology 1997;17 (6) 1098-1105.

[60] Stampfer MJ, Sacks FM, Salvini S, Willett WC, Hennekens CH. A Prospective Study of Cholesterol, Apolipoproteins, and the Risk of Myocardial Infarction. The New England Journal of Medicine 1991;325 (6) 373-381.

[61] Yu S, Yarnell JWG, Sweetnam P, Bolton CH. High Density Lipoprotein Subfractions and the Risk of Coronary Heart Disease: 9-Years Follow-up in the Caerphilly Study. Atherosclerosis 2003;166 (2) 331-338.

[62] Morgan J, Carey C, Lincoff A, Capuzzi D. High-Density Lipoprotein Subfractions and Risk of Coronary Artery Disease. Current Atherosclerosis Reports 2004;6 (5) 359-365.

[63] Bosello O, Cominacini L, Zocca I, Garbin U, Ferrari F, Davoli A. Effects of Guar Gum on Plasma Lipoproteins and Apolipoproteins C-Ii and C-Iii in Patients Affected by Familial Combined Hyperlipoproteinemia. The American Journal of Clinical Nutrition 1984;40 (6) 1165-1174.

[64] McIvor ME, Cummings CC, Van Duyn MA, Leo TA, Margolis S, Behall KM, Michnowski JE, Mendeloff AI. Long-Term Effects of Guar Gum on Blood Lipids. Atherosclerosis 1986;60 (1) 7-13.

[65] Anderson JW, O'Neal DS, Riddell-Mason S, Floore TL, Dillon DW, Oeltgen PR. Postprandial Serum Glucose, Insulin, and Lipoprotein Responses to High- and Low-Fiber Diets. Metabolism: Clinical and Experimental 1995;44 (7) 848-854.

[66] Behall KM, Scholfield DJ, Hallfrisch J. Effect of Beta-Glucan Level in Oat Fiber Extracts on Blood Lipids in Men and Women. Journal of the American College of Nutrition 1997;16 (1) 46-51.

[67] Williams PT, Krauss RM, Vranizan KM, Stefanick ML, Wood PDS, Lindgren FT. Associations of Lipoproteins and Apolipoproteins with Gradient Gel Electrophoresis

Estimates of High Density Lipoprotein Subfractions in Men and Women. Arteriosclerosis and Thrombosis 1992;12 (3) 332-340.

[68] Krauss RM. Lipoprotein Subfractions and Cardiovascular Disease Risk. Current Opinion in Lipidology 2010;21 (4) 305-311.

[69] Ozawa H, Kobayashi T, Sakane H, Imafuku S, Mikami Y, Homma Y. Effects of Dietary Fiber Polydextrose Feeding on Plasma Lipids Levels and Diurnal Change in Plasma Sugar, Insulin, and Blood Pressure Levels. Nippon Eiyo Shokuryo Gakkaishi 1993;46 (5) 395-399.

[70] Lefebvre P, Cariou B, Lien F, Kuipers F, Staels B. Role of Bile Acids and Bile Acid Receptors in Metabolic Regulation. Physiological Reviews 2009;89 (1) 147-191.

[71] Wang DQ. Regulation of Intestinal Cholesterol Absorption. Annual Review of Physiology 2007;69 221-248.

[72] Ridlon JM, Kang DJ, Hylemon PB. Bile Salt Biotransformations by Human Intestinal Bacteria. Journal of Lipid Research 2006;47 (2) 241-259.

[73] Chiang JYL. Bile Acids: Regulation of Synthesis. Journal of Lipid Research 2009;50 (10) 1955-1966.

[74] Charlton-Menys V, Durrington PN. Human Cholesterol Metabolism and Therapeutic Molecules. Experimental Physiology 2008;93 (1) 27-42.

[75] Lia A, Hallmans G, Sandberg AS, Sundberg B, Aman P, Andersson H. Oat B-Glucan Increases Bile Acid Excretion and a Fiber-Rich Barley Fraction Increases Cholesterol Excretion in Ileostomy Subjects. American Journal of Clinical Nutrition 1995;62 (6) 1245-1251.

[76] Theuwissen E, Mensink RP. Water-Soluble Dietary Fibers and Cardiovascular Disease. Physiology and Behavior 2008;94 (2) 285-292.

[77] Hengst C, Ptok S, Roessler A, Fechner A, Jahreis G. Effects of Polydextrose Supplementation on Different Faecal Parameters in Healthy Volunteers. International Journal of Food Sciences and Nutrition 2008;60 (5) 96-105.

[78] Zacherl C, Eisner P, Engel K-H. In Vitro Model to Correlate Viscosity and Bile Acid-Binding Capacity of Digested Water-Soluble and Insoluble Dietary Fibres. Food Chemistry 2011;126 (2) 423-428.

[79] Murphy O. Non-Polyol Low-Digestible Carbohydrates: Food Applications and Functional Benefits. British Journal of Nutrition 2001;85 (Suppl 1) S47-S53.

[80] Satoh H, Hara T, Murakawa D, Matsuura M, Takata K. Soluble Dietary Fiber Protects against Nonsteroidal Anti-Inflammatory Drug-Induced Damage to the Small Intestine in Cats. Digestive Diseases and Sciences 2010;55 (5) 1264-1271.

[81] Ogata S, Fujimoto K, Iwakiri R, Matsunaga C, Ogawa Y, Koyama T, Sakai T. Effect of Polydextrose on Absorption of Triglyceride and Cholesterol in Mesenteric Lymph-Fistula Rats. Proceedings of the Society for Experimental Biology and Medicine 1997;215 (1) 53-58.

[82] Watanabe K, Iwata K, Tandai Y, Nishizawa M, Yamagishi T, Yoshizawa I. Effects of Soluble Sodium Alginates on the Excretion of Cholesterol, Trp-P-1 and Aflatoxin B 1 in Rats. Japanese Journal of Toxicology and Environmental Health 1992;38 (3) 258-262.

[83] MacDonald IA, Bokkenheuser VD, Winter J. Degradation of Steroids in the Human Gut. Journal of Lipid Research 1983;24 (6) 675-700.

[84] Litvak DA, Hwang KO, Evers BM, Townsend CM, Jr. Induction of Apoptosis in Human Gastric Cancer by Sodium Butyrate. Anticancer Research 2000;20 (2A) 779-784.

[85] Mariadason JM, Corner GA, Augenlicht LH. Genetic Reprogramming in Pathways of Colonic Cell Maturation Induced by Short Chain Fatty Acids: Comparison with Trichostatin a, Sulindac, and Curcumin and Implications for Chemoprevention of Colon Cancer. Cancer Research 2000;60 (16) 4561-4572.

[86] Wong JM, de SR, Kendall CW, Emam A, Jenkins DJ. Colonic Health: Fermentation and Short Chain Fatty Acids. Journal of Clinical Gastroenterology 2006;40 (3) 235-243.

[87] Alvaro A, Solà R, Rosales R, Ribalta J, Anguera A, Masana L, Vallvé JC. Gene Expression Analysis of a Human Enterocyte Cell Line Reveals Downregulation of Cholesterol Biosynthesis in Response to Short-Chain Fatty Acids. IUBMB Life 2008;60 (11) 757-764.

[88] Lin Y, Vonk RJ, Slooff JH, Kuipers F, Smit MJ. Differences in Propionate-Induced Inhibition of Cholesterol and Triacylglycerol Synthesis between Human and Rat Hepatocytes in Primary Culture. British Journal of Nutrition 1995;74 (2) 197-207.

[89] Layden BT, Yalamanchi SK, Wolever TMS, Dunaif A, Lowe Jr WL. Negative Association of Acetate with Visceral Adipose Tissue and Insulin Levels. Diabetes, Metabolic Syndrome and Obesity: Targets and Therapy 2012;5 49-55.

[90] Boila RJ, Salomons MO, Milligan LP, Aherne FX. The Effect of Dietary Propionic Acid on Cholesterol Synthesis in Swine. Nutrition Reports International 1981;23 (6) 1113-1121.

[91] Nishina PM, Freedland RA. Effects of Propionate on Lipid Biosynthesis in Isolated Rat Hepatocytes. Journal of Nutrition 1990;120 (7) 668-673.

[92] Wright RS, Anderson JW, Bridges SR. Propionate Inhibits Hepatocyte Lipid Synthesis. Proceedings of the Society for Experimental Biology and Medicine 1990;195 (1) 26-29.

[93] Illman RJ, Topping DL, McIntosh GH, Trimble RP, Storer GB, Taylor MN, Cheng BQ. Hypocholesterolaemic Effects of Dietary Propionate: Studies in Whole Animals and Perfused Rat Liver. Annals of Nutrition and Metabolism 1988;32 (2) 97-107.

[94] Adam A, Levrat-Verny MA, Lopez HW, Leuillet M, Demigné C, Rémésy C. Whole Wheat and Triticale Flours with Differing Viscosities Stimulate Cecal Fermentations and Lower Plasma and Hepatic Lipids in Rats. Journal of Nutrition 2001;131 (6) 1770-1776.

[95] Venter CS, Vorster HH, Cummings JH. Effects of Dietary Propionate on Carbohydrate and Lipid Metabolism in Healthy Volunteers. American Journal of Gastroenterology 1990;85 (5) 549-553.

[96] Beaulieu KE, McBurney MI. Changes in Pig Serum Lipids, Nutrient Digestibility and Sterol Excretion During Cecal Infusion of Propionate. Journal of Nutrition 1992;122 (2) 241-245.

[97] Wolever TMS, Spadafora P, Eshuis H. Interaction between Colonic Acetate and Propionate in Humans. American Journal of Clinical Nutrition 1991;53 (3) 681-687.

[98] Todesco T, Rao AV, Bosello O, Jenkins DJA. Propionate Lowers Blood Glucose and Alters Lipid Metabolism in Healthy Subjects. American Journal of Clinical Nutrition 1991;54 (5) 860-865.

[99] Vogt JA, Wolever TMS. Fecal Acetate Is Inversely Related to Acetate Absorption from the Human Rectum and Distal Colon. Journal of Nutrition 2003;133 (10) 3145-3148.

[100] Mäkivuokko H, Kettunen H, Saarinen M, Kamiwaki T, Yokoyama Y, Stowell J, Rautonen N. The Effect of Cocoa and Polydextrose on Bacterial Fermentation in Gastrointestinal Tract Simulations. Bioscience Biotechnology and Biochemistry 2007;71 (8) 1834-1843.

[101] Makelainen HS, Makivuokko HA, Salminen SJ, Rautonen NE, Ouwehand AC. The Effects of Polydextrose and Xylitol on Microbial Community and Activity in a 4-Stage Colon Simulator. Journal of Food Science 2007;72 (5) M153-M159.

[102] Hernot DC, Boileau TW, Bauer LL, Middelbos IS, Murphy MR, Swanson KS, Fahey GC. In Vitro Fermentation Profiles, Gas Production Rates, and Microbiota Modulation as Affected by Certain Fructans, Galactooligosaccharides, and Polydextrose. Journal of Agricultural and Food Chemistry 2009;57 (4) 1354-1361.

[103] Beloshapka AN, Wolff AK, Swanson KS. Effects of Feeding Polydextrose on Faecal Characteristics, Microbiota and Fermentative End Products in Healthy Adult Dogs. British Journal of Nutrition 2011;1-7.

[104] Stowell JD. Prebiotic Potential of Polydextrose. In: Charalampopoulos D, Rastall RA (ed.) Prebiotics and Probiotics Science and Technology, Reading: Springer; 2009. p337-352.

[105] Wang X, Gibson GR. Effects of the in-Vitro Fermentation of Oligofructose and Inulin by Bacteria Growing in the Human Large-Intestine. Journal of Applied Bacteriology 1993;75 (4) 373-380.

[106] Vester Boler BM, Hernot DC, Boileau TW, Bauer LL, Middelbos IS, Murphy MR, Swanson KS, Fahey GC, Jr. Carbohydrates Blended with Polydextrose Lower Gas Production and Short-Chain Fatty Acid Production in an in Vitro System. Nutrition Research 2009;29 (9) 631-639.

[107] Vester Boler BM, Rossoni Serao MC, Bauer LL, Staeger MA, Boileau TW, Swanson KS, Fahey GC. Digestive Physiological Outcomes Related to Polydextrose and Soluble Maize Fibre Consumption by Healthy Adult Men. British Journal of Nutrition 2011;106 (12) 1864-1871.

[108] Makivuokko H, Nurmi J, Nurminen P, Stowell J, Rautonen N. In Vitro Effects on Polydextrose by Colonic Bacteria and Caco-2 Cell Cyclooxygenase Gene Expression. Nutrition and Cancer-An International Journal 2005;52 (1) 94-104.

[109] Mäkeläinen H, Ottman N, Forssten S, Saarinen M, Rautonen N, Ouwehand AC. Synbiotic Effects of Galacto-Oligosaccharide, Polydextrose and Bifidobacterium Lactis Bi-07 in Vitro. International Journal of Probiotics and Prebiotics 2010;5 (4) 203-210.

[110] Bäckhed F, Ding H, Wang T, Hooper LV, Gou YK, Nagy A, Semenkovich CF, Gordon JI. The Gut Microbiota as an Environmental Factor That Regulates Fat Storage. Proceedings of the National Academy of Sciences of the United States of America 2004;101 (44) 15718-15723.

[111] Martínez I, Wallace G, Zhang C, Legge R, Benson AK, Carr TP, Moriyama EN, Walter J. Diet-Induced Metabolic Improvements in a Hamster Model of Hypercholesterolemia Are Strongly Linked to Alterations of the Gut Microbiota. Applied and Environmental Microbiology 2009;75 (12) 4175-4184.

[112] Cheng S, Munukka E, Wiklund P, Pekkala S, Völgyi E, Xu L, Lyytikäinen A, Marjomäki V, Alen M, Vaahtovuo J, Keinänen-Kiukaanniemi S. Women with and without Metabolic Disorder Differ in Their Gut Microbiota Composition. Obesity 2012;20 (5) 1082-1087.

[113] Patrone V, Ferrari S, Lizier M, Lucchini F, Minuti A, Tondelli B, Trevisi E, Rossi F, Callegari ML. Short-Term Modifications in the Distal Gut Microbiota of Weaning Mice Induced by a High-Fat Diet. Microbiology 2012;158 (4) 983-992.

[114] Hooda S, Boler Vester BM, Serao Rossoni MC, Brulc JM, Staeger MA, Boileau TW, Dowd SE, Fahey GC, Jr., Swanson KS. 454 Pyrosequencing Reveals a Shift in Fecal Microbiota of Healthy Adult Men Consuming Polydextrose or Soluble Corn Fiber. Journal of Nutrition 2012;

[115] Probert HM, Apajalahti JHA, Rautonen N, Stowell J, Gibson GR. Polydextrose, Lactitol, and Fructo-Oligosaccharide Fermentation by Colonic Bacteria in a Three-Stage Continuous Culture System. Applied and Environmental Microbiology 2004;70 (8) 4505-4511.

[116] Truswell AS. Cereal Grains and Coronary Heart Disease. European Journal of Clinical Nutrition 2002;56 (1) 1-14.

[117] Salas-Salvadó J, Bulló M, Pérez-Heras A, Ros E. Dietary Fibre, Nuts and Cardiovascular Diseases. British Journal of Nutrition 2006;96 Suppl 2 S46-51.

[118] Lairon D, Play B, Jourdheuil-Rahmani D. Digestible and Indigestible Carbohydrates: Interactions with Postprandial Lipid Metabolism. Journal of Nutritional Biochemistry 2007;18 (4) 217-227.

[119] Ford ES, Liu S. Glycemic Index and Serum High-Density Lipoprotein Cholesterol Concentration among Us Adults. Archives of Internal Medicine 2001;161 (4) 572-576.

[120] Liu S, Manson JE, Stampfer MJ, Holmes MD, Hu FB, Hankinson SE, Willett WC. Dietary Glycemic Load Assessed by Food-Frequency Questionnaire in Relation to Plasma High-Density-Lipoprotein Cholesterol and Fasting Plasma Triacylglycerols in Postmenopausal Women. American Journal of Clinical Nutrition 2001;73 (3) 560-566.

[121] Ravid Z, Bendayan M, Delvin E, Sane AT, Elchebly M, Lafond J, Lambert M, Mailhot G, Levy E. Modulation of Intestinal Cholesterol Absorption by High Glucose Levels: Impact on Cholesterol Transporters, Regulatory Enzymes, and Transcription Factors. American Journal of Physiology - Gastrointestinal and Liver Physiology 2008;295 (5) G873-G885.

[122] Silbernagel G, Lütjohann D, MacHann J, Meichsner S, Kantartzis K, Schick F, Häring HU, Stefan N, Fritsche A. Cholesterol Synthesis Is Associated with Hepatic Lipid Content and Dependent on Fructose/Glucose Intake in Healthy Humans. Experimental Diabetes Research 2012;2012

[123] Foster-Powell K, Holt SH, Brand-Miller JC. International Table of Glycemic Index and Glycemic Load Values: 2002. American Journal of Clinical Nutrition 2002;76 (1) 5-56.

[124] Shimomura Y, Nagasaki M, Matsuo Y, Maeda K, Murakami T, Sato J, Sato Y. Effects of Polydextrose on the Levels of Plasma Glucose and Serum Insulin Concentrations in Human Glucose Tolerance Test. Journal of Japanese Association for Dietary Fiber Research 2004;8 (2) 105-109.

[125] Tappy L, Le KA. Metabolic Effects of Fructose and the Worldwide Increase in Obesity. Physiological Reviews 2010;90 (1) 23-46.

[126] Knapp BK, Parsons CM, Swanson KS, Fahey GC. Physiological Responses to Novel Carbohydrates as Assessed Using Canine and Avian Models. Journal of Agricultural and Food Chemistry 2008;56 (17) 7999-8006.

[127] Wilson T, Luebke JL, Morcomb EF, Carrell EJ, Leveranz MC, Kobs L, Schmidt TP, Limburg PJ, Vorsa N, Singh AP. Glycemic Responses to Sweetened Dried and Raw Cranberries in Humans with Type 2 Diabetes. Journal of Food Science 2010;75 (8) H218-223.

[128] Kurotobi T, Fukuhara K, Inage H, Kimura S. Glycemic Index and Postprandial Blood Glucose Response to Japanese Strawberry Jam in Normal Adults. Journal of Nutritional Science and Vitaminology 2010;56 (3) 198-202.

[129] Kovacs EMR, Westerterp-Plantenga MS, Saris WHM, Melanson KJ, Goossens I, Geurten P, Brouns F. The Effect of Guar Gum Addition to a Semisolid Meal on Appetite Related to Blood Glucose, in Dieting Men. European Journal of Clinical Nutrition 2002;56 (8) 771-778.

[130] King NA, Craig SAS, Pepper T, Blundell JE. Evaluation of the Independent and Combined Effects of Xylitol and Polydextrose Consumed as a Snack on Hunger and Energy Intake over 10 D. British Journal of Nutrition 2005;93 (6) 911-915.

[131] Monsivais P, Carter BE, Christiansen M, Perrigue MM, Drewnowski A. Soluble Fiber Dextrin Enhances the Satiating Power of Beverages. Appetite 2011;56 (1) 9-14.

[132] Willis HJ, Eldridge AL, Beiseigel J, Thomas W, Slavin JL. Greater Satiety Response with Resistant Starch and Corn Bran in Human Subjects. Nutrition Research 2009;29 (2) 100-105.

[133] Ranawana V, Muller A, Henry JK. Polydextrose: Its Effects on Short-Term Food Intake and Subjective Feelings of Satiety: A Randomized Controlled Study. European Journal of Nutrition 2012;

[134] Saarinen M, Olli K, Hull S, Re R, Stowell J, Tiihonen K. The Effects of Polydextrose on Satiety in Humans. In 2nd Swiss Food Tech Day 2011, "Micronutrients & Functional Ingredients", 11th May 2011. Sisseln, Switzerland.

[135] Hull S, Re R, Tiihonen K, Viscione L, Wickham M. Consuming Polydextrose in a Mid-Morning Snack Increases Acute Satiety Measurements and Reduces Subsequent Energy Intake at Lunch in Healthy Human Subjects. 2012 Manuscript in Preparation.

[136] Lin HV, Frassetto A, Kowalik EJ, Jr., Nawrocki AR, Lu MM, Kosinski JR, Hubert JA, Szeto D, Yao X, Forrest G, Marsh DJ. Butyrate and Propionate Protect against Diet-Induced Obesity and Regulate Gut Hormones Via Free Fatty Acid Receptor 3-Independent Mechanisms. PLoS One 2012;7 (4) e35240.

[137] Leuvenink HGD, Bleumer EJB, Bongers LJGM, Van Bruchem J, Van Der Heide D. Effect of Short-Term Propionate Infusion on Feed Intake and Blood Parameters in

Sheep. American Journal of Physiology - Endocrinology and Metabolism 1997;272 (6 35-6) E997-E1001.

[138] Oba M, Allen MS. Intraruminal Infusion of Propionate Alters Feeding Behavior and Decreases Energy Intake of Lactating Dairy Cows. Journal of Nutrition 2003;133 (4) 1094-1099.

[139] Karaki SI, Tazoe H, Hayashi H, Kashiwabara H, Tooyama K, Suzuki Y, Kuwahara A. Expression of the Short-Chain Fatty Acid Receptor, Gpr43, in the Human Colon. Journal of Molecular Histology 2008;39 (2) 135-142.

[140] Tolhurst G, Heffron H, Lam YS, Parker HE, Habib AM, Diakogiannaki E, Cameron J, Grosse J, Reimann F, Gribble FM. Short-Chain Fatty Acids Stimulate Glucagon-Like Peptide-1 Secretion Via the G-Protein-Coupled Receptor Ffar2. Diabetes 2012;61 (2) 364-371.

[141] Vanhoutvin SA, Troost FJ, Hamer HM, Lindsey PJ, Koek GH, Jonkers DM, Kodde A, Venema K, Brummer RJ. Butyrate-Induced Transcriptional Changes in Human Colonic Mucosa. PLoS ONE 2009;4 (8) e6759.

[142] Bassaganya-Riera J, DiGuardo M, Viladomiu M, de Horna A, Sanchez S, Einerhand AWC, Sanders L, Hontecillas R. Soluble Fibers and Resistant Starch Ameliorate Disease Activity in Interleukin-10-Deficient Mice with Inflammatory Bowel Disease. Journal of Nutrition 2011;141 (7) 1318-1325.

[143] Wachtershauser A, Loitsch SM, Stein J. Ppar-Gamma Is Selectively Upregulated in Caco-2 Cells by Butyrate. Biochemical and Biophysical Research Communications 2000;272 (2) 380-385.

[144] Putaala H, Makivuokko H, Tiihonen K, Rautonen N. Simulated Colon Fiber Metabolome Regulates Genes Involved in Cell Cycle, Apoptosis, and Energy Metabolism in Human Colon Cancer Cells. Molecular and Cellular Biochemistry 2011;357 (1-2) 235-245.

[145] Bunger M, van den Bosch HM, van der Meijde J, Kersten S, Hooiveld GJEJ, Muller M. Genome-Wide Analysis of Ppar{Alpha} Activation in Murine Small Intestine. Physiological Genomics 2007;15 (4) 837-845.

[146] de Vogel-van den Bosch HM, Bunger M, de Groot PJ, Bosch-Vermeulen H, Hooiveld GJ, Muller M. Pparalpha-Mediated Effects of Dietary Lipids on Intestinal Barrier Gene Expression. BMC.Genomics 2008;9 231.

[147] Ranhotra HS. Long-Term Caloric Restriction up-Regulates Ppar Gamma Co-Activator 1 Alpha (Pgc-1α) Expression in Mice. Indian Journal of Biochemistry and Biophysics 2010;47 (5) 272-277.

[148] Rera M, Bahadorani S, Cho J, Koehler Christopher L, Ulgherait M, Hur Jae H, Ansari William S, Lo Jr T, Jones DL, Walker David W. Modulation of Longevity and Tissue Homeostasis by the Drosophila Pgc-1 Homolog. Cell Metabolism 2011;14 (5) 623-634.

[149] Finck BN, Gropler MC, Chen Z, Leone TC, Croce MA, Harris TE, Lawrence, Jr., Kelly DP. Lipin 1 Is an Inducible Amplifier of the Hepatic Pgc-1[Alpha]/Ppar[Alpha] Regulatory Pathway. Cell Metabolism 2006;4 (3) 199-210.

[150] Suviolahti E, Reue K, Cantor RM, Phan J, Gentile M, Naukkarinen J, Soro-Paavonen A, Oksanen L, Kaprio J, Rissanen A, Salomaa V, Kontula K, Taskinen MR, Pajukanta P,

Peltonen L. Cross-Species Analyses Implicate Lipin 1 Involvement in Human Glucose Metabolism. Human Molecular Genetics 2006;15 (3) 377-386.

[151] Yao-Borengasser A, Rasouli N, Varma V, Miles LM, Phanavanh B, Starks TN, Phan J, Spencer Iii HJ, McGehee Jr RE, Reue K, Kern PA. Lipin Expression Is Attenuated in Adipose Tissue of Insulin-Resistant Human Subjects and Increases with Peroxisome Proliferator-Activated Receptor Γ Activation. Diabetes 2006;55 (10) 2811-2818.

[152] Kruit JK, Groen AK, van Berkel TJ, Kuipers F. Emerging Roles of the Intestine in Control of Cholesterol Metabolism. World Journal of Gastroenterology 2006;12 (40) 6429-6439.

[153] Field FJ, Watt K, Mathur SN. Origins of Intestinal Abca1-Mediated Hdl-Cholesterol. Journal of Lipid Research 2008;49 (12) 2605-2619.

[154] Brunham LR, Kruit JK, Iqbal J, Fievet C, Timmins JM, Pape TD, Coburn BA, Bissada N, Staels B, Groen AK, Hussain MM, Parks JS, Kuipers F, Hayden MR. Intestinal Abca1 Directly Contributes to Hdl Biogenesis in Vivo. Journal of Clinical Investigation 2006;116 (4) 1052-1062.

[155] Boadu E, Choi HY, Lee DWK, Waddington EI, Chan T, Asztalos B, Vance JE, Chan A, Castro G, Francis GA. Correction of Apolipoprotein a-I-Mediated Lipid Efflux and High Density Lipoprotein Particle Formation in Human Niemann-Pick Type C Disease Fibroblasts. Journal of Biological Chemistry 2006;281 (48) 37081-37090.

[156] De Preter V, Falony G, Windey K, Hamer HM, De Vuyst L, Verbeke K. The Prebiotic, Oligofructose-Enriched Inulin Modulates the Faecal Metabolite Profile: An in Vitro Analysis. Molecular Nutrition and Food Research 2010;54 (12) 1791-1801.

[157] Dullens SPJ, Mensink RP, Mariman ECM, Plat J. Differentiated Caco-2 Cells as an in-Vitro Model to Evaluate De-Novo Apolipoprotein a-L Production in the Small Intestine. European Journal of Gastroenterology and Hepatology 2009;21 (6) 642-649.

[158] Gylling H. Cholesterol Metabolism and Its Implications for Therapeutic Interventions in Patients with Hypercholesterolaemia. International Journal of Clinical Practice 2004;58 (9) 859-866.

[159] Sviridov DD, Safonova IG, Talalaev AG. Regulation of Cholesterol Synthesis in Isolated Epithelial Cells of Human Small Intestine. Lipids 1986;21 (12) 759-763.

[160] Dietschy JM, Siperstein MD. Effect of Cholesterol Feeding and Fasting on Sterol Synthesis in Seventeen Tissues of the Rat. Journal of Lipid Research 1967;8 (2) 97-104.

[161] Dietschy JM, Wilson JD. Regulation of Cholesterol Metabolism. New England Journal of Medicine 1970;282 (21) 1179-1183.

[162] Hara H, Haga S, Aoyama Y, Kiriyama S. Short-Chain Fatty Acids Suppress Cholesterol Synthesis in Rat Liver and Intestine. Journal of Nutrition 1999;129 (5) 942-948.

Chapter 12

Spent Brewer's Yeast and Beta-Glucans Isolated from Them as Diet Components Modifying Blood Lipid Metabolism Disturbed by an Atherogenic Diet

Bożena Waszkiewicz-Robak

Additional information is available at the end of the chapter

http://dx.doi.org/10.5772/51530

1. Introduction

In the report of the Experts of the World Health Organisation and the Food and Agriculture Organisation [1] which reviewed research results concerning the influence of lifestyle, particularly diet components on the risk level of diet-dependent diseases, beta-glucan was acknowledged as a substance limiting the risk of many the so-called civilisation diseases. Simultaneously, it was recognized that the physiological influence of dietary fibre and interactions with other diet components are not fully known, therefore, further research within the scope is reasonable. Among various fractions of dietary fibre, β-glucans from cereals are especially significant, as they are considered safe and at the same time recommended for intake as food components lowering total cholesterol concentration in blood. Unlike widely-known fractions of dietary fibre, recommended as a factor modifying and preventing the risk of circulatory system and digestive system diseases, beta-glucans show multidirectional and still not entirely recognized health influence [2].

β-glucans discovered so far have been used in the pharmaceutical industry as substances strengthening the immune system, preparations of antiviral and antibacterial activity, and as natural adjuvants, which resulted in them being called "biological response modifiers" (BRMs). It is assumed that substances of this type cannot do harm, they help the body to adjust to various environmental and biological stresses and have a regulating and multi-directed influence on the body, most of all, supporting the immune system, but also showing another positive influence on some functions of the body, e.g. correcting lipid metabolism, correcting glycemic index in people with type 2 diabetes, or exhibiting antitumor activity [3].

2. Sources and general properties of β-glucans

β-glucans are long-chain, multidimensional polymers of glucose, in which particular particles of glucopyranose are linked with glycosidic bonds of β type, linearly, in (1→3) and/or (1→4) structure or in a branched way, i.e. with side chains of varied length, linked to the main core with glycosidic bonds of β-(1→6) type. They are structural components of plant cell walls (mostly cereals – oats and barley), yeast (*Saccharomyces cerevisiae, Saccharomyces fragilis, Candida tropicalis, Candida utilis* among others), as well as the so-called Chinese or Japanese fungi. Also beta glucans constituting the components of cell walls, or being the excretion of various bacteria (e.g. *Alcaligenes faecalis* var. *Myxogenes, Cellulomonas flavigena Bacillus* or *Micromonospora)* [4] are known. The presence of β-glucans have also been confirmed in the cell walls of some vegetables (carrot, radish, soybean) and fruit (bananas) [5].

β-glucans isolated from fungi seem to be the most advantageous, i.e. of greatest pro-health influence. β-glucans from cereals are quite well-known. Present interest in isolating β-glucans takes into account new sources of β-glucans, e.g. baker's yeast *Sacharomyces cerevisiae*, considered a better source than cereals or fungi in terms of economics.

The pro-health influence of beta glucans on the body depends on their physicochemical properties. The physicochemical properties of *β*-glucans differ depending on characteristics of their primary structure, including linkage type, degree of branching, molecular weight, and conformation (e.g. triple helix, single helix, and random coil structures) [3,4].

Native β-glucans, depending on their origin contain different bonds, show varied solubility degree and varied direction of pro-health influence. Beta glucans from:

- cereals – containing (1→3)-(1→4)-β bonds and constituting main soluble fractions, serve as dietary fibre, of a particularly important function aiming to lower cholesterol concentration and triacyloglycerols in blood,
- yeast - containing (1→3)-(1→6)-β bonds and constituting usually insoluble forms. They are known for their enhancing the immune system, by activating first of all macrofags. They also stimulate the skin cell response to combat free radicals and defend against the environmental pollution, significantly delaying aging process, and act anti-inflammatory.
- fungi – contain both (1→3)/(1→6)-β and (1→3)/(1→4)-β type bonds, from which 53-83% constitute insoluble fractions and 16-46% - soluble fractions. They are called heteroglucans showing universal immunostimulating and immunomodulating activity of antiviral, antibacterial and antiallergic character. They also have the ability to lower high blood cholesterol, inhibit excessive cholesterol synthesis and remove the excess of glucose from peripheral blood. Beta glucan activity as an anti-tumour factor concerns mostly (1→3)-(1→6)-β forms.

A lower level of branching and lower polymerisation degree are characterised by better solubility (Fig. 1). It is believed that insoluble β-glucans are those whose degree of polymerisation (DP) is higher than 100 [6]. Insoluble or slightly soluble beta glucans contain very long, multi-branched side chains in the particle (Fig. 2).

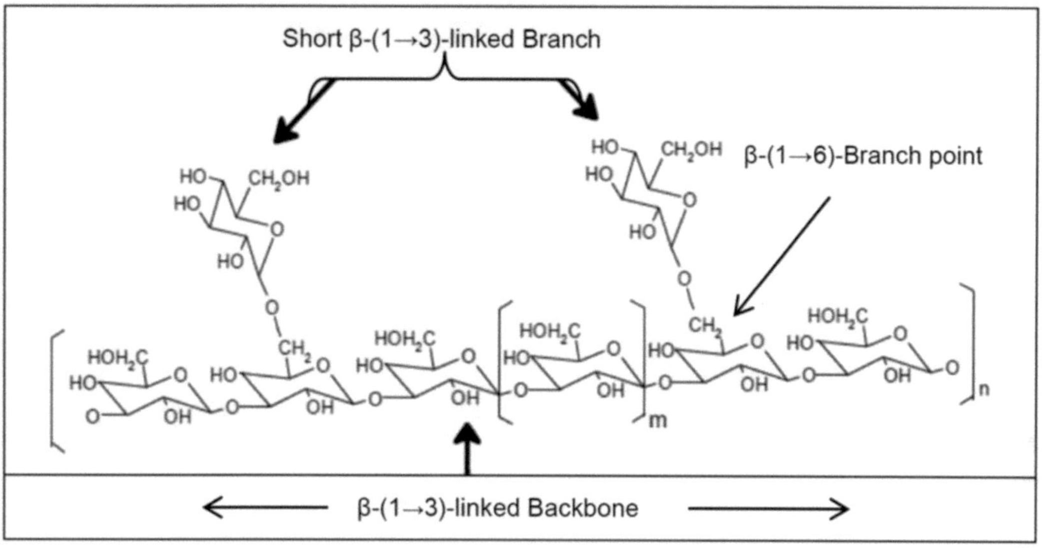

Figure 1. An example of the molecular structure of soluble yeast β-glucan.

Molecular weight of beta glucans obtained from various sources differs within a wide range of values from 0,2 x 10^1 kDa to 4 x 10^4 kDa. From technological point of view, beta glucans of high molecular weight (> 3 x 10^3 kDa) are characterised by high viscosity, and those of low molecular weight (about 9 kDa) constitute gels. Hydrolysed beta-glucans are soluble, but not very viscous and do not constitute gels.

Physicochemical properties of β-glucans might be modified through the use of various technologies during their isolation. Used chemical or enzymatic methods, leading to the hydrolysis of long-chain β-glucans, allow to lower the degree of depolymerisation and their particle mass in relation to native form, which simultaneously increases their solubility and lowers viscosity in liquids [7].

Among many methods leading to depolymerisation of long-chained and multi-branched β-glucans, it is essential to distinguish other chemical modifications, e.g. esterification [8], phosphorylation [9], sulphonation [10], chlorosulphonation [11], or carboxylmethylation [12]. This last method is considered to be one of the most effective methods transforming insoluble forms into soluble fractions [13]. All authors state, however, that introducing an additional functional group to β-glucan chain might lead to simultaneous growth of glucan particle size, which in turn leads to excessive increase in their viscosity in water solution, and therefore, shows different than expected physiological influence [14]. There is also research published showing that viscosity of β-gluccans depends to a large extent on the degree of purification during their isolation [15].

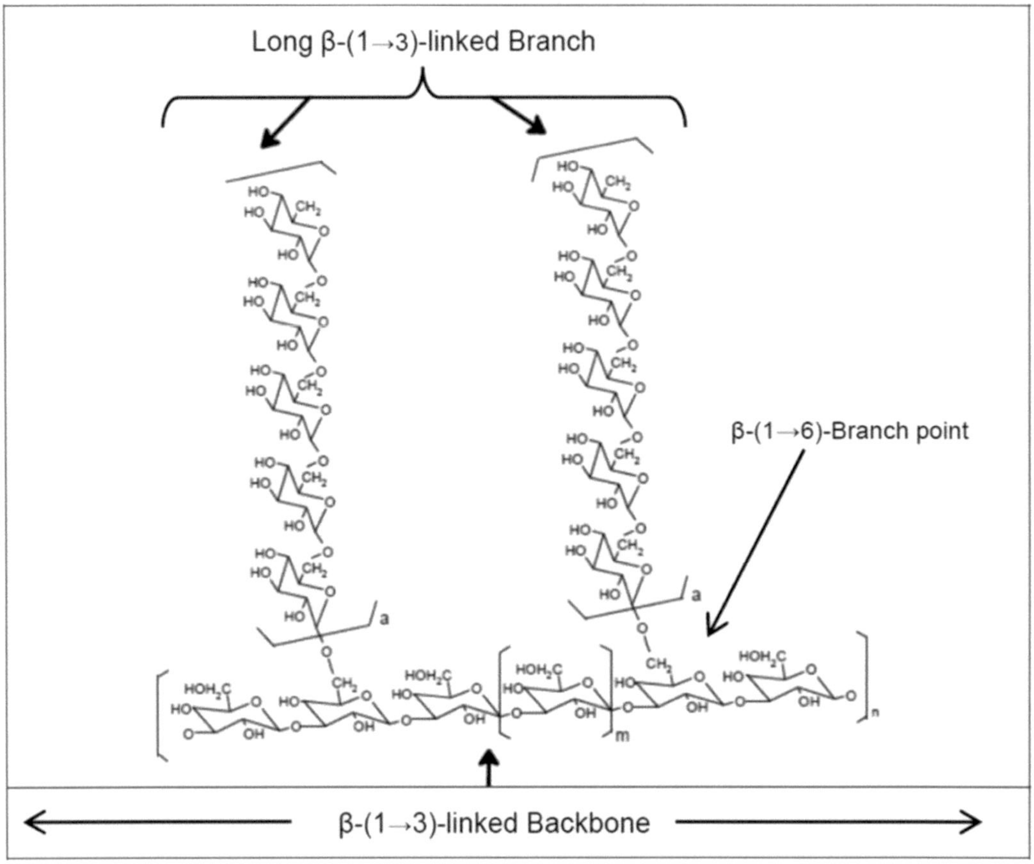

Figure 2. An example of the molecular structure of insoluble yeast β-glucan.

2.1. β-glucans isolated from cereals

Among cereals, the greatest amount of β-glucan in relations to dry mass can be found in barley grains (3-11%) and oat grains (3-7%). Small quantities of β-glucans are also found in rice (about 2%), wheat (about 1%) and sorghum (0.2-0.5%) [11]. In case of oat, β-glucans are present mostly in external layers of the grain, whilst in barley grain, these substances are spread evenly in the entire grain.

Unlike insoluble cellulose, whose glucose particles are linked linearly with β-D-(1→4) bonds, β-glucans contained in the endosperm of cereals grains are the mixture of β-D-glucose unbranched chains linked with β-(1→3) and β-(1→4) glycosidic bonds (Fig. 3) [16].

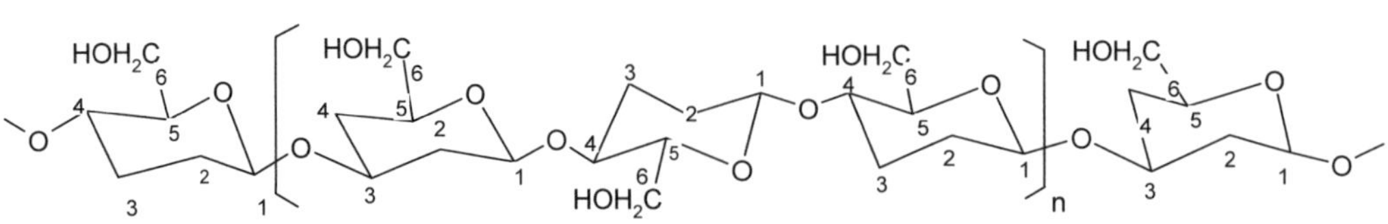

Figure 3. Primary molecular structure of (1-3)/(1-4)-β-glucan from barley grain.

Slightly different properties are characteristic of β-glucans isolated from sorghum, in which all three types of chains, i.e. both β-(1→3)-, β-(1→ 4)-, and β-(1→ 6) [17] have been found. In β-glucans isolated from most cereals β-(1→3) bonds constitute about 30%, whilst β-(1→4) bonds - about 70% of all bonds, with slight deviations characteristic of particular cereals [18].

β-glucans from oat are known as substances of pro-health influence comparable to β-glucans isolated from barley [19], particularly in the ability to lower glucose concentration in blood [20], total cholesterol and triacylglycerols in blood [21,22].

β-glucans extracted from cereals, which mainly contain β-(1,3-1,4)-d-glucan, have been demonstrated to reduce blood lipid levels, including cholesterol and triacylglycerols levels. The mechanisms by which β-glucans from cereals reduce blood lipid levels have been shown to include prevention of cholesterol reabsorption by adsorption, elimination of bile acid by adsorption, an increase in bile acid synthesis, and suppression of hepatic cholesterol biosynthesis by short-chain fatty acids produced by fermentation with intestinal bacteria [23,24].

2.2. β-glucans isolated from fungi

There are "medicinal" fungi, used in traditional medicine of the countries of the East [25], such as Chinese Reishi (*Ganoderma lucidum),* or Japanese Shiitake *(Lentinula edodes)* and Maitake (*Grifola frondosa*), arboreal fungi: Chaga (*Inonotus obliquus),* Turkey Tail (*Trametes versicolor),* Split Gill (*Schizophyllum commune),* Mulberry Yellow Polypore (*Phellinus linteus)* and cultivated, e.g. Hiratake (*Pleurotus ostreatus, Oyster mushroom*). The concentration of β-glucans in Basidiomycota fungi is relatively low and ranges from 0.21 to 0.53 g/100 g of dry mass [26].

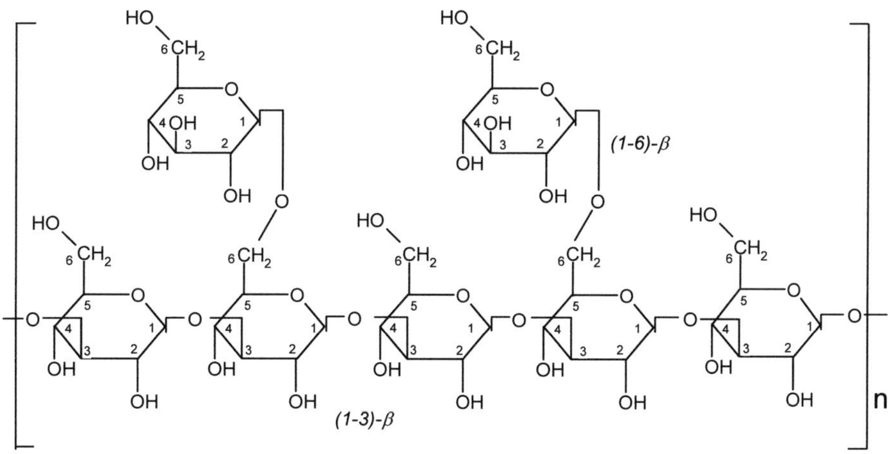

Figure 4. Primary molecular structure of lentinan from *Lentinus edodes.*

β-glucans isolated from fungi are heteroglucans containing both (1→3)/(1→4)-β and (1→3)/(1→6)-β bonds. They usually constitute the mixture of insoluble (about 53-83%

participation) and soluble (about 16-46%) fractions [40] of varied properties. They are mostly known as factors stimulating the immune system, having antiviral, antimicrobial and antiallergic properties [27,28]. They also have the ability to lower high blood pressure, slow down the excessive cholesterol synthesis and lower glucose concentration in blood [29], as well as show antioxidating properties [23]. They are also known as substances of anti-tumour properties [4]. β-glucans well-known in terms of structure and biological activity are identified in accordance with their names, e.g.: lentinan (Fig. 4) obtained from *Lentinus edodes*, schizophyllan (SPG) (Fig. 5A) from *Schizophyllum commune*, pleuran from *Pleurotus ostreatus or* pullulans (AP-FBG) (Fig. 5B) from *Aureobasidium pullulans*, scleroglucan (SGG) (Fig. 6) from *Sclerotium* rolfsii, grifolan (GRN) from *Grifola frondosa*, krestin (PSK - polysaccharide-K and PSP - polysaccharopeptide) from *Coriolus versicolor* [30-34].

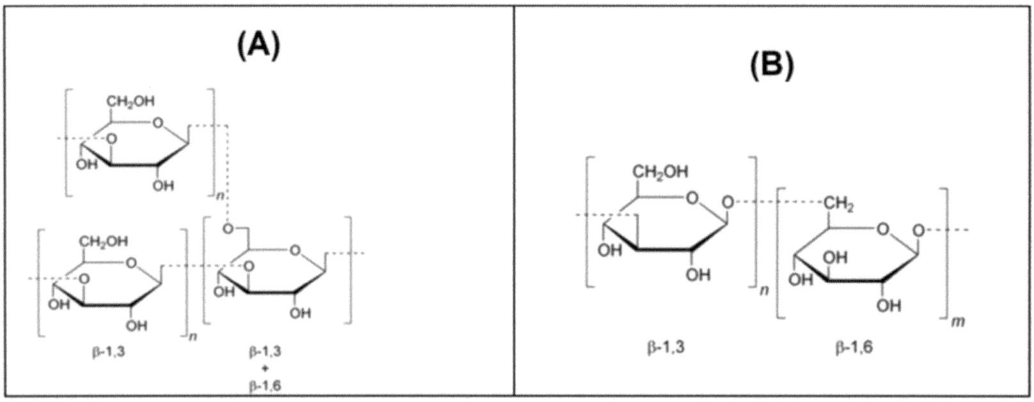

Figure 5. Primary molecular structure of Schizophyllan (A) from *Schizophyllum commune* and pleuran (B) from *Aureobasidium pullulans.*

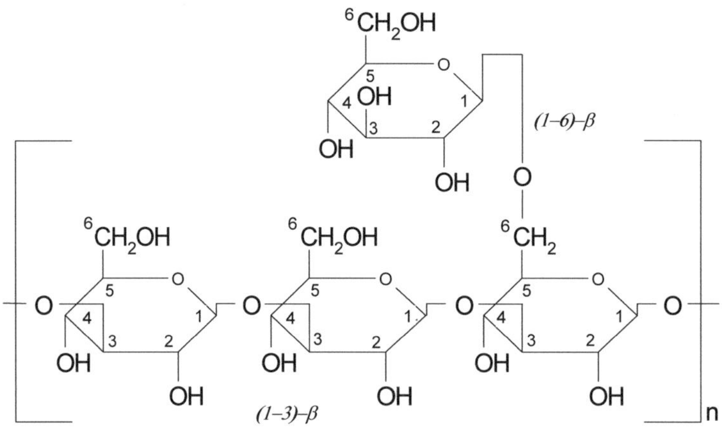

Figure 6. Primary molecular structure of scleroglucan from *Sclerotium rolfsii.*

Recently characterized structure of a novel water-soluble polysaccharide (ZPS - Zhuling polysaccharide) from the fruit bodies of medicinal mushroom *Polyporus umbellatus* and investigate its immunobiological function [35].

2.3. β-glucans isolated from bacteria

Polysaccharides of bacterial origin are known and widely used in food industry mostly as additives. They are often called bacterial egzopolisaccharides and constitute the ingredient of the cell wall, or can be excretions of various microorganisms, such as: *Cellulomonas flavigena* of KU strain [36], *Bacillus curdlanolyticus* and *Bacillus kobensis* [37], *Bacillus* and *Micromonospora* [38] *Agrobacterium* spp. ATCC31749 [39], *Bradyrhizobium, Rhizobium* spp. *Sarcina ventriculi* [40].

The ones mass produced and used are: xanthan, dextran, pullulan or gellan. β-glucans of bacterial origin have the structure similar to mannans, but glucose constitutes their basic unit building block. Mucilages called xanthans produced by *Xanthomonas campestris* bacteria pathogenic for plants are widely used. Beta glucans produced as a result of microbiological fermentation called curdlan (Fig. 7) and laminarin are known from technological point of view.

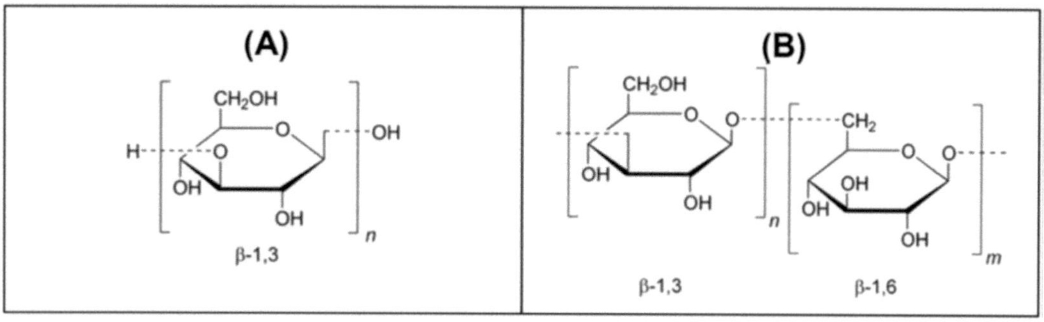

Figure 7. Primary molecular structure of (1-3)-β-glukan (A – curdlan; B - laminarin).

Dextran is a glucan synthesized from saccharose by *Leuconostoc mesenteroides* and *Streptococcus,* containing glucose particles connected most often with (1→6) bonds of α type [41].

Microorganisms used in food industry, mostly lactid acid bacteria (LAB) are a rich source of egzopolisaccharides [42].

2.4. β-glucans isolated from Saccharomyces cerevisiae

Yeast, both baker's and spent brewer's yeast, are characterised by high concentration of beta glucans, amounting on average to 7.7%, located in the cell wall. Cell wall (constituting 15-30% of dry mass of yeast cells), is a complex, multi-particle structure, consisting in 50-60% of β-glucans and in about 40% of mannoproteins. Natural β-glucans isolated from yeast are insoluble in water, and their insolubility is caused by chitin, a polisaccharid consisting of residues of N-acetyl-glucosamine, linked with (1→4)-β-glycosidic bonds (chitin amounts to about 1% of cell wall mass). Chitin complex–(1→3)-β-glucan (about 3-9% of cell wall mass), is located on the inside of cell wall (1→6)-β β-glucan branches, link particular components of cell wall with the use of mannoproteins and covalent bonds. Mannoproteins are located on the outside of yeast cell wall [43].

Sparse research on β-glucans isolated in the laboratory from cell walls of baker's yeast *Saccharomyces cerevisiae,* shows varied biological activity depending on the used technology of their isolation. They can strengthen the immune system, show antioxidant properties, and delay the process of cell aging [23,44].

Due to a high content of β-glucans in spent brewer's yeast *Saccharomyces cerevisiae,* remaining after alcohol fermentation in the process of beer production, it seems that they can be an effective and inexpensive material for obtaining β-glucan preparations.

Fig. 8 presents the diagram showing the use of spent brewer's yeast, which constitute troublesome waste for the brewing industry.

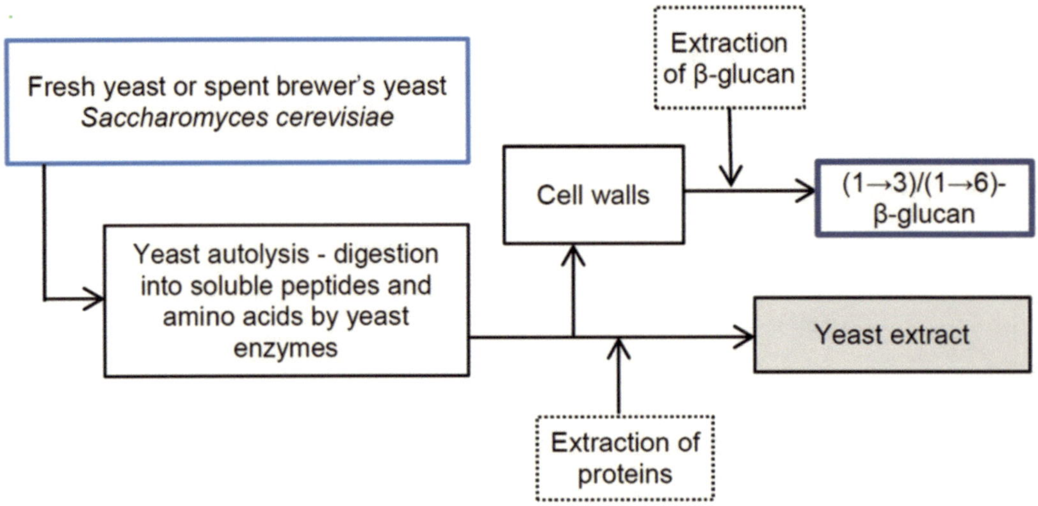

Figure 8. The possibilities of using spent brewer's yeast *Saccharomyces cerevisiae.*

Beta glucans might be obtained as a byproduct in the production of preparations enhancing flavour (yeast extracts), and the remains after fibre extraction constitute a good material for obtaining beta glucans.

So far no research has been conducted on pro-health β-glucans obtained from spent brewer's yeast *Saccharomyces cerevisiae,* which constitute a natural, often a troublesome byproduct of the brewing industry, waste product after alcohol fermentation in beer production. Sparse research on β-glucans obtained from this type of material is conducted on a laboratory scale and aims mostly to examine their technological properties, conditioning their usage as additional substances of thickening, gelling and/or water binding properties.

3. The purpose and scope of work

This work has aimed to assess pro-health activity of β-glucans isolated from a new, uninvestigated within this scope source, i.e. spent brewer's yeast *Saccharomyces cerevisiae.*

Functional properties, i.e. physico-chemical properties of dried spent brewer's yeast and β-glucans isolated from them have been characterized. In order to determine the influence of glucan preparations (soluble BG-CMG and native - insoluble BG-HP) and spent brewer's yeast on the lipid metabolism of the rat body, examined preparations have been added to atherogenic diet of animals (1% of cholesterol and 20% of fat) in such an amount so as to obtain the following levels:

a. for β-glucans: 10 and 100 mg/kg of body mass - the dose of 10 mg/kg body mass is the amount calculated for an adult weighing 70 kg - 700 mg per day, the dose 100 mg/kg body mass – 7 g per day,
b. Spent brewer's yeast were added in the amount 100 mg daily (0.5% of diet components, which is about 500 mg/kg body weight). This amount corresponded to the intake of beta-glucans from spent brewer's yeast in an amount of 10 mg/kg body weight.

The research has been conducted in relation to control group, which has not been given yeast preparation additive.

4. Research material and conditions of biological experiment

Material consisted of:

- dried, spent brewer's yeast *Saccharomyces cerevisiae* - from INTER YEAST company, constituted the research material (Content: Protein - 43.5%, fat - 4% Total Carbohydrates - 25%, squalene - 125 mg per 100 g of powder, beta-glucan - 1.9%),
- commercial, pure beta glucans isolated from spent brewer's yeast (from the yeast cell walls): insoluble BG-HP (Beta HP(1/3)-(1/6)-β-D-Glucane Powder),
- and soluble carboxymethylglucan BG-CMG (Beta CMG: 92% β-1,3/1,6-D-glucan concentration, 1.2% protein, <0.6% of mannans and <0.5% chitin), were provided by German company LEIBER GmbH - INTER YEAST.

4.1. Biological experiment and its progress

The experimental animals were growing male rats (Wistar) with an initial body weight of about 100 g. Prior to the start of the experiment, animals were given water and commercial, standard rat food LSM® ad libitum for 7 days to adapt them to the experimental conditions. Later the animals were randomly divided into 6 groups (7 rats in one group) in relation with diet composition:

a. Control - without β-glucans,
b. BG-CMG - with carboxymethylglucan:
    - $BG\text{-}CMG_{10}$ (10 mg/kg of body mass),
    - $BG\text{-}CMG_{100}$, (100 mg/kg of body mass),
c. BG-HP - with insoluble beta glucan:
    - $BG\text{-}HP_{10}$ (10 mg/kg of body mass),
    - $BG\text{-}HP_{100}$ (100 mg/kg of body mass),
d. and SBY – with dried spent brewer's yeast.

The average body mass of rats in each group was similar. Diets (semisynthetic, isocaloric) were prepared in accordance with the recommendations of the American Institute of Nutrition [45]. Mineral mixture AIN-93G-MX and vitamin mixture AIN-93G-MV were used. The composition of experimental diets is presented in Table 1.

The research was conducted on control group, which did not receive beta glucan additive. Diet intake and body weight growth of research animals were controlled during the research. Ethics Committee approved of the research. Energy derived from fat, protein and carbohydrates was 40.1; 15.8 and 44.1%, respectively.

Components	Diet					
	Control	BG-CMG10	BG-CMG100	BG-HP10	BG-HP100	SBY100
Wheat starch, g	49.0	49.0	49.0	49.0	49.0	48.5
Casein, g	20.0	20.0	20.0	20.0	20.0	20.0
Soya oil, g	20.0	20.0	20.0	20.0	20.0	20.0
α-cellulose, g	5.0	5.0	5.0	5.0	5.0	5.0
DL-methionine, g	0.3	0.3	0.3	0.3	0.3	0.3
Choline bitartrate, g	0.2	0.2	0.2	0.2	0.2	0.2
Mineral mix, g	3.5	3.5	3.5	3.5	3.5	3.5
Vitamin mix, g	1.0	1.0	1.0	1.0	1.0	1.0
Cholesterol[a/], g	1.0	1.0	1.0	1.0	1.0	1.0
Spent brewer's yeast, g	0	0	0	0	0	0,5
β-glucans from spent brewer's yeast, mg/kg of body mass/day[b/]:	0	10	100	10	100	0
Protein, g/100 g of diet (% of EV)	18.0 (15.8%)					18.1 (15.9)
Fat, g/100 g of diet (% of EV)	20.3 (40.1%)					20.3 (40.2)
Carbohydrates, g/100 g of diet (% of EV)	50.2 (44.1%)					49.9 (43.9)
Energy value (EV), kJ (kcal)	1904 (455,5)					1900.5 (454.7)

Table 1. Composition of 100 g control and model diet enriched with β-glucans.
[a/] Sample weight of prepared earlier diet were mixed with fresh cholesterol in the proportion 99:1, directly before being served to animals; [b/] β-glucans were weighed in the amounts adequate for each rat's body mass, then mixed with small diet portions (5 g) and given to each animal individually. After having eaten, the animals were served diet and water *ad libitum.*

During the whole experimental period (6 weeks) rats were housed in individual cages with 24 h access to water. The premises, in which the experimental rats were housed had a 12:12h light cycle with temperature of 21-22°C and humidity of 55-65%. The proper experiment lasted 6 weeks, after which blood from myocardium was collected. Animals were put to sleep with the peritoneal injection of Thiopental.

4.2. Research methods

4.2.1. Particle size and swelling ability

The size of particles was analysed with the method of laser difraction with the use of Mastersizer S analyser of Malvern Instruments Ltd., Malvern, Great Britain. Particle size distribution of examined preparations was measured using the wet process in oil emulsions and/or water solutions of concentration within the range of 0.01 – 0.05%.

4.2.2. Viscosity of water solutions

Rheometric measurements were conducted with the use of rheo-viscometer of Brookfield DV III+ using ULA spindle and DIN-82. Measurement device was coupled with RHEOCALC for Windows version 2.1. computer programme, from which dynamic viscovity values were read at varied shear velocity.

4.2.3. Antioxidant properties of preparations with in vitro method

Antioxidant properties of preparations were marked with spectrophotometric method with the use of synthetic radicals $ABTS^{\bullet +}$ [46]. Antioxidant activity of examined preparations was expressed as the ability of an examined preparation to de-activation of cation radicals $ABTS^{\bullet +}$ and as TEAC (Trolox Equivalent Antioxidant Capacity), i.e. μM of Trolox for 1g of preparation.

4.2.4. Lipid content

Total lipid content was marked with a modified method of Folch et al. [47].

Total cholesterol - methyl esters have been prepared, from which 0.5% of the solution has been made using toluene as solvent. 1μl was collected from prepared solutions, which was dosed with a μ-syringe on the Hewelett-Packard HP 6890 Series GC System Plus gas chromatographer with a flame ionization detector (FID) and capilary column with polar stationary phase of 30 m length. Stigmasterol produced by Sigma was used as a standard.

Lipid fractions - particular lipid fractions: HDL-cholesterol, and triacylglycerols (TG) in the plasma (mmol/L) were enzymatically measured with INTEGRA analyser. The concentrations of LDL cholesterol (mg/dL) were calculated as LDL cholesterol = total cholesterol – HDL cholesterol - (triacylglycerols/5). Cholesterol was converted from mg/dL to mmol/L by multiplying by 0.0259. VLDL-cholesterol was calculated as 1/5 TG [48]. In order to calculate the amount of cholesterol expressed in mg/dl for mmol/l, 0.0258 multiplier was used.

Atherogenic index - atherogenic index was calculated as the relation of assessed lipid fraction (HDL-Chol or LDL-Chol) to total cholesterol content (Total-Chol). This index allowed for defining the changes of these fraction participation in relation to total cholesterol content.

4.2.5. Statistical analysis

Data is presented as means ± standard deviation (SD). Obtained results were statistically analysed with STATGRAPHIC programme for Windows (v. 4.1.). The data was analysed using one-way analysis of variance (ANOVA). When a significant F ratio was found, Tukey's multiple-comparison tests were conducted. Differences were considered significant at $P<0.05$.

5. Results and discussion

5.1. Characteristics of physico-chemical properties of used preparations

Preparations of pure β-glucans and the preparation of dried spent brewer's yeast examined in this work have proven to be efficient in correcting blood lipid metabolism, which has been shown in biological experiment on rats, which were given atherogenic diet, containing 20% of fat and 1% of cholesterol, and at the same time preparations of beta glucans: soluble (BG-CMG) and insoluble (BG-HP) or dried, spent brewer's yeast (SBY).

These preparations differed in physico-chemical properties, i.e. particle size, solubility, the ability of water absorption and viscosity. These properties had a significant influence on the final effects obtained after their use in the experiment.

During the examination of distribution of particle size of powdered β-glucans in comparison with spent brewer's yeast preparations, it has been established that BG-HP preparation contained 60% of all particles of 59.4 μm in diameter and only about 5% of about 5 μm in diameter. The preparation of soluble β-glucan BG-CMG contained at least three clusters of particles of varied size, i.e. appropriately 0.2 μm, 3.5 μm and 90.2 μm, whereas the majority of particles (about 20% of all) had a diameter of 90.2 μm. Dried spent brewer's yeast were characterised by three groups of varied size, and their greatest share (over 40%) had the size of about 63.6 μm. Dried spent brewer's yeast particles were similar in size to particles of β-glucan BG-HP preparation.

Table 2 presents the percentage cumulated participation of particles in preparation content (e.g. d_5 means that 5% of particles has the size below the value shown in the table, d_{50} = 50% of particles has the size not exceeding the value presented in the table, etc.).

Particles of all examined preparations absorbed water during hydration. Preparation of native β-glucan BG-HP from brewer's yeast and dried spent brewer's yeast did not dissolve or dissolved only partially creating unstable water solutions with the tendency to create residue. Water solutions of β-glucan BG-CMG preparations were very viscid (65.2 mPas for

1% water solution and 574.9 mPas for 3% solution), whereas the preparations of β-glucan HP preparations and dried spent brewer's yeast, dissolved in water only partially, creating nonviscid or only slightly viscid solutions (0.4-1.4 mPas) - tab. 3.

Preparations	The size of particles in cumulated values (d) [μm]							$X_{śr.}$ [μm]
	d_5	d_{10}	d_{25}	d_{50}	d_{75}	d_{90}	d_{95}	
HP β-glucan	5.2	16.8	32.7	50.14	70.74	93.4	107.3	52.98
CM β-glucan	0.2	0.48	2.24	17.0	67.7	133.6	174.6	44.62
SBY	6.61	16.26	34.8	64.5	169.5	325	396.9	119.4

Table 2. The comparison of cumulated distribution of particle size of examined β-glucans and powdered spent brewer's yeast.

β-glucan particles isolated from spent brewer's yeast, in the initial phase of hydration increased their volume from 3 (soluble BG-CMG) to about 5 times (insoluble BG-HP). These glucans were characterised by the fact that in the final stage of hydration, these particles decreased. The increasing, and then decreasing sizes of particles in the initial stage of hydration, may constitute the proof of tearing hydrogen and covalency bindings of helix of pre-hydrated β-glucans.

Preparation	Viscosity for 10 RPM [mPas]		The level of adjustment reliance [%]	
	1%	3%	1%	3%
β-glucan BG-CMG	$65.2^a \pm 7.5$	$574.9^a \pm 36.3$	96.0 ± 2.1	94.4 ± 4.7
β-glucan BG-HP	$1.4^c \pm 0.2$	$1.9^c \pm 0.1$	90.0 ± 1.3	93.6 ± 0.9
SBY	$0.4^d \pm 0.04$	$1.5^d \pm 0.04$	84.6 ± 4.7	90.9 ± 1.6

Table 3. The characteristics of viscosity[a]/ of 1% and 3% water solutions of β-glucan preparations in comparison with 1% and 3% viscosity of water solutions of spent brewer's yeast.
[a]/ identical letter signs in columns equal the lack of a significant difference between compared mean values

Limited solubility in water of native β-glucan HP might be explained with the presence in the structure of long, side chains with bindings β-(1→6), which can cause high crystality and insolubility of this β-glucan [6].

Weak hydration of complex structure of helix of high molecular weight β-glucans is the reason for their mutual intermolecular interactions between β-(1→3)-D and β-(1→6)-D-glucan bindings, of strenght exceeding the interactions between bindings of β-glucan and water particle bindings or another solvent. Lowering of degree of polymerisation of beta glucans with β-(1→3)/(1→6)-D-glucan bindings to DP below 20, results in the weakening of intermolecular interactions, therefore, creating new bindings between β-glucan particles and solvent, causing its dissolution [2,4].

The apparent improvement of β-glucan solubility in water solutions, without polymer degradation, can be achieved by activities stabilizing their scattering in water environment. [49]. It is possible to achieve stable scattering of β-glucans in water solutions, e.g. through microwave heating, with temperature range 100-121°C and increased pressure within 4-10 min. Quite advantageous effects in the modification of physico-chemical properties of β-glucans are also obtained while using ultrasounds, as the method does not change the chemical structure of polymer's particle size, resulting only in the decrease in the particle size, through breaking of the most sensitive chemical bindings. This method is used to obtain the so-called micronized β-glucan preparations. The process of micronization improves the distribution and stability of slightly soluble powders in water environment. The method also leads to permanent reduction of solution viscosity. According to the definition in the Polish Pharmacopoeia, micronized powders should contain particles of average diameter below 10 μm, at admissible 20% particle content of up to 50 μm diameter.

CMG β-glucan preparation of modified chemical properties is the example of β-glucan examined in this work. HP native beta-glucan obtained from spent brewer's yeast underwent the process of carboxymethylation, and in turn led to obtaining BG-CMG β-glucan preparation of modified viscosity, dozen times higher than the viscosity of HP native β-glucan (tab. 3).

Carboxymethylated β-glucan CMG strongly absorbed water creating solutions of very high viscosity and stability, but also not showing properties of sedimentation. Native HP β-glucan did not dissolve in water, created nonviscous solutions, and moreover, strongly sedimented. Higher viscosity of carboxymethylated CMG β-glucan than native HP β-glucan, despite comparable particle size, might be explained by the fact that carboxymethylated CMG β-glucan might be characterised by higher particle mass resulting from additional methyl groups contained in their structure, which in turn enabled ist stronger hydration and viscosity increase.

Many biological experiments showed that the change of physicochemical parameters of β-glucans as a result of chemical or enzymatic modification might lead to the change of their pro-health influence, changes in sensoric quality [50, 51], therefore, it is extremely important to conduct research in case of each newly obtained preparation.

During the evaluation of bioactive substance properties very often the evaluation of antioxidant properties is conducted, which are also checked for native β-glucan HP and β-glucan BG-CMG modified through carboxymethylation. The preparations of these β-glucans were characterised by varied antioxidant activity expressed as TEAC (the number of Trolox milimols for each 1 g of preparation) - Fig. 9.

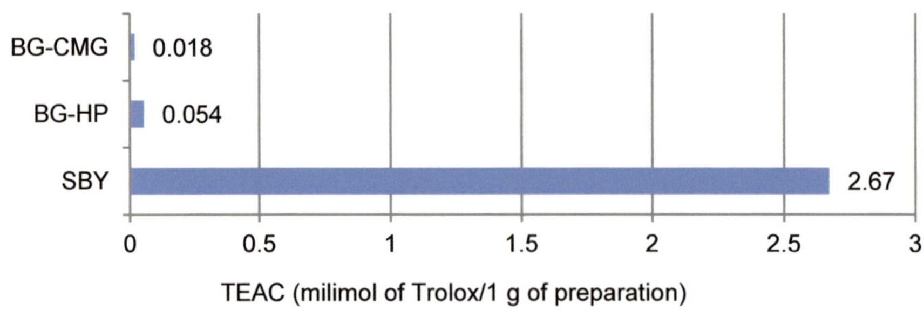

Figure 9. The antioxidant activity of β-glucan preparations in comparison with spent brewer's yeast.

The preparation of spent brewer's yeast showed over 50-100 times higher antioxidant activity than β-glucan BG-HP isolated from them and β-glucan BG-CMG subject to chemical modification. Such high antioxidant activity of spent dried yeast preparation might result from squalene contained in the preparation, whose presence was confirmed in parallel research at the rate of 125 mg per 100 g of powder.

5.2. Blood lipid metabolism

In numerous research conducted on animals and in clinical research on people, hypocholesterolemic influence of β-glucans of cereal origin containing (1→3)/(1→4)-β bindings has been proven. This influence has been confirmed in case of β-glucans isolated from fungi, containing (1→3)/(1→6)-β bindings, however, it has been weaker in comparison with cereal β-glucans. However, there is no literature data on the influence of β-glucans from spent brewer's yeast on the lipid metabolism of both experimental animals and people [52, 53].

During biological experiment, animals given diets supplemented with β-glucans HP and CMG and dried spent brewer's yeast grew at a comparable pace. Body mass of animals after the experiment ranged from 390.8 to 412.3 g, and daily growth ranged from 6.5 to 7.2 g. Slight differences between particular groups were not statistically significant. In the groups of animals receiving β-glucans or spent brewer's yeast, feed efficiency ratio (FER) did not differ significantly and ranged from 0.36 to 0.38 (tab. 4).

Group – experimental factor		Diet intake [g/day]	Feed efficiency ratio FER[4/]
CONTROL		$18.1^{a} \pm 0.4$	$0.38^{a} \pm 0.03$
β-glucans	BG-CMG10	$18.0^{a} \pm 04$	$0.38^{a} \pm 0.03$
	BG-CMG100	$17.7^{a} \pm 0.5$	$0.36^{a} \pm 0.03$
	BG-HP10	$17.7^{a} \pm 0.7$	$0.37^{a} \pm 0.04$
	BG-HP100	$17.9^{a} \pm 0.4$	$0.38^{a} \pm 0.02$
SBY – spent brewer's yeast		$17.9^{a} \pm 0.9$	$0.38^{a} \pm 0.03$
	SEM [2/] (*p*[3/])	0.067 (0.710)	0.004 (0.874)

Table 4. The comparison of intake and nutritious efficiency of diets supplemented with β-glucan preparations and spent brewer's yeast[1/] (n=63).
[1/] mean values ± standard deviation for n = 7 or 8, [2/] *SEM* – standard error mean; [3/] ANOVA, $p < 0.05$, [4/] Feed efficiency ratio: body mass growth (g/day) x diet intake^{-1} (g/day)$^{-1}$, identical letter signs in columns equal the lack of a significant difference between compared mean values

Table 5 and Fig. 10-11 show the results determing the influence of β-glucans and dried spent brewer's yeast on total cholesterol concentrationm HDL and LDL fraction cholesterol and triacylglycerols in rat blood plasma.

Total cholesterol concentration in the blood of rats in control group, given a model atherogenic diet (1% cholesterol, 20% fat) amounted to 3.79 mmol/l and was significantly higher than in all experimental groups. A significantly higher (p=0.043) concentration of LDL fractions (1.8 mmol/l) was also observed in the control group. Total cholesterol concentration in the blood of rats given β-glucans preparations from spent brewer's yeast in the daily amount equalling 100 mg/kg of bady mass or preparation of spent brewer's yeast ranged from 2.82 to 2.97 mmol/l.The differences between these three groups were, however, insignificant statistically. The concentration of LDL-cholesterol fraction ranged in these groups respectively from 1.09 to 1.11 mmol/l (tab. 5).

Group – experimental factor		Total cholesterol [mmol/l]	Cholesterol fractions		
			HDL [mmol/l]	LDL [mmol/l]	VLDL [mmol/l]
	Control	3.79^{a} ± 0.13	1.58^{a} ± 0.15	1.80^{a} ± 0.12	0.41^{a} ± 0.03
β-glucans	BG-CMG$_{10}$	3.23^{bc} ± 0.23	1.52^{ab} ± 0.14	1.35^{bc} ± 0.14	0.26^{bc} ± 0.04
	BG-CMG$_{100}$	2.95^{bc} ± 0.17	1.51^{ab} ± 0.12	1.11^{de} ± 0.15	0.33^{bc} ± 0.03
	BG-HP$_{10}$	3.20^{b} ± 0.38	1.56^{ab} ± 0.15	1.31^{bc} ± 0.23	0.31^{bc} ± 0.05
	BG-HP$_{100}$	2.82^{bc} ± 0.38	1.38^{ab} ± 0.19	1.10^{e} ± 0.19	0.30^{ab} ± 0.16
SBY		2.97^{bc} ± 0.36	1.39^{b} ± 0.13	1.29^{bce} ± 0.26	0.30^{bc} ± 0.04
SEM		*p = 0.0065*	*p = 0.415*	*p=0.043*	*p=0.0295*

Table 5. Selected lipid parameters of peripheral blood in experimental animals given atherogenic diets, supplemented with β-glucan preparations and spent brewer's yeast preparation[1/] (n=63).
[1/] mean values ± standard deviation for n = 7 or 8; [2/] SEM – standard error mean; [3/] ANOVA, $p < 0.05$; identical letter signs in columns equal the lack of significant difference between compared mean values

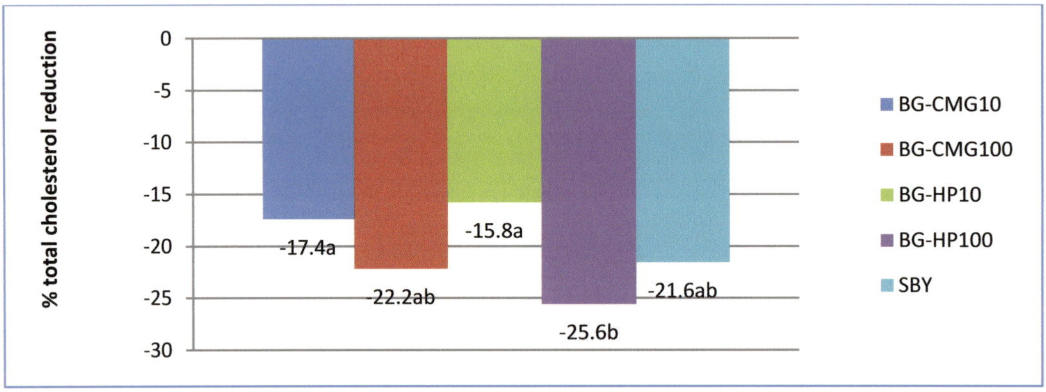

Figure 10. The degree of total cholesterol reduction in peripheral blood of experimental animals on atherogenic diets caused by diet supplementation with β-glucan preparations and spent brewer's yeast (*/ identical letters indicate no significant difference).

It was concluded that diet supplementation with spent brewer's yeast preparation, contributed to achieving lower concentration of total cholesterol of 21.6%. In groups of animals given diets containing β-glucans in a daily dosage of 10 and 100 mg/kg of body mass, the concentration of total cholesterol in blood was lower than in control group of

22.2% (in the group with β-glucan BG-CMG_{100}) and of 25.6% (in the group with β-glucan BG-HP_{100}) – Fig. 10. In these groups, LDL-cholesterol fraction was respectively lower of 38.3 to 39.1% in comparison with control group (Fig. 11).

The type of β-glucans from spent brewer's yeast (BG-CMG and BG-HP) did not influence significantly the level of total cholesterol in blood ($p = 0.638$), whereas their dosage ($p = 0.002$) had a significant influence. In rats from control group on a model athrogenic diet (1% cholesterol, 20% fat), cholesterol of HDL fraction amounted to 41.7% of total cholesterol, and LDL fraction cholesterol – 47.5%. The use of examined preparations in diet supplementation caused changes in the configuration of these fractions leading to lowering the LDL fraction participation and increasing percentage participation of HDL fraction cholesterol. Changes of these fractions in total cholesterol (LDL-cholesterol fraction below 40% of total cholesterol), were particularly visible in groups of rats given CMG and HP β-glucan preparations from spent brewer's yeast in the amount equalling 100 mg/kg of body mass daily.

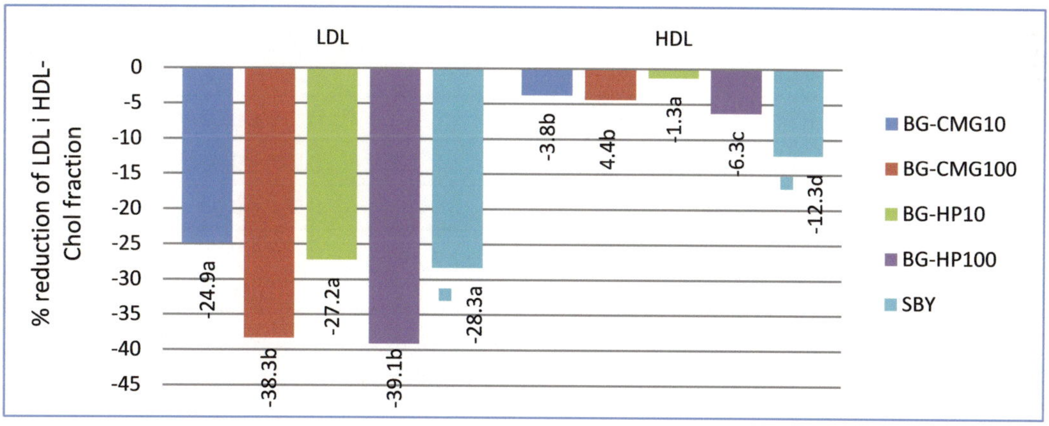

Figure 11. Reduction ratio of LDL and HDL-cholesterol fractions and triacylglycerols in peripheral blood of experimental animals on atherogenic diets caused by diet supplementation with β-glucan preparations and dried spent brewer's yeast (*/ identical letters indicate no significant difference).

Table 6 presents the ratios of atherogenic factors of examined preparations. The ratio of HDL fraction to Chol-C and HDL to LDL fractions, after the experiment completion was in each case significantly higher in comparison with control group, which suggests that each of the examined preparations, regardless of the type and dosage, significantly improves the lipid metabolism of animals given atherogenic diet.

In groups with beta glucan participation, the concentration of triacylglycerols ranged from 0.67 to 0.76 mmol/l plasma, i.e. was lower in the control group from 14.8 to 25.6% (tab. 7, Fig. 10).

Dried spent brewer's yeast given to animals in a daily dosage of 100 mg/kg of body mass contributed to lower the concentration of TG in blood in relation to control group of 27.2% ($p = 0,008$) – tab. 7, Fig. 12.

Group – experimental factor		Atherogenic factors	
		HDL/Chol-C	HDL/LDL
CONTROL		$0.42^{a} \pm 0.03$	$0.88^{a} \pm 0.12$
β-glucans	BG-CMG10	$0.49^{bc} \pm 0.03$	1.16 ± 0.15^{b}
	BG-CMG100	$0.52^{cd} \pm 0.04$	$1.39^{c} \pm 0.29$
	BG-HP10	$0.49^{bc} \pm 0.02$	$1.23^{bc} \pm 0.12$
	BG-HP100	$0.52^{d} \pm 0.03$	$1.36^{c} \pm 0.15$
SBY		$0.47^{b} \pm 0.03$	$1.09^{b} \pm 0.15$
SEM[2/] (p[3/])		*0.006 (0.0001)*	*0.035 (0.0001)*

Table 6. The comparison of atherogenic factors characteristic of blood of experimental animals given atherogenic diets with β-glucan additive and spent brewer's yeast[1/].
[1/] mean values ± standard deviation for n = 7 or 8; [2/] *SEM* – standard error mean; [3/] ANOVA, $p < 0.05$; identical letter signs in columns equal the lack of significant difference between compared mean values

Group – experimental factor		TG – triacylglycerols [mmol/l]
CONTROL		$0.90^{a} \pm 0.07$
β-glucans	β-glucan BG-CMG10	$0.72^{b} \pm 0.06$
	β-glucan BG-CMG100	$0.67^{b} \pm 0.04$
	β-glucan BG-HP10	$0.74^{b} \pm 0.02$
	β-glucan BG-HP100	$0.76^{b} \pm 0.04$
SBY – spent brewer's yeast		$0.66^{b} \pm 0.09$
SEM[2] (p[3])		*0.019 (0.008)*

Table 7. Selected lipid parameters of peripheral blood of test animals on atherogenic diets, supplemented with β-glucans and the preparation of dried brewer's yeast [1/].
[1/] mean values ± standard deviation for n = 7 or 8; [2/] *SEM* – standard error mean; [3/] ANOVA, $p < 0.05$; identical letter signs in columns equal the lack of a significant difference between compared mean values

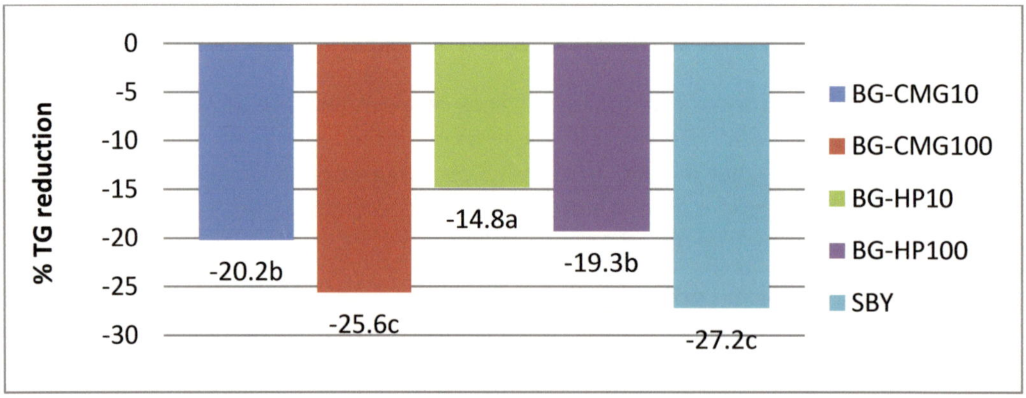

Figure 12. The percentage of lowered (with regard to the control group) the concentration of triacylglycerols (TG) in blood plasma in rats on atherogenic diets supplemented with β-glucans and dried spent brewer's yeast (*/ identical letters indicate no significant difference).

Two-factor analysis showed the lack of significant influence of the type of β-glucan (soluble and insoluble) ($p=0.091$). Also the dosage of these beta glucans did not influence the reduction ratio of TG in rat blood ($p=0.786$).

Table 8 compiles the total content of lipids and cholesterol in liver of rats on atherogenic diets supplemented with β-glucans and dried spent brewer's yeast. The content of lipids was presented both in the equivalent of the so-called wet tissue and dry mass, whereas cholesterol content was presented in the equivalent of wet tissue and in reference to total lipid content.

Group – experimental factor		Lipids		Total cholesterol	
		g/100 g of wet tissue	g/100 g s.m. of the liver	mg/1 g of wet tissue	mg/g of lipids
Control		$20.9^{a} \pm 2.8$	$47.3^{bc} \pm 1.3$	$82.5^{a} \pm 7.5$	$432.1^{ab} \pm 23.7$
β-glucans	BG-CMG10	$19.5^{a} \pm 3.3$	$42.0^{ab} \pm 2.7$	$69.9^{b} \pm 6.0$	$352.1^{c} \pm 42.6$
	BG-CMG100	$18.6^{a} \pm 3.5$	$39.6^{a} \pm 4.1$	$67.5^{bc} \pm 6.5$	$340.9^{c} \pm 26.4$
	BG-HP10	$18.4^{a} \pm 1.9$	$42.5^{ab} \pm 3.9$	$66.0^{bc} \pm 1.1$	$361.4^{c} \pm 28.1$
	BG-HP100	$18.7^{a} \pm 34$	$39.1^{a} \pm 3.7$	$65.\ 1^{bc} \pm 5.4$	$348.3^{c} \pm 38.8$
SBY		$19.1^{a} \pm 2.7$	$43.4^{ab} \pm 4.4$	$65.1^{bc} \pm 5.0$	$369.1^{bc} \pm 30.1$
SEM[2/] (p[3])		*0.110 (0.62)*	*0.513 (0.007)*	*14.4 (0.05)*	*8.16 (0.001)*

Table 8. The content of lipids and cholesterol in the liver of rats on atherogenic diets supplemented with β-glucans and dried spent brewer's yeast.
[1/] mean values ± standard deviation for $n = 5$ or 6; [2/] *SEM* – standard error mean; [3/] ANOVA, $p < 0.05$, identical letter signs in columns equal the lack of a significant difference between compared mean values

Total lipid content in fresh liver mass of rats did not differ significantly ($p=0.110$) in all groups and ranged from 18.4 to 20.9 g/100 g of wet tissue. Statistical analysis showed that the type of tested β-glucans ($p=0.287$) did not influence the concentration of lipids in the liver, whereas significantly better effects were observed when a higher dosage ($p=0.003$) was used.

In comparison with cholesterol level, it has been stated that neither the type ($p=0,444$) nor the amount of β-glucans ($p=0.720$) in the diet, significantly influence the cholesterol concentration in the liver.

Table 9 presents the percentage participation of saturated fatty acids (SFA), monounsaturated fatty acids (MUFA) and polyunsaturated fatty acids (PUFA) in total lipid pool in livers. The concentration of these groups of fatty acids was not influenced by the used β-glucans, but by their dosage ($p=0.018$).

The type of β-glucan from spent brewer's yeast did not significantly influence the ratio of blood lipid parameters metabolism in rats on atherogenic diet containing 1% of cholesterol. The concentration of HDL-cholesterol fraction and triacylglycerols in rat blood in this case depended neither on the type of β-glucan nor its dosage.

Literature data shows that hypolipemic activity of cereal β-glucans depends on the particle size and therefore, particle mass [54]. Using beta glucans of higher viscosity and higher particle mass in diet supplementation gives a better hypocholesterolemic effect [55]. Particle mass is a significant factor influencing hypocholesterolemic effect of β-glucans, but also it is essential to pay attention to the method of its designation [56]. Due to the variety of methods used by different researchers, it is difficult to compare experiment results presented by various authors. Hypocholesterolemic effect in people, resulting from cereal β-glucan intake also depends on the dosage, diet supplementation period and even the age of tested people. β-glucan intake in the dosage of 3 g daily for 4 weeks, reduced the cholesterol concentration in the blood of children and teenagers with mild hypercholesterolemia of about 6-7% [57]. After 40 days of consuming diet containing from 1 to 5% of β-glucan from barley, total cholesterol concentration was reduced of 39%, LDL cholesterol fraction of 61% and triacylglycerols of 21%.

Group – experimental factor		% fatty acids in total pool of lipids		
		Saturated SFA	Monounsaturated MUFA	Polyunsaturated PUFA
Control		$20.8^{a} \pm 2.9$	$26.7^{a} \pm 2.2$	$48.6^{ab} \pm 3.7$
β-glucans	BG-CMG10	$19.1^{abc} \pm 1.9$	$26.7^{a} \pm 0.6$	$44.8^{bc} \pm 2.4$
	BG-CMG100	$15.4^{c} \pm 1.0$	$31.7^{b} \pm 1.4$	$51.4^{a} \pm 0.7$
	BG-HP10	$19.2^{ab} \pm 4.2$	$28.7^{ab} \pm 4.0$	$44.6^{c} \pm 4.1$
	BG-HP100	$15.9^{bc} \pm 0.6$	$29.6^{ab} \pm 2.5$	$45.1^{bc} \pm 0.1$
SBY		$15.9^{bc} \pm 0.4$	$27.0^{a} \pm 1.2$	$50.5^{a} \pm 0.7$
SEM[2/] (*p*[3/])		*0.578 (0.023)*	*0.856 (0.0001)*	*0.841 (0.0001)*

Table 9. The percentage participation of fatty acids in total lipid pool of livers in experimental rats given β-glucan preparations and spent brewer's yeast.
[1/] mean values ± standard deviation for n = 5 or 6; [2/] *SEM* – standard error mean; [3/] ANOVA, $p < 0.05$; identical letter signs in columns equal the lack of a significant difference between compared mean values

Significant results were obtained also as a result of 5% supplementation of rats' diet with β-glucan from oyster mushroom (*Ostreatus Pleurotus*). Such a level in the low- and high-cholesterol diet lowered the concentration of cholesterol, including LDL and VLDL cholesterol fractions, in both cases of about 30% in blood plasma and of about 50% in the liver, which was simultaneously connected with lowering of HMG - CoA reductase activity [58].

This work has not confirmed significant differencies between hypocholesterolemic effect of carboxymethylated β-glucan (soluble, of higher particle mass) and native β-glucan (insoluble).

The influence of β-glucans on lipid metabolism depends to a large extent on the size of their particles. The carboxymethylated β-glucan isolated in the laboratory from baker's yeast *Saccharomyces cerevisiae,* had a very low hipocholesterolemic activity despite its good solubility and high viiscosity. It has been explained by authors by the fact that apart from the process of carboxymethylation, β-glucan underwent additional depolymerisation of particles through the use of ultrasounds. It led to a significant lowering of its particle mass, and therefore, the direction of its pro-health influence was changed.

In the research on humans using cereal β-glucans in the diet, an atherogenic factor was expressed as the ratio of HDL cholesterol to LDL cholesterol, in almost every case was increased in comparison with control group. A similar effect was obtained in the research described in this work. Diet supplementation with β-glucan isolated from spent brewer's yeast and preparation of dried yeast influenced the value of HDL/Chol-total ratio and HDL/LDL ratio. In each case of diet supplementation, these ratios were significantly more advantageous than in control group, which used only atherogenic diet [59].

Dried spent brewer's yeast given to animals in the diet in the amount of 0.5% diet, were as efficient as β-glucan preparations prepared from them and helped to lower the concentration in blood of: total cholesterol of 21.6%, LDL fraction – of 28.2% and triacylogliceroles of 27.2% in relation to control group.

Available literature data concerning the influence of diet supplementation with yeast preparations as the source of dietary fibre concerns in most cases other types or species of yeast. In the research on obese men with hypercholesterolemia have shown that intake of 15 g of fibre from spent brewer's yeast (containing β-glucan) advantageously lowered the concentration of total cholesterol in blood, increasing the concentration of HDL fraction cholesterol. Simultaneously, the changes in the concentration of triacylogliceroles in blood were not observed. Authors, however, did not give the exact consitution of yeast fibre, which made it difficult to compare these results with the results obtained in this work [60].

Lowering of the concentration of total cholesterol in blood of experimental animals, as a result of diet supplementation with yeast, might be the result of not only β-glucan contained in them, but also the presence of squalens [61]. The ability of correcting blood lipid metabolism as a result of diet supplementation with yeast might result from the prebiotic properties of both the whole dried yeast cells and beta glucans contained in them, thanks to which the composition of natural bacterial flora can be additionally corrected [62].

As the research results show, the degree of liver fatness was significantly influenced by the dosage of beta glucans from spent brewer's yeast, whereas the solubility did not matter statistically. Both examined β-glucan preparations were given in daily dosage of 100 mg/kg of body mass, efficiently protected the liver against excessive fat layering.

The type of β-glucans from spent brewer's yeast and their amount used in the diet did not, however, influence the cholesterol concentration in the livers. In comparison with the control group, the participation of cholesterol in liver lipids was in each case significantly lower. Two-factor analysis of variance showed that the higher dosage of β-glucans in the diet, i.e. 100 mg/kg of body mass daily, contributed to higher concentration of polyunsaturated fatty acids (PUFA) in livers and simultaneously lower concentration of saturated fatty acids (SFA). The dosage of β-glucans did not significanlty influence the concentration of monounsaturated fatty acids (MUFA). The concentration of all these groups of fatty acids was not influenced by the type of used β-glucans. Dried spent brewer's yeast, like β-glucans, also contributed to obtaining lower concentration of cholesterol in calculation for the wet tissue of the liver.

Beta glucans, regardless of origin, serve as dietary fibre in the body of mammals, therefore, their hipocholesterolemic effect might be associated with the mechanism recognised for dietary fibre. The influence of soluble fractions of dietary fibre on the cholesterol concentration in the body is known, by binding bile acids in the intestine and consequently increases the amount of bile acids excreted in the feces. It results in decreasing the pool of bile salt able to take part in the synthesis of cholesterol in liver and disregulation of micellas in intestines, which hampers lipid absorption. Cholesterol is used in the synthesis of bile acids instead of lipoproteid synthesis, therefore, speeding its circulation, and its concentration in plasma lowers [63,64].

Hipocholesterolemic effect of tested β-glucans might be also compared with the activity of known prebiotic (inulin) and oat fibre. Inulin while undergoing fermentation in large intestine influences the proportions of produced SCFA [65], decreasing the amount of produced octan, and increasing the level of propionic and butyric acid. It is especially advantageous, as octan acts as a simulator and propionian as inhibitor of cholesterol synthesis [66]. Research *in vitro* showed that propionic acid hampers cholesterol and fatty acid synthesis in the liver. It seems that the combination of increased excretion of bile acid with faeces and slight lowering of cholesterol synthesis in liver aims to lower total cholesterol concentration and LDL fraction in blood [67].

Supplementation of rat diets with β-glucan preparations from spent brewer's yeast examined in this work and the preparation of dried brewer's yeast contributes to adventegous lowering of cholesterol concentration in blood, at simultaneous achieving a more adventegous in relations to control group content of bowel microflora, connected particularly with increased numer of *Bifidobacterium* bacteria of lactid acid, which was shown in parallelly conducted research.

It is quite difficult to explain the estimated mechanism of lowering cholesterol concentration under the influence of prebiotics. However, increased excretion of cholesterol with faeces through hampering the creation of easily digested fatty micellas has been suggested. In rats, increased excretion of cholesterol in faeces has been confirmed, and similar research presents this mechanism also in people. It is possible that some bacteria of lactid acid can assimilate cholesterol directly. There is proof that fructooligosaccharides (FOS) lower the synthesis of triacylglycerols in liver, however, so far the mechanism has not been identified.

Similar significance to probiotics is also attributed to prebiotics. Prebiotics arouse even greater interest due to practical means – they are characterised by greater durability than probiotics, their activity is not conditioned by micorbe viability after intake and they might be added to many food products as one of the ingredients. There is little research available concerning the research on people, therefore, most conclusions have been drawn based on the research on animals. In rats, for example, after a 5-week inulin administration a significant lowering of triacyloglicerole concentration was observed. In people, however, oligofructose administration for 4 weeks did not lead to lowering triacyloglicerole and cholesterol [68]. Especially strong influence of prebiotics on lowering VLDL fraction is suggested [69].

6. Conclusions

No significant differences have been observed in hypocholesterolemic effect of soluble β-glucan – (CMG) and insoluble native β-glucan (HP). The results showed that after hydration, carboxymethylated β-glucan CMG was characterised by higher viscosity and mean particle size amounting to about 90 μm, whereas particles of insoluble HP β-glucan, established nonviscous solutions of particle size amounting to about 50 μm and about 320 μm. Examined β-glucans showed an effective hypocholesterolemic effect. It has been proven that they influenced lipid metabolism advantageously, especially in case of LDL fraction cholesterol and triacylglycerols (TG). An advantageous HDL/Chol-total factor and HDL/LDL factor has also been confirmed. Dried spent brewer's yeast were given to animals in a daily dosage of 100 mg/kg of body mass were as efficient as β-glucans isolated from them and they lowered the concentration in blood of: total cholesterol of 21.6%, LDL fraction – of 28.2% and triacylglycerols of 27.2% in relation to control group. The research also proves that advantageous influence of yeast on lipid metabolism and their level in blood might be linked with prebiotic properties of yeast on lipid metabolism, as in the research simultaneously conducted by the Author, the advantageous composition of intestine microflora was observed (a higher number of lactid acid bacteria of *Bifidobacterium* type was obtained).

High nucleic acid content in yeast (supplying from 12% to 25% of total nitrogen content) [70] limits their use as a traditional ingredient in human nutrition. It has been stated that the excess of nucleic acid in the diet of people and most monogastric animals is toxic and results in excessive accumulation of uric acid in organism, leading to arthritis. Therefore, it is recommended to consume their little portions as diet supplement supplying mainly vitamins from B group.

Numerous research on fish proved that diet supplementation with yeast to a particular level (in the amount providing no more than 50% of proteins in the diet), does not show disadvantageous health effects, such as abnormal growth, improper nitrogen balance or liver diseases [71]. However, only lower diet intake was observed when spent brewer's yeast constituted more than 25% of the diet [70]

It seems that diet supplementation with dried spent brewer's yeast *S.cerevisiae* in the amount of 0.5% of the diet contributed significantly to correcting possible disorders in lipid metabolism of rats on an atherogenic diet – it enhances lipid changes in organism, enhancing their parameters.

During the research on hypocholesterolemic activity of 81 different yeast strains, showed hypocholesterolemic activity of spent brewer's yeast of male Wistar rats with their

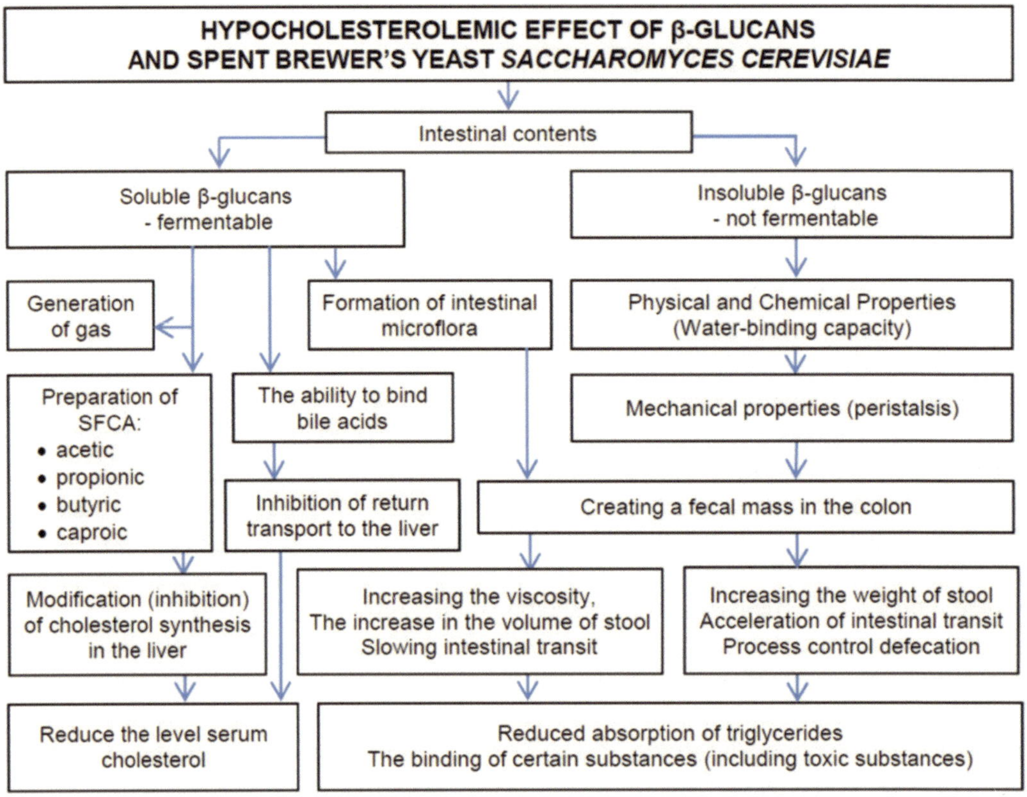

Figure 13. Probable mechanism of hypocholesterolemic effect of beta-glucans and spent brewer's yeast Saccharomyces cerevisiae.

participation of 10% in the diet [72]. The hypocholesterolemic activities of the yeast varied remarkably between strains. In contrast, brewer's yeast and baker's yeast, which have been predominantly used for food, did not exhibit hypocholesterolemic activity even when administered at concentration of 10%. Whereas, during the research on obese men with hypocholesterolemy it has been shown that the intake of spent brewer's yeast considerably lowers the concentration of total cholesterol, increasing the concentration of advantageous fraction of HDL cholesterol when consumed in the amount supplying 15 g of fiber daily. Triacylglycerol concentration in blood did not change considerably [60]. The yeast-derived b-glucan fiber significantly lowered total cholesterol concentrations and was well tolerated; HDL-cholesterol concentrations rose, but only 4 weeks after the fiber was stopped. Described varied hypocholesterolemic activity of various spent brewer's yeast results among others from the kind of yeast and the amount of their supplementation in the diet. Advantageous lowering of cholesterol concentration in the blood of test animals due to diet supplementation with yeast can be caused by prebiotic properties of yeast, which corrects natural content of bacterial flora [61] or considerably high amount of squalens in yeast lipids [62].

A probable mechanism of HP beta glucan and insoluble, dried brewer's yeast influence presented in the diagram (Fig. 13) is associated with their advantageous influence on testine peristlsis and lowering HMG (3-hydroxy-3-methylglutaryl) CoA reductase activity, since also lowering of cholesterol concentration in liver was obtained.

The influence of soluble beta glucan fractions (CMG) on cholesterol concentration in the body was associated with the ability to bind bile acids in a small testine. It might have led to a decrease in bile salt pool able to participate in cholesterol synthesis in liver and disregulation of micellas creation in testine, which hampered lipid absorption. Cholesterol was then used to a larger extent in bile acid synthesis rather than lipoproteid synthesis, therefore, its concentration in blood plasma was decreased. CMG and HP β-glucans given in a higher dosage (100 mg/kg of body mass daily), protected the liver more efficiently against excessive fat layering. Dried spent brewer's yeast also contributed to obtaining lower cholesterol concentration in liver in comparison with control group.

7. Requests

Present interest of consumers to a large extent concerns food that can be used in prevention of many diet-dependent diseases, whereas the interest of food industry is directed at the search for new ingredients of pro-health influence. The knowledge of functional properties of preparations containg β-glucans might be used to shape proper quality of food products for special purposes.

β-Glucan is a valuable functional ingredient and various extraction techniques are available for its extraction. Choice of an appropriate extraction technique is important as it may affect the quality, structure, rheological properties, molecular weight, and other functional properties of the extracted β-glucan. These properties lead to the use of β-glucan into various food systems and have important implications in human health.

Diet supplementation with β-glucans from spent brewer's yeast and preparation of dried spent brewer's yeast contributed to advantageous lowering of cholesterol concentration in blood and lowering lipid concentration in liver. The results described above allow for the formulation of the following conclusions:

1. β-glucan preparations obtained from spent brewer's yeast and dried spent brewer's yeast show efficient biological activity, connected with the improvement of blood lipid profile and liver of experimental animals.
2. Spent brewer's yeast show a similar pro-health influence to β-glucans isolated from them, therefore, they can be a valuable and much cheaper diet suplement, correcting blood lipid metabolism disturbed by atherogenic diet.
3. β-glucan preparations from spent brewer's yeast (CMG and HP) given in higher doses (100 mg/kg of body mass daily), efficiently protect liver against excessive fat layering.

Results obtained in the experiment described above with various yeast preparations are valuable, since they point out that β-glucans obtained from a new source, i.e. spent brewer's yeast have a hypocholesterolemic effect, similarly to other glucans described in literature. Moreover, it has been shown that each of examined β-glucans isolated from spent brewer's yeast was as efficient. Final effect correcting lipid metabolism, particularly various fractions of lipids, was more connected with the dose, rather than physic-chemical properties.

Health advantages contributing to significant cholesterol reduction in blood obtained in experiments on animals, might constitute the basis for assuming that similar influence will be observed in case of a human body. Therefore, it would be recommended to supplement human diet with β-glucans, particularly for people whose diet is abundant in fat and cholesterol. Spent brewer's yeast constituting a serious problem for brewing plants (waste material), can be used successfully as a valuable source of beta glucans, which can be used as diet supplements or as food additives, e.g. in yoghurts, breakfast desserts or snacks.

Currently conducted research is the continuation of a presented experiment. It shows that atherogenic diet supplementation with beta-glucans or spent brewer's yeast contributed to simultaneous obtaining more advantageous content of testine microflara in relation to control group, connected with the increased number of lactid acid bacteria *Bifidobacterium* and *Lactobacillus* and limited growth frequency of disadvantageous yeast fungi *Candida albicans*. Conducted research on functional properties and biological experiment proves the complexity of β-glucan and other fibre preparation influence on experimental animals.

Author details

Bożena Waszkiewicz-Robak
Warsaw University of Life Sciences (WULS-SGGW),
Faculty of Human Nutrition and Consumer Sciences,
Department of Functional Foods and Commodity, Warsaw, Poland

8. References

[1] Report of the Joint WHO/FAO export consultation. Geneva, 2002. Diet, nutrition and prevention of chronic disease.

[2] Ahmad A, Anjum FM, Zahoor T, Nawaz H, Dilshad SM.. Beta glucan: a valuable functional ingredient in foods. Crit Rev Food Sci Nutr. 2012;52(3) 201-12.

[3] Tada R, Tanioka A, Iwasawa H, Hatashima K, Shoji Y, Ishibashi K, Adachi Y, Yamazaki M, Tsubaki K, Ohno N. Structural characterisation and biological activities of a unique type beta-D-glucan obtained from Aureobasidium pullulans. Glycoconj J. 2008;25(9) 851-61.

[4] Sandeep Rahar, Gaurav Swami, Navneet Nagpal, Manisha A. Nagpal, Gagan Shah Singh. Preparation, characterization, and biological properties of β-glucans. J Adv Pharm Technol Res. 2011;2(2) 94-103.

[5] Peumans W.J., Barre A., Derycke V., Rougé P., Zhang W., May G.D., Delcour J.A., Van Leuven F., Van Damme E. J. M. Purification, characterization and structural analysis of an abundant β-(1,3)-glucanase from banana fruit. Eur. J. Biochem. 2000;267(4) 1188-95.

[6] Zeković D.B., Kwiatkowski S. Natural and Modified (1→3)-β-D-Glucans in Health Promotion and Disease Alleviation. Crit. Rev. Biotechnol. 2005;25 205-30.

[7] Hromadkova Z., Ebringerova A., Sasinkov V., Sandula J., Hrıbalova V., Omelkova J. Influence of the drying method on the physical properties and immunomodulatory activity of the particulate (1→3)-b-D-glucan from *Saccharomyces cerevisiae.* Carbohyd. Polym. 2003;51(1) 9-15.

[8] Kuniak L., Karácsonyi S., Augusti J., Ginterová A., Széchényl S., Kravarik D., Dubaj J., Varjú J. A new fungal glucan and its preparation. 1993. World Patent number 9312243.

[9] Williams D.L., Browder I., DiLuzio N.R. Soluble phosphorylated glucan: methods and compositions for wound healing. 1990. U.S. Patent number 4975421.

[10] Petrus H.A., Ensley H.E., McNamee R.B., Jones E.L., Browder I.W., Williams D.L. Isolation, physicochemical characterization and preclinical efficacy evaluation of soluble scleroglucan. Am. Society for Pharma. and Experim. 1991;257(1) 500-10.

[11] Ohno N., Uchiyama M., Tsuzuki A., Tokunaka K., Miura N.N., Adachi Y., Aizawa M.W., Tamura H., Tanaka S., Yadomae T. Solubilization of yeast cell-wall β-(1→3)-D-glucan by sodium hypochlorite oxidation and dimethyl sulfoxide extraction. Carbohyd. Res. 1999;316(1-4) 161-72.

[12] Takuma Sasaki, Yukio Sugino. Carboxymethylated derivatives of beta-1,3-glucan. 1984. US Patent number: 4454315.

[13] Šoltés L., Alföldi J., Sandula J. HPLC and C-NMR study of carboxymethyl-β-(1→6)-D-gluco-β-(1→3)-D-glucan derived from *Saccharomyces cerevisiae.* J. Appl. Polym. Sci. 1993;48 1313-19.

[14] Zhang P., hang L., Cheng S. Solution properties of an alpha-(1→3)-D-glucan from *Lentinus edodes* and its sulfated derivatives. Carbohyd. Res. 2002;337(2) 155-60.

[15] Colleoni-Sirghie M., Kovalenko I.V., Briggs J.L., Fulton B., White P.J. Rheological and molecular properties of water soluble (1,3)/(1,4)-β-D-glucans from high-β-glucan and traditional oat lines. Carbohyd. Polym. 2003;52(4) 439-47.

[16] Bednarski W., Reps A. Food Biotechnology (in Polish). Scientific and Technical Publishing House (WNT), Warsaw; 2001.

[17] Onwurah I.N.E., 2001. Crystallinity and polysaccharide chains of β-glucan in white sorghum, SK5912. Int. J. Biol. Macromol. 29, 281-286.

[18] Charles S., Brennan C.S., Cleary L.J. The potential use of cereal (1/3,1/4)-β-D-glucans as functional food ingredients. J. Cereal Sci. 2005;42(1) 1-13.

[19] Smith K.N., Queenan K., Thomas, W., Fulcher, G., Slavin, J. Cholesterol-lowering effect of barley beta glucan in hypercholesterolemic subjects. FASEB J., 2004;18 A149.

[20] Poyhonen U.L. Control of blood glucose through oat soluble fibre beta-glucan. Agro-Food-Industry Hi-Tech. 2004;15 10-1.

[21] FDA. Food labeling: Health claims; soluble dietary fiber from certain foods and coronary heart disease. Interim final rule. Fed Register. 2002;67(191) 61773-83.

[22] Kerckhoffs D.A.J.M., Hornstra G., Mensink R.P. Cholesterol lowering effect of β-glucan from oat bran in mildly hypercholersterolemic subjects may decrease when β-glucan is incorporated into bread and cookies. Am. J. Clin. Nutr. 2004;(78) 221-27.

[23] Kofuji K., Aoki A., Tsubaki K., Konishi M., Isobe T., Murata Y. Antioxidant Activity of β-Glucan. ISRN Pharm., 2012.

[24] Talati R., Baker W.L., Pabilonia M.S., White C.M., Coleman C.I. The Effects of Barley-Derived Soluble Fiber on Serum Lipids. Ann Fam Med. 2009;7(2) 157–63.

[25] Lull C., Wichers H.J., Savelkoul H.F.J. Antiinflammatory and Immunomodulating Properties of Fungal Metabolitem. Mediat. Inflamm. 2005;(2), 63-80.

[26] Manzi P., Pizzoferrato L. Beta glucans in edible mushrooms. Food Chem., 2000;(68) 315-18.

[27] Ishibashi K.I., Miura N.N., Adachi Y., Tamura H., Tanaka S., Ohno N. The solubilization and biological activities of *Aspergillus* β-(1/3)-D-glucan. FEMS Immunol. Med. Mic. 2004;(42) 155-66.

[28] Kumar C.G., Joo H.S., Choi J.W., Koo Y.M., Chang C.S. Purification and characterisation of an extracellular polysaccharide from haloalkalophilic Bacillus sp. I-450. Enzyme Microb. Tech. 2004;34(7) 673-81.

[29] Ding X., Hang J., Jiang P., Xu X., Liu Z. Structural features and hypoglycaemic activity of an exopolysaccharide produced by Sorangium cellulosum. Lett. Appl. Microbiol. 2004;38(3) 223-28.

[30] Kony D.B., Damm W., Stoll S., van Gunsteren W.F., Hünenberger P.H. Explicit-Solvent Molecular Dynamics Simulations of the Polysaccharide Schizophyllan in Water. Biophys J. 2007;93(2) 442–55.

[31] Standish L.J., Wenner A.A., Sweet E.S., Bridge C., Nelson A., Martzen M., Novack J., Torkelson C. *Trametes versicolor* Mushroom Immune Therapy in Breast Cancer. J. Soc. Integr Oncol. 2008;6(3)122–28.

[32] Oba K, Kobayashi M, Matsui T, Kodera Y, Sakamoto J. Individual patient based meta-analysis of lentinan for unresectable/recurrent gastric cancer. Anticancer Res. 2009;29(7) 2739-45.

[33] Schmid J., Müller-Hagen D., Bekel T., Funk L., Stahl U., Sieber V., Meyer V. Transcriptome sequencing and comparative transcriptome analysis of the scleroglucan producer *Sclerotium rolfsii*. BMC Genomics. 2010;11 329.

[34] Jong Suk Lee, Su-Young Park, Dinesh Thapa, Mi Kyoung Choi, Ill-Min Chung, Young-Joon Park, Chul Soon Yong, Han Gon Choi, Jung-Ae Kim. *Grifola frondosa* water extract alleviates intestinal inflammation by suppressing TNF-α production and its signaling. Exp Mol Med. 2010;42(2)143–54.

[35] Dai H, Han XQ, Gong FY, Dong H, Tu PF, Gao XM. Structure elucidation and immunological function analysis of a novel β-glucan from the fruit bodies of Polyporus umbellatus (Pers.) Fries. Glycobiology, 2012. DOI: 10.1093/glycob/cws099.

[36] Kenyon W.J., Esch S.W., Buller C.S. The curdlan-type exopolysaccharide produced by Cellulomonas flavigena KU forms part of an extracellular glycocalyx involved in cellulose degradation. Anton. Leeuw. 2005;87(2) 143-48.

[37] Kanzawa Y., Harada A., Takeuchi M., Yokota A., Harada T. *Bacillus curdlanolyticus sp.* nov. and *Bacillus kobensis sp.* nov., which hydrolyze resistant curdlan. Int. J. Syst. Bacteriol. 1995;45(3) 515-21.

[38] Obst M., Sallam A., Luftmann H., Steinbuchel A. Isolation and characterization of gram-positive cyanophycin-degrading bacteria-kinetic studies on cyanophycin depolymerase activity in aerobic bacteria. Biomacromolecules. 2004;5(1) 153-61.

[39] Stasinopoulos S.J., Fisher P.R., Stone B.A., Stanisich V.A., 1999. Detection of two loci involved in (1→3)-β-glucan (curdlan) biosynthesis by Agrobacterium sp. ATCC31749, and comparative sequence of the putative curdlan synthase gene. Glycobiology, 1999;9(1) 31-41.

[40] Ross P., Mayer R., Benziman M. Cellulose biosynthesis and function in bacteria. Microbiol. Rev. 1991;55 35-58.

[41] Khalikova E., Susi P., Korpela T. Microbial Dextran-Hydrolyzing Enzymes: Fundamentals and Applications. Microbiol Mol Biol Rev. 2005;69(2) 306–25.

[42] Blättel V., Larisika M., Pfeiffer P., Nowak C., Eich A., Eckelt J., König H. β-1,3-Glucanase from *Delftia tsuruhatensis* Strain MV01 and Its Potential Application in Vinification. Appl Environ Microbiol. 2011;77(3) 983–90.

[43] Lesage G., Bussey H. Cell Wall Assembly in *Saccharomyces cerevisiae.* Microbiol Mol Biol Rev. 2006;70(2) 317–43.

[44] Cross G.G., Jennings H.J., Whitfield D.M., Penney C.L., Zacharie B., Gagnon L. Immunostimulant oxidized β-glucan conjugates. Int. Immunopharmacol. 2001;1(3) 539-50.

[45] Reeves P.G., Nielsen F.H., Fahey G.C. AIN-93 purified diets for laboratory rodents: final report of the American Institute of Nutrition ad hoc writing committee on the reformulation of the AIN-76A rodent diet. J. Nutr. 1993;123 1939-51.

[46] Re R., Pellegrini N., Proteggente A., Pannala A., Yang M., Rice-Evans C. Antioxidant activity applying an improved ABTS radical cation decolorization assay. Free Radical Bio. Med. 1999;26 1231-37.

[47] Folch J., Lees M., Stanley G.H.S. A simple method for the isolation and purification of total lipids from animal tissues. J. Biol. Chem.1957;226(1) 497-09.

[48] Friedewald W.T., Levy R., Fredrickson D.S. Estimation of the concentration of low-density lipoprotein cholesterol in plasma, without use of the preparative ultracentrifuge. Clin. Chem. 1972;(18) 499-02.

[49] Wang Q., Wood P.J., Cui W. Microwave assied dissolution of β-glucan in water – implications for the characterisatotion of his polmer. Carbohyd. Polym. 2002;47(1) 35-8.

[50] Hozová B., Kuniak Ł., Kelemenová B. Application of β-D-Glucans Isolated from Mushrooms *Pleurotus ostreatus* (Pleuran) and *Lentinus edodes* (Lentinan) for Increasing the Bioactivity of Yoghurts. Czech. J. Food Sci. 2004;22(6) 204-14.

[51] Volikakis P., Biliaderis C.G., Vamavakas C., Zerfiridis G.K. Effects of a commercial oat-β-glucan concentrate on the chemical, physico-chemical and sensory attributes of a low-fat white-brined cheese produkt. Food Res. Int. 2004;37(1) 83-94.

[52] Othman R.A., Moghadasian M.H., Jones P.J. Cholesterol-lowering effects of oat β-glucan. Nutr Rev. 2011;69(6) 299-09.

[53] Wolever TM, Gibbs AL, Brand-Miller J, Duncan AM, Hart V, Lamarche B, Tosh SM, Duss R. Bioactive oat β-glucan reduces LDL cholesterol in Caucasians and non-Caucasians. Nutr J. 2012;25(10) 130.

[54] Brown G.D., Gordon S., 2003. Fungal beta-glucans and mammalian immunity. Immunity. 2003;19(3) 311-15.

[55] Vetvicka V., Yvin J.C. Effects of marine β-1,3 glucan on immune reactions. Int. Immunopharmacol. 2004;4 721-30.

[56] Biörklund M., van Rees A, Mensink R.P., Onning G. Changes in serum lipids and postprandial glucose and insulin concentrations after consumption of beverages with β-glucan from oats or barley: a randomised dose-controlled trial. Eur. J. Clin. Nutr. 2005;59(11) 1272-81.

[57] Maki K.C., Davidson M.H., Ingram K.A., Veith P.E., Bell M., Gugger E. Lipid responses to consumption of a beta-glucan containing ready-to-eat cereal in children and adolescents with mild-to-moderate primary hypercholesterolemia. Nutr. Res. 2003; 23(11) 1527-35.

[58] Bobek P, Hromadova M, Ozdin L. Oyster mushroom (*Pleurotus ostreatus)* reduces the activity of 3-hydroxy-3-methylglutaryl CoA reductase in rat liver microsomes. Cell. Mol. Life Sci. 1995;51(6) 589-91.

[59] Clevidence B.A., Judo J.T., Schatzkin A., Muesing R.A., Campbell W.S., Brown C.C., Taylor P.R. Plasma lipid and lipoproteid concentration of men consuming a law FAT, high fiber diet. Am. J. Clin. Nutr. 1992;(55) 689-94.

[60] Nicolosi R., Bell S.J., Bistrian B.R., Greenberg I., Forse R.A., Blackburn G.K. Plasma lipid changes after supplementation with β-glucan fiber from yeast. Am. J. Clin. Nut. 1999;(70) 208-12.

[61] Blagović B., Rupčić J., Mesarić M., Georgiú K., Marić V. Lipid Composition of Brewer's Yeast. Food Technol. Biotechnol. 2001;39(3) 175-81

[62] Blaut M. Relationship of prebiotics and food to intestinal microflora. Eur. J. Nutr. 2002;41(S) 11-16.

[63] Andersson M., Ellegård L., Andersson, H. Oat bran stimulates bile acid synthesis within 8 h as measured by 7α-hydroxy-4-cholesten-3-one. Am. J. Clin. Nutr. 2002;76(5) 1111-16.

[64] Kahlon T.S., Woodruff C.L. In vitro Binding of Bile Acids by Rice Bran, Oat Bran, Barley and β-Glucan Enriched Barley. Cereal Chem. 2003;80(3) 260-63.

[65] Wang X., Gibson G.R. Effects of the in vitro fermentation of oligofructosenand inulin by bacteria growing in the human large intestine. J. Appl. Bacteriol. 1993;75 373-80.

[66] Wolever T.M.S., Brighenti F., Royall D. Effect of rectal infusion of short chain fatty acids in human subjects. Am. J. Gastroenterd.1990;84 1027.

[67] Wright R.S., Anderson J.W., Bridges S.R. Priopionate inhibits hepatocyte lipid synthesis. Proc. Soc. Exp. Biol. Med. 1990;195 26.

[68] Luo J., Rizkalla S.W., Alamowitch C. Chronic consumption of short-chain fructooligosaccharides by healthy subjects decreased basal hepatic glucose production but had no effect on insulin-stimulated glucose metabolism. Am. J. Clin. Nutr. 1996;(63) 939-45.

[69] Canzi, E., Guglielmetti, S., Mora, D., Tamagnini, I. and Parini, C. Conditions affecting cell surface properties of human intestinal bifidobacteria. Antonie van Leeuwenhoek. 2005;(88) 207–19.

[70] Rumsey G.L., Winfree R.A., Hughes S.G., Nutritional values of dietary nucleic acids and purine bases to rainbow trout. Aquaculture. 1992;108 97-110.

[71] Oliva-Teles A., Goncalves P. Partial replacement of fishmeal by brewers yeast Saccaromyces cerevisae in diets for sea bass Dicentrarchus labrax juveniles, Aquaculture. 2001;202 269-78.

[72] Yoshida Y., Yokoi W., Wada Y., Ohishi K., Ito M., Sawada H. Potent hypocholesterolemic activity of the yeast *Kluyveromyces marxianus* YIT 8292 in rats fed a high cholesterol diet. Biosci. Biotechnol. Biochem. 2004;68 1185-92.

Chapter 13

Lipid Involvement in Viral Infections: Present and Future Perspectives for the Design of Antiviral Strategies

Miguel A. Martín-Acebes, Ángela Vázquez-Calvo, Flavia Caridi, Juan-Carlos Saiz and Francisco Sobrino

Additional information is available at the end of the chapter

http://dx.doi.org/10.5772/51068

1. Introduction

Viruses constitute important pathogens that can infect animals, including humans and plants. Despite their great diversity, viruses share as a common feature the dependence on host cell factors to complete their replicative cycle. Among the cellular factors required by viruses, lipids play an important role on viral infections [1-4]. The involvement of lipids in the infectious cycle is shared by enveloped viruses (those viruses whose infectious particle is wrapped by one or more lipid membranes) and non-enveloped viruses [1-4]. Apart from taking advantage on cellular lipids that are usually located inside cells, viruses induce global metabolic changes on infected cells, leading to the rearrangement of the lipid metabolism to facilitate viral multiplication [1,5-11]. In some cases, these alterations produce the reorganization of intracellular membranes of the host cell, building the adequate microenvironment for viral replication [12,13]. All these findings highlight the intimate connections between viruses and lipid metabolism. Along this line, modulation of cellular lipid metabolism to interfere with virus multiplication is currently raising as a feasible antiviral approach [6,14].

2. A lipid perspective of the virus life cycle

Inherent to their condition of obligate intracellular parasites, viruses have to invade a cell to complete their replicative cycle. During this step, viruses express their own proteins and also co-opt host cell factors for multiplication, including lipids [15]. A schematic view of a virus replication cycle is shown in Figure 1. Initial steps of viral infection include the attachment of the virus particle to a specific receptor located on the cell surface, in some cases a specific lipid (section 2.1.1). The viral genome has to entry into the host cell to reach the replication sites. Different lipids, located either on plasma and/or endosomal membranes, can contribute to these processes by enabling receptor clustering, virus internalization, or membrane fusion (sections 2.1.2 and 2.1.3). Replication of viral genome can take place associated to cellular membranes or other lipid structures, like lipid droplets, forming structures termed replication complexes (section 2.2). Newly synthesized viral genomes are enclosed inside *de novo* synthesized viral particles, a process in which several lipids can play, again, an important role (section 2.3), especially in the case of viruses containing a lipid envelope as an integral component of their infectious particle. Then, viral particles maturate to render infectious particles that are released from host cell to initiate a new infection cycle.

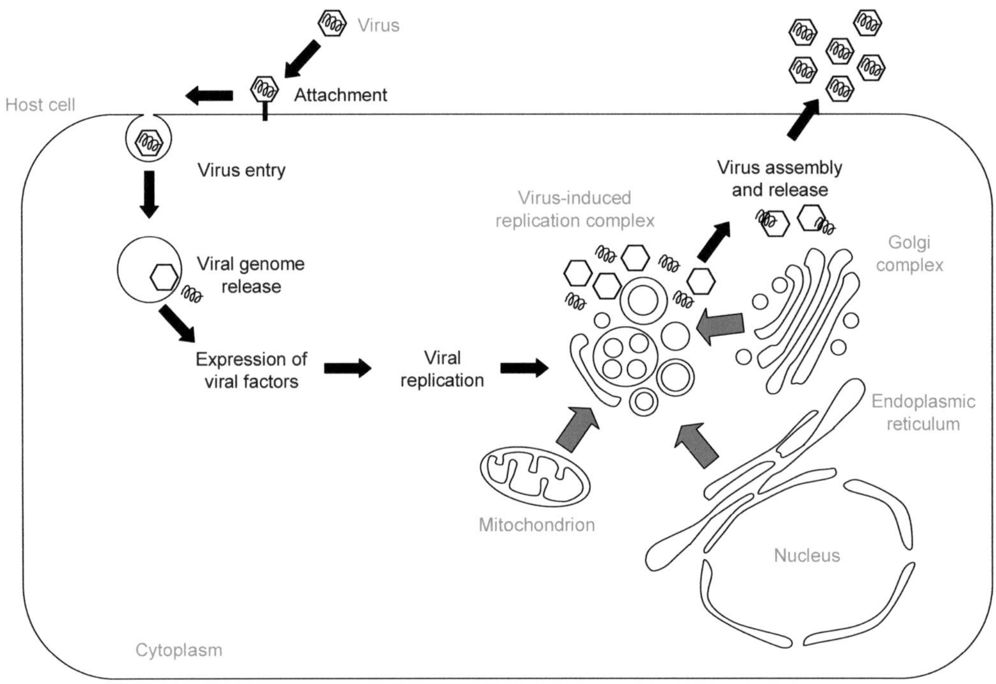

Figure 1. Schematic view of a virus replication cycle. For a detailed description of the different roles of lipids during virus infection see the text.

2.1. Lipids and viral entry

The viral entry into a host cell to start their replicative cycle involves the attachment of the virus particle to a specific receptor(s) located on the cell surface, prior to the introduction of the viral genome within the host cell. The latter can take place by internalization of the whole viral particle, constituting a sort of minute Trojan horse [16], or by direct penetration of viral genome from plasma membrane. During these processes, a variety of specific lipids play multiple roles, which may vary between viruses (Table 1).

Virus	Lipid	Function	Refs.
VSV	phosphatidylserine	Cellular receptor	[17]
	LBPA	Cofactor for membrane fusion	[18,19]
SV40	GM1	Cellular receptor	[20]
	cholesterol	Lipid raft-caveola mediated endocytosis	[21]
DENV	LBPA	Cofactor for membrane fusion	[22]
VACV	phosphatidylserine	Induction of viral internalization	[23]

Abbreviations used in this Table: DENV, dengue virus; LBPA, lysobisphosphatidic acid; SV40, simian virus 40; VACV, vaccinia virus; VSV, vesicular stomatitis virus.

Table 1. Examples of lipids required for viral entry

2.1.1. Lipids and viral attachment

The first event of virus infection comprises the recognition of the target cell, which generally occurs through the interaction between the virus and a specific receptor on the cell surface. Receptors exploited by viruses include different macromolecules like proteins, carbohydrates and lipids. An increasing number of viruses is known to attach to lipid-containing molecules. For instance, members of the *Polyomaviridae* family use gangliosides, being the binding highly specific [24]. The simian virus 40 (SV40) employs exclusively the ganglioside GM1, whereas the mouse polyomavirus can use GD1a and GT1b, and BK virus can utilize GD1b and GT1b [25-28]. Other important human pathogens, such as influenza virus (*Orthomyxoviridae*) and Human immunodeficiency virus, HIV (*Retroviridae*), can also bind to different gangliosides [29,30].

Another example of a virus whose receptor is supposed to be a lipid is the rhabdovirus vesicular stomatitis virus (VSV), which seems to gain cell entry through interaction with negatively charged phospholipids, like phosphatidylserine [17]. VSV particles interact very strongly with membranes containing phosphatidylserine through viral glycoprotein G [31], and although it is not actually clear whether phosphatidylserine is the viral receptor [32], a direct interaction between the G protein and this lipid could take place in the membrane [31].

On the other hand, some members of the *Flaviviridae* family -hepatitis C virus (HCV), GB virus C/hepatitis G virus and bovine viral diarrhea virus (BVDV)-, use the low-density lipoprotein receptor (LDL-R) [33], which is a cholesterol receptor. An interesting case is hepatitis C virus (HCV) that requires the interaction with the low-density lipoprotein receptor (LDL-R) and with glycosaminoglycans to entry into the cell [8]. The component of the virion that interacts with LDL-R likely is a cell-derived lipoprotein, i. e. a viral-lipoprotein (section 2.3.1).

2.1.2. Lipids and viral internalization

Cells use a broad spectrum of mechanisms to internalize substances from their environment. Endocytosis is a general term for the internalization of particles, solutes, fluids, and membrane components by invagination of the plasma membrane and internalization of the resulting membrane vesicles [24,34-36]. The plasma membrane does not present a continuous or homogeneous composition. It contains lipid microdomains termed lipid rafts [37], characterized by their high content of cholesterol, glycosphinglolipids, glycophosphatidylinositol (GPI), anchored proteins like the GPI-anchored, myristoylated and palmytoylated proteins, as well as transmembrane proteins [38]. Lipid rafts have been associated with various endocytic mechanisms to internalize these membrane regions [39-42], being the formation of cave-shaped invaginations, termed caveolae, the predominant mechanism [24,34]. Lipid rafts have been related to the entry of a number of viruses, for example the coronavirus severe acute respiratory syndrome (SARS), murine leukemia virus, herpes simplex virus, Japanese encephalitis virus, SV40, and echovirus 1 [34,43-48]. In addition, some viruses require cholesterol-enriched microdomains in the viral membrane for efficient virus entry, for example influenza virus A, human herpes virus 6, and Canine distemper virus [49-51]. On the other hand, some viruses that enter into the cells using mechanisms independent of lipid rafts require cholesterol for an efficient internalization. This is the case of foot-and-mouth disease virus (FMDV) and human rhinovirus type 2, whose entry into cells, by clathrin-mediated endocytosis, requires the presence of plasma membrane cholesterol [52,53]. In other viruses such as HIV-1, a requirement of cholesterol for viral entry has been documented [47] and related to the clustering of viral receptors, thus enabling viral internalization [54]. This role of cholesterol and lipid-rafts has also been documented for coxsackievirus B3 (CVB3) infection [55].

The plasma membrane also exhibits clusters of other lipids like phosphatidylinositol 4,5-bisphosphate ($PI(4,5)P_2$) [56], which is a minor lipid of the inner leaflet of the plasma membrane with an important role in the clathrin-mediated endocytosis [57-60]. Even when the number of viruses that use clathrin-mediated endocytosis to entry into the cells is wide [61], the importance of this lipid in viral entry has not been analyzed in depth yet. However, it has been reported that $PI(4,5)P_2$ production by a specific lipid kinase is crucial for HIV-1 entry in permissive lymphocytes [62]. Likewise, foot-and-mouth disease virus (FMDV) and VSV require the presence of this phospholipid in the plasma membrane for internalization (Vázquez-Calvo *et al.*, submitted).

As commented before, specific lipids located in the viral particles can also play a role on viral entry of enveloped viruses [8], including 'those located in' lipid rafts [49-51]. Vaccinia virus provides another example of the relationships between lipids located on the viral particle and viral entry. In this case, the presence of exposed phosphatidylserine in the viral envelope is critical to induce blebs on cellular membrane that promote virus internalization [23].

2.1.3. Lipids and viral genome delivery

Viruses have to release their genome from the particle to enable proper expression of viral proteins and genome replication within host cell. In the case of enveloped viruses, fusion between viral envelope and cellular membranes is a generalized strategy to facilitate these events. This process is assisted by viral proteins termed fusion proteins, and results in lipid mixing between the viral envelope and the target cellular membrane

[63-66]. Viral fusion occurs either with the plasma membrane for pH-independent viruses, or, in the case of viruses entering through receptor-mediated endocytosis, with membranes of endocytic organelles in which particles are internalized. There is evidence showing that both groups of viruses use fusion proteins that, via hydrophobic segments, interact with membrane lipids, leading to conformational changes that make them able for fusion [63-66]. Compelling evidence indicates that specific lipids can influence the compartment of virus uncoating and viral genome delivery into the cytosol [22,67,68]. A number of enveloped viruses take advantage of the low pH inside endosomes to promote endosome fusion, permitting viral genome release [69]. Thus, utilization of specific lipids allows the virus to ensure membrane fusion at the proper cellular compartment. For instance, DENV takes advantage of the anionic late endosome-specific lipid bis(monoacylglycero)phosphate (BMP), also named lysobisphosphatidic acid (LBPA), to promote virus fusion with the late endosomal membrane [22]. A relevant role of LBPA in promoting membrane fusion and lipid mixing has also been shown in VSV infection [70]. Initially, VSV envelope fuses with intraluminal vesicles inside multivesicular bodies, which later fuse with external membrane of the multivesicular body, allowing the release of viral nucleocapsid to the cytosol [18,19]. However, fusion of other viruses, such as influenza virus, does not rely on these lipids [70]. Cholesterol, a major and vital constituent of eukaryotic cellular membranes, has been implicated in promoting lipid transfer and fusion pore expansion in the virus-cell membrane fusion mediated by the haemagglutinin of influenza virus [68]. The presence of cholesterol on the target membrane also promotes West Nile virus (WNV) membrane fusion activity [71], and both cholesterol and sphingolipids, but not lipid-rafts, are required for alphavirus fusion [67].

Regarding the entry of non-enveloped viruses, it is generally believed that the mechanism(s) involved does not include membrane fusion activity. Nevertheless, recent data obtained from biochemical and structural studies indicate that the overall mechanisms of entry of certain non-enveloped viruses are similar to those of enveloped ones, and that capsid proteins can function in these activities in a manner similar to that of the membrane viral proteins [72]. For instance, the outer capsid protein VP5 of the non-enveloped rotaviruses and orbiviruses, shares secondary structural features with fusion proteins of enveloped viruses [73], like the capacity to associate with lipid rafts in cellular membranes [72]. These findings indicate that VP5 may be responsible for membrane penetration [74]. Post-translational modifications of viral proteins, i.e. myristoylation of capsid protein VP4 in poliovirus (PV) and VP2 of polyomavirus, have been related to the ability of these proteins to induce pores on cellular membranes for genome release [75,76].

2.2. Lipids and viral multiplication

Following entry into the host cell, viruses have to produce accurate self-copies to generate new infectious viral particles. To this end, viruses use to recruit cellular factors, including lipids and enzymes involved in their metabolism.

2.2.1. Cellular membranes and viral replication complex assembly

Viruses co-opt host cell factors to develop the most adequate environment for their replication, a feature that is especially highlighted by the viral replication complex found assembled inside cells infected with positive strand RNA viruses [2,15,77]. Viruses belonging to this group share as a common feature a viral genome consisting of one or more RNA molecules of positive polarity that mimic the characteristics of cellular messenger RNA (mRNA) to be translated into viral proteins. Positive strand RNA viruses comprise several viral families that include important animal (including human) and plant pathogens such as *Picornaviridae* (i.e. PV, FMDV), *Flaviviridae* (i.e. DENV, WNV, HCV), *Caliciviridae* (i.e. Nowalk virus), *Coronaviridae* (i.e. SARS coronavirus), or *Togaviridae* (i.e. rubella virus). Replication of positive-strand RNA viruses is tightly associated to intracellular lipid membranes derived from different organelles: endoplasmic reticulum, Golgi complex, mitochondria, chloroplasts, peroxisomes, vacuoles, endosomes, or lysosomes [2]. Besides membranes derived from cellular organelles, these viruses can also usurp cytoplasmic lipid droplets for their replication [78,79]. In this way, viral replication results in the induction of marked alterations of the intracellular architecture mainly characterized by the remodelling of cellular membranes. These alterations include intracellular membrane proliferation and changes on shape and size of membranous structures. Consequently, viral replication originates a variety of structures that may rely on different mechanisms for their generation [12,15]. Examples of these structures (Figure 2) include the formation of convoluted membranes and vesicle packets as a result of flavivirus replication [80-82], the development of heterogeneous vesicular structures that conform the membranous web found in HCV-infected cells [83], or the proliferation of vesicular structures (including double membrane vesicles) in cells infected by enteroviruses (a genus within the *Picornaviridae* family) like PV [84,85].

Morphological changes on membrane shape induced by viral infections are accompanied by an enrichment in the viral and cellular components, including specific proteins and lipids [1-3,12]. Despite the diversity of the membrane alterations induced, these changes provide the physical scaffold for viral replication, thus offering the most suitable platform for viral replication complex assembly, and hence increasing the local concentration of specific cellular and viral factors necessary for replication [1,12]. In addition, membrane remodelling can also improve viral multiplication by hiding viral components from the innate immune system [1,12,86]. In flaviviruses (DENV and WNV) the evasion of interferon response has been shown to depend on the expression of hydrophobic viral proteins involved in membrane rearrangements [87-89]; in particular, the cholesterol content of these membranes is important to down regulate the interferon-stimulated antiviral signalling response to infection [90]. Related to this, antiviral interferon response also involves down regulation of sterol biosynthesis [91]. Likewise, lipid droplets, which can constitute platforms for viral replication, also play important roles on the coordination of immune responses [92].

All these changes in the membrane morphology and composition result in the formation of customized cellular microenvironments that support viral replication and can be actually considered novel virus-induced organelles [93-95]. Regarding the lipid composition of these structures, great progresses have been recently made (see below) that have uncovered the

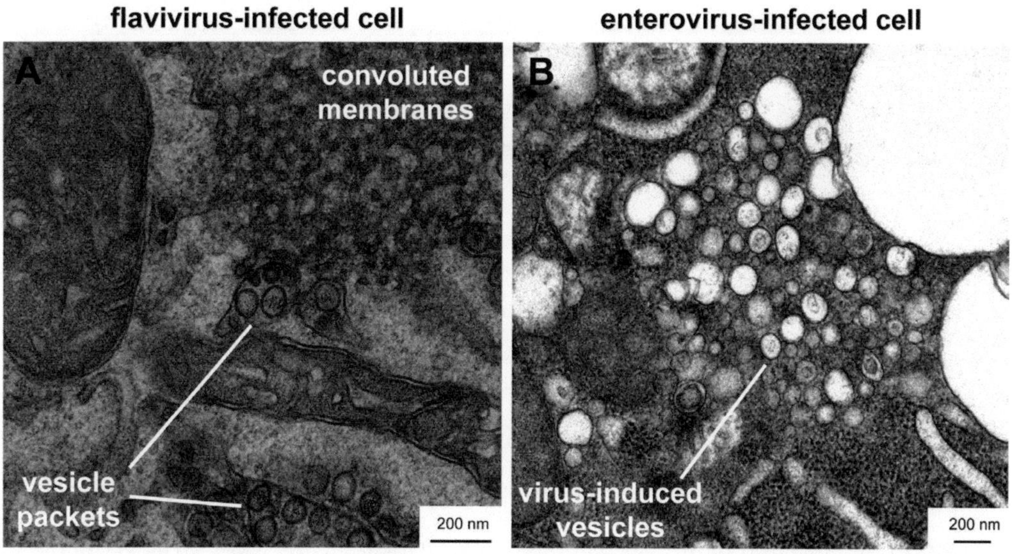

Figure 2. Distinct alterations on intracellular membrane architecture induced by the infection of positive strand RNA viruses. A) Induction of convoluted membranes and vesicle packets in flavivirus infected cells. Image corresponds to Vero cells infected with WNV, fixed and processed for transmission electron microscopy at 24 h post-infection. B) Proliferation of vesicular structures in enterovirus-infected cells. Porcine cells (IBRS-2) were infected with the enterovirus swine vesicular disease virus (SVDV), fixed, and processed for transmission electron microscopy at 7 h post-infection. For technical details related to virus infection and sample preparation see references [81,84].

dependence on different cellular lipids for replication complex organization, although their roles and importance vary between viruses.

2.2.2. *Cellular lipids involved in viral replication complex assembly*

To render the specific lipid microenvironment adequate for multiplication, viruses co-opt cellular machinery for their replication, including host factors involved in different aspects of lipid metabolism, i.e. sterol biosynthesis, fatty acid metabolism and synthesis of specific phosphoinositides [15]. For instance, a marked alteration of cellular metabolism and an increase in fatty acid biosynthetic pathway have been described upon human cytomegalovirus (HCMV), DENV or HCV infection [1,5,6,11]. The association of viral multiplication with modulation of host cell factors involved in lipid metabolism is not an exclusive feature of animal viruses, thus, replication and recombination of the plant pathogens tombusviruses has been revealed to rely on host genes involved in lipid metabolism [96-99]. Representative examples of cellular factors related to lipid metabolism and associated to viral replication are summarized in Table 2.

Several studies have highlighted the role of the cholesterol and the cholesterol biosynthetic pathway in the replication of viruses, including important human pathogens belonging to the *Flaviviridae* family -WNV [90], DENV [110], and HCV [8,111-113]- and to the *Caliciviridae* -Nowalk virus [114]-families. In addition, the cholesterol biosynthetic pathway has also been

Virus	Host factor	Function	Refs.
BMV	Ole1	Fatty acid desaturation	[100,101]
DENV	FASN	Fatty acid synthesis	[102]
DCV	SREBP	Fatty acid synthesis	[103]
WNV	3-HMG-CoA reductase	Cholesterol synthesis	[90]
TBSV	Erg25, SMO1, SMO2	Sterol synthesis	[104]
	INO2	Regulation of phospholipid synthesis	[105]
HCV	PI4KIIIα	Synthesis of PI4P	[106,107]
PV, CVB3, AiV	PI4KIIIβ	Synthesis of PI4P	[93,108,109]

Abbreviations used in this Table: AiV, Aichi virus; BMV: brome mosaic virus, CVB3, coxsackievirus B3; DCV, Droshophila C virus; DENV, Dengue virus; Erg25, ergosterol enzyme 25; FASN, fatty acid synthase; HCV, Hepatitis C virus; 3-HMG-CoA reductase, 3-hydroxy-methyglutaryl-CoA reductase; INO2, inositol-1-phosphate synthase 2; Ole1, Delta(9) fatty acid desaturase; PI4KIIIα and β, phosphatidylinositol 4-kinase class III α and β; PI4P, phosphatidylinositol 4-phosphate; PV, poliovirus; SMO1 and 2, sterol4α-methyl-oxidase 1 and 2; SREBP, sterol regulatory element binding protein; TBSV, tomato bushy stunt virus; WNV, West Nile virus.

Table 2. Examples of host cell genes associated to lipid metabolism and involved in viral replication

associated to the infection of animal pathogens like African swine fever virus [115]. On the other hand, sterols have been involved in the replication of plant pathogens, for example tomato bushy stunt virus (TBSV) [104]. Due to the high diversity of viruses that exploit the cholesterol biosynthetic pathway for replication, this could consider a common requirement. However, replication of viruses may rely on lipids other than cholesterol, as described for the alphanodavirus flock house virus (FHV) [116].

Another major class of lipids that has been related to viral replication are the fatty acids, whose metabolism has been shown to be required for the multiplication of viruses such as brome mosaic virus (BMV) [100,101], Droshophila C virus (DCV) [103], CVB3 [117], and PV [118]. In some cases, in addition to the dependence of cholesterol (discussed in the previous paragraph), viral multiplication is also dependent on fatty acid synthesis. Examples of viruses sharing both cholesterol and fatty acid requirements include DENV [102], WNV [81,102], and HCV [8,112]. Indeed, during DENV infection, the key enzyme responsible for fatty acid synthesis, the fatty acid synthase (FASN), is recruited to the viral replication complex by direct interaction with the viral protein NS3, enhancing its activity [102]. Dependence of DENV replication on fatty acids is shared by mammalian and mosquito host cells [9]. Even more, DENV modulates lipid metabolism through induction of a form of autophagy that targets lipid droplet stores, promoting the depletion of cellular triglycerides and the release of fatty acids. This results on an increase in β-oxidation and ATP production that stimulate viral replication [1,5]. Infection with other viruses (HCV or CVB3) also relies on fatty acids and results in an increase on FASN expression [117,119], a phenomenon that does not occur upon DENV or WNV infection [81,102].

Besides cholesterol and fatty acids, specific phospholipids can also play a key role in viral replication. For instance, replication of TBSV and FHV is dependent on phospholipid biosynthesis [105]. Replication of FHV was initially associated to glycerophospholipids, being independent of cholesterol or sphingomyelin (a membrane phospholipid that is not derived from glycerol) [116]. However, recent advances on the biology of FHV indicate that its replication is based on the outer mitochondrial membrane and is dependent on the anionic phospholipid cardiolipin, which is almost exclusive of these membranes [120]. In this regard, more than 20 years ago, phospholipids were already associated to the replication of PV, a member of the *Picornaviridae* family [121]. More recently, this relationship has been confirmed after the identification of a specific phospholipid, the phosphatidylinositol 4 phosphate (PI4P), as a key component of PV replication complexes [93]. Requirement of PI4P is shared by other members of the *Picornaviridae* family - CVB3, Aichi virus (AiV), bovine kubovirus, and human rhinovirus 14 [93,108,109,122]- and also by viruses from other families, i.e. HCV [93,106,107,123-126]. All these viruses can specifically recruit different isoforms of the enzyme that drives the formation of PI4P from phosphatidylinositol, the phosphatidylinositol 4-kinase class III (PI4KIII) α or β, to their replication complexes. For instance, HCV recruits the lipid kinase PI4KIIIα by direct interaction with viral protein NS5A [125,127], while in picornaviruses, the recruitment of PI4KIIIβ can be mediated by the interaction of viral protein 3A with a third cellular partner associated to the viral replication complex, ABC3D (acyl-coenzyme A binding domain containing 3) [108] or other proteins implicated in the secretory pathway [93]. The dependence on either PI4KIIIα or β isoforms varies between viruses. Replication of picornaviruses is specifically associated to PI4P synthesized by PI4KIIIβ [93,108,109,122], while replication of HCV has been mainly associated to the function of PI4KIIIα [106,107], and in a lower extent to PI4KIIIβ [93,126]. In any case, PI4P is not universally required among viruses, since the replication of the flaviviruses (WNV and DENV), and the pestivirus bovine viral diarrhea virus (all members of the *Flaviviridae* family, like HCV) has been shown to be independent of PI4P [81,106,125].

2.2.3. *Lipid functions associated to viral genome replication*

The presence of specific lipids in the viral replication complex can accomplish with several missions. For instance, post-translational modification of viral proteins by lipids is associated to viral replication functions [128,129]. Table 3 displays representative examples of lipid functions during viral replication.

Virus	Lipid	Function	Refs.
BMV	fatty acids	Increase in membrane plasticity and fluidity	[100,101]
DENV	fatty acids	Energy production to support viral replication	[5]
PV	PI4P	Anchor of viral replicase to replication complex	[93]
FHV	cardiolipin	Anchor of viral replicase to replication complex	[120]
HCV	sphingomyelin	Activation of RNA polymerase activity	[130]
WNV	cholesterol	Innate immune evasion	[90]

Abbreviations used in this table: BMV, brome mosaic virus; HCV, hepatitis C virus; DENV, Dengue virus; FHV, flock house virus; PI4P, phosphatidylinositol 4-phosphate; PV, poliovirus; WNV, West Nile virus.

Table 3. Examples of lipid roles during viral replication

Lipids can contribute to viral replication by acting as scaffolding molecules to anchor viral proteins. In PV, location of specific phospholipids (PI4P) to the viral replication sites mediates direct recruitment of the RNA dependent RNA polymerase (the enzyme that replicates the viral genome), which specifically interacts with this lipid [93]. The RNA polymerase of FHV also interacts with a specific phospholipid, the cardiolipin located on the outer mitochondrial membrane, where its replication takes place [120]. In addition to these examples, different events related to the replication of viral genomes are also influenced by specific phospholipids [131,132]. The activation of HCV replication due to a direct binding of sphingomyelin to HCV RNA polymerase has also been documented [130].

Proper topology of viral replication complexes usually depends on the induction of a membrane curvature, which may require the presence of specific proteins [133]. Membrane curvature can also be induced by modification of its lipid structure, either through changes in the polar head group or in the acyl chain composition [2,134]. Thus, during BMV infection, the function of an allele of delta9 fatty acid desaturase, an enzyme that introduces double bond in unsaturated fatty acids, has been associated to viral replication complex assembly to increase membrane fluidity and plasticity [100,101]. The accumulation of cone-shaped lipids, such as lysophospholipids, which contain single acyl chain per phospholipid molecule, and of special lipids like cholesterol or cardiolipin, has been associated with alterations on the membrane curvature and plasticity that can contribute to replication complex assembly [1,2,135].

As commented before, the membrane rearrangements resulting from replication complex assembly can also contribute to evade the cellular immune response by hiding viral components from pathogen sensors of the innate immune machinery. Thus, WNV-induced redistribution of cellular cholesterol contributes to down regulate the interferon-stimulated antiviral signalling response to infection [90].

Finally, the reorganization of cellular lipid metabolism during infection can also contribute to the generation of ATP in order to provide energy to support robust viral replication [1,5].

2.3. Lipids and viral morphogenesis

Most enveloped-viruses acquire their lipid membrane by budding through a cellular membrane that can be provided by different sources. For instance, flaviviruses (i.e. DENV or WNV) bud into the endoplasmic reticulum for acquisition of their envelope [80,82], while VSV (Figure 3), influenza, or HIV acquire their envelope by budding from plasma membrane [136-139]. In other cases, different cellular organelles can contribute with distinct membranes to virus envelopment, is reported for herpersvirus and poxvirus [140-142]. Viruses can take advantage of specific parts of the membrane for their assembly. Cholesterol and lipid raft microdomains play an important role on the assembly of a variety of viruses [136-138,143]. In HIV, the presence of $PI(4,5)P_2$ on the membrane is also necessary for assembly and budding of viral particles, and the viral protein Gag localizes to assembly sites via the interaction with this lipid [144]. The synthesis of fatty acids has also been associated to the envelopment of viruses [6].

Other cellular lipid structures play a role on the assembly of a number of viruses. Thus, of intracellular lipid droplets have been associated with the assembly and morphogenesis

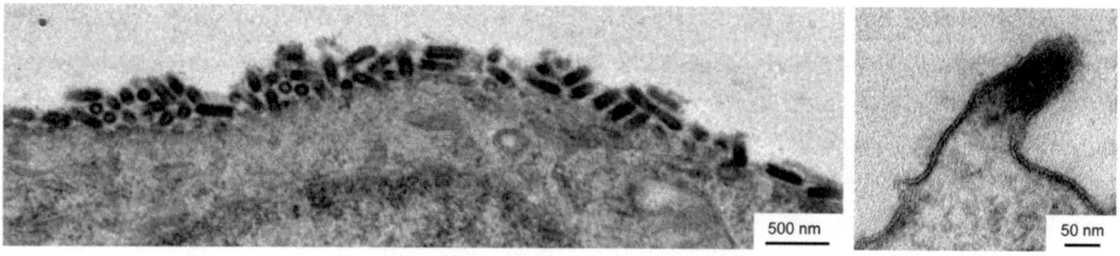

Figure 3. Virus budding through the plasma membrane. Images correspond to BHK-21 cells infected with the rhabdovirus VSV, fixed, and processed for transmission electron microscopy at 7 h post-infection. For technical details related to virus infection and sample preparation see [145].

of DENV and HCV [78,79,146]. Assembly of HCV particles occurs on the surface of lipid droplets and, as mentioned earlier, it is related to the very low density lipoprotein (VLDL) pathway, a phenomenon that leads to the formation of unique lipo-viro-particles [4,147]. The lipoprotein component associated to HCV particles is essential for their infectivity [148], since one of its functions is to interact with LDL-R, thus contributing to viral attachment (section 2.1.1).

Lipids incorporated to viral proteins due to post-translational modifications are also involved in crucial steps of enveloped virus assembly [149,150]. Regarding morphogenesis of non-enveloped viruses, myristoylation of VP4 protein of PV and FMDV has been shown necessary for proper capsid assembly [151,152].

2.3.1. Lipid composition of enveloped viruses

Differences on the lipid composition of the viral membranes may reflect their different origin. Despite that the lipid content of enveloped viruses has been studied for decades [153-155], quantitative analyses of viral lipidomes (the entire content of lipids) at the individual molecular species level have not been possible until recently, by means of the improvement of mass spectrometry [3,139]. Following this approach, several studies have extended the knowledge on viral lipid composition. Nevertheless, drawbacks associated to the purification of cellular membranes, in particular the plasma membrane, still complicate the analysis of lipid sorting during viral budding [3].

As commented above, viral membranes can be originated from varied cellular sources (section 2.3). The lipid composition of both Semliki Forest virus (SFV) and VSV is indistinguishable and only displays slight differences with that of the plasma membrane [139]. Being SFV and VSV from different viral families (*Togaviridae* and *Rhabdoviridae,* respectively), these viruses constitute an example of little selection of the lipids included in their envelopes. Since the composition of the viral envelopes of both viruses is similar to that of the plasma membrane, the small differences observed between plasma membrane and these viral envelopes could be explained by the enrichment in specific lipids to facilitate the membrane curvature required for viral budding [139].

In the case of retroviruses (i.e. HIV and murine leukaemia virus), the overall lipid composition of viral envelopes resembles that of detergent-resistant membrane microdomains [156,157]. An enrichment in PI(4,5)P_2 has also been documented in HIV envelope, which is compatible with the dependence on the interaction between the viral protein Gag and this lipid to promote HIV budding from plasma membrane [157]. Another virus that buds from membrane rafts is influenza virus [138]. The lipidome of this virus has been analyzed for viruses budding from the apical membrane of polarized cells [158]. This study revealed that that the apical cellular membrane was enriched in sphingolipids and cholesterol, whereas glycerophospholipids were reduced, and storage lipids were depleted compared with the whole-cell membranes. These results are consistent with an accumulation of lipid rafts at the membranes where the virus buds. In addition, the virus membrane exhibited a further enrichment of sphingolipids and cholesterol when compared with the donor membrane at the expense of phosphatidylcholines [158].

In other cases, major differences in lipid content between viral envelopes and host cell membranes have been found. An interesting example is the envelope of HCMV, which contains more phosphatidylethanolamines and less phosphatidylserines than the host cell membranes, resembling the synaptic vesicle lipidome [159]. Another virus with marked differences with cellular membranes is HCV, whose particles show a unique lipid composition in comparison with all other viruses analyzed to date. In addition, the lipid content of the HCV envelope is also different from that of the cells in which it was produced (cholesteryl esters comprise almost half of the total HCV lipids), resembling the composition of VLDL and LDL [160]. This finding is compatible with the association of HCV assembly with the VLDL pathway that leads to the formation of lipo-viro-particles [4,147].

3. Targeting lipid metabolism, a novel antiviral strategy

Specific lipids are essential for multiple steps of the viral replication cycle and, therefore, different strategies can be used to interfere with virus infection. As a first approach to inhibit enveloped virus multiplication, the functions of lipids incorporated into the viral particle can be targeted by chemical compounds or even by antibodies [161]. This is the case of broad-spectrum antivirals, – some of them already licensed for human use, such as arbidol [162-164] –, or inhibitors of membrane fusion [3]. Impairment of viral fusion can be achieved also by targeting viral machinery involved in this process, a strategy currently assayed for HIV treatment [165].

An alternative, non-excluding lipid-targeted strategy to prevent viral multiplication is based on inhibitors of enzymes that catalyse lipid metabolic fluxes upregulated by viral infections [6]. Examples of compounds that act at distinct points of lipid metabolism and with reported antiviral activity *in vitro* are given in Table 4. Targeting lipid metabolism as an antiviral strategy raises important concerns. On one hand, alteration of such important metabolic pathway for cellular homeostasis may resemble a non-specific strategy, which could result in deleterious effects for the host. However, it should be also considered that currently antiviral compounds also target other major metabolic pathways, i.e. that of nucleic acids metabolism [166-169]. On the other hand, targeting host factors to avoid viral replication could also carry advantages. Drugs that target host factors seem to be less susceptible to the development of viral resistance than strategies focused on viral proteins. Another advantage of this approach is that compounds targeting a specific group of lipids can successfully inhibit replication of different unrelated viruses (Table 4), thus constituting candidates for broad-spectrum antiviral drugs. These facts make that the use of drugs that impair different aspects of lipid metabolism has been proposed as a feasible antiviral approach [1,6,14].

Target lipid	Inhibitor	Antiviral activity against	Refs.
Cholesterol	Statins	HIV, HCV, influenza	[170-176]
	U18666A	DENV, HCV	[113,177]
Fatty acids	TOFA	HCMV, Influenza	[6]
	C75	HCMV, DENV, YFV, WNV, Influenza, HCV, CVB3	[6,9,81,102,117,119]
	Cerulenin	DENV, WNV, PV, CVB3	[81,102,117,121]
	Arachidonate	HCV	[178]
	Oleic acid	PV	[118]
PI4P	Enviroxime-like	PV, AiV	[108,109]
	PIK93	PV, CVB3, CVB5	[81,93,109]
	AL-9	HCV	[179]
Sphingolipids	Myriocin	Hepatitis B virus, HCV	[180-182]
Multiple	Valproic acid	VACV, WNV, SFV, SINV, ASFV, VSV, LCMV, USUV	[145]

Abbreviations used in this table: AiV, Aichi virus; ASFV, African swine fever virus; CVB, coxsackievirus B; C75, trans-4-carboxy-5-octyl-3-methylene-butyrolactone; DENV, Dengue virus; HCMV, human cytomegalovirus; HCV, hepatitis C virus; HIV, human immunodeficiency virus; LCMV, lymphocytic chioriomeningitis virus; PV, poliovirus; SINV, Sindbis virus; SFV, Semliki Forest virus; TOFA, 5-tetradecyloxy-2-furoic acid; USUV, Usutu virus; VACV, vaccinia virus; VSV, vesicular stomatitis virus; WNV, West Nile virus; YFV, yellow fever virus

Table 4. Examples of drugs targeting lipid metabolism with reported antiviral activity

3.1. Targeting cholesterol as an antiviral strategy

Cholesterol is involved in multiple steps of the viral cycle. Impairment of cholesterol biosynthetic pathway by inhibitors of 3-hydroxy-3-methyl-glutaryl-CoaA reductase (3-HMG-CoA reductase) like statins, commonly used in treatment of cardiovascular disease, constitutes a novel antiviral approach [174,175,183]. The clinical success of these inhibitors for human disorders also indicates that inhibitors of lipid metabolism can be safe and effective for human therapy. An additional effect of the treatment with statins, unrelated to the inhibition of 3-HMG-CoA reductase, is the inhibition of the binding of leukocyte function-associated antigen-1 (LFA-1) to the intercellular adhesion molecule (ICAM-1) [184], thus being immunomodulators and anti-inflammatory agents [185,186]. These properties can carry additional advantages for fighting HIV [174-176].

The infection with the paramyxovirus respiratory syncitial virus (RSV) is dependent on the isoprenylation at the carboxy terminus of the cellular protein RhoA by geranylgeranyltransferase. Lovastatin, which blocks prenylation pathways in the cell by directly inhibiting 3-HMG-CoA reductase, inhibits RSV infection both in cultured cells and in mice [183]. Treatment of patients with different statins (i.e. lovastatin, simvastin, or fluvastin) resulted in diverse effects on HCV infection, ranging from an absence of antiviral effect to a modest improvement of sustained antiviral response, or a reduction of viremia [172,173,187-189]. Beneficial effects derived from treatment with statins of infection with diverse influenza strains have also been reported in animal models and human studies [170,171], although other studies do not support these conclusions [190].

Targeting cholesterol in viral infection can be achieved using drugs other than statins, for instance U18666A. This is an intracellular cholesterol transport inhibitor widely used to block the intracellular trafficking of cholesterol and mimic Niemann-Pick type C disease, which also blocks cholesterol biosynthesis by inhibiting oxidosqualene cyclase and desmosterol reductase [191]. Treatment with U18666A inhibits DENV infection in cultured cells, and the effect of this compound is additive to the inhibitory effect of C75 (an inhibitor of FASN), which shows that both, cholesterol and fatty acids, are required for successful DENV replication [177]. U18666A also displays an antiviral effect against HCV infection and a synergistic effect has been reported when combined with interferon [113].

3.2. Inhibitors of fatty acid biosynthesis as potential antiviral compounds

The biosynthesis of fatty acids plays an important role for multiplication of a wide variety of viruses [6,9,81,102]. Pharmacological inhibition of this metabolic pathway can be achieved using 5-tetradecyloxy-2-furoic acid (TOFA), an inhibitor of acetyl-CoA carboxylase (ACC) [192]. Treatment with this compound has been shown to block replication of HCMV and influenza A virus [6]. Although the results derived from these experiments performed in model cell culture systems need to be further reproduced using animal models, the concentrations of TOFA that successfully inhibit HCMV infection in cultured cells are in the range of plasma concentrations found in rats treated with this inhibitor [6]. In HCV, treatment with TOFA attenuates the enhancement of replication of HCV induced by ethanol [193].

On the other hand, treatment with trans-4-carboxy-5-octyl-3-methylene-butyrolactone (C75) – an inhibitor of FASN, the key enzyme of fatty acid biosynthetic pathway – also resulted in inhibition of the replication of both HCMV and influenza A virus [6]. These experiments were performed in cultured cells, and the concentrations of the inhibitor tested did not induce host cell toxicity or apoptosis [6]. Similar results have been obtained for DENV, yellow fever virus (YFV), WNV, and HCV using the FASN inhibitor C75 [9,81,102,119], or cerulenin, another FASN inhibitor [81,102,111]. HMCV, influenza A, DENV, YFV, and WNV are enveloped viruses. The antiviral effect of either cerulenin or C75 has also been probed for the non-enveloped viruses CVB3 and PV [117,121], enlarging the potential antiviral spectrum of FASN inhibitors. However, it should be noted that blockage of FASN by C75 can cause severe anorexia and weight loss in animal models [194]. This makes of C75 a drug not aimed for human use, although it has aided to the identification of potential pathways to target obesity [195], and is also contributing to the understanding of the relationship between biosynthetic fatty acid synthesis and viral multiplication [6,9,81,102,117]. For DENV, a direct interaction between the viral protein NS3 and FASN has been reported

[102]. Inhibition of this interaction could contribute to the design of antivirals to fight this important human disease.

Infection of HCV is intimately connected to lipid metabolism, including the fatty acid biosynthetic pathway [4,8], and its replication can be inhibited by C75 [119]. Indeed, fatty acids can either stimulate or inhibit HCV replication, depending on their degree of saturation [112]. Arachidonate, a polyunsaturated fatty acid, also inhibits HCV replication [112] via the lipid peroxidation induced by reactive oxygen species (ROS) derived from HCV replication that converts polyunsaturated fatty acids into reactive carbonyls that inactivate proteins [178]. These events can be prevented by treatment with the antioxidant vitamin E [178]. As a result of the connections between fatty acids and cholesterol biosynthetic pathways, inhibition of fatty acid synthesis can be also related to the reduction of the infection of HCV, through inhibition of the geranylgeranylation of cellular factors required for HCV replication [112,196]. The use of unsaturated fatty acids has also been applied to block myristoylation of HIV Gag protein to prevent virus budding [150].

3.3. Phosphlipids as antiviral targets

Viral replication also relies on phospholipid biosynthesis [105,121]. This makes drugs interfering this pathway candidates for antiviral design. Along this line, the antiviral properties of valproic acid - a short chain fatty acid commonly used for the treatment of epilepsy and bipolar disorder that impairs multiple aspects of phosphoinositide metabolism [197-199] - against a broad panel of enveloped viruses have been reported (Table 4) [145].

Treatment with a chimeric antibody directed against phospahtidylserine can cure arenavirus and cytomegalovirus infections in animal models [200]. The mechanism of action of this therapy is based on the exposure of phosphatidylserine on the external leaflet of the plasma membrane, a preapoptotic event in cells infected by a broad variety of viruses. The safety and pharmacokinetics of this antibody have been already evaluated in clinical trials for treatment of other human disorders [201]. Another example of the use of anti-phospholipidantibodies to combat a viral disease is provided by HIV, since different anti-phospholipid antibodies have shown a broad neutralizing activity against this virus [161].

Recent reports have highlighted the role of a specific phospholipid species, PI4P, in the replication of enteroviruses (PV, CVB3) and HCV (section 2.2.2). The synthesis of PI4P associated to viral replication relies on the function of the cellular enzymes PI4KIIIα and β. This makes both lipid kinases potential drug targets for antiviral design. An inhibitor of PI4KIIIβ, PIK93 [202], has been shown to impair replication of enteroviruses [81,93,109]. Related reports have also uncovered that this enzyme is the cellular target of known antiviral compounds against enteroviruses [109]. This is so for some enviroxime-like compounds – T-00127-HEV1 and GW5074 [93] – that integrate a group of antivirals that inhibits enterovirus replication, for which mutations conferring drug resistance mapped to the same region of the enteroviral protein 3A [109,203-205]. The recruitment of PI4KIIIβ to viral replication complexes requires the participation of cellular partners like the Golgi adaptor protein acyl coenzyme A (acyl-CoA) binding domain protein 3 (ACBD3/GPC60), as described for AiV [108,122]. In this way, modulation of the interaction between these proteins could also constitute a novel antiviral strategy [122].

In HCV infection the isoform of the enzyme involved in viral replication is mainly PI4KIIIα [106,107], although a role of the β isoform in the inhibition of HCV replication due to treatment with PIK93 has also been reported [126]. Consistent with these findings, specific compounds that successfully inhibit PV replication through blockage of PI4KIIIβ (GW5074 and T-00127-HEV1) do not affect HCV replication, although other enviroxime-like compounds can affect both enteroviral and HCV replication [109]. On the other hand, 4-anilino quinazolines were first reported to have antiviral activity against HCV, although the mechanism was not well defined. However, a recent study has associated the antiviral activity of a representative 4-anilino quinazoline (AL-9) with the inhibition of PI4KIIIα during HCV infection, which opens new therapeutic approaches [179]. Since the viral protein NS5A directly interacts with PI4KIIIα during HCV infection [125,127], modulation of this interaction also raises novel possibilities for antiviral research.

Overall, these examples of drugs targeting different enzymes related to phosphoinositide metabolism support this strategy as a feasible approach for antiviral drug discovery. In this line, related phosphoinositide kinases constitute an important emerging class of drug targets [202].

3.4. Sphingolipids as antiviral targets

Sphingolipids constitute a major component of lipid rafts [37,38], which, as commented before, are involved in different steps of viral infection, making sphingolipids potential antiviral targets. Along this line, ebolavirus requires the activity of acid sphingomyelinase, the enzyme that converts sphingomyelin to phosphocholine and ceramide for infection, and depletion of sphingomyelin reduces its infection [206]. A dependence on sphingomyelin for HCV replication has also been documented [130]. Inhibition of serine palmitoyltransferase, the enzyme that catalyzes the first step on sphingolipid biosynthesis, using myriocin has also been assayed against HCV or hepatitis B virus, either alone or in combination with interferon [180-182]. However, a certain controversy exists regarding whether the inhibitory effect of myriocin on HCV replication is attributable to the specific inhibition of serine palmitoyltransferase, since FTY720, a compound that like myriocin is structurally similar to sphingosine but does not inhibit serine palmitoyltransferase, also inhibits HCV replication [207].

4. Conclusion

The analysis of the functions of cellular factors in viral infections has highlighted the role of different lipid species in these infections. Viruses can use cellular lipids like bricks to build viral particles or to develop viral replication complexes, thus facilitating its multiplication. But viruses can also manipulate host cell metabolism towards the production of specific lipid species, unveiling an intimate relationship between viruses and host cell lipid metabolism. Indeed, great progresses have been recently made in this area due to the identification of specific lipids as key factors for viral multiplication. However, the specific function of most of these lipids remains to be determined. A better understanding of the interactions between viral infections and lipid metabolism is desirable to asses the roles of lipids in viral multiplication. This knowledge could lead to the identification of lipid targets and druggable metabolic pathways suitable for antiviral development. Lipid candidates for these interventions have already been identified, for instance fatty acids, cholesterol or specific phospholipids. Indeed, initial lipid-based antiviral approaches have been already started, even at clinical level (i.e. statins). This example has probed that drugs already licensed for humans that act at different points of lipid metabolism can constitute potential candidates to fight viral diseases. These lipid-targeted antiviral approaches could be exclusive or could also be complementary to other antiviral therapies already available.

As recently remarked, 'if RNA ruled the last decade and DNA dominated the previous one, could the next decade be the one for lipids?' [208]. The new advances on the knowledge of the interplay between viruses and lipids evidence that the answer to this question could be 'Yes' in the case of virology [1]. Hopefully, we are now assisting to the promising birth of a novel lipid-based branch of antiviral research focused on this challenging and still poorly explored field for drug discovery.

Author details

Miguel A. Martín-Acebes, Ángela Vázquez-Calvo, Flavia Caridi and Francisco Sobrino
Department of Virology and Microbiology, Centre for Molecular Biology "Severo Ochoa" (CBMSO) (UAM/CSIC), Cantoblanco, Madrid, Spain

Juan-Carlos Saiz
Department of Biotechnology, National Institute for Food Science and Technology (INIA), Madrid, Spain

Acknowledgement

Work at CBMSO was supported by grants from Ministerio de Ciencia e Innovación (MICINN, Spain) BIO2008-0447-C03-01, and BIO2011-24351, and by an institutional grant from the "Fundación Ramón Areces".

Work at INIA was supported by grants RTA2011-00036 from the Spanish Ministerio de Ciencia e Innovación (MICINN) and the Network of Animal Disease Infectiology and Research-European Union NADIR-EU-228394. MAMA is the recipient of a JAE-Doc fellowship from Spanish Research Council (CSIC).

5. References

[1] Heaton NS, Randall G (2011) Multifaceted roles for lipids in viral infection. Trends Microbiol 19: 368-375.

[2] Stapleford KA, Miller DJ (2010) Role of cellular lipids in positive-sense RNA virus replication complex assembly and function. Viruses 2: 1055-1068.

[3] Lorizate M, Krausslich HG (2011) Role of lipids in virus replication. Cold Spring Harb Perspect Biol 3: a004820.

[4] Alvisi G, Madan V, Bartenschlager R (2011) Hepatitis C virus and host cell lipids: an intimate connection. RNA Biol 8: 258-269.

[5] Heaton NS, Randall G (2010) Dengue virus-induced autophagy regulates lipid metabolism. Cell Host Microbe 8: 422-432.

[6] Munger J, Bennett BD, Parikh A, Feng XJ, McArdle J, Rabitz HA, Shenk T, Rabinowitz JD (2008) Systems-level metabolic flux profiling identifies fatty acid synthesis as a target for antiviral therapy. Nat Biotechnol 26: 1179-1186.

[7] Blackham S, Baillie A, Al-Hababi F, Remlinger K, You S, Hamatake R, McGarvey MJ (2010) Gene expression profiling indicates the roles of host oxidative stress, apoptosis, lipid metabolism, and intracellular transport genes in the replication of hepatitis C virus. J Virol 84: 5404-5414.

[8] Targett-Adams P, Boulant S, Douglas MW, McLauchlan J (2010) Lipid metabolism and HCV infection. Viruses 2: 1195-1217.

[9] Perera R, Riley C, Isaac G, Hopf-Jannasch AS, Moore RJ, Weitz KW, Pasa-Tolic L, Metz TO, Adamec J, Kuhn RJ (2012) Dengue virus infection perturbs lipid homeostasis in infected mosquito cells. PLoS Pathog 8: e1002584.

[10] Rodgers MA, Saghatelian A, Yang PL (2009) Identification of an overabundant cholesterol precursor in hepatitis B virus replicating cells by untargeted lipid metabolite profiling. J Am Chem Soc 131: 5030-5031.

[11] Diamond DL, Syder AJ, Jacobs JM, Sorensen CM, Walters KA, Proll SC, McDermott JE, Gritsenko MA, Zhang Q, Zhao R, Metz TO, Camp DG, 2nd, Waters KM, Smith RD, Rice CM, Katze MG (2010) Temporal proteome and lipidome profiles reveal hepatitis C virus-associated reprogramming of hepatocellular metabolism and bioenergetics. PLoS Pathog 6: e1000719.

[12] Miller S, Krijnse-Locker J (2008) Modification of intracellular membrane structures for virus replication. Nat Rev Microbiol 6: 363-374.

[13] den Boon JA, Diaz A, Ahlquist P (2010) Cytoplasmic viral replication complexes. Cell Host Microbe 8: 77-85.

[14] Bassendine MF, Sheridan DA, Felmlee DJ, Bridge SH, Toms GL, Neely RD (2011) HCV and the hepatic lipid pathway as a potential treatment target. J Hepatol 55: 1428-1440.

[15] Nagy PD, Pogany J (2012) The dependence of viral RNA replication on co-opted host factors. Nat Rev Microbiol 10: 137-149.

[16] Sandvig K, van Deurs B (2008) Cell biology: Viruses in camouflage. Nature 453: 466-467.

[17] Schlegel R, Tralka TS, Willingham MC, Pastan I (1983) Inhibition of VSV binding and infectivity by phosphatidylserine: is phosphatidylserine a VSV-binding site? Cell 32: 639-646.

[18] Matsuo H, Chevallier J, Mayran N, Le Blanc I, Ferguson C, Faure J, Blanc NS, Matile S, Dubochet J, Sadoul R, Parton RG, Vilbois F, Gruenberg J (2004) Role of LBPA and Alix in multivesicular liposome formation and endosome organization. Science 303: 531-534.

[19] Le Blanc I, Luyet PP, Pons V, Ferguson C, Emans N, Petiot A, Mayran N, Demaurex N, Faure J, Sadoul R, Parton RG, Gruenberg J (2005) Endosome-to-cytosol transport of viral nucleocapsids. Nat Cell Biol 7: 653-664.

[20] Campanero-Rhodes MA, Smith A, Chai W, Sonnino S, Mauri L, Childs RA, Zhang Y, Ewers H, Helenius A, Imberty A, Feizi T (2007) N-glycolyl GM1 ganglioside as a receptor for simian virus 40. J Virol 81: 12846-12858.

[21] Anderson HA, Chen Y, Norkin LC (1996) Bound simian virus 40 translocates to caveolin-enriched membrane domains, and its entry is inhibited by drugs that selectively disrupt caveolae. Mol Biol Cell 7: 1825-1834.

[22] Zaitseva E, Yang ST, Melikov K, Pourmal S, Chernomordik LV Dengue virus ensures its fusion in late endosomes using compartment-specific lipids. PLoS Pathog 6: e1001131.

[23] Mercer J, Helenius A (2008) Vaccinia virus uses macropinocytosis and apoptotic mimicry to enter host cells. Science 320: 531-535.

[24] Ewers H, Helenius A (2011) Lipid-mediated endocytosis. Cold Spring Harb Perspect Biol 3: a004721.

[25] Low JA, Magnuson B, Tsai B, Imperiale MJ (2006) Identification of gangliosides GD1b and GT1b as receptors for BK virus. J Virol 80: 1361-1366.

[26] Tsai B, Gilbert JM, Stehle T, Lencer W, Benjamin TL, Rapoport TA (2003) Gangliosides are receptors for murine polyoma virus and SV40. Embo J 22: 4346-4355.

[27] Magaldi TG, Buch MH, Murata H, Erickson KD, Neu U, Garcea RL, Peden K, Stehle T, Dimaio D (2012) Mutations in the GM1 Binding Site of SV40 VP1 Alter Receptor Usage and Cell Tropism. J Virol.

[28] Tsai B, Qian M (2010) Cellular entry of polyomaviruses. Curr Top Microbiol Immunol 343: 177-194.

[29] Meisen I, Dzudzek T, Ehrhardt C, Ludwig S, Mormann M, Rosenbruck R, Lumen R, Kniep B, Karch H, Muthing J (2012) The human H3N2 influenza viruses A/Victoria/3/75 and A/Hiroshima/52/2005 preferentially bind to alpha2,3-sialylated monosialogangliosides with fucosylated poly-N-acetyllactosaminyl chains. Glycobiology.

[30] Izquierdo-Useros N, Lorizate M, Contreras FX, Rodriguez-Plata MT, Glass B, Erkizia I, Prado JG, Casas J, Fabrias G, Krausslich HG, Martinez-Picado J (2012) Sialyllactose in Viral Membrane Gangliosides Is a Novel Molecular Recognition Pattern for Mature Dendritic Cell Capture of HIV-1. PLoS Biol 10: e1001315.

[31] Carneiro FA, Lapido-Loureiro PA, Cordo SM, Stauffer F, Weissmuller G, Bianconi ML, Juliano MA, Juliano L, Bisch PM, Da Poian AT (2006) Probing the interaction between vesicular stomatitis virus and phosphatidylserine. Eur Biophys J 35: 145-154.

[32] Coil DA, Miller AD (2004) Phosphatidylserine is not the cell surface receptor for vesicular stomatitis virus. J Virol 78: 10920-10926.

[33] Agnello V, Abel G, Elfahal M, Knight GB, Zhang QX (1999) Hepatitis C virus and other flaviviridae viruses enter cells via low density lipoprotein receptor. Proc Natl Acad Sci U S A 96: 12766-12771.

[34] Marsh M, Helenius A (2006) Virus entry: open sesame. Cell 124: 729-740.

[35] Conner SD, Schmid SL (2003) Regulated portals of entry into the cell. Nature 422: 37-44.

[36] Mayor S, Pagano RE (2007) Pathways of clathrin-independent endocytosis. Nat Rev Mol Cell Biol 8: 603-612.

[37] Simons K, Ikonen E (1997) Functional rafts in cell membranes. Nature 387: 569-572.

[38] Jacobson K, Mouritsen OG, Anderson RG (2007) Lipid rafts: at a crossroad between cell biology and physics. Nat Cell Biol 9: 7-14.

[39] Chinnapen DJ, Chinnapen H, Saslowsky D, Lencer WI (2007) Rafting with cholera toxin: endocytosis and trafficking from plasma membrane to ER. FEMS Microbiol Lett 266: 129-137.

[40] Martin-Belmonte F, Martinez-Menarguez JA, Aranda JF, Ballesta J, de Marco MC, Alonso MA (2003) MAL regulates clathrin-mediated endocytosis at the apical surface of Madin-Darby canine kidney cells. J Cell Biol 163: 155-164.

[41] Rollason R, Korolchuk V, Hamilton C, Schu P, Banting G (2007) Clathrin-mediated endocytosis of a lipid-raft-associated protein is mediated through a dual tyrosine motif. J Cell Sci 120: 3850-3858.

[42] Stoddart A, Dykstra ML, Brown BK, Song W, Pierce SK, Brodsky FM (2002) Lipid rafts unite signaling cascades with clathrin to regulate BCR internalization. Immunity 17: 451-462.

[43] Bender FC, Whitbeck JC, Ponce de Leon M, Lou H, Eisenberg RJ, Cohen GH (2003) Specific association of glycoprotein B with lipid rafts during herpes simplex virus entry. J Virol 77: 9542-9552.

[44] Damm EM, Pelkmans L, Kartenbeck J, Mezzacasa A, Kurzchalia T, Helenius A (2005) Clathrin- and caveolin-1-independent endocytosis: entry of simian virus 40 into cells devoid of caveolae. J Cell Biol 168: 477-488.

[45] Das S, Chakraborty S, Basu A Critical role of lipid rafts in virus entry and activation of phosphoinositide 3' kinase/Akt signaling during early stages of Japanese encephalitis virus infection in neural stem/progenitor cells. J Neurochem 115: 537-549.

[46] Glende J, Schwegmann-Wessels C, Al-Falah M, Pfefferle S, Qu X, Deng H, Drosten C, Naim HY, Herrler G (2008) Importance of cholesterol-rich membrane microdomains in the interaction of the S protein of SARS-coronavirus with the cellular receptor angiotensin-converting enzyme 2. Virology 381: 215-221.

[47] Liao Z, Cimakasky LM, Hampton R, Nguyen DH, Hildreth JE (2001) Lipid rafts and HIV pathogenesis: host membrane cholesterol is required for infection by HIV type 1. AIDS Res Hum Retroviruses 17: 1009-1019.

[48] Lu X, Xiong Y, Silver J (2002) Asymmetric requirement for cholesterol in receptor-bearing but not envelope-bearing membranes for fusion mediated by ecotropic murine leukemia virus. J Virol 76: 6701-6709.

[49] Huang H, Li Y, Sadaoka T, Tang H, Yamamoto T, Yamanishi K, Mori Y (2006) Human herpesvirus 6 envelope cholesterol is required for virus entry. J Gen Virol 87: 277-285.

[50] Imhoff H, von Messling V, Herrler G, Haas L (2007) Canine distemper virus infection requires cholesterol in the viral envelope. J Virol 81: 4158-4165.

[51] Sun X, Whittaker GR (2003) Role for influenza virus envelope cholesterol in virus entry and infection. J Virol 77: 12543-12551.

[52] Martin-Acebes MA, Gonzalez-Magaldi M, Sandvig K, Sobrino F, Armas-Portela R (2007) Productive entry of type C foot-and-mouth disease virus into susceptible cultured cells requires clathrin and is dependent on the presence of plasma membrane cholesterol. Virology 369: 105-118.

[53] Snyers L, Zwickl H, Blaas D (2003) Human rhinovirus type 2 is internalized by clathrin-mediated endocytosis. J Virol 77: 5360-5369.

[54] Yi L, Fang J, Isik N, Chim J, Jin T (2006) HIV gp120-induced interaction between CD4 and CCR5 requires cholesterol-rich microenvironments revealed by live cell fluorescence resonance energy transfer imaging. J Biol Chem 281: 35446-35453.

[55] Coyne CB, Bergelson JM (2006) Virus-induced Abl and Fyn kinase signals permit coxsackievirus entry through epithelial tight junctions. Cell 124: 119-131.

[56] Kwiatkowska K (2010) One lipid, multiple functions: how various pools of PI(4,5)P(2) are created in the plasma membrane. Cell Mol Life Sci 67: 3927-3946.

[57] Antonescu CN, Aguet F, Danuser G, Schmid SL (2011) Phosphatidylinositol-(4,5)-bisphosphate regulates clathrin-coated pit initiation, stabilization, and size. Mol Biol Cell 22: 2588-2600.

[58] De Matteis MA, Godi A (2004) PI-loting membrane traffic. Nat Cell Biol 6: 487-492.

[59] James DJ, Khodthong C, Kowalchyk JA, Martin TF (2008) Phosphatidylinositol 4,5-bisphosphate regulates SNARE-dependent membrane fusion. J Cell Biol 182: 355-366.

[60] Zoncu R, Perera RM, Sebastian R, Nakatsu F, Chen H, Balla T, Ayala G, Toomre D, De Camilli PV (2007) Loss of endocytic clathrin-coated pits upon acute depletion of phosphatidylinositol 4,5-bisphosphate. Proc Natl Acad Sci U S A 104: 3793-3798.

[61] Mercer J, Schelhaas M, Helenius A (2010) Virus entry by endocytosis. Annu Rev Biochem 79: 803-833.

[62] Barrero-Villar M, Barroso-Gonzalez J, Cabrero JR, Gordon-Alonso M, Alvarez-Losada S, Munoz-Fernandez MA, Sanchez-Madrid F, Valenzuela-Fernandez A (2008) PI4P5-kinase Ialpha is required for efficient HIV-1 entry and infection of T cells. J Immunol 181: 6882-6888.

[63] Teissier E, Pecheur EI (2007) Lipids as modulators of membrane fusion mediated by viral fusion proteins. Eur Biophys J 36: 887-899.

[64] Harrison SC (2008) Viral membrane fusion. Nat Struct Mol Biol 15: 690-698.

[65] Puri A, Paternostre M, Blumenthal R (2002) Lipids in viral fusion. Methods Mol Biol 199: 61-81.

[66] Rey FA (2006) Molecular gymnastics at the herpesvirus surface. EMBO Rep 7: 1000-1005.

[67] Kielian M, Chanel-Vos C, Liao M (2010) Alphavirus Entry and Membrane Fusion. Viruses 2: 796-825.
[68] Biswas S, Yin SR, Blank PS, Zimmerberg J (2008) Cholesterol promotes hemifusion and pore widening in membrane fusion induced by influenza hemagglutinin. J Gen Physiol 131: 503-513.
[69] Vazquez-Calvo A, Saiz JC, McCullough KC, Sobrino F, Martin-Acebes MA (2012) Acid-dependent viral entry. Virus Res. In press
[70] Roth SL, Whittaker GR (2011) Promotion of vesicular stomatitis virus fusion by the endosome-specific phospholipid bis(monoacylglycero)phosphate (BMP). FEBS Lett 585: 865-869.
[71] Moesker B, Rodenhuis-Zybert IA, Meijerhof T, Wilschut J, Smit JM (2010) Characterization of the functional requirements of West Nile virus membrane fusion. J Gen Virol 91: 389-393.
[72] Bhattacharya B, Roy P (2010) Role of lipids on entry and exit of bluetongue virus, a complex non-enveloped virus. Viruses 2: 1218-1235.
[73] Trask SD, Guglielmi KM, Patton JT (2010) Primed for Discovery: Atomic-Resolution Cryo-EM Structure of a Reovirus Entry Intermediate. Viruses 2: 1340-1346.
[74] Hassan SH, Wirblich C, Forzan M, Roy P (2001) Expression and functional characterization of bluetongue virus VP5 protein: role in cellular permeabilization. J Virol 75: 8356-8367.
[75] Danthi P, Tosteson M, Li QH, Chow M (2003) Genome delivery and ion channel properties are altered in VP4 mutants of poliovirus. J Virol 77: 5266-5274.
[76] Krauzewicz N, Streuli CH, Stuart-Smith N, Jones MD, Wallace S, Griffin BE (1990) Myristylated polyomavirus VP2: role in the life cycle of the virus. J Virol 64: 4414-4420.
[77] Mackenzie J (2005) Wrapping things up about virus RNA replication. Traffic 6: 967-977.
[78] Samsa MM, Mondotte JA, Iglesias NG, Assuncao-Miranda I, Barbosa-Lima G, Da Poian AT, Bozza PT, Gamarnik AV (2009) Dengue virus capsid protein usurps lipid droplets for viral particle formation. PLoS Pathog 5: e1000632.
[79] Miyanari Y, Atsuzawa K, Usuda N, Watashi K, Hishiki T, Zayas M, Bartenschlager R, Wakita T, Hijikata M, Shimotohno K (2007) The lipid droplet is an important organelle for hepatitis C virus production. Nat Cell Biol 9: 1089-1097.
[80] Welsch S, Miller S, Romero-Brey I, Merz A, Bleck CK, Walther P, Fuller SD, Antony C, Krijnse-Locker J, Bartenschlager R (2009) Composition and three-dimensional architecture of the dengue virus replication and assembly sites. Cell Host Microbe 5: 365-375.
[81] Martin-Acebes MA, Blazquez AB, Jimenez de Oya N, Escribano-Romero E, Saiz JC (2011) West nile virus replication requires Fatty Acid synthesis but is independent on phosphatidylinositol-4-phosphate lipids. PLoS One 6: e24970.
[82] Mackenzie JM, Westaway EG (2001) Assembly and maturation of the flavivirus Kunjin virus appear to occur in the rough endoplasmic reticulum and along the secretory pathway, respectively. J Virol 75: 10787-10799.

[83] Moradpour D, Gosert R, Egger D, Penin F, Blum HE, Bienz K (2003) Membrane association of hepatitis C virus nonstructural proteins and identification of the membrane alteration that harbors the viral replication complex. Antiviral Res 60: 103-109.

[84] Martin-Acebes MA, Gonzalez-Magaldi M, Rosas MF, Borrego B, Brocchi E, Armas-Portela R, Sobrino F (2008) Subcellular distribution of swine vesicular disease virus proteins and alterations induced in infected cells: a comparative study with foot-and-mouth disease virus and vesicular stomatitis virus. Virology 374: 432-443.

[85] Suhy DA, Giddings TH, Jr., Kirkegaard K (2000) Remodeling the endoplasmic reticulum by poliovirus infection and by individual viral proteins: an autophagy-like origin for virus-induced vesicles. J Virol 74: 8953-8965.

[86] Hoenen A, Liu W, Kochs G, Khromykh AA, Mackenzie JM (2007) West Nile virus-induced cytoplasmic membrane structures provide partial protection against the interferon-induced antiviral MxA protein. J Gen Virol 88: 3013-3017.

[87] Ambrose RL, Mackenzie JM (2011) West Nile virus differentially modulates the unfolded protein response to facilitate replication and immune evasion. J Virol 85: 2723-2732.

[88] Munoz-Jordan JL, Laurent-Rolle M, Ashour J, Martinez-Sobrido L, Ashok M, Lipkin WI, Garcia-Sastre A (2005) Inhibition of alpha/beta interferon signaling by the NS4B protein of flaviviruses. J Virol 79: 8004-8013.

[89] Munoz-Jordan JL, Sanchez-Burgos GG, Laurent-Rolle M, Garcia-Sastre A (2003) Inhibition of interferon signaling by dengue virus. Proc Natl Acad Sci U S A 100: 14333-14338.

[90] Mackenzie JM, Khromykh AA, Parton RG (2007) Cholesterol manipulation by West Nile virus perturbs the cellular immune response. Cell Host Microbe 2: 229-239.

[91] Blanc M, Hsieh WY, Robertson KA, Watterson S, Shui G, Lacaze P, Khondoker M, Dickinson P, Sing G, Rodriguez-Martin S, Phelan P, Forster T, Strobl B, Muller M, Riemersma R, Osborne T, Wenk MR, Angulo A, Ghazal P (2011) Host defense against viral infection involves interferon mediated down-regulation of sterol biosynthesis. PLoS Biol 9: e1000598.

[92] Saka HA, Valdivia RH (2012) Emerging Roles for Lipid Droplets in Immunity and Host-Pathogen Interactions. Annu Rev Cell Dev Biol.

[93] Hsu NY, Ilnytska O, Belov G, Santiana M, Chen YH, Takvorian PM, Pau C, van der Schaar H, Kaushik-Basu N, Balla T, Cameron CE, Ehrenfeld E, van Kuppeveld FJ, Altan-Bonnet N (2010) Viral reorganization of the secretory pathway generates distinct organelles for RNA replication. Cell 141: 799-811.

[94] den Boon JA, Ahlquist P (2010) Organelle-like membrane compartmentalization of positive-strand RNA virus replication factories. Annu Rev Microbiol 64: 241-256.

[95] Kopek BG, Perkins G, Miller DJ, Ellisman MH, Ahlquist P (2007) Three-dimensional analysis of a viral RNA replication complex reveals a virus-induced mini-organelle. PLoS Biol 5: e220.

[96] Jiang Y, Serviene E, Gal J, Panavas T, Nagy PD (2006) Identification of essential host factors affecting tombusvirus RNA replication based on the yeast Tet promoters Hughes Collection. J Virol 80: 7394-7404.

[97] Serviene E, Jiang Y, Cheng CP, Baker J, Nagy PD (2006) Screening of the yeast yTHC collection identifies essential host factors affecting tombusvirus RNA recombination. J Virol 80: 1231-1241.

[98] Panavas T, Serviene E, Brasher J, Nagy PD (2005) Yeast genome-wide screen reveals dissimilar sets of host genes affecting replication of RNA viruses. Proc Natl Acad Sci U S A 102: 7326-7331.

[99] Serviene E, Shapka N, Cheng CP, Panavas T, Phuangrat B, Baker J, Nagy PD (2005) Genome-wide screen identifies host genes affecting viral RNA recombination. Proc Natl Acad Sci U S A 102: 10545-10550.

[100] Lee WM, Ahlquist P (2003) Membrane synthesis, specific lipid requirements, and localized lipid composition changes associated with a positive-strand RNA virus RNA replication protein. J Virol 77: 12819-12828.

[101] Lee WM, Ishikawa M, Ahlquist P (2001) Mutation of host delta9 fatty acid desaturase inhibits brome mosaic virus RNA replication between template recognition and RNA synthesis. J Virol 75: 2097-2106.

[102] Heaton NS, Perera R, Berger KL, Khadka S, Lacount DJ, Kuhn RJ, Randall G (2010) Dengue virus nonstructural protein 3 redistributes fatty acid synthase to sites of viral replication and increases cellular fatty acid synthesis. Proc Natl Acad Sci U S A 107: 17345-17350.

[103] Cherry S, Kunte A, Wang H, Coyne C, Rawson RB, Perrimon N (2006) COPI activity coupled with fatty acid biosynthesis is required for viral replication. PLoS Pathog 2: e102.

[104] Sharma M, Sasvari Z, Nagy PD (2010) Inhibition of sterol biosynthesis reduces tombusvirus replication in yeast and plants. J Virol 84: 2270-2281.

[105] Sharma M, Sasvari Z, Nagy PD (2011) Inhibition of phospholipid biosynthesis decreases the activity of the tombusvirus replicase and alters the subcellular localization of replication proteins. Virology 415: 141-152.

[106] Vaillancourt FH, Pilote L, Cartier M, Lippens J, Liuzzi M, Bethell RC, Cordingley MG, Kukolj G (2009) Identification of a lipid kinase as a host factor involved in hepatitis C virus RNA replication. Virology 387: 5-10.

[107] Berger KL, Cooper JD, Heaton NS, Yoon R, Oakland TE, Jordan TX, Mateu G, Grakoui A, Randall G (2009) Roles for endocytic trafficking and phosphatidylinositol 4-kinase III alpha in hepatitis C virus replication. Proc Natl Acad Sci U S A 106: 7577-7582.

[108] Sasaki J, Ishikawa K, Arita M, Taniguchi K (2011) ACBD3-mediated recruitment of PI4KB to picornavirus RNA replication sites. Embo J 31: 754-766.

[109] Arita M, Kojima H, Nagano T, Okabe T, Wakita T, Shimizu H (2011) Phosphatidylinositol-4 kinase III beta is a target of enviroxime-like compounds for anti-poliovirus activity. J Virol 85: 2364-2372.

[110] Rothwell C, Lebreton A, Young Ng C, Lim JY, Liu W, Vasudevan S, Labow M, Gu F, Gaither LA (2009) Cholesterol biosynthesis modulation regulates dengue viral replication. Virology 389: 8-19.

[111] Sagan SM, Rouleau Y, Leggiadro C, Supekova L, Schultz PG, Su AI, Pezacki JP (2006) The influence of cholesterol and lipid metabolism on host cell structure and hepatitis C virus replication. Biochem Cell Biol 84: 67-79.

[112] Kapadia SB, Chisari FV (2005) Hepatitis C virus RNA replication is regulated by host geranylgeranylation and fatty acids. Proc Natl Acad Sci U S A 102: 2561-2566.

[113] Takano T, Tsukiyama-Kohara K, Hayashi M, Hirata Y, Satoh M, Tokunaga Y, Tateno C, Hayashi Y, Hishima T, Funata N, Sudoh M, Kohara M (2011) Augmentation of DHCR24 expression by hepatitis C virus infection facilitates viral replication in hepatocytes. J Hepatol 55: 512-521.

[114] Chang KO (2009) Role of cholesterol pathways in norovirus replication. J Virol 83: 8587-8595.

[115] Quetglas JI, Hernaez B, Galindo I, Munoz-Moreno R, Cuesta-Geijo MA, Alonso C Small rho GTPases and cholesterol biosynthetic pathway intermediates in African swine fever virus infection. J Virol 86: 1758-1767.

[116] Wu SX, Ahlquist P, Kaesberg P (1992) Active complete in vitro replication of nodavirus RNA requires glycerophospholipid. Proc Natl Acad Sci U S A 89: 11136-11140.

[117] Rassmann A, Henke A, Jarasch N, Lottspeich F, Saluz HP, Munder T (2007) The human fatty acid synthase: a new therapeutic target for coxsackievirus B3-induced diseases? Antiviral Res 76: 150-158.

[118] Guinea R, Carrasco L (1991) Effects of fatty acids on lipid synthesis and viral RNA replication in poliovirus-infected cells. Virology 185: 473-476.

[119] Yang W, Hood BL, Chadwick SL, Liu S, Watkins SC, Luo G, Conrads TP, Wang T (2008) Fatty acid synthase is up-regulated during hepatitis C virus infection and regulates hepatitis C virus entry and production. Hepatology 48: 1396-1403.

[120] Stapleford KA, Rapaport D, Miller DJ (2009) Mitochondrion-enriched anionic phospholipids facilitate flock house virus RNA polymerase membrane association. J Virol 83: 4498-4507.

[121] Guinea R, Carrasco L (1990) Phospholipid biosynthesis and poliovirus genome replication, two coupled phenomena. Embo J 9: 2011-2016.

[122] Greninger AL, Knudsen GM, Betegon M, Burlingame AL, Derisi JL (2012) The 3A protein from multiple picornaviruses utilizes the golgi adaptor protein ACBD3 to recruit PI4KIIIbeta. J Virol 86: 3605-3616.

[123] Tai AW, Benita Y, Peng LF, Kim SS, Sakamoto N, Xavier RJ, Chung RT (2009) A functional genomic screen identifies cellular cofactors of hepatitis C virus replication. Cell Host Microbe 5: 298-307.

[124] Tai AW, Salloum S (2011) The role of the phosphatidylinositol 4-kinase PI4KA in hepatitis C virus-induced host membrane rearrangement. PLoS One 6: e26300.

[125] Reiss S, Rebhan I, Backes P, Romero-Brey I, Erfle H, Matula P, Kaderali L, Poenisch M, Blankenburg H, Hiet MS, Longerich T, Diehl S, Ramirez F, Balla T, Rohr K, Kaul A, Buhler S, Pepperkok R, Lengauer T, Albrecht M, Eils R, Schirmacher P, Lohmann V, Bartenschlager R (2011) Recruitment and Activation of a Lipid Kinase by Hepatitis C Virus NS5A Is Essential for Integrity of the Membranous Replication Compartment. Cell Host Microbe 9: 32-45.

[126] Borawski J, Troke P, Puyang X, Gibaja V, Zhao S, Mickanin C, Leighton-Davies J, Wilson CJ, Myer V, Cornellataracido I, Baryza J, Tallarico J, Joberty G, Bantscheff M, Schirle M, Bouwmeester T, Mathy JE, Lin K, Compton T, Labow M, Wiedmann B, Gaither LA (2009) Class III phosphatidylinositol 4-kinase alpha and beta are novel host factor regulators of hepatitis C virus replication. J Virol 83: 10058-10074.

[127] Lim YS, Hwang SB (2011) Hepatitis C virus NS5A protein interacts with phosphatidylinositol 4-kinase type IIIalpha and regulates viral propagation. J Biol Chem 286: 11290-11298.

[128] Levental I, Grzybek M, Simons K (2010) Greasing their way: lipid modifications determine protein association with membrane rafts. Biochemistry 49: 6305-6316.

[129] Yu GY, Lee KJ, Gao L, Lai MM (2006) Palmitoylation and polymerization of hepatitis C virus NS4B protein. J Virol 80: 6013-6023.

[130] Weng L, Hirata Y, Arai M, Kohara M, Wakita T, Watashi K, Shimotohno K, He Y, Zhong J, Toyoda T (2010) Sphingomyelin activates hepatitis C virus RNA polymerase in a genotype-specific manner. J Virol 84: 11761-11770.

[131] Ahola T, Lampio A, Auvinen P, Kaariainen L (1999) Semliki Forest virus mRNA capping enzyme requires association with anionic membrane phospholipids for activity. Embo J 18: 3164-3172.

[132] Saito K, Nishijima M, Kuge O (2006) Phosphatidylserine is involved in gene expression from Sindbis virus subgenomic promoter. Biochem Biophys Res Commun 345: 878-885.

[133] Graham TR, Kozlov MM (2010) Interplay of proteins and lipids in generating membrane curvature. Curr Opin Cell Biol 22: 430-436.

[134] Szule JA, Fuller NL, Rand RP (2002) The effects of acyl chain length and saturation of diacylglycerols and phosphatidylcholines on membrane monolayer curvature. Biophys J 83: 977-984.

[135] Fuller N, Rand RP (2001) The influence of lysolipids on the spontaneous curvature and bending elasticity of phospholipid membranes. Biophys J 81: 243-254.

[136] Ono A (2010) Relationships between plasma membrane microdomains and HIV-1 assembly. Biol Cell 102: 335-350.

[137] Waheed AA, Freed EO (2010) The Role of Lipids in Retrovirus Replication. Viruses 2: 1146-1180.

[138] Nayak DP, Balogun RA, Yamada H, Zhou ZH, Barman S (2009) Influenza virus morphogenesis and budding. Virus Res 143: 147-161.

[139] Kalvodova L, Sampaio JL, Cordo S, Ejsing CS, Shevchenko A, Simons K (2009) The lipidomes of vesicular stomatitis virus, semliki forest virus, and the host plasma membrane analyzed by quantitative shotgun mass spectrometry. J Virol 83: 7996-8003.

[140] Mettenleiter TC, Klupp BG, Granzow H (2009) Herpesvirus assembly: an update. Virus Res 143: 222-234.

[141] Condit RC, Moussatche N, Traktman P (2006) In a nutshell: structure and assembly of the vaccinia virion. Adv Virus Res 66: 31-124.

[142] Sodeik B, Krijnse-Locker J (2002) Assembly of vaccinia virus revisited: de novo membrane synthesis or acquisition from the host? Trends Microbiol 10: 15-24.

[143] Chazal N, Gerlier D (2003) Virus entry, assembly, budding, and membrane rafts. Microbiol Mol Biol Rev 67: 226-237, table of contents.

[144] Ghanam RH, Samal AB, Fernandez TF, Saad JS (2012) Role of the HIV-1 Matrix Protein in Gag Intracellular Trafficking and Targeting to the Plasma Membrane for Virus Assembly. Front Microbiol 3: 55.

[145] Vazquez-Calvo A, Saiz JC, Sobrino F, Martin-Acebes MA (2011) Inhibition of enveloped virus infection of cultured cells by valproic Acid. J Virol 85: 1267-1274.

[146] Roingeard P, Hourioux C, Blanchard E, Prensier G (2008) Hepatitis C virus budding at lipid droplet-associated ER membrane visualized by 3D electron microscopy. Histochem Cell Biol 130: 561-566.

[147] Bartenschlager R, Penin F, Lohmann V, Andre P (2011) Assembly of infectious hepatitis C virus particles. Trends Microbiol 19: 95-103.

[148] Shimizu Y, Hishiki T, Ujino S, Sugiyama K, Funami K, Shimotohno K (2011) Lipoprotein component associated with hepatitis C virus is essential for virus infectivity. Curr Opin Virol 1: 19-26.

[149] Majeau N, Fromentin R, Savard C, Duval M, Tremblay MJ, Leclerc D (2009) Palmitoylation of hepatitis C virus core protein is important for virion production. J Biol Chem 284: 33915-33925.

[150] Lindwasser OW, Resh MD (2002) Myristoylation as a target for inhibiting HIV assembly: unsaturated fatty acids block viral budding. Proc Natl Acad Sci U S A 99: 13037-13042.

[151] Moscufo N, Simons J, Chow M (1991) Myristoylation is important at multiple stages in poliovirus assembly. J Virol 65: 2372-2380.

[152] Goodwin S, Tuthill TJ, Arias A, Killington RA, Rowlands DJ (2009) Foot-and-mouth disease virus assembly: processing of recombinant capsid precursor by exogenous protease induces self-assembly of pentamers in vitro in a myristoylation-dependent manner. J Virol 83: 11275-11282.

[153] Aloia RC, Jensen FC, Curtain CC, Mobley PW, Gordon LM (1988) Lipid composition and fluidity of the human immunodeficiency virus. Proc Natl Acad Sci U S A 85: 900-904.

[154] Hirschberg CB, Robbins PW (1974) The glycolipids and phospholipids of Sindbis virus and their relation to the lipids of the host cell plasma membrane. Virology 61: 602-608.

[155] Klenk HD, Choppin PW (1971) Glycolipid content of vesicular stomatitis virus grown in baby hamster kidney cells. J Virol 7: 416-417.

[156] Brugger B, Glass B, Haberkant P, Leibrecht I, Wieland FT, Krausslich HG (2006) The HIV lipidome: a raft with an unusual composition. Proc Natl Acad Sci U S A 103: 2641-2646.

[157] Chan R, Uchil PD, Jin J, Shui G, Ott DE, Mothes W, Wenk MR (2008) Retroviruses human immunodeficiency virus and murine leukemia virus are enriched in phosphoinositides. J Virol 82: 11228-11238.

[158] Gerl MJ, Sampaio JL, Urban S, Kalvodova L, Verbavatz JM, Binnington B, Lindemann D, Lingwood CA, Shevchenko A, Schroeder C, Simons K (2012) Quantitative analysis of the lipidomes of the influenza virus envelope and MDCK cell apical membrane. J Cell Biol 196: 213-221.

[159] Liu ST, Sharon-Friling R, Ivanova P, Milne SB, Myers DS, Rabinowitz JD, Brown HA, Shenk T (2011) Synaptic vesicle-like lipidome of human cytomegalovirus virions reveals a role for SNARE machinery in virion egress. Proc Natl Acad Sci U S A 108: 12869-12874.

[160] Merz A, Long G, Hiet MS, Brugger B, Chlanda P, Andre P, Wieland F, Krijnse-Locker J, Bartenschlager R (2011) Biochemical and morphological properties of hepatitis C virus particles and determination of their lipidome. J Biol Chem 286: 3018-3032.

[161] Moody MA, Liao HX, Alam SM, Scearce RM, Plonk MK, Kozink DM, Drinker MS, Zhang R, Xia SM, Sutherland LL, Tomaras GD, Giles IP, Kappes JC, Ochsenbauer-Jambor C, Edmonds TG, Soares M, Barbero G, Forthal DN, Landucci G, Chang C, King SW, Kavlie A, Denny TN, Hwang KK, Chen PP, Thorpe PE, Montefiori DC, Haynes BF (2010) Anti-phospholipid human monoclonal antibodies inhibit CCR5-tropic HIV-1 and induce beta-chemokines. J Exp Med 207: 763-776.

[162] Teissier E, Zandomeneghi G, Loquet A, Lavillette D, Lavergne JP, Montserret R, Cosset FL, Bockmann A, Meier BH, Penin F, Pecheur EI (2011) Mechanism of inhibition of enveloped virus membrane fusion by the antiviral drug arbidol. PLoS One 6: e15874.

[163] Boriskin YS, Leneva IA, Pecheur EI, Polyak SJ (2008) Arbidol: a broad-spectrum antiviral compound that blocks viral fusion. Curr Med Chem 15: 997-1005.

[164] Wolf MC, Freiberg AN, Zhang T, Akyol-Ataman Z, Grock A, Hong PW, Li J, Watson NF, Fang AQ, Aguilar HC, Porotto M, Honko AN, Damoiseaux R, Miller JP, Woodson SE, Chantasirivisal S, Fontanes V, Negrete OA, Krogstad P, Dasgupta A, Moscona A, Hensley LE, Whelan SP, Faull KF, Holbrook MR, Jung ME, Lee B (2010) A broad-spectrum antiviral targeting entry of enveloped viruses. Proc Natl Acad Sci U S A 107: 3157-3162.

[165] Berkhout B, Eggink D, Sanders RW (2012) Is there a future for antiviral fusion inhibitors? Curr Opin Virol 2: 50-59.

[166] Andrei G, De Clercq E, Snoeck R (2008) Novel inhibitors of human CMV. Curr Opin Investig Drugs 9: 132-145.

[167] Graci JD, Cameron CE (2006) Mechanisms of action of ribavirin against distinct viruses. Rev Med Virol 16: 37-48.

[168] De Clercq E (2009) The history of antiretrovirals: key discoveries over the past 25 years. Rev Med Virol 19: 287-299.

[169] Olschlager S, Neyts J, Gunther S (2011) Depletion of GTP pool is not the predominant mechanism by which ribavirin exerts its antiviral effect on Lassa virus. Antiviral Res 91: 89-93.

[170] Liu Z, Guo Z, Wang G, Zhang D, He H, Li G, Liu Y, Higgins D, Walsh A, Shanahan-Prendergast L, Lu J (2009) Evaluation of the efficacy and safety of a statin/caffeine combination against H5N1, H3N2 and H1N1 virus infection in BALB/c mice. Eur J Pharm Sci 38: 215-223.

[171] Brett SJ, Myles P, Lim WS, Enstone JE, Bannister B, Semple MG, Read RC, Taylor BL, McMenamin J, Nicholson KG, Nguyen-Van-Tam JS, Openshaw PJ (2011) Pre-admission statin use and in-hospital severity of 2009 pandemic influenza A(H1N1) disease. PLoS One 6: e18120.

[172] Mihaila R, Nedelcu L, Fratila O, Rezi EC, Domnariu C, Ciuca R, Zaharie AV, Olteanu A, Bera L, Deac M (2009) Lovastatin and fluvastatin reduce viremia and the pro-inflammatory cytokines in the patients with chronic hepatitis C. Hepatogastroenterology 56: 1704-1709.

[173] Bader T, Fazili J, Madhoun M, Aston C, Hughes D, Rizvi S, Seres K, Hasan M (2008) Fluvastatin inhibits hepatitis C replication in humans. Am J Gastroenterol 103: 1383-1389.

[174] Gilbert C, Bergeron M, Methot S, Giguere JF, Tremblay MJ (2005) Statins could be used to control replication of some viruses, including HIV-1. Viral Immunol 18: 474-489.

[175] Giguere JF, Tremblay MJ (2004) Statin compounds reduce human immunodeficiency virus type 1 replication by preventing the interaction between virion-associated host intercellular adhesion molecule 1 and its natural cell surface ligand LFA-1. J Virol 78: 12062-12065.

[176] Montoya CJ, Jaimes F, Higuita EA, Convers-Paez S, Estrada S, Gutierrez F, Amariles P, Giraldo N, Penaloza C, Rugeles MT (2009) Antiretroviral effect of lovastatin on HIV-1-infected individuals without highly active antiretroviral therapy (The LIVE study): a phase-II randomized clinical trial. Trials 10: 41.

[177] Poh MK, Shui G, Xie X, Shi PY, Wenk MR, Gu F (2012) U18666A, an intra-cellular cholesterol transport inhibitor, inhibits dengue virus entry and replication. Antiviral Res 93: 191-198.

[178] Huang H, Chen Y, Ye J (2007) Inhibition of hepatitis C virus replication by peroxidation of arachidonate and restoration by vitamin E. Proc Natl Acad Sci U S A 104: 18666-18670.

[179] Bianco A, Reghellin V, Donnici L, Fenu S, Alvarez R, Baruffa C, Peri F, Pagani M, Abrignani S, Neddermann P, De Francesco R (2012) Metabolism of phosphatidylinositol

4-kinase IIIalpha-dependent PI4P Is subverted by HCV and is targeted by a 4-anilino quinazoline with antiviral activity. PLoS Pathog 8: e1002576.

[180] Tatematsu K, Tanaka Y, Sugiyama M, Sudoh M, Mizokami M (2011) Host sphingolipid biosynthesis is a promising therapeutic target for the inhibition of hepatitis B virus replication. J Med Virol 83: 587-593.

[181] Umehara T, Sudoh M, Yasui F, Matsuda C, Hayashi Y, Chayama K, Kohara M (2006) Serine palmitoyltransferase inhibitor suppresses HCV replication in a mouse model. Biochem Biophys Res Commun 346: 67-73.

[182] Amemiya F, Maekawa S, Itakura Y, Kanayama A, Matsui A, Takano S, Yamaguchi T, Itakura J, Kitamura T, Inoue T, Sakamoto M, Yamauchi K, Okada S, Yamashita A, Sakamoto N, Itoh M, Enomoto N (2008) Targeting lipid metabolism in the treatment of hepatitis C virus infection. J Infect Dis 197: 361-370.

[183] Gower TL, Graham BS (2001) Antiviral activity of lovastatin against respiratory syncytial virus in vivo and in vitro. Antimicrob Agents Chemother 45: 1231-1237.

[184] Weitz-Schmidt G, Welzenbach K, Brinkmann V, Kamata T, Kallen J, Bruns C, Cottens S, Takada Y, Hommel U (2001) Statins selectively inhibit leukocyte function antigen-1 by binding to a novel regulatory integrin site. Nat Med 7: 687-692.

[185] Weitz-Schmidt G (2003) Lymphocyte function-associated antigen-1 blockade by statins: molecular basis and biological relevance. Endothelium 10: 43-47.

[186] Weitz-Schmidt G (2002) Statins as anti-inflammatory agents. Trends Pharmacol Sci 23: 482-486.

[187] Harrison SA, Rossaro L, Hu KQ, Patel K, Tillmann H, Dhaliwal S, Torres DM, Koury K, Goteti VS, Noviello S, Brass CA, Albrecht JK, McHutchison JG, Sulkowski MS (2010) Serum cholesterol and statin use predict virological response to peginterferon and ribavirin therapy. Hepatology 52: 864-874.

[188] Mihaila RG, Nedelcu L, Fratila O, Retzler L, Domnariu C, Cipaian RC, Rezi EC, Beca C, Deac M (2011) Effects of simvastatin in patients with viral chronic hepatitis C. Hepatogastroenterology 58: 1296-1300.

[189] Patel K, Lim SG, Cheng CW, Lawitz E, Tillmann HL, Chopra N, Altmeyer R, Randle JC, McHutchison JG (2011) Open-label phase 1b pilot study to assess the antiviral efficacy of simvastatin combined with sertraline in chronic hepatitis C patients. Antivir Ther 16: 1341-1346.

[190] Kwong JC, Li P, Redelmeier DA (2009) Influenza morbidity and mortality in elderly patients receiving statins: a cohort study. PLoS One 4: e8087.

[191] Cenedella RJ (2009) Cholesterol synthesis inhibitor U18666A and the role of sterol metabolism and trafficking in numerous pathophysiological processes. Lipids 44: 477-487.

[192] Halvorson DL, McCune SA (1984) Inhibition of fatty acid synthesis in isolated adipocytes by 5-(tetradecyloxy)-2-furoic acid. Lipids 19: 851-856.

[193] Seronello S, Ito C, Wakita T, Choi J (2010) Ethanol enhances hepatitis C virus replication through lipid metabolism and elevated NADH/NAD+. J Biol Chem 285: 845-854.

[194] Loftus TM, Jaworsky DE, Frehywot GL, Townsend CA, Ronnett GV, Lane MD, Kuhajda FP (2000) Reduced food intake and body weight in mice treated with fatty acid synthase inhibitors. Science 288: 2379-2381.

[195] Kuhajda FP, Landree LE, Ronnett GV (2005) The connections between C75 and obesity drug-target pathways. Trends Pharmacol Sci 26: 541-544.

[196] Wang C, Gale M, Jr., Keller BC, Huang H, Brown MS, Goldstein JL, Ye J (2005) Identification of FBL2 as a geranylgeranylated cellular protein required for hepatitis C virus RNA replication. Mol Cell 18: 425-434.

[197] Shaltiel G, Shamir A, Shapiro J, Ding D, Dalton E, Bialer M, Harwood AJ, Belmaker RH, Greenberg ML, Agam G (2004) Valproate decreases inositol biosynthesis. Biol Psychiatry 56: 868-874.

[198] Tokuoka SM, Saiardi A, Nurrish SJ (2008) The mood stabilizer valproate inhibits both inositol- and diacylglycerol-signaling pathways in Caenorhabditis elegans. Mol Biol Cell 19: 2241-2250.

[199] Xu X, Muller-Taubenberger A, Adley KE, Pawolleck N, Lee VW, Wiedemann C, Sihra TS, Maniak M, Jin T, Williams RS (2007) Attenuation of phospholipid signaling provides a novel mechanism for the action of valproic acid. Eukaryot Cell 6: 899-906.

[200] Soares MM, King SW, Thorpe PE (2008) Targeting inside-out phosphatidylserine as a therapeutic strategy for viral diseases. Nat Med 14: 1357-1362.

[201] Gerber DE, Stopeck AT, Wong L, Rosen LS, Thorpe PE, Shan JS, Ibrahim NK (2011) Phase I safety and pharmacokinetic study of bavituximab, a chimeric phosphatidylserine-targeting monoclonal antibody, in patients with advanced solid tumors. Clin Cancer Res 17: 6888-6896.

[202] Knight ZA, Gonzalez B, Feldman ME, Zunder ER, Goldenberg DD, Williams O, Loewith R, Stokoe D, Balla A, Toth B, Balla T, Weiss WA, Williams RL, Shokat KM (2006) A pharmacological map of the PI3-K family defines a role for p110alpha in insulin signaling. Cell 125: 733-747.

[203] Arita M, Wakita T, Shimizu H (2009) Cellular kinase inhibitors that suppress enterovirus replication have a conserved target in viral protein 3A similar to that of enviroxime. J Gen Virol 90: 1869-1879.

[204] De Palma AM, Thibaut HJ, van der Linden L, Lanke K, Heggermont W, Ireland S, Andrews R, Arimilli M, Al-Tel TH, De Clercq E, van Kuppeveld F, Neyts J (2009) Mutations in the nonstructural protein 3A confer resistance to the novel enterovirus replication inhibitor TTP-8307. Antimicrob Agents Chemother 53: 1850-1857.

[205] Heinz BA, Vance LM (1995) The antiviral compound enviroxime targets the 3A coding region of rhinovirus and poliovirus. J Virol 69: 4189-4197.

[206] Miller ME, Adhikary S, Kolokoltsov AA, Davey RA (2012) Ebolavirus requires acid sphingomyelinase activity and plasma membrane sphingomyelin for infection. J Virol. 86:7473-7483.

[207] Ciesek S, Steinmann E, Manns MP, Wedemeyer H, Pietschmann T (2008) The suppressive effect that myriocin has on hepatitis C virus RNA replication is independent of inhibition of serine palmitoyl transferase. J Infect Dis 198: 1091-1093.

[208] Doucleff M (2010) Select: Lipids out loud. Cell 143: 853-855.

Chapter 14

The Role of Altered Lipid Metabolism in Septic Myocardial Dysfunction

Luca Siracusano and Viviana Girasole

Additional information is available at the end of the chapter

http://dx.doi.org/10.5772/51001

1. Introduction

Despite the novel pathogenetic and therapeutic acquisitions sepsis remains the main cause of death in the critically ill patient (p.). The incidence of sepsis is increasing, with more than 750 000 cases occurring in the United States every year; sepsis is complicated by organ dysfunction giving rise to severe sepsis which causes more than 200 000 deaths each year [1]. The cardiovascular syndrome is the cause of the major part of the fatalities leading to the picture of the septic shock with 90,000 deaths annually. The myocardial dysfunction in sepsis has been widely studied and many causes of heart dysfunction have been described. The presence of a metabolic compromise is well known in chronic heart failure and has been considered as a basis for contractile failure, interestingly similar alterations have been recently described also in sepsis. The purpose of this study is to examine the current available data on this topic.

Sepsis has been defined as the systemic host reaction to an infection [2]. The typical immune response in sepsis presents a first stage, characterized by an increased production of proinflammatory Interleukins (ILs) by monocytes, macrophages. lymphocytes and endothelial cells in response to a few molecules, common to all virulent pathogens, called pathogen-associated molecular patterns (PAMPs) [3]. They are recognized by receptors on the surface of the immune cells, named Pattern Recognition Receptors (PRP) the most important being the Toll-like Receptors (TLRs), existing in 13 different types each recognizing a different microbial constituent. TLR are an important component of immune activity programmed to respond quickly to the infectious challenges by recognizing PAMP. Lipopolysaccharide (LPS) in particular is recognized by the complex TLR4-CD14 in the plasma membrane and the inflammatory signal is transduced by the recruitment of the adaptor molecules that associate with the intracellular Toll/interleukin-1 receptor (TIR) domain of the TLR to initiate signal transduction. Of these adaptor molecules myeloid differentiation primary- response protein 88 (MyD88) is associated with all TLRs except TLR3 while the TIR-domain containing adaptor inducing interferon (IFN)-β (TRIF) is only associated to TLR3 [3]. Both of them lead to nuclear factor-κB (NF-kB) activation and induction of over 150 inflammatory and procoagulant genes with increased expression of the proinflammatory ILs tumor necrosis factor α(TNFα), IL1β, IL6, interferon γ (IFNγ), chemokines and cell adhesion molecules. This phase, named Systemic Inflammatory Reaction Syndrome (SIRS) is followed by a second phase, the compensatory anti- inflammatory response syndrome (CARS), that modulates SIRS through death by apoptosis of immune cells, gene silencing of the pro-inflammatory genes and increased production of the contra-inflammatory ILs IL10, IL4 and TGFβ [4-6] Through this biphasic reaction in the largest part of the cases the homeostasis is re-established. It is possible however that during the proinflammatory phase because of the "cytokine storm"-induced organ damage, further increased through the release by the injured tissue of the endogenous damage-associated molecular pattern (DAMPs or alarmins such as hig mobility group protein B1(HMBG1), hyaluronan, HSP, proteins S100 etc), as more frequently occurs in young and reactive people, or during the contra-inflammatory phase, due to immunosuppression and diffuse infection, death may ensue [4]. The normal biphasic reaction may be altered when sepsis is present in very old and diseased persons that frequently present a mild phase of SIRS or do not present it at all; in the later stages it seems that immunosuppression is almost always present [7]. Indeed from what has been described it seems that in both the cases sepsis is characterized by an "altered immune response", unbalanced [8] with prevalence of an excessive proinflammatory reaction in the early phase and a prevalent immunosuppression in the late phase [8.] The definition of sepsis based on the recent achievement on this topic could be reconsidered focusing more on the immune status, we propose the sequent definition: " sepsis is the altered immune response to an infectious challenge, either increased or decreased, and followed by a compromised organ function". The passage from the SIRS to the CARS is marked by the phenomenon of LPS tolerance [9]: the prolonged stimulation of TLR4, the specific receptor for endotoxin, by LPS leads to the silencing of proinflammatory genes and to the stimulation of the contra-inflammatory ones through a process of gene reprogramming [10] with increased expression of IL-10, TGF-β, and type I IFNs. Neutrophil function is seriously impaired in sepsis with the development of a decreased ability to migrate into the infection site, related to the severity of the disease [for review see 11]. During this stage macrophages exhibit an increased phagocytic ability but an altered capacity of antigen presentation due to reduced expression of several major histocompatibility complex (MHC) Class II molecules (e.g. HLA-DRs) with impaired T-cell proliferation as well as reduced production of IFNγ. This phase corresponds also to a stage of ischemic tolerance caused by the reduced production of NF-kB responsible for the amplification of the damage induced by ischemia [12]. TLRs are indeed involved in the tissue damage caused by non-infectious challenges such as ischemia-reperfusion injury (IRI), burns, surgery, trauma etc. because they mediate the inflammatory reaction to the alarmins released by these noxae: the deletion of TLR2 and TLR4 may reduce the cellular damage in these settings [13-14].The mitochondrial DNA released after tissue damage may be recognized by TLRs, behaving as a DAMP for its far origin by bacteria according to endosymbiotic theory; its experimental infusion may cause a picture similar to the ARDS [15]. TLRs are also important to explain the link between inflammation and metabolic alterations [16] and the state of low grade inflammation present for so far unknown reasons in obesity, metabolic syndrome, diabetes and in chronic myocardial ischemia; moreover they may also be involved in the adipose tissue dysfunction described during sepsis [17,18]. One of the main problems in the study of sepsis has been its experimental reproduction: the LPS infusion method, used also at low doses in human volunteers, is not reliable because it reproduces only the proinflammatory phase and led in the past to misunderstand the complex regulation of immunity in sepsis, moreover in this model is lacking an infectious focus. The availability of successive different models such as the infusion of living bacteria and the cecal ligation and puncture (CLP), at present considered a good reproduction of human septic peritonitis, allowed further progress supplying models similar to human sepsis [19].

2. Metabolic response in sepsis and injury

The first phase of sepsis, coincident with SIRS and also called flow phase, is characterized by a state of hypercatabolism with negative nitrogen balance induced by the increase in proinflammatory ILs and stress hormones, while the anabolic ones are reduced. This phase is also marked by hyperglycemia, hyperlactatemia and increased energy expenditure varying with the nature of the injurious stress (15-20% after surgery, 20-40% in sepsis and up to 120% in burns [20]). Injury in general and sepsis in particular are associated with an increased protein breakdown (mainly derived by the muscle representing the main store of proteins in the body, up to 40% of total body proteins), protein catabolism in sepsis may reach 260 gr\day [21] corresponding to a loss of 1 Kg muscle, with negative nitrogen balance, an increased blood pool of amino acids (a.a.), used in the liver for neoglucogenesis and the production of acute phase proteins, and reduced uptake of a.a. by the muscle. The protein utilization as a fuel is opposite to the normal and rapidly depletes body lean mass. The increased production of IL-1β, IL-6 and TNFα causes protein catabolism both directly and indirectly through the stimulation of the Hypothalamus–Pituitary-Adrenal (HPA) axis [22]. The increased protein catabolism may be reproduced by counter-regulatory hormones infusion.

2.1. Glucose metabolism and insulin sensitivity in sepsis

Insulin resistance may be defined as the inability of insulin to adequately stimulate glucose uptake in the muscle or to inhibit gluconeogenesis in the liver [23]. The pathogenesis of the insulin resistance is no more interpreted on the basis of the glucocentric but of the lipocentric theory [24] stating that the excess of circulating free fatty acids (FFA), the main competitive inhibitors of glucose utilization in the cell, when present in excess in plasma because of increased lipolysis, decreased fat storing capacity of adipose tissue or reduced fatty acid oxydation (FAO) may accumulate in the organs (liver, myocardium, pancreas etc) giving origin to reduced sensitivity to insulin, increased hepatic glucose output and to the phenomenon of lipotoxicity, syndrome characterized by accumulation of FFA in the cell, increased production of reactive oxygen species (ROS), activation of apoptosis (lipoapoptosis) and organ dysfunction [25]. The etiology of insulin resistance in sepsis is related to the increase of the contra-insular substances (glucagon, TNFα, growth hormone, cortisol) and to the reduced expression of the insulin-sensitizing adiponectin while the endogenous insulin secretion in the critically ill p. is increased as occurs in the early phase of type II diabetes mellitus, on the contrary of what was suggested in the past [26]. The consequences of the metabolic storm in sepsis are an increased hepatic production of glucose, a reduced glucose uptake by insulin-dependent tissues, increased levels of FFA- consequence of the increased lipolysis- reduced FAO and reduced insulin sensitivity at the muscular and hepatic level [27]. The high levels of blood glucose allow a high uptake by the non-insulin-dependent cells because of the increased expression of the stress- and Ils-dependent glucose transporter GLUT1 [27]. In this way a high rate of glucose oxidation through mitochondria is made possible leading to an enhanced production of ROS: the increased oxidative and nitrosative stress, chiefly in presence of a reduction in ROS scavengers, -mainly glutathione[28]- typical of the critical states, may damage mainly the Complexes I and III of the electron transport chain (ETC) initiating the mitochondrial dysfunction. Insulin is provided with an anti-inflammatory action that is missing if a reduced sensitivity to its action is present, such as in critical illness, further increasing inflammation [27]. Proinflammatory ILs interfere with insulin activity through multiple mechanisms ; 1) TNFα and other cytokines activate Jun-N-terminal kinase (JNK) responsible for serine phosphorylation of the insulin receptor substrate 1 (IRS-1) at Ser 307, so disrupting insulin signalling [29] 2) furthermore JNK activation has been showed, in LPS-induced experimental sepsis, to depress PPARα expression reducing FFA oxidation [30]; JNK inhibition prevented cardiac dysfunction, despite continued induction of inflammatory markers, demonstrating that there is a dysmetabolic basis for LPS-induced cardiac dysfunction in this experimental setting [30]. An important clinical application of the role played by the altered glucose metabolism in the critically ill p. derived from the Leuven Study [31] that showed a striking reduction from 8% to 4,6% in the mortality of critically ill surgical p. receiving mechanical ventilation by maintaining glycemia between 80 and 110 mg% with intensive insulin therapy. However in 2009 the NICE SUGAR Study showed that a blood glucose target of 180 mg% or less per deciliter resulted in lower mortality than did a target of 81 to 108 mg range, probably by reducing the incidence of hypoglycaemia [32]. A diffuse coverage of this matter is beyond the scope of this report (for review see reference [33]).

Hyperlactatemia in sepsis has been considered as a consequence of the establishment of an hypoxic environment, this concept is however no longer tenable, except for the p. in septic shock, because in many organs an increased oxygen saturation has been showed both in clinical sepsis and after LPS infusion [34]. Currently the cause of hyperlactatemia is considered to be the increased expression of Hypoxia-inducible factor1 (HIF-1)- and of cytokines activating PDHK4, an enzyme inhibiting PDH (pyruvate dehydrogenase) through phosphorylation so preventing the transformation of pyruvate into acetyl-CoA and its oxidation through the TCA (Tricarboxilic acid Cycle); the excess of pyruvate is transformed into lactate by Lactate dehydrogenase (LDH) through a process called accelerated aerobic glycolysis [35-38]. The plasma levels of lactate seems to be related to the outcome [35].

2.2. TG and FFA utilization in the normal heart

In a physiological environment rich in oxygen but also in pathophysiological conditions (like diet rich in lipids, starvation or diabetes) the heart can utilize all metabolites but it prefers FFA oxidation, from which it gets 60-90% of the necessary energy, obtaining the remaining part from the oxidation of glucose and ketone bodies [39]. The myocardiocyte gets FFA mainly taking up tryglicerides (TG)-rich lipoproteins (LP) (chylomicrons and very low-density lipoprotein, VLDL) through the endothelial lipoprotein lipase (LPL), enzyme present in the capillary endothelium and bound to it through a proteoglycan, the Glycosylphosphatidyl-inositol high density lipoprotein-binding protein 1 (GPIHBP1), which anchors LPL to endothelium and serves as a bridge allowing LP uptake[40]. The myocardial cells may take up FFA also from the albumin-bound pool (10 time less abundant). FFA obtained from hydrolysis of TG by LPL or transported by albumin are then taken up by the myocardiocyte, through transporters, mainly FAT\CD36 (50-60%) but also by fatty acid binding protein (FABP) and fatty acid transport plasma membrane (FATPpm), only a very small part is taken up by diffusion [41]. Once transported into the cytosol, FFAs are esterified to long chain acyl CoA by fatty acyl CoA synthase (FACS) and transported for FFA oxidation(FAO) across mitochondrial membrane. This process is carried out in three steps: at first acyl-CoA is metabolized into acyl-carnitine by the enzyme carnitine palmitoyl transferase-1 (CPT-1), located on the outer mitochondrial membrane. Acyl-carnitine is hence transported across the inner mitochondrial membrane by carnitine translocase (CAT) and again transformed into long chain Acyl-CoA and carnitine by CPT- 2 (carnitine shuttle) [42]. The step catalyzed by CPT-1 is the rate-limiting reaction of FAO and the activity of this enzyme is strictly regulated by malonyl-CoA (the product of carboxylation of acetyl-CoA), whose levels are controlled by a balance between the activity of the enzymes involved in its metabolism, the acetyl CoA carboxylase (ACC) and malonyl CoA decarboxylase. AMP-activated protein kinase (AMPK), a fundamental energy sensor in the cell, controls this reaction phosphorylating and inhibiting ACC whenever it senses a decrease in the ATP\AMP ratio [42]. In the normal heart, 75% of the fatty acids taken up are immediately oxidized. Acetyl-CoA has a central role in the regulation of the utilization of the substrates: it is the metabolic product of both glucose (through pyruvate) and fatty acid utilization. It may be utilized for oxidation in the Krebs cycle or, if the cellular level of ATP is high, used for FFA synthesis. Acetyl-CoA may also be transformed into pyruvate and lactate by LDH in the presence of hypoxia but also when it is produced in huge quantities. More than 40 years ago Randle described the reciprocal inhibition exercised by glucose and FFA utilization [43]. He displayed in the isolated heart and in a skeletal muscle preparation that the oxidation of one substrate inhibited directly, without hormonal intermediation, the use of the other (Randle cycle). So an increase in FAO causes a proportional decrease in glucose oxidation and uptake leading to hyperglycemia. The actual interpretation of Randle cycle is that an increase in serum concentration and uptake of FFA activates FAO and causes accumulation of its byproducts as ROS, ceramides, diacylglycerol, acyl-carnitine and fatty acyl-CoAs inside the skeletal muscle so depressing glucose uptake, whereas in the liver they inhibit insulin-mediated suppression of glycogenolysis and gluconeogenesis [44-45]. Also the increased lipolysis present in many conditions (fasting, exercise, inflammatory conditions, diabetes and obesity) leading to an increased FAO may downregulate glucose utilization through increased serum FFA and reduced insulin sensitivity. All these signals, particularly diacylglycerol, interfere with insulin signalling activating PKC novel isoforms ($\delta,\varepsilon,\eta,\theta$) causing a reduced tyrosine phosphorylation of the IRS-1 which is normally responsible for the activation through phosphatidyl inositol 3-kinase (PI3K) and Akt of the membrane translocation of the insulin-dependent glucose transporter 4 (GLUT4)[46]. So an increase in FAO causes a proportional decrease in glucose uptake and oxidation with hyperglycemia. This mechanism has been considered important in the pathophysiology of diabetes mellitus type2 (T2DM). Conversely glucose uptake and oxidation to acetyl CoA and pyruvate involves the conversion to malonylCoA by ACC leading to inhibition of CPT-1 and consequently of FAO; moreover insulin decreases lipolysis and the level of FFA. During starvation increased lipolysis raises FFA uptake and oxidation inhibiting glucose oxidation and favouring accumulation of pyruvate and lactate redirected to glycogen synthesis allowing also glucose sparing for the brain. Conversely after a glucose rich meal the increased uptake and utilization of glucose inhibit the utilization of FFA through the accumulation of malonylCoA. The normal heart responds to an increase in workload by switching from FFA to preferential glucose utilization. The Randle cycle explains how the heart regulates the fuel selection in the short term to face physiologic challenges however the long-term adaptation to physiologic and pathophysiologic conditions is mediated by translational and post-translational modifications rather than by the metabolic ones. A fitting example is the metabolic switch occurring after birth. During the fetal life the heart, probably because of the relatively hypoxic medium, relies more on carbohydrate metabolism, whereas in the adult myocardiocyte glycogen occupies less than 2% of the cell volume, in the fetal cells it represents more than 30% of the cell volume [47]. After birth the heart, due probably to the increased availability of oxygen, prefers FFA oxidation because of the discontinuous availability of metabolites and the elevated fat content of mother's milk; the metabolic shift is accompanied by increased expression of the enzymes involved in FAO. The utilization of both lipid and carbohydrates has advantages and drawbacks: the complete oxidation of a molecule of palmitic acid (molecular mass 256,43) yields more ATP (105 molecules vs 31) but consumes much more oxygen (46 atoms vs 12) than the oxidation of a molecule of glucose. Moreover the oxidation of lipid produces more oxidative stress, a drawback partially corrected by the increased production of the uncoupling protein 3(UCP3) and differently from anaerobic glycolysis it is not available in hypoxic or ischemic settings. Such long term substrate modifications are transcriptionally regulated and the switch to carbohydrate utilization is due to a downregulation of the nuclear receptors PPARα involved in the transcription of the enzymes of FFA transport and utilization.

The key enzyme in the regulation of pyruvate metabolism is the PDH. The activity of cardiac PDH is mainly modulated by the PDH kinase (PDHK4), an isoform of the kinase phosphorylating and transforming PDH from the active to the inactive form. Short-term metabolic inhibition of PDHK4 is affected by pyruvate while its activation is affected by acetyl CoA and NADH. The long-term regulation is determined by many conditions characterized by insulin deficiency (diabetes) or resistance (starvation, high-fat diet, and hyperthyroidism) that increase PDHK expression, while insulin suppresses its production [35,36,38].

3. The metabolic myocardial switch

In pathological conditions a long term modification in substrate preference may be present: the diabetic heart relies almost exclusively on FAO [48], on the contrary the myocardium submitted to mechanical, ischemic\hypoxic or inflammatory stress switches to the anaerobic glycolysis, which can also continue in an environment poor in oxygen. Even though glycolysis allows a much lesser production of energy (2 molecules of ATP instead of 36 per molecule of glucose oxidized) through the transformation of pyruvate into lactate by LDH it presents the advantage to go on also in a hypoxic setting; however this process, which in the short-term is adaptive, in the long-term becomes maladaptive because of the reduced energy production [49]. The better the heart defends itself in the presence of stressful events, the more easily it is able to switch to the type of metabolism more efficient in that situation and the more it is provided with metabolic flexibility. Thus the survival of the myocardium depends, in these conditions, on an increased supply of glucose that is assured by the augmentation of the main transmembrane glucose transporters, GLUT1 and GLUT4. GLUT1 is present ubiquitously, augments in presence of reduced glucose levels and during inflammatory, metabolic and osmotic stress [50]; GLUT4 is present in the adipose tissue, heart, liver and in the striated muscle and is the typical insulin-dependent transporter. The increase in glucose transporters, mainly in GLUT1, has an adaptive meaning in the stressed heart; its overexpression protects against experimental ventricular hypertrophy, at least until cardiac failure appears, causing its downregulation [51].

This metabolic remodelling seems to be controlled by the fetal gene program, so called because it is present in the fetal environment, relatively hypoxic, and is reactivated whenever a stressful situation is present [47,52]. It modifies the expression of contractile proteins switching the expression of heavy myosin chain (HMC) from the more efficient but more energy expensive alpha to the slower but less energy consuming beta isoform, and increases the production of some humoral factors (brain natriuretic peptide, BNP) and of several protective proteins (heat shock proteins, HSP). The cardioprotective pathway of the PI3K and Akt, activated during pre- and post-conditioning, is also activated by the fetal gene program supplying an antiapoptotic protection and leading to an overlapping between cardioprotection in chronic ischemia and ischemic preconditioning [52]. The metabolic component is mainly regulated by the enzyme pyruvate deydrogenase kinase (PDHK4) phosphorylating and inactivating pyruvate deydrogenase (PDH) and inhibiting the transformation into Acetyl-CoA that could enter the TCA; it is instead transformed into lactate by LDH allowing a continued production of ATP also in low oxygen settings. This activation of glycolysis, such as the dependent increase in GLUT1,4, in LDH and glycolytic enzymes is mainly controlled by the transcription factor HIF-1 that is upregulated in the settings of ischemia\hypoxia but also in non-hypoxic conditions such as during inflammatory states and tumours because its expression is increased through a cross-talk with NF-kB [53]. On the other hand hypoxia and inflammation are not completely separated conditions as showed by the induction of TLR4 and TLR6 by HIF-1 during hypoxia [54]. HIF-1 is composed by a constitutively expressed HIF-1β subunit and an oxygen-sensitive HIF-1α subunit, target under normoxic conditions of three prolyl hydroxilases 1,2,3(PDH1,2,3), the hydroxylation allows the binding of the von Hippel-Lindau protein (VHL) and the consequent ubiquitination and proteasome degradation of HIF-1α. On the contrary during hypoxia PDH2 activity is reduced with accumulation of HIF-1α, its dimerization with HIF-1β and the expression of many target genes [55].

The increased expression of HIF-1 causes at the same time a downregulation of mitochondrial lipid oxidation depressing the expression of the transcription factor PPARα (possessing a DNA consensus motif for HIF-1)[56] and an upregulation of PPARγ activating fatty acid uptake and glycerolipid biosynthesis so leading to lipotoxicity [57]. HIF-1 stimulates also mitochondrial autophagy to rebalance the reduced oxidation with mitochondrial mass[58]. The stimulation of glycolysis by HIF-1 has an important role in sepsis because the phagocytes use huge quantities of glucose through glycolysis in the hypoxic environment of the inflamed tissues either for cell migration either for phagocytosis and bacterial killing [59]. The activity of HIF-1 is regulated by acetylation performed by CBP\p300 and inhibited by deacetylation by SIRT1. The inverse shift to mitochondrial lipid oxidation is controlled by SIRT1 which increases the expression of PGC-1α with simultaneous activation of both mitochondrial biogenesis and lipid oxidation through PPARα upregulation. SIRT1 and HIF-1 are reciprocally regulated so that in the hypoxic\inflammatory setting HIF-1α is activated while Sirt1 is decreased due to NAD^+ scarcity so inhibiting HIF-1α deacetylation and inactivation while in normoxic environment HIF-1α is inactivated by oxygen-dependent prolyl hydroxylases PHD2 activated by SIRT1.

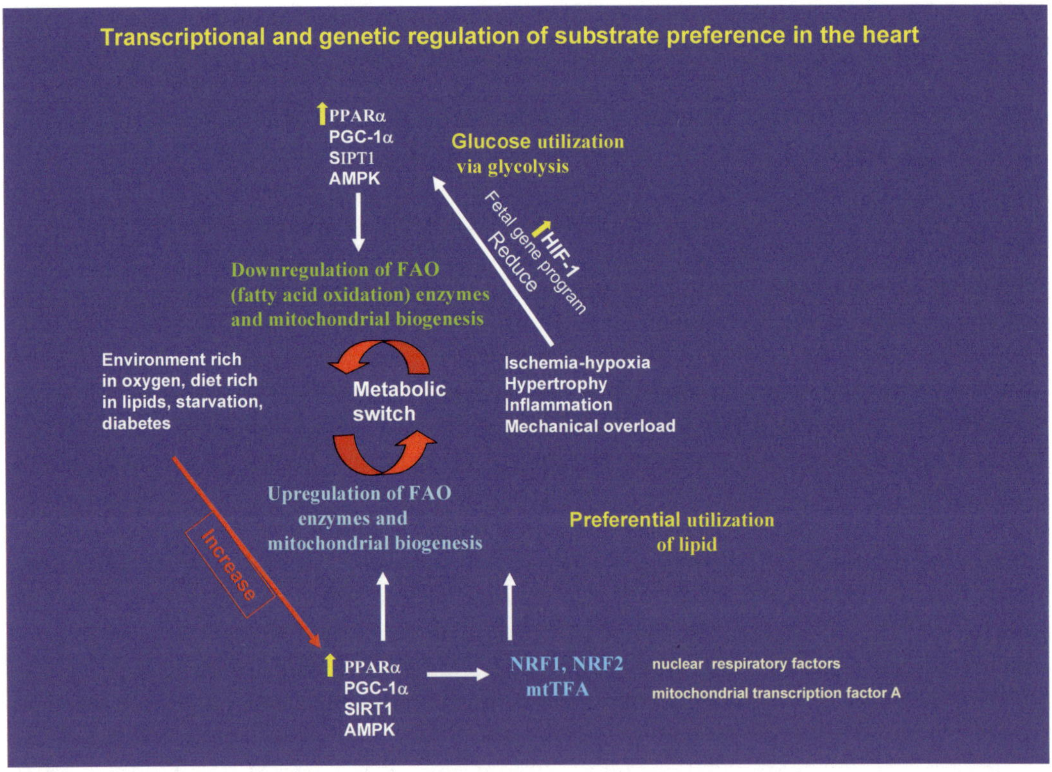

Figure 1. Metabolic switch. See text for explanation.

Sirtuins are class III NAD^+-dependant histone deacetylases (HDAC) targeting histones, transcription factors and enzymes regulating in this way gene expression and metabolic function in relation to the energy status of the cell [60-64]. They have been related to the regulation of metabolism, apoptosis and inflammation, to extending life span and to the healthy aging. Sirtuins exist in seven forms with different subcellular localization: SIRT1,6,7 present in nucleus, SIRT2 in cytoplasm, SIRT3,4,5 in the mitochondria. Because they are mainly regulated by the levels of NAD^+, the AMPK that increases its concentration upregulates their expression while the DNA-repairing enzyme poly(ADP-ribose) polymerase 1 (PARP), activated whenever there is an oxidative stress and consuming for its activity high quantities of NAD^+, downregulates sirtuin expression . SIRT1 is able to deacetylate and activate a series of transcription factors involved in many steps of metabolism (AMPK, FOXO, HIF-1, PGC-1α, p53, NF-κB, PPARα and β, LXR,FXR,ERR). Mitochondrial sirtuins are in a critical location to regulate metabolism and biogenesis of the organelles controlling oxidative phosphorylation (OXPHOS), intracellular Calcium and the production of ROS [65]. SIRT1 is also regulated via microRNA: microRNA34a downregulates its expression metabolically and microRNA199a in the hypoxic setting [66,67]. Statins have been showed to upregulate SIRT1 expression in endothelial cells contributing possibly to improve clinically endothelial function [68].

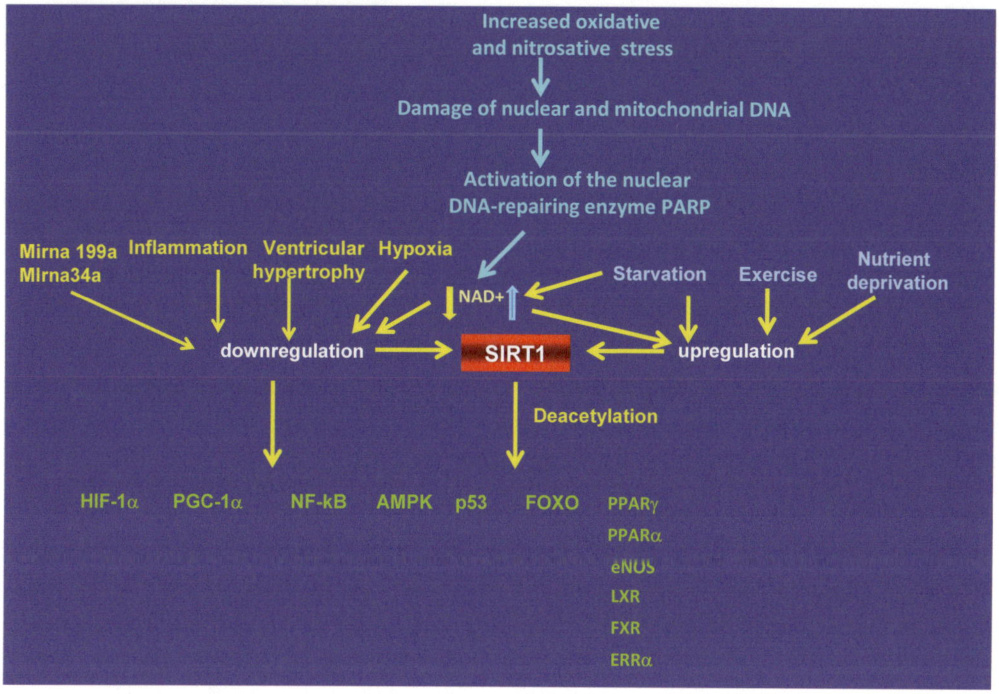

Figure 2. Regulation of SIRT1 expression. See text for explanation.

4. Transcriptional regulation of FFA transport, uptake and oxidation

Transport, uptake and oxidation of FFA in the cell is a process tightly regulated by several transcription factors belonging to the nuclear hormone receptor superfamily. The nuclear receptors involved include the peroxisome proliferator-activated receptors (PPARs), liver X receptors (LXRs), farnesoid X receptor (FXR) and ERR (estrogen related receptor), which bind and are activated by lipids, acting as sensors of endocrine signals and of dietary components and planners of the physiological response to nutrients. PPARs, the most important of them, are present in three types (alpha, beta and gamma), besides their action as lipids sensors, they are involved in the regulation of lipid and glucose metabolism, insulin sensitivity and modulation of inflammation (for review see [69-71]); their actions are partially overlapping with a certain degree of redundancy but they are not coincident. In elucidating the function of PPARs an important role has been played by the studies in genetically modified mice with overexpression or deletion of these nuclear receptors. PPARs are activated by endogenous ligands, FFA or their derivatives (arachidonic acid, eicosanoids, leukotrienes and oxidized lipoproteins) but there are also known exogenous ligands, used as drugs, for PPARα (fibrates) and PPARγ (thiazolidinediones) or for both PPARα and γ (muraglitazar) [72].

The PPARs form heterodimers with retinoid X receptors (RXR) and bind to consensus DNA sequences in the promoter of the target genes, the PPAR response binding element (PPRE), formed by two hexameric nucleotides sequences separated by one base pair. In the absence of ligands the heterodimer binds with the co-repressors, blocking gene transcription; when activated by ligands, the complex, because of a change of conformation, releases the co-repressors and recruits the co-activators and the RNA polymerase giving rise to transcription. PPARα are expressed mainly in tissues with high oxidative metabolism such as heart, muscle and liver. PPARγ are expressed at high levels only in adipose tissue where they regulate the maturation and fat deposition in adipocytes so indirectly regulating, through the plasma level of FFA, the insulin sensitivity; they are however expressed at low level in many organs among which the heart [73]. Whereas PPARα and γ share the ability to activate the transcription of proteins involved in FFA uptake, storage and oxidation, PPARβ only activate the proteins involved in FFA oxidation. Also different are the effects on glucose metabolism: PPARα depress glucose oxidation whereas PPARβ activate glycolysis (through PDHK4 activation) and glucose uptake; PPARγ activate only glucose uptake [69,74].

PPARβ\δ are expressed in various tissues where they regulate lipid but even glucose metabolism. PPARγ also regulate mitochondrial biogenesis through interaction with the PPARγ coactivator 1 (PGC-1) network (see below)[74]. Because FAO takes mainly place in mitochondria (only the breakdown of very long chain fatty acids, subsequently converted to medium chain fatty acids and shuttled to mitochondria, takes place in the peroxisomes) there is a common regulatory mechanism for FAO and mitochondrial biogenesis controlled by PPARs and by the network of PGC-1. The PPARγ mainly but also the PPARα, have been showed, in several model systems, to modulate inflammation by transrepressing target genes of the transcription factors NF-κB, nuclear factor of activated T cells (NFAT), activator protein 1 (AP1) and signal transducers and activators of transcription (STATs) through a process called transrepression [75-77] so modulating the action of lymphocytes, macrophages and dendritic cells. This process has twofold importance, on the one side it may regulate the inflammation induced by tissue macrophages, involved in the low grade inflammation and important in dysmetabolic conditions such as reduced insulin sensitivity, metabolic syndrome and atherosclerosis on the other side it may be of critical interest in regulating inflammatory reaction in sepsis [78]. LXRs and FXR heterodimerize also with RXR and are activated respectively by oxysterol and bile acids: both exist in the isoforms α and β, contribute to lipid and lipoprotein regulation and modulate inflammation. In the regulation of FAO a fundamental role is also played by the orphan receptor (transcription factors without an identified endogenous ligand) ERR (estrogen related receptor) involved also in the regulation of mitochondrial biogenesis, gluconeogenesis and oxidative phosphorylation by interacting with PPARα and γ and PGC-1 [79].

5. TG delivery: Lipolysis

The amount of lipid in the myocardial cell is regulated by the balance between TG delivery to the heart through the VLDL- regulated by lipolysis- and the oxidation of TG in the myocardiocyte. Considering their importance in cellular signalling, lipid synthesis and as energy substrates, the level of circulating TG and FFA is tightly regulated [80]. Adipocytes are the only cells able to hydrolize TG giving rise to FFA and glycerol utilized by other tissues. This process is initiated by the adipose triglyceride lipase (ATGL) catalysing the hydrolysis of triglycerides to diglycerides followed by the hydrolysis of diglycerides to monoglycerides by the hormone-sensitive lipase (HSL) able also to catalyse the first phase and of monoglycerides to TG and glycerol by the monoglyceride lipase (MGL)[81-83]. ATGL deficiency is associated with fat deposition in all tissues indicating that ATGL is rate limiting in the catabolism of cellular fat depots [84]. Lipolysis is also regulated by perilipin , a protein coating the lipid droplets, that exposes TG of a lipid droplet to the action of the lipases [85].

Many substances may activate physiologically and in diseases HSL, the more important enzyme for its sensitivity to the hormonal regulation but also for its action modulating adipogenesis and adipose metabolism [86]. Catecholamines acting through β_1, β_2 and also β_3 receptors coupled to a G stimulating (G_s) protein are the main stimulators of HSL; the $alpha_2$ receptors inhibit instead lipolysis through a G inhibitory (G_i) protein, this effect may be antagonized by administration of beta-blockers. Also natriuretic peptides are able to enhance lipolysis by activating guanylyl cyclase and increasing cGMP [83]. TNFα, IL1β and IL6 increase HSL activity through the stimulation of several kinases of the MAP kinase cascade (janus kinases (JNK), p44\42 and extracellular signal-regulated kinase-1/2 (ERK1/2) and the consequent increase in cAMP [87,88]. These kinases phosphorylate perilipin allowing HSL and ATGL to access and hydrolyse TG; this effect was prevented by metformin [89].

LPS may activate lipolysis by increasing ILs level, the demonstration however that the inhibition of TNF-alpha, IL1 and cathecolamines could not prevent lipolysis in endotoxemic rats, led to show a direct lipolytic action carried out by low-dose endotoxin [90].This action is not mediated by an increase in cAMP, activation of PKA or PKC or inhibition of NFkB but through phosphorylation of perilipin by LTR4 and ERK1/2.

The main inhibitor of lipolysis is insulin through the insulin-like receptor substrates 1and 2(IRS-1and 2) that activate the phosphaditYl inositol 3-kinase(PI3K) complex and phosphorylate and activate the phosphodiesterase 3(PDE-3) [80]. Insulin acts also via an Akt-Independent PI3K-dependent signalling pathway which modifies PKA phosphorylation of perilipin [91]. The reduction in insulin activity is responsible for increased lipolysis in diabetes and obesity together with the reduction in the insulin-sensitizing activity of adiponectin [92] probably linked to the adipose tissue dysfunction described in sepsis [17,18]. Moreover adiponectin may reduce fat deposition in visceral adipose tissue increasing the deposit in the subcutaneous compartment through PPARγ upregulation [18]. The lipolytic activity is differently regulated in subcutaneous and visceral fat: the former, more important for the basal activity, is more sensitive to the antilipolytic action of insulin, the latter is mainly activated during hormonal stimulation and provides FFA directly to the liver through the portal circulation in physiological and pathophysiological situations. In sepsis seems to be present a failure of adipocytes differentiation leading to a decreased storage ability of the subcutaneous tissue allowing FFA to be accumulated in visceral fat (with an increase in the metabolic and cardiovascular risk) and in organs giving rise to lipotoxicity for the concomitant reduction of FAO [18]. Lipolysis is increased in sepsis [14] due to a raised activity of the lipases of the adipose tissue, mainly the HSL, because of the increased plasma level of catecholamines, ILs and natriuretic peptides and the reduced activity of insulin and adiponectin (fig 3).

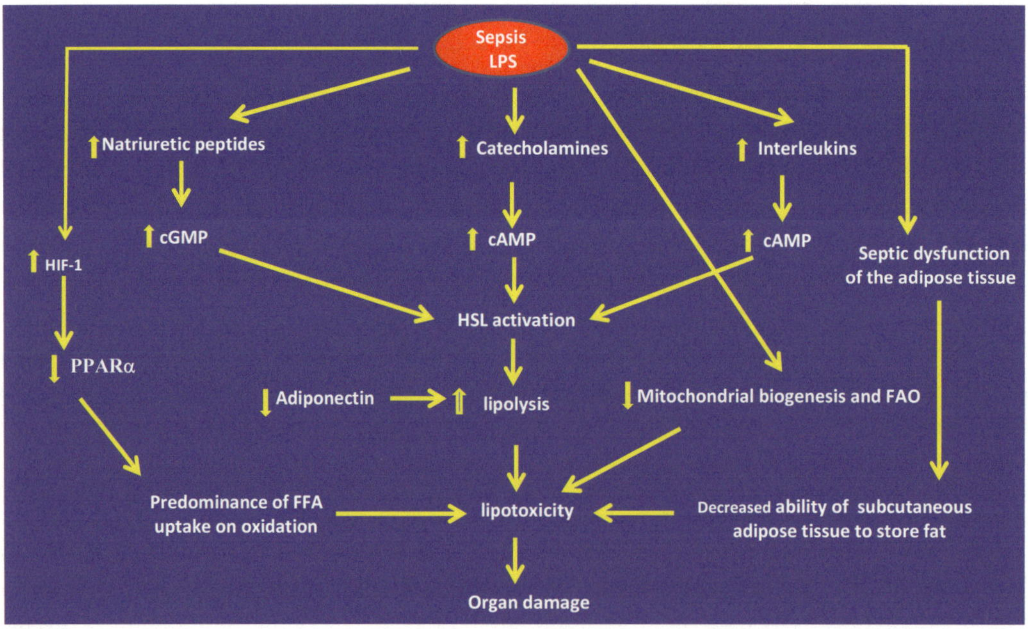

Figure 3. Lipolysis in sepsis. See text for explanation.

5.1. Lipoprotein metabolism in sepsis

Sepsis and inflammation reproduce an atherogenic picture of serum lipoproteins [93] with an early reduction -preceding even the change in leukocytes- of total HDL- and LDL-cholesterol, an increase in VLDL and TG justified by augmented liver synthesis and lipolysis, a reduction in HDL phospholipids compensated by an increase in VLDL phospholipids.

5.2. HDL in sepsis

Until recently HDL were considered as devoted only to reverse cholesterol transport (RCT), a process through which the cholesterol is transferred from the cells to the acceptor apolipoproteinA-1 by the specific transporter A binding cassette 1(ABC1) and delivered to the liver where it is finally secreted and eliminated in the bile, the only way of its removal from the body. The recent application in this field of the Gel Filtration Chromatography based proteomics revealed that HDL contain not only apo-A1, apo-A2 and some enzymatic and transfer protein involved in cholesterol transport but more than 50 other associated proteins [94]. Many of the proteins isolated carry out functions completely different from RCT belonging to the complement proteins (C3,C1 inhibitor, factor H) and to serine protease inhibitors (SERPIN) [95-97]. The recent attainments point to an important role of HDL in immunity and in the modulation of the inflammatory response but they are also involved in a lot of disparate functions ranging from glucose metabolism to endothelial protection displaying also an antithrombotic action (for review see [98,99]). Of main importance in sepsis is the property of HDL to bind and neutralize LPS, mediated through its content in phospholipids.

HDLs may carry out anti-inflammatory actions in many ways: they downregulate the proinflammatory transcription factor NF-kB through a not yet completely understood mechanism -probably by the reduced degradation of Inhibitor kappa-B-a (IkB-a) [100]-, moreover they reduce the expression of the adhesion molecules CD11b and MCP-1 on human monocytes [97] and may curtail TNF-alpha production and upregulate IL-10 production by lymphocytes. The normal anti-inflammatory function of HDLs turns into a proinflammatory one during the acute phase reaction (APR) when they become dysfunctional [101]. The reasons for this change are manifold: there is a reduction in ApoA-1 levels, partially substituted by serum amyloid A apolipoprotein (Apo-SAA), their size is smaller because of a reduced activity of lecytin cholesterol acyl transferase (LCAT), enzyme deputed to esterification of cholesterol that allows the enlargement of HDL, HDLs become poorer in the antioxidant enzymes paraoxanase [102,103].

The interference with the function of the inflammatory cells may be direct or mediated by the effect of the HDL on the reduction of cellular cholesterol and of cholesterol-enriched microdomains or rafts of their plasma membrane; this is also showed by the increased lethality and inflammatory response observed during sepsis in transgenic null mice for critical receptors involved in cholesterol efflux as SR-BI and ACBA1 [104].

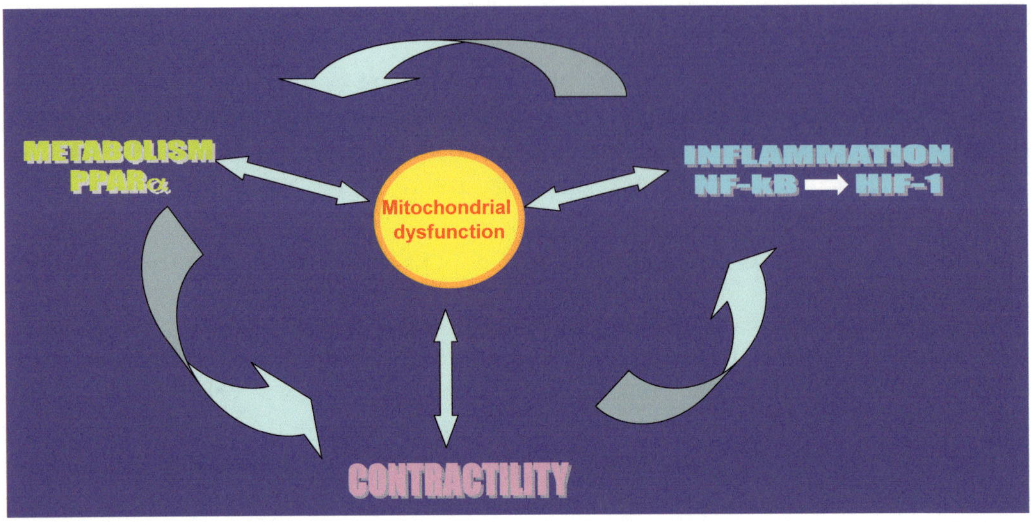

Figure 4. Relationships among mitochondrial dysfunction, metabolism, and contractility. See text for explanation.

HDL may bind and inactivate LPS mainly through their phospholipid component [105,106], in sepsis and inflammation because of the HDL reduction their LPS inhibiting function is assumed by the VLDL phospholipids.

Also the endothelial function is modified through an increased production of nitric oxide (NO) by the stimulation of endothelial nitric oxide synthase (eNOS) mediated by the activation of the protective PI3K\Akt pathway leading to vasodilation, antiadhesion and anti-inflammatory effects [107]. A similar cardioprotective and antiapoptotic action of HDL have been shown through the activation of Stat3 mediated by sphingosine 1 phosphate (S1P), one of their common component [108]. The recombinant HDL(rHDL) or HDL mimetics, currently under clinical trial, are provided with the same actions attributed to the HDL [109,110]. The level of total, HDL- and LDL-cholesterol is decreased in septic and critically ill patients, as well as in experimental animals infused with LPS and proinflammatory cytokines and the decrease is negatively related to IL6 and TNFa concentrations [111]; HDL reduction is also related to mortality and severity of the disease [105,106].

The reduced level of serum HDL and cholesterol in sepsis is explained by a reduced RCT [112] mediated by the LPS-induced downregulation of the scavenger receptors SR-B1 and ABCA1 [113]. The sequestration of the cholesterol into the cell may be useful in the short term, due to the increased delivery to the immune cells, but harmful in the long run because of the decreased delivery to the steroidogenetic and liver cells and to the atherogenic picture it induces.

5.3. VLDL

VLDL are a circulant reservoir of TG and FFA able to activate PPARα and γ [114]. In clinical sepsis and experimental endotoxemia the serum level of VLDL, FFA and TG is increased due to the upregulation of the hepatic synthesis of TG, FFA and apoB, to the increased lipolysis, decreased lipid oxidation and inhibition of LPL [103]. The increased lipolysis in sepsis is due to the activation of the hormone-sensitive lipase (HSL) by catecholamines acting through PKA stimulation and cAMP increase. To the increased lipolysis contribute also the increased level of ILs, of natriuretic peptides and the reduction in insulin and adiponectin activity (see paragraph on lipolysis).

Feingold, in mice, showed that LPS reduced in the heart, diaphragm and kidneys [115-117] the levels of many enzymes involved in the fatty acid metabolism (FATP1,MCAD, CD36, CPT1β etc) through the reduced expression of many transcription factors: PPARα and γ, LXRα, FXRα, pregnane X receptors and their coactivators PPARγ coactivator 1α and β (PGC-1α and β), steroid coactivator receptor 1 and 2 (SRC1-2) and ERRα. The downregulation of the nuclear receptors can be reproduced by IL-1 and TNFα administration. Maitra and colleagues described an important role for IRAK1, a signalling component downstream of TLR4, in the downregulation of these transcription factors in sepsis showing that IRAK1 $^{-/-}$ mice were protected against alterations in lipid metabolism [118]. Because all these factors are deacetylated and activated by SIRT1 their downregulation in sepsis may play an important causative role [68] (see the paragraphs on metabolic switch and mitochondrial dysfunction).

The increase in VLDL during sepsis, traditionally considered as a reaction mobilizing lipid stores to delivery an increased amount to the immune cells, may also have a protective meaning: the increased level of serum VLDL and of their content in phospholipids can substitute for the HDL in binding and neutralizing LPS [119,120].

6. Mitochondrial dysfunction play an important role in septic cardiomyopathy

Mitochondrial dysfunction -present in sepsis but also in many other pathological states such as chronic heart failure, diabetes mellitus, metabolic syndrome and several neurodegenerative diseases- is a syndrome characterized by a picture of reduced oxygen consumption, ineffective ATP production, increased accumulation of ROS and calcium in the organelle leading to the opening in the internal mitochondrial membrane of a high conduction pore allowing the entry of solutes until a molecular weight of 1.500, with mitochondrial swelling, collapse of the electron gradient, release of proapoptotic proteins and death of the organelle (mitoptosis) followed by mitophagy: this phenomenon called mitochondrial permeability transition pore (MPTP) has an important role in sepsis and its inhibition may experimentally improve septic myocardial dysfunction [28,121-123].

Mitochondrial functionality is regulated by the equilibrium between de novo mitochondrial formation (mitochondrial biogenesis) and mitochondrial autophagy (mitophagy), frequently preceding whole cell autophagy. This latter process, taking place only in deenergized organelles, is very important for cell survival because it allows the elimination of dysfunctional mitochondria, producing too much radical oxygen species(ROS) and assures the high quality of the mitochondria provided with a high membrane potential and resistant to MPTP [124]. Moreover autophagy has been shown to be protective in ischemia-reperfusion injury (IRI) and inflammation by inhibiting the exposition of mtDNA and the consequent activation of the inflammasome NALP3 [125]. Autophagy involves a complex molecular machinery including more than 30 Atg (AutophaGy-related) proteins and 50 lysosomal hydrolases [126].

The mitochondrial biogenesis is orchestrated by PPARα and β\δ, by the ERRα and above all by the network PGC-1α, PGC1– β and PGC-1 related coactivator (PRC), factors enriched in tissues with high oxidative capacity (heart, muscle, brown adipose tissue and kidneys) and highly inducible by starvation, exercise and cold acclimation (126-128); PGC1-β is also induced by Ils [129]. Mice with single deficiency in PGC-1α or PGC1-β display only minimal alteration under nonstressed conditions and have a normal mitochondrial mass [130,131] whereas mice with double deletion of both PGC-1 forms died shortly after birth with small hearts, bradycardia, intermittent heart block, and a markedly reduced cardiac output [132], allowing to think that one isoform may compensate for the other. Mitochondrial biogenesis to take place needs the transcription of the genes controlled by mitochondrial DNA, a process activated by the mitochondrial transcription factor A (Tfam), a nuclear-encoded transcription factor essential for replication, maintenance and transcription of mitochondrial DNA [133]. The majority of the genes codifying mitochondrial proteins are however present in nuclear DNA and are activated, such as Tfam, by the nuclear respiratory factors 1 and 2 (NRF1 and NRF2). PGC-1 coordinates the function of NRF1, NRF2 and Tfam, regulating mitochondrial biogenesis and, through the complex PPARs-ERRs, controls FAO such that a prompt adaptive response to physiological events as cold acclimation, exercise, starvation etc may be possible with selection of the most suitable level of FFA oxidation needed in the particular situation.

Cardiac contractile activity is linked to the mitochondrial biogenesis because an increase in intracellular calcium increases the expression of PGC-1 via calcineurin (CaN) -activating also PPARα promoter and FAO- and Ca-calmodulin dependent kinase (CaMK), a process requiring cAMP response element-binding protein (CREB)(126,133): in this way the contractile activity is strictly linked to the metabolism and to the mitochondrial oxidative function.

PGC-1 expression is also controlled hormonally by tyroid hormones (TH), metabolically via adrenergic system and cAMP, by AMPK and p38 MAPK through phosphorylation [126,133] and by eNOS-produced NO. The cellular mitochondrial content is proportional to the energy requirement [75], mitochondrial biogenesis is therefore controlled by the two main energy sensors in the cell: Sirt1(silent mating type information regulator 2 homolog 1) and AMPK act coordinately to control PGC-1 activity respectively through deacetylation and phosphorylation. Sirtuins are class III histone deacetylating enzymes supplied by AMPK with the adequate level of the NAD^+, essential activator of Sirt1 that in turn deacetylates PGC-1 and activates its gene expression [75]. Sirt1 is also an important in vivo regulator of mitophagy by deacetylation of the autophagy genes Atg5, Atg7 and Atg8 [134], linking this protective mechanism, devoted to the clearance of depotentiated mitochondria, with PGC-

1a mediated biogenesis. For biogenesis to occur it is necessary mitochondria undergo the processes of fusion and fission regulated respectively by mitofusins (Mfn1-2) and by dynamin-related protein(DRP1 and OPA1) [126].

The first description of mitochondrial dysfunction in sepsis dates back to 1970′ [135,136], but the initial studies were not reliable due to inadequate techniques to test mitochondrial function. More recent studies however linked the altered oxygen utilization and ATP production in sepsis to mitochondrial dysfunction (137,138), even though there are substantial differences among the sepsis model induced by LPS administration in which is present a widespread mitochondrial damage and the CLP model characterized by a less evident mitochondrial pathology because damaged organelles undergo autolysis and autophagy [139]. Several alterations have been described in mitochondria in experimental and human sepsis both morphological (swelling, destruction of cristae, decreased electron density, breaks in membrane and altered outer membrane integrity) and biochemical (release of cytochrome c, decreased mtDNA copy number, reduced activity of Complexes I and III) [28,140,141]; their extent has been related to outcome [142]. Several studies showed an initial increase of mitochondrial activity in sepsis, followed by a reduction. Singer [132] hypothesized that, after a metabolic stimulation of mitochondrial function. caused by the excessive inflammatory response, in the successive phase there is a metabolic downregulation determined by the mitochondrial dysfunction. In this latter phase a stimulation of oxygen consumption (VO2) would be harmful because it forces mitochondria, adapted to a reduction of metabolism, to overwork without being prepared for it. The restorative phase of sepsis is linked to the activation of mitochondrial biogenesis; also LPS may have a role in inducing this process [140,143]. The absence of relevant cell death by apoptosis or necrosis in parenchymatous organs and the ability also of the tissues with less regenerative capacity to recover led to think that multiple organ dysfunction syndrome (MODS) were related mainly to a functional compromise mediated by endocrine and metabolic alterations and provided with a protective role [144-146]. In sepsis a paradoxical increase has been observed, in some tissue, in blood oxygen saturation [147], related to outcome and linked to an altered mitochondrial oxygen utilization (cytopathic hypoxia) [148], which has been attributed to nitric oxide (NO) overproduction by mitochondrial nitric oxide synthase (mtNOS) [149,150] or other NOS isoforms: NO competitively inhibits oxygen binding to cytochrome c oxydase (COX) determining a tonic inhibition of mitochondrial oxygen consumption, reversible on inhibiting its excessive production [151]. The exact role of NO inhibition by COX in vivo in physiologic and pathologic conditions is however an unsettled problem [152]. Other gaseous molecules share with NO the ability to interact with COX, to inhibit it competitively and to regulate at this level the body oxygen consumption [153,154]; they are called gasotransmitters and include carbon monoxide (CO) and Hydrogen Sulphide (H_2S), this latter molecule was first shown able to induce experimentally in mice, but not in pigs and superior mammals, a particular state of depression of the metabolism and of the resistance to hypoxia, called "suspended animation" (155]. A similar observation has been made with NO and CO in Drosophila [156,157]. Exploiting this property of gasotransmitters in the treatment of myocardial and cerebral hypoxia\ischemia is tempting, considered also the limitations of the current treatment with hypothermia of the hypoxic organ injury, even though they also have a high toxicity [158]. To the picture of metabolic hibernation may contribute, besides NO, also CO and H_2S increased during sepsis [159-161].

In addition to the antagonism against COX the higher levels of NO, in presence of an increased oxidative stress, by reacting with superoxide, may further injure mitochondria determining the formation of the toxic peroxynitrite able to damage the Complex I and III of the ETC, the membrane lipid and mitochondrial and nuclear DNA. The available data however cannot be explained only by this mechanism; the metabolic ebb phase, coincident with CARS and silencing of proinflammatory genes, is characterized by a profound state of mitochondrial depression, reduced oxidative metabolism and oxygen consumption leading to a state of metabolic hibernation responsible for the depressed cell function during MODS in sepsis; mitochondrial depression is however completely reversible on recovery from sepsis. Recently Schilling and colleagues showed that LPS administration through TLR4 stimulation may induce a fuel switch from preferential myocardial use of lipid to glycolysis, similar to the one observed in the failing heart, with decreased mitochondrial oxidation, lipid accumulation within them and a suppression of the genes encoding PGC-1α and β: the genetic overexpression of PGC-1β may restore mitochondrial function independently of the inflammatory response [162]. Smeding and colleagues [163], on the other hand, observed that the sirtuin activator resveratrol protect mitochondria in a mice model of CLP improving myocardial dysfunction, preserving energy production but without improving survival. At this point some question should be raised: could we think that the mitochondrial dysfunction is a reversible event even in the presence of a continuing sepsis? Which may be the correct link and the ordinated succession among all the alterations described?

We try to reconstruct the successive steps leading to mitochondrial dysfunction and to metabolic hibernation in sepsis (fig. 5). The first step is the hypercatabolic phase with the transient activation of mitochondrial oxidative phosphorylation (OXPHOS) activated by the acute hormonal stress response in the very early phase, with increased oxidative and nitrosative stress damaging ETC and inducing a downregulation of many of its proteins. Immediately after, in the inflammatory setting of sepsis, occurs the shift to glycolysis and the activation of mito autophagy. SIRT1 is rapidly deactivated by the reduced function of AMPK, the decreased NAD^+ levels due to the activation of PARP and by the increased expression of miR199a [66]. The stimulation of this enzyme in sepsis was first showed by Fink [148]; recently Zhang and colleagues, after LPS administration in mice, observed that the plasma levels of ATP, SIRT1 and AMPK decline precipitously after 10′ and remain below the detection level for up to 12 h while HIF-1 increases contemporarily along with an increase in mitochondrial autophagy. Importantly all these effects are absent in wild type mice treated with resveratrol but not in Sirt1 liver knockout mice [164]. This study further confirm the critical role of SIRT1 that would be downregulated in sepsis for many causes: increased HIF-1 expression, increased miR199a expression, drastic reduction of NAD^+ by activation of PARP consuming it and reduced activity of AMPK supplying it. The main consequence of these modifications are the reduced deacetylation by SIRT1 and phosphorylation by AMPK of PGC-1α, also PGC1$-\beta$ seems to be reduced in muscle during sepsis [162,165] making impossible a compensation. The role of PARP has also been showed by Soriano in the setting of human septic myocardiopathy [166], where the degree of myocardial compromise related well with the staining for the product of activated PARP [poly(ADP-ribose) (PAR)], and in many experimental model of cardiovascular diseases[167] in which PARP inhibitors provide significant benefits. Interestingly the metabolic hibernation in sepsis according to our hypothesis has a different starting point from the true mammals hibernation in which the scarcity of nutrients leads to increased levels of NAD+ and AMP with AMPK and SIRT1 activation and deacetylation of clock protein BMAL1 and the opposite switch from glucose to lipid metabolism [168]. The connection between bioenergetics impairment and inflammation in sepsis has also been studied by Liu and colleagues [169-170] that underline the role of Sirt1 in reprogramming immune response through the silencing of the proinflammatory genes and the coordination of the metabolic response. In the experimental setting many attempts have been made to treat mitochondrial dysfunction by supplying substrates, cofactors, mitochondrial-targeted antioxidants, scavengers of mitochondrial ROS and membrane stabilizers displaying improvements at many levels: ATP production, reduced production of ROS in mitochondrial ETC, reduction of apoptosis and prevention of MPTP opening [171-174]. Apoptosis may also have a role in septic mitochondrial dysfunction as it has in CHF. Lancel and colleagues demonstrated in cardiomyocytes isolated 4 hours after endotoxin injection in rats, an increase in the release of caspase-3, -8, and -9-like activities, associated with destruction of the sarcomeric structure and cleavage of components of the cardiac myofilament [175]. Simvastatin, whose use has been proposed in sepsis, may protect against apoptosis induced by Staphylococcus aureus alpha-toxin [176].

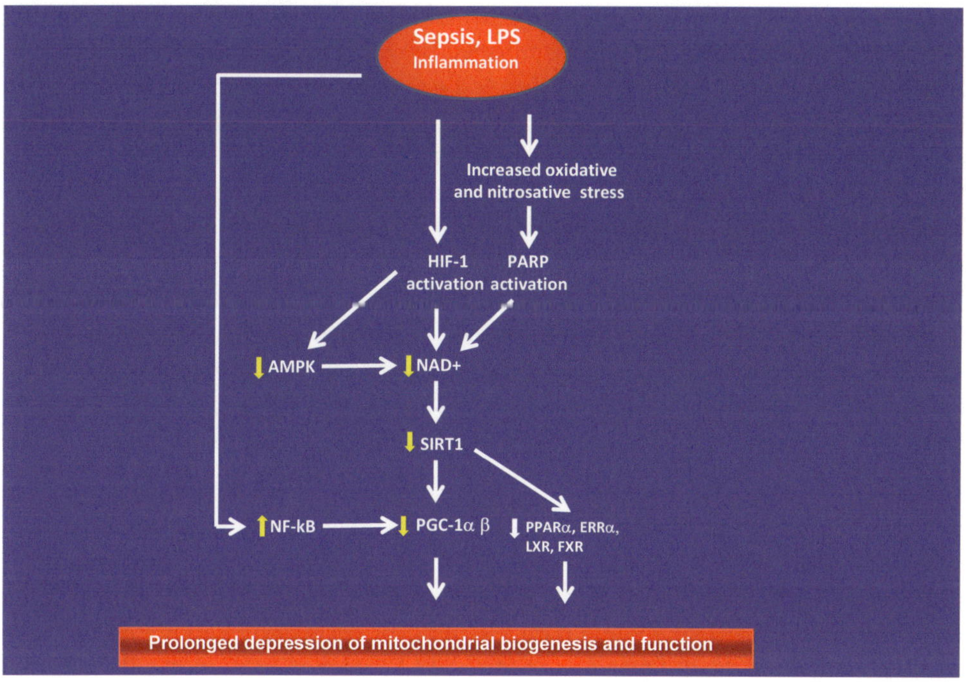

Figure 5. Mitochondrial dysfunction in sepsis. See text for explanation

6.1. Cardiac function in sepsis

The pathogenesis of the myocardial dysfunction in sepsis is not definitively explained and is probably caused by a myriad of alterations. The morphological picture recognized in sepsis was formerly considered unspecific but more recently many interesting alterations have been described even though certainly some of them are not the cause but the consequence of the acute cardiac damage. Beside not specific alterations such as cell edema, the already described mitochondrial lesions, damage of cytoplasmic membrane and myofibrils, inflammatory cells infiltration [139,177], more definite biochemical and microscopic changes have been observed with lipid infiltration [178], increased deposits of glycogen and increased levels of glucose uptake, GLUT1 and GLUT4 [141], increased sarcolemmal permeability [179], disruption of sarcolemmal dystrophin and beta-dystroglycan [180].

6.2. Hemodynamic pattern

Parker and colleagues in 20 p. in septic shock [181], adequately resuscitated, with the combined use of radionuclide-gated cardiac cineangiography and thermodilution observed important differences in the hemodynamic pattern of survivors and non survivors. Both groups had a hyperdynamic pattern with high cardiac index (CI) and low systemic vascular resistance (SVR) but survivors had an important LV dilatation and a reduced left ventricle ejection fraction (LVEF) normalizing in 7-10 days while non survivors paradoxically showed higher LVEF but did not show ventricular dilatation. On the basis of these data Parker thought that LV dilatation were an adaptive mechanism apt to increase systolic stroke through a better utilization of Starling mechanism (early preload adaptation). Successive studies by echocardiography have not confirmed however a significant LV dilatation while observing an altered biventricular relaxation and a systolic dysfunction of the right ventricle in 41% of the p, isolated or in conjunction with a LV dysfunction [182-185].The apparently better cardiac function in non survivors is currently perceived as a consequence of the persistent septic hemodynamic pattern with decreased SVR causing higher CI and LVEF, both being heavily load-dependent indexes [186]. A LV depressed contractile performance is constant in human and experimental sepsis [187] if related to pre and after-load, it is explained by the global ventricular hypokinesia observed in 60% of the p. in septic shock [188]: the impairment of LV contractility may be unravelled also by the reduction of CI in response to norepinephrine infusion [181]. A feature of septic myocardiopathy is the absence of the increased LV filling pressure, characteristic of cardiogenic shock, due to the dysfunction of the right ventricle [189] and to the slightly increased LV compliance [190]

Currently the hyperkinetic syndrome (small left ventricle, supranormal ejection fraction, tachycardia, high cardiac index) had a 100% mortality rate [186]. In contrast with the majority of other reports Jianhui and colleagues (describe in mice infused with intraperitoneal LPS and studied with left ventricular (LV) pressure-volume catheters significant drop in LV stroke volume with a significant decrease in LVEF with no apparent change in LV afterload. load-dependent indexes of LV function were markedly reduced at 6 h, including EF, stroke work, and dP/dtmax. In contrast, there was no reduction of load-independent indexes of LV contractility leading the authors to think that the depressed contractility after LPS infusion was due only to loading conditions [191].

6.3. Pathophysiological mechanism

The infusion of small doses of LPS in healthy volunteers may reproduce the features of the septic circulatory dysfunction with low systemic resistances and a depressed myocardial function [187]. The mechanism of the altered myocardial function, at first attributed to a myocardial depressant factor (MDF) [192], began to be understood when in 1985 Parrillo [193] showed that the serum of septic humans during the acute phase may depress the contractile function of isolated myocardiocytes; this effect may be prevented, as subsequently demonstrated by Kumar, by immunoadsorption of IL-1β and TNFα [194]. Ils may cause myocardial depression both directly or through the NO produced by the induction of iNOS [195]. In the recent years the focus of the research has been turned on the upstream mediators of ILs, the TLRs, that have been shown to be main mediators of myocardial damage in sepsis models of both LPS infusion and CLP and in human sepsis [196]. Their effect as already seen is due to the release, consequent to the inflammatory reaction and to the tissue damage, of DAMP further increasing tissue injury. The main TLRs types expressed in the heart are TLR2 (recognizing lipoteichoic acid) and TLR4 (LPS receptor) but also TLR 3 and 9 are present [196]. Both TLR2 and TLR4 have been demonstrated as essential mediators of the septic myocardial damage: in mice with their genetic deficiency there was a better preservation of cardiac function and a decreased mortality[14,197,198]. Also TLR5, receptor for bacterial flagellin, TLR9 (endocellular recognizing bacterial DNA) and very recently TLR3, endocellular receptor recognizing viral double stranded RNA, have been showed to play a deleterious role in mediating cardiac dysfunction in sepsis [199,200]. This depression of myocardial function is linked to the response of myocardiocytes to the release of alarmins with increased production of pro- and anti-inflammatory ILs, of chemokines and cell adhesion molecules [196]. The connection with the reduced contractile function is represented by the increased production of the 2 small calcium regulated molecules (S100A8 and S100A9) that have been showed with coimmunoprecipitation, able to suppress calcium flux interacting with the RAGE receptor [201]. TLRs lead to iNOS stimulation, NF-kB upregulation and to increased expression of TNFα, IL1β, IL6, IFNγ, chemokines and cell adhesion molecules responsible for the cellular damage but also for the initiation of the reparative process [202]. The inflammatory reaction, as already seen, is modulated by the appearance of LPS tolerance and proinflammatory genes silencing. As already said, a long term stimulation with LPS or a TLR4 ligand (such as HMBG1) may induce preconditioning [9] and in decreased brain infarct size in mice that were subjected to focal cerebral ischaemia/reperfusion injury [10].

In sepsis there is an increased production of NO by inflammatory cells infiltrating myocardium but also by endothelial and smooth muscle vascular cells due to stimulation of iNOS. The increased NO production causes an impressive vasodilation, a reduced sensitivity to the vasoconstrictors and an increase in capillary permeability. NO has also a depressive action upon the myocardium mediated by the production of cGMP. In fact NO behaves as a double-edged sword because if on one hand depresses myocardial contractility increasing cGMP production, reduces oxygen consumption by antagonizing COX and may induce apoptosis on the other hand it supports relaxation normalizing the stiffness of the septic myocardium, antagonizes the action of the increased endothelin and has a cardioprotective effect through the induction of preconditioning [203]: unselective antagonism of NOS with NNMA is harmful in sepsis because even though it raises blood pressure it decreases cardiac, hepatic and renal blood flow [204]. Many other alterations have been described in septic myocardium: an altered phosphorylation of Troponin I (TnI) in serin 23-24 by Protein Kinase A (PKA), activated by β receptors or an upregulation of Protein Phosphatase 2A (PP2A). dephosphorylating TnI [205,206]. The cause of the increased phosphorylation of Tn seems to be the increased β-adrenergic activity during the early phases of sepsis followed by a reduction during the late phase characterized by the hypodynamic cardiac pattern. A calcium leak from sarcoplasmic reticulum has been also described in sepsis similar to that observed in CHF and determined also by PKA activation and increased phosphorylation of the calstabin, a protein maintaining in its stable form the sarcoplasmic ATPase assigned to the re-entry of Calcium in sarcoplasmic reticulum after systole [207,208]. Such an alteration could justify both diastolic dysfunction due to the diastolic calcium leak and the systolic dysfunction showing itself in the late phase as expression of depletion of Calcium reserves. An altered autonomic tone with increased in sympathetic activity in the early phases of sepsis and decreased heart rate variability has been described [209].

Levy and colleagues [141], as already seen, showed in the septic myocardium important alterations (reduced cardiac performances, increased glucose uptake, increased myocardial glucose transmembrane transporters GLUT1 and GLUT4, increased deposits of glycogen). Because these modifications have been described as typical of the myocardial hibernation, Levy proposed that this latter may take part in the septic cardiac dysfunction. It is however debatable that the "true" ischemic myocardial hibernation is responsible for cardiac dysfunction in sepsis for several reasons: 1)myocardial hibernation is no longer considered as a down-regulation of the contractile and metabolic activity aiming at reducing the oxygen consumption and at adapting it to the reduced blood supply (smart heart hypothesis). It is instead attributed to repetitive episodes of myocardial stunning [210] 2) reduced myocardial perfusion has never been demonstrated in sepsis [211], the biochemical modifications showed in septic myocardium are not features of hibernating myocardium, they are instead present in the fetal heart and also in the stressed myocardium as expressions of the reactivation of the fetal gene program [47,52]. The alterations described in septic myocardium would therefore be unspecific and their presence could be explained in sepsis by the inflammatory state that characterizes it. The picture of metabolic hibernation present in sepsis should therefore be separated from that of the true myocardial ischemic hibernation whose existence, in our opinion, has not been convincingly demonstrated in sepsis.

Myocardial injury in sepsis is also shown by the increase of many markers such as troponin (Tn) and natriuretic peptides. Whereas Tn I and TnT levels are good indicators for cardiac function in sepsis relating well with left ventricular dysfunction and a poor prognosis, BNP is related to the outcome but only weakly with cardiac filling pressures [212]. A high level of BNP >144 pg/ml predicts cardiac dysfunction with high sensitivity (92%) and high specificity (86%)[213]. BNP upregulation takes part in the reactivation of the fetal gene program and its production has been shown to be increased during inflammatory processes related to the ability of inflammatory ILs and of p38MAPK to increase its secretion increasing its promoter activity [214]. Differently from the regulation of the similar molecule ANP, BNP secretion is regulated more by inflammation than by hemodynamic compromise.

7. Metabolic dysfunction in chronic heart failure

The chronically failing heart is certainly energy-deprived [215], as has been ascertained by studies with ^{31}P magnetic resonance (MR) spectroscopy [216] showing the reduced phosphocreatine: ATP ratio, important index of the energetic state of the heart correlated with the indexes of systolic and diastolic function [217]. The cardiac contractile function is inextricably linked to the metabolic function so that the alterations of cardiac metabolism observed in chronic heart failure must affect also the contractile function. As heart failure progresses mithocondrial respiration is gradually compromised preventing that a normal level of FAO may take place. In samples taken from explanted hearts, during transplantation in patients with advanced heart failure, the level of the enzymes of FAO was low compared to the non-failing hearts [218]. The reduction of mitochondrial biogenesis and of FFA oxidation in the advanced phase of CHF is, as already seen, caused by the reactivation of the fetal gene program through the upregulation of HIF-1 and the downregulation of PPARα, β\δ, ERRα,, of SIRT1 and of the PGC-1α network demonstrated in myocardial samples of patients with end-stage heart failure compared with explanted non failing hearts [219]. The expression of these transcription factors and coactivators is reduced in pathological hypertrophy and heart failure whereas it is upregulated in physiological forms of hypertrophy related to postnatal growth or exercise training [220] so furnishing a precise boundary between physiologic and pathologic cardiac growth. Interestingly also a constitutive cardiospecific overexpression of PGC-1α in mice (MHC–PGC-1α mice) may damage the heart leading to myocardiopathy with uncontrolled mitochondrial proliferation but only in the neonatal period, whereas the overexpression in adult mice provoked only modest mitochondrial proliferation [221,222]. PGC-1α -\- mice show a reduced capacity both of exercising and of acclimating to cold temperature [223].

The fetal gene program is mediated by an incompletely known but modified expression of various microRNA [224-226]: Sucharov described that changes in the expression level of miR 100 and 133b contribute to the regulation of the fetal gene program [225]. The reduced expression of SIRT1 underlies the depressed mitochondrial biogenesis and FAO in the chronically failing heart. SIRT1 seems to be expressed at higher levels in the first phases of hypertrophy, the first physiologic response to the overload of the heart, as a response to the stressing event inducing it but begins to be downregulated when PARP activation takes place, due to the increased oxidative stress [227], reducing NAD^+ availability. The reduction in SIRT1, provided with an antiapoptotic function, and the compromised mitochondrial activity may contribute to the increased cellular death in chronically failing myocardium [228,229]. Overall we may conclude that some similarities exist between the metabolic and morphological alterations observed in sepsis and CHF.

8. Cardiac lipotoxicity in chronic heart failure and sepsis

In 1858 Virchow first reported intramyocyte lipid accumulation in patients with congestive heart failure, he referred to it as "lipid atrophy" of the myocardium [230]. At present the presence in the myocardial cell of neutral lipid droplets is ascribed to the altered glucose and lipid metabolism and to a mismatch between lipid delivery and oxidation. In normal conditions TG are stored only in adipocytes, under the control of PPARγ, with minimal presence of lipids in other tissues [231,232]; in this way adipocytes play indirectly a key role in the control of systemic glucose, lipid homeostasis and insulin sensitivity through the regulation of the serum level of FFA. In congenital lipodystrophy, a disease characterized by a decreased capacity of lipid storage in adipose tissue, the non-adipose organs accumulate TG and there is a premature cardiomyopathy [233]. When an overload of cellular FFA takes place caused by increased lipolysis or increased uptake (evident in clinical settings as in diabetes, in the experimental CD36 and LPL overexpression [234,235] or in settings of reduced FAO), lipid deposits in the myocardium and other organs may occur giving rise to the already seen phenomenon of lipotoxicity [236]. The contractile dysfunction caused by intramyocardial lipid accumulation is mediated at least partly by an altered expression of Sarco/Endoplasmic Reticulum Calcium ATPasi (SERCA2) as showed in specimen taken intraoperatively in patients with aortic stenosis and metabolic syndrome [237]. A diastolic dysfunction is also present, frequently preceding the systolic derangement and associated with interstitial fibrosis. Lipid accumulation is present in the heart of patients with CHF mainly in people with obesity, diabetes and metabolic syndrome. The relationship is bidirectional, insulin resistance predisposes to CHF and CHF increases insulin resistance. A reduced insulin sensitivity is observed in many patients with CHF, moreover its presence represents a risk factor for the eventual development of heart failure. Therefore the lipid accumulation alone without a reduced insulin sensitivity, obesity or metabolic syndrome can cause lipotoxicity. The importance of the cardiac isolated steatosis has been showed in the experimental context by demonstrating that myocardial overexpression of both PPARα and γ is associated with lipid accumulation and contractile dysfunction [238,239] probably because they stimulate more the uptake than the oxidation of FFA; moreover the PPARα activator fenofibrate can prevent the contractile dysfunction and the reduced calcium sensitivity in a rat model of LPS infusion further demonstrating the tight relationships between metabolic and contractile compromise [240]. Lipid deposits in the cardiomyocytes as TG in CHF is only a marker of an imbalance between the uptake and oxidation of FFA and not necessarily relates to toxic lipid byproducts formation. The chronic accumulation of neutral lipids is probably not, per se, immediately harmful for the myocardial cell in CHF but represents a mechanism of defence against the excess of the FFAs, more metabolically reactive, reaching it [241]. In the long term however lipid store may behaves as a time bomb because when a critical point is reached, either by accumulation of excessive quantity of lipid or by some event triggering an increased FAO, the accumulation of toxic byproducts such as ceramides, diacylglycerol, fatty acyl-CoAs and acyl-carnitine ensues damaging the myocardial cell.

The lipid accumulation in the heart during infections has been described since the '90 of the last century [242] however the only complete study in sepsis is the article by Rossi and colleagues [169]. They showed in septic myocardium an increased staining by the dye oil red O, specific for lipid, and attributed it to an altered metabolism of the myocardium.

These alterations are the morphological expression of the switch from lipid to glucose utilization in a setting in which lipolysis is increased and FAO reduced by PPARα downregulation and by acute mitochondrial dysfunction.

Very little is known about the significance of lipid accumulation in the septic myocardium; initially interpreted as a degenerative marker in infectious diseases it could have in the setting of the acute septic myocardiopathy a meaning considerably different from the chronic lipid accumulation in CHF even though the microscopic aspect is similar.

Certainly a lipidomic approach to the problem may be of great help.

In conclusion notwithstanding similar morphological aspects and the involvement of many common biochemical pathways the cardiac dysfunction in sepsis and in CHF may have different meanings and consequences.

9. Conclusions

In the recent years the strict relationships between myocardial contractility and metabolism have been ascertained and a metabolic basis for cardiac contractile dysfunction verified in many clinical and experimental settings. Several metabolic alterations have been showed in CHF and septic myocardial dysfunction, their relationship with cardiac contractile dysfunction is not completely understood. They are probably a marker of the complex transcriptional and posttranscriptional alterations induced by the inflammatory, mechanical and metabolic stress the heart undergoes in both conditions and particularly of the coordinated compromise of mitochondrial function and of lipid oxidation but they represent also a direct inducer and amplifier of cellular damage. The significance of the morphological and metabolic alterations could be remarkably different in the slowly-evolving setting of CHF and in the acute one of the septic myocardial dysfunction, moreover the malignancy of the noxae underlying similar microscopic aspects may be very dissimilar. To understand in deep this aspect more thorough studies are needed. We currently do not know if they may represent a target for therapy because of the uncertain efficacy of the drugs until now used for this purpose but perhaps the light shed on the pathophysiological mechanism may give us an important help in the search for a future effective treatment.

Author details

Luca Siracusano* and Viviana Girasole
Department of Neuroscience, Psychiatric and Anesthesiological Sciences, University of Messina, School of Medicine, Policlinico Universitario G. Martino, Italy

10. References

[1] Angus DC, Linde-Zwirble WT, Lidicker J, Clermont G, Carcillo J, Pinsky MR. Epidemiology of severe sepsis in the United States: analysis of incidence, outcome and associated costs of care. Crit Care Med. 2001;29:1303–1310.
[2] Levy MM, Fink MP, Marshall JC, Abraham E, Angus D, Cook D, Cohen J, Opal SM, Vincent JL, Ramsay G; SCCM/ESICM/ACCP/ATS/SIS: 2001 SCCM/ESICM/ACCP /ATS/SIS International Sepsis Definitions Conference. Crit Care Med. 2003 Apr;31(4):1250-6.
[3] Cinel I, Opal SM: Molecular biology of inflammation and sepsis: a primer. Crit Care Med. 2009 Jan;37(1):291-304.
[4] Boomer JS, To K, Chang KC, Takasu O, Osborne DF, Walton AH, Bricker TL, Jarman SD 2nd, Kreisel D, Krupnick AS, Srivastava A, Swanson PE, Green JM, Hotchkiss RS: Immunosuppression in patients who die of sepsis and multiple organ failure. JAMA. 2011 Dec 21;306(23):2594-605.
[5] Skrupky LP, Kerby PW, Hotchkiss RS: Advances in the management of sepsis and the understanding of key immunologic defects. Anesthesiology. 2011 Dec;115(6):1349-62
[6] Shubin NJ, Monaghan SF, Ayala A: Anti-inflammatory mechanisms of sepsis. Contrib Microbiol. 2011;17:108-24.
[7] Lorne E, Dupont H, Abraham E: Toll-like receptors 2 and 4: initiators of non-septic inflammation in critical care medicine? Intensive Care Med. 2010 Nov;36(11):1826-35.
[8] Skrupky LP, Kerby PW, Hotchkiss RS: Advances in the management of sepsis and the understanding of key immunologic defects. Anesthesiology. 2011 Dec;115(6):1349-62.
[9] van der Poll T, van Zoelen MA, Wiersinga WJ: Regulation of pro-and anti-inflammatory host responses. Contrib Microbiol. 2011;17:125-36.
[10] Biswas SK, Lopez-Collazo E: Endotoxin tolerance: new mechanisms, molecules and clinical significance. Trends Immunol. 2009 Oct;30(10):475-87.
[11] McCall CE, Yoza B, Liu T, El Gazzar M: Gene-specific epigenetic regulation in serious infections with systemic inflammation. J Innate Immun. 2010;2(5):395-405
[12] Alves-Filho JC, Spiller F, Cunha FQ: Neutrophil paralysis in sepsis. Shock. 2010 Sep;34 Suppl 1:15-21.
[13] Vartanian K, Stenzel-Poore M: Toll-like receptor tolerance as a mechanism for neuroprotection. Transl Stroke Res. 2010 Dec 1;1(4):252-260.
[14] Frantz S, Ertl G, Bauersachs J: Mechanisms of disease: Toll-like receptors in cardiovascular disease. Nat Clin Pract Cardiovasc Med. 2007 Aug;4(8):444-54.

---

* Corresponding Author

[15] Zhao P, Wang J, He L, Ma H, Zhang X, Zhu X, et al: Deficiency in TLR4 signal transduction ameliorates cardiac injury and cardiomyocyte contractile dysfunction during ischemia. J Cell Mol Med 2009;13:1513–25.
[16] Calfee CS, Matthay MA: Clinical immunology: Culprits with evolutionary ties. Nature. 2010 Mar 4;464(7285):41-2.
[17] Könner AC, Brüning JC: Toll-like receptors: linking inflammation to metabolism. Trends Endocrinol Metab. 2011 Jan;22(1):16-23.
[18] Langouche L, Perre SV, Thiessen S, Gunst J, Hermans G, D'Hoore A, Kola B, Korbonits M, Van den Berghe G: Alterations in adipose tissue during critical illness: An adaptive and protective response? Am J Respir Crit Care Med. 2010 Aug.
[19] Siracusano L, Girasole V: Sepsis and Adiponectin. In: Masayoshi Y (Ed): Adiponectin: Production, Regulation and Roles in Disease. Nova Publishers At Press.
[20] van der Poll T: Experimental human sepsis models. Drug Discovery Today: Disease Models, 2012:9;e3-e9.
[21] Weissman C: The metabolic response to stress: an overview and update. Anesthesiology. 1990 Aug;73(2):308-27.
[22] Biolo G, Toigo G, Ciocchi B, Situlin R, Iscra F, Gullo A, Guarnieri G: Metabolic response to injury and sepsis: changes in protein metabolism. Nutrition. 1997 Sep;13(9 Suppl):52S-57S.
[23] Tappy L, Chioléro R: Substrate utilization in sepsis and multiple organ failure. Crit Care Med 2007; 35[Suppl.]:S531–S534.
[24] Li L, Messina JL: Acute insulin resistance following injury. Trends Endocrinol Metab. 2009 Nov;20(9):429-35.
[25] Mittra S, Bansal VS, Bhatnagar PK: From a glucocentric to a lipocentric approach towards metabolic syndrome. Drug Discov Today. 2008 Mar;13(5-6):211-8.
[26] Unger RH, Clark GO, Scherer PE, Orci L: Lipid homeostasis, lipotoxicity and the metabolic syndrome. Biochim Biophys Acta. 2010 Mar;1801(3):209-14.
[27] Duska F, Andel M: Intensive blood glucose control in acute and prolonged critical illness: endogenous secretion contributes more to plasma insulin than exogenous insulin infusion. Metabolism. 2008 May;57(5):669-71.
[28] Van den Berghe G: How does blood glucose control with insulin save lives in intensive care? J Clin Invest 2004; 114:1187–1195.
[29] Crouser ED: Mitochondrial dysfunction in septic shock and multiple organ dysfunction syndrome. Mitochondrion. 2004 ; 4:729-41.
[30] Karpac J, Jasper H: Insulin and JNK: optimizing metabolic homeostasis and lifespan. Trends Endocrinol Metab. 2009 Apr;20(3):100-6.
[31] Drosatos K, Drosatos-Tampakaki Z, Khan R, Homma S, Schulze PC, Zannis VI, Goldberg IJ: Inhibition of c-Jun-N-terminal kinase increases cardiac peroxisome proliferator-activated receptor alpha expression and fatty acid oxidation and prevents lipopolysaccharide-induced heart dysfunction. J Biol Chem. 2011 Oct 21;286(42):36331-9.
[32] van den Berghe G, Wouters P, Weekers F, Verwaest C, Bruyninckx F, Schetz M, Vlasselaers D, Ferdinande P, Lauwers P, Bouillon R: Intensive insulin therapy in critically ill patients. N Engl J Med. 2001 Nov 8;345(19):1359-67.

[33] NICE-SUGAR Study Investigators, Finfer S, Chittock DR, Su SY, Blair D, Foster D, Dhingra V, Bellomo R, Cook D, Dodek P, Henderson WR, Hébert PC, Heritier S, Heyland DK, McArthur C, McDonald E, Mitchell I, Myburgh JA, Norton R, Potter J, Robinson BG, Ronco JJ: Intensive versus conventional glucose control in critically ill patients.

[34] N Engl J Med. 2009 Mar 26;360(13):1283-97.

[35] Egi M, Finfer S, Bellomo R: Glycemic control in the ICU. Chest. 2011 Jul;140(1):212-20.

[36] Dyson A, Stidwill R, Taylor V, Singer M: Tissue oxygen monitoring in rodent models of shock. Am J Physiol Heart Circ Physiol. 2007 Jul;293(1):H526-33.

[37] Levy B: Lactate and shock state: the metabolic view. Curr Opin Crit Care. 2006 ;12:315-21.

[38] Holness MJ, Sugden MC: Regulation of pyruvate dehydrogenase complex activity by reversible phosphorylation. Biochem Soc Trans. 2003 ;31 :1143-51.

[39] Alamdari N, Constantin-Teodosiu D, Murton AJ, Gardiner SM, Bennett T, Layfield R, Greenhaff PL: Temporal changes in the involvement of pyruvate dehydrogenase complex in muscle lactate accumulation during lipopolysaccharide infusion in rats. J Physiol. 2008 15;586:1767-75.

[40] Siracusano L, Girasole V: Glucose and lipid metabolism in sepsis and endotoxemia. Acta Anaesthesiol Scand. 2009 Mar;53(3):413-14.

[41] Stanley WC, Recchia F, Lopaschuk GD: Myocardial Substrate Metabolism in the Normal and Failing Heart. Physiol Rev 2005; 85:1093–1129.

[42] Davies BS, Beigneux AP, Fong LG, Young SG: New wrinkles in lipoprotein lipase biology. Curr Opin Lipidol. 2012 Feb;23(1):35-42.

[43] Koonen, D.P., Glatz, J.F., Bonen, A., Luiken, J: Long-chain fatty acid uptake and FAT/CD36 translocation in heart and skeletal muscle. Biochim. Biophys. Acta, Mol. Cell Biol. Lipids2005: 1736;163–180.

[44] Lopaschuk GD, Ussher JR, Folmes CD, Jaswal JS, Stanley WC: Myocardial fatty acid metabolism in health and disease. Physiol Rev. 2010 Jan;90(1):207-58.

[45] Randle PJ, Garland PB, Hales CN, Newsholme EA. The glucose-fatty acid cycle: its role in insulin sensitivity and the metabolic disturbances of diabetes mellitus. Lancet 1963; 1:785–789.

[46] Hue L, Taegtmeyer H. The Randle cycle revisited: a new head for an old hat. Am J Physiol Endocrinol Metab. 2009;297:E578–E591.

[47] Shuldiner AR, McLenithan JC: Genes and pathophysiology of type 2 diabetes: more than just the Randle cycle all over again. J Clin Invest 2004;114: 1414–1417.

[48] Watson RT, Pessin JE: Bridging the GAP between insulin signaling and GLUT4 translocation. Trends Biochem Sci. 2006 Apr;31(4):215-22.

[49] Rajabi M, Kassiotis EC, Razeghi P, Taegtmeyer H: Return to the fetal gene program protects the stressed heart: a strong hypothesis. Heart Fail Rev 2007; 12:331–343.

[50] van de Weijer T, Schrauwen-Hinderling VB, Schrauwen P: Lipotoxicity in type 2 diabetic cardiomyopathy. Cardiovasc Res. 2011 Oct 1;92(1):10-8.

[51] Taegtmeyer H, Wilson CR, Razeghi P, Sharma S: Metabolic energetics and genetics in the heart. Ann NY Acad Sci 2005; 1047:208-18.

[52] Sheperd PR, Kahn BB: Glucose transporters and insulin action. Implications for Insulin Resistance and Diabetes Mellitus. N Engl J Med 2003; 341:248–257.
[53] Friehs I, Moran AM, Stamm C, Colan SD, Takeuchi K, Cao-Danh H, Rader CM, McGowan FX, del Nido PJ: Impaired glucose transporter activity in pressure-overload hypertrophy is an early indicator of progression to failure.
[54] Circulation 1999; 100:II187–II193.
[55] Taegtmeyer H, Sen S, Vela D: Return to the fetal gene program: a suggested metabolic link to gene expression in the heart. Ann N Y Acad Sci. 2010 Feb; 1188:191-8.
[56] van Uden P, Kenneth NS, Rocha S: Regulation of hypoxia-inducible factor-1alpha by NF-kappaB. Biochem J. 2008 Jun 15;412(3):477-84.
[57] Kuhlicke J, Frick JS, Morote-Garcia JC, Rosenberger P, Eltzschig HK: Hypoxia inducible factor (HIF)-1 coordinates induction of Toll-like receptors TLR2 and TLR6 during hypoxia. PLoS One. 2007 Dec 26;2(12):e1364.
[58] Semenza GL. Regulation of oxygen homeostasis by hypoxia-inducible factor 1. Physiology (Bethesda) 2009;24:97–106.
[59] Narravula S, Colgan SP: Hypoxia-inducible factor 1-mediated inhibition of peroxisome proliferator-activated receptor alpha expression during hypoxia. J Immunol. 2001 Jun 15;166(12):7543-8.
[60] Krishnan J, Suter M, Windak R, Krebs T, Felley A, Montessuit C, Tokarska-Schlattner M, Aasum E, Bogdanova A, Perriard E, Perriard JC, Larsen T, Pedrazzini T, Krek W: Activation of a HIF1alpha-PPARgamma axis underlies the integration of glycolytic and lipid anabolic pathways in pathologic cardiac hypertrophy. Cell Metab. 2009 Jun;9(6):512-24.
[61] Cadenas S, Aragonés J, Landázuri MO: Mitochondrial reprogramming through cardiac oxygen sensors in ischaemic heart disease. Cardiovasc Res. 2010 Nov 1;88(2):219-28.
[62] Kominsky DJ, Campbell EL, Colgan SP: Metabolic shifts in immunity and inflammation. J Immunol. 2010 Apr 15;184(8):4062-8.
[63] Haigis MC, Sinclair DA: Mammalian sirtuins: biological insights and disease relevance. Annu Rev Pathol. 2010;5:253-95.
[64] Rahman S, Islam R: Mammalian Sirt1: insights on its biological functions. Cell Commun Signal. 2011 May 8;9:11.
[65] Cantó C, Auwerx J: Targeting sirtuin 1 to improve metabolism: all you need is NAD(+)? Pharmacol Rev. 2012 Jan;64(1):166-87.
[66] Cantó C, Auwerx J: PGC-1alpha, SIRT1 and AMPK, an energy sensing network that controls energy expenditure. Curr Opin Lipidol. 2009 Apr;20(2):98-105.
[67] Borradaile NM, Pickering JG: NAD(+), sirtuins, and cardiovascular disease. Curr Pharm Des. 2009;15(1):110-7.
[68] Menzies KJ, Hood DA: The role of SirT1 in muscle mitochondrial turnover. Mitochondrion. 2012 Jan;12(1):5-13.
[69] Rane S, He M, Sayed D, Vashistha H, Malhotra A, Sadoshima J, Vatner DE, Vatner SF, Abdellatif M: Downregulation of miR-199a derepresses hypoxia-inducible factor-1alpha and Sirtuin 1 and recapitulates hypoxia preconditioning in cardiac myocytes. Circ Res. 2009 Apr 10;104(7):879-86.

[70] Lee J, Kemper JK: Controlling SIRT1 expression by microRNAs in health and metabolic disease. Aging (Albany NY). 2010 Aug;2(8):527-34.

[71] Tabuchi T, Satoh M, Itoh T, Nakamura M: MicroRNA-34a regulates the longevity-associated protein SIRT1 in coronary artery disease: effect of statins on SIRT1 and microRNA-34a expression. Clin Sci (Lond). 2012 Aug 1;123(3):161-71.

[72] Lopaschuk GD, Ussher JR, Folmes CD, Jaswal JS, Stanley WC. Myocardial fatty acid metabolism in health and disease. Physiol Rev. 2010 Jan;90(1):207-58.

[73] Desvergne B, Michalik L, Wahli W: Transcriptional regulation of metabolism. Physiol Rev 86: 465–514, 2006.

[74] Huss JM, Kelly DP: Nuclear receptor signaling and cardiac energetics. Circ Res 95: 568–578, 2004.

[75] Schupp M, Lazar MA: Endogenous ligands for nuclear receptors: digging deeper. J Biol Chem. 2010 Dec 24; 285(52):40409-15.

[76] Grimaldi PA: Metabolic and nonmetabolic regulatory functions of peroxisome proliferator-activated receptor beta. Curr Opin Lipidol. 2010 Jun;21(3):186-91.

[77] Finck BN, Kelly DP. Peroxisome proliferator-activated receptor gamma coactivator-1 (PGC-1) regulatory cascade in cardiac physiology and disease. Circulation 2007;115:2540–2548.

[78] Huang W, Glass CK: Nuclear receptors and inflammation control: molecular mechanisms and pathophysiological relevance. Arterioscler Thromb Vasc Biol. 2010 Aug;30(8):1542-9.

[79] Glass CK, Ogawa S: Combinatorial roles of nuclear receptors in inflammation and immunity. Nature Rev. Immunol. 2006;6,44–55.

[80] Bensinger SJ, Tontonoz P: Integration of metabolism and inflammation by lipid-activated nuclear receptors. Nature. 2008 Jul 24;454(7203):470-7.

[81] von Knethen A, Soller M, Brüne B: Peroxisome proliferator-activated receptor gamma (PPAR gamma) and sepsis. Arch Immunol Ther Exp 2007; 55:19-25.

[82] Eichner LJ, Giguère V: Estrogen related receptors (ERRs): a new dawn in transcriptional control of mitochondrial gene networks. Mitochondrion. 2011 Jul;11(4):544-52.

[83] Arner P: Human fat cell lipolysis: biochemistry, regulation and clinical role. Best Pract Res Clin Endocrinol Metab. 2005;19:471-82.

[84] Lass A, Zimmermann R, Oberer M, Zechner R: Lipolysis - a highly regulated multi-enzyme complex mediates the catabolism of cellular fat stores. Prog Lipid Res. 2011 Jan;50(1):14-27.

[85] Ahmadian M, Wang Y, SulHS: Lipolysis in adipocytes. Int J Biochem Cell Biol. 2010 May;42(5):555-9.

[86] Lafontan M, Langin D: Lipolysis and lipid mobilization in human adipose tissue. Prog Lipid Res. 2009;48:275-97.

[87] Haemmerle G, Lass A, Zimmermann R, Gorkiewicz G, Meyer C, Rozman J, Heldmaier G, Maier R, Theussl C, Eder S, Kratky D, Wagner EF, Klingenspor M, Hoefler G, Zechner R: Defective lipolysis and altered energy metabolism in mice lacking adipose triglyceride lipase. Science. 2006 May 5;312(5774):734-7.

[88] Lampidonis AD, Rogdakis E, Voutsinas GE, Stravopodis DJ: The resurgence of Hormone-Sensitive Lipase (HSL) in mammalian lipolysis. Gene. 2011 May 15;477(1-2):1-11.
[89] Shen WJ, Yu Z, Patel S, Jue D, Liu LF, Kraemer FB: Hormone-sensitive lipase modulates adipose metabolism through PPARγ. Biochim Biophys Acta. 2011 Jan;1811(1):9-16.
[90] Chen X, Xun K, Chen L, Wang Y. TNF-alpha, a potent lipid metabolism regulator. Cell Biochem. Funct. 2009;27:407–416.
[91] Cawthorn WP, Sethi JK: TNF-alpha and adipocyte biology. FEBS Lett. 2008 Jan 9;582(1):117-31.
[92] Zhang T, He J, Xu C, Zu L, Jiang H, Pu S, Guo X, Xu G: Mechanisms of metformin inhibiting lipolytic response to isoproterenol in primary rat adipocytes. J Mol Endocrinol. 2009 Jan;42(1):57-66.
[93] Zu L, He J, Jiang H, Xu C, Pu S, Xu G: Bacterial endotoxin stimulates adipose lipolysis via toll-like receptor 4 and extracellular signal-regulated kinase pathway. J Biol Chem. 2009 Feb 27;284(9):5915-26.
[94] Choi SM, Tucker DF, Gross DN, Easton RM, DiPilato LM, Dean AS, Monks BR, Birnbaum MJ: Insulin regulates adipocyte lipolysis via an Akt-independent signaling pathway. Mol Cell Biol. 2010 Nov;30(21):5009-20.
[95] Qiao L, Kinney B, Schaack J, Shao J: Adiponectin inhibits lipolysis in mouse adipocytes. Diabetes. 2011 May;60(5):1519-27.
[96] W. Khovidhunkit, R.A. Memon, K.R. Feingold, C. Grunfeld, Infection and inflammation-induced proatherogenic changes of lipoproteins, J. Infect.Dis. 181 (2000) 462–472.80
[97] Davidsson P, Hulthe J, Fagerberg B, Camejo G. Proteomics of apolipoproteins and associated proteins from plasma high-density lipoproteins. Arterioscler Thromb Vasc Biol 2010;30:156–63.
[98] Gordon,S.M. et al.:Proteomic characterization of human plasma high density lipoprotein fractionated by gel filtration chromatography. 2010:J. Proteome.Res. 9, 5239–5249 68.
[99] Gordon S, Deng J, Lu LJ, Davidson WS: High-density lipoprotein proteomics: Identifying new drug targets and biomarkers by understanding functionality. Curr. Cardio.RiskRep. 2010:4, 1–8.
[100] Murphy,A.J. et al. High-density lipoprotein reduces the human monocyte inflammatory response. Arterioscler. Thromb. Vasc. Biol. 2008;28, 2071–2077.
[101] Gordon SM, Hofmann S, Askew DS, Davidson WS: High density lipoprotein: it's not just about lipid transport anymore. Trends Endocrinol Metab. 2011;22:9-15.
[102] Säemann MD, Poglitsch M, Kopecky C, Haidinger M, Hörl WH, Weichhart T:The versatility of HDL: a crucial anti-inflammatory regulator. Eur J Clin Invest. 2010 ;40(12):1131-43.
[103] Galbois A, Thabut D, Tazi KA, Rudler M, Mohammadi MS, Bonnefont- Rousselot D et al: Ex vivo effects of high-density lipoprotein exposure on the lipopolysaccharide-induced inflammatory response in patients with severe cirrhosis. Hepatology 2009;49:175–84.

[104] Hima Bindu G, Rao VS, Kakkar VV: Friend Turns Foe: Transformation of Anti-Inflammatory HDL to Proinflammatory HDL during Acute-Phase Response. Cholesterol, vol. 2011, no. 19, Article ID 274629, 6 pages, 2011.

[105] Esteve E, Ricart W, Fernández-Real JM: Dyslipidemia and inflammation: an evolutionary conserved mechanism. Clin Nutr. 2005 Feb;24(1):16-31.

[106] Khovidhunkit W, Kim MS, Memon RA, Shigenaga JK, Moser AH, Feingold KR, Grunfeld C: Effects of infection and inflammation on lipid and lipoprotein metabolism: mechanisms and consequences to the host. J Lipid Res 45 : 1169 –1196,2004.

[107] Zhu X, Lee JY, Timmins JM, Brown JM, Boudyguina E, Mulya A et al: Increased cellular free cholesterol in macrophage-specific Abca1 knock-out mice enhances pro-inflammatory response of macrophages. J Biol Chem 2008;283:22930–41.

[108] Murch O, Collin M, Hinds CJ, Thiemermann C: Lipoproteins in inflammation and sepsis. I. Basic science. Intensive Care Med. 2007;33:13-24.

[109] Wendel M, Paul R, Heller AR: Lipoproteins in inflammation and sepsis. II. Clinical aspects. Intensive Care Med. 2007 Jan;33(1):25-35.

[110] Mineo C, Shaul PW: HDL stimulation of endothelial nitric oxide synthase: a novel mechanism of HDL action. Trends Cardiovasc Med. 2003 Aug;13(6):226-31.

[111] Theilmeier,G. et al. (2006) High-density lipoproteins and their constituent, sphingosine-1-phosphate, directly protect the heart against ischemia/reperfusion injury in vivo via the S1P3 lysophospholipid receptor. Circulation 114,1403–1409.

[112] Frias MA., Lang U, Gerber-Wicht C, James RW: Native and reconstituted HDL protect cardiomyocytes from doxorubicin-induced apoptosis. Cardiovasc. Res. (2010):85, 118–126 51.

[113] Frias MA, Lang U, Gerber-Wicht C, James RW: Emerging high-density lipoprotein infusion therapies: fulfilling the promise of epidemiology? J Clin Lipidol. 2010 Sep-Oct;4(5):399-404.

[114] Chien JY, Jerng JS, Yu CJ, Yang PC: Low serum level of high-density lipoprotein is a poor prognostic factor for severe sepsis. 2005 Crit Care Med 33:1688–1693.

[115] Feingold KR, Grunfeld C: The acute phase response inhibits reverse cholesterol transport. J Lipid Res. 2010 Apr;51(4):682-4. Epub 2010 Jan 13.

[116] Baranova I, Vishnyakova T, Bocharov A, Chen Z, Remaley AT, Stonik J, Eggerman TL, Patterson AP: Lipopolysaccharide down regulates both scavenger receptor B1 and ATP binding cassette transporter A1 in RAW cells. Infect Immun. 2002 Jun;70(6):2995-3003.

[117] Ziouzenkova O, Perrey S, Asatryan L, Hwang J, MacNaul KL, Moller DE, Rader DJ, Sevanian A, Zechner R, Hoefler G, Plutzky J: Lipolysis of triglyceride-rich lipoproteins generates PPAR ligands: evidence for an antiinflammatory role for lipoprotein lipase. Proc Natl Acad Sci U S A. 2003 Mar 4;100(5):2730-5

[118] Feingold K, Kim MS, Shigenaga J, Moser A, Grunfeld C: Altered expression of nuclear hormone receptors and coactivators in mouse heart during the acute-phase response. Am J Physiol Endocrinol Metab. 2004;286(2):E201-7.

[119] Feingold KR, Wang Y, Moser A, Shigenaga JK, Grunfeld C: LPS decreases fatty acid oxidation and nuclear hormone receptors in the kidney. J Lipid Res.2008; 49:2179-87.

[120] Feingold KR, Moser A, Patzek SM, Shigenaga JK, Grunfeld C: Infection decreases fatty acid oxidation and nuclear hormone receptors in the diaphragm. J Lipid Res. 2009;50:2055-63.

[121] Maitra U, Chang S, Singh N, Li L: Molecular mechanism underlying the suppression of lipid oxidation during endotoxemia. Mol Immunol. 2009;47:420-5.

[122] Halestrap AP: What is the mitochondrial permeability transition pore? J Mol Cell Cardiol. 2009 Jun;46(6):821-31.

[123] Andrews DT, Royse C, Royse AG: The mitochondrial permeability transition pore and its role in anaesthesia-triggered cellular protection during ischaemia-reperfusion injury. Anaesth Intensive Care. 2012 Jan;40(1):46-70.

[124] Larche J, Lancel S, Hassoun SM, Favory R, Decoster B, Marchetti P, Chopin C, Neviere R: Inhibition of mitochondrial permeability transition prevents sepsis-induced myocardial dysfunction and mortality. J Am Coll Cardiol. 2006 Jul 18;48(2):377-85.

[125] Lee J, Giordano S, Zhang J: Autophagy, mitochondria and oxidative stress: cross-talk and redox signalling. Biochem J. 2012 Jan 15;441(2):523-40.

[126] Nakahira K, Haspel JA, Rathinam VA, Lee SJ, Dolinay T, Lam HC, Englert JA, Rabinovitch M, Cernadas M, Kim HP, Fitzgerald KA, Ryter SW, Choi AM: Autophagy proteins regulate innate immune responses by inhibiting the release of mitochondrial DNA mediated by the NALP3 inflammasome. Nat Immunol. 2011 Mar;12(3):222-30.

[127] Ventura-Clapier R, Garnier A, Veksler V: Transcriptional control of mitochondrial biogenesis: the central role of PGC-1alpha. Cardiovasc Res. 2008 Jul 15;79(2):208-17.

[128] Scarpulla RC: Metabolic control of mitochondrial biogenesis through the PGC-1 family regulatory network. Biochim Biophys Acta. 2011 Jul;1813(7):1269-78.

[129] Scarpulla RC: Transcriptional paradigms in mammalian mitochondrial biogenesis and function. Physiol Rev. 2008 Apr;88(2):611-38.

[130] Vats D, Mukundan L, Odegaard JI, Zhang L, Smith KL, Morel CR, et al. Oxidative metabolism and PGC-1beta attenuate macrophage-mediated inflammation. Cell Metab: 2006;4:13–24.

[131] Lin J, Wu P-H, Tarr PT, Lindenberg KS, St-Pierre J,Zhang C-Y, Mootha VK, Jãger S, Vianna, CR, Reznick, R.M., et al. 2004. Defects in adaptive energy metabolism with CNS-linked hyperactivity in PGC-1 null mice. Cell119: 121–135.

[132] Leone, T.C., Lehman, J.J., Finck, B.N., Schaeffer, P.J., Wende, A.R., Boudina, S., Courtois, M., Wozniak, D.F., Sambandam, N., Bernal-Mizrachi, C., et al. PGC-1 deficient mice exhibit multi-system energy metabolic derangements: Muscle dysfunction, abnormal weight control, and hepatic steatosis. PLoS Biol. 2005 3: 672–687.

[133] Lai L, Leone TC, Zechner C, Schaeffer PJ, Kelly SM, Flanagan DP, Medeiros DM, Kovacs A, Kelly DP: Transcriptional coactivators PGC-1alpha and PGC-lbeta control overlapping programs required for perinatal maturation of the heart. Genes Dev. 2008 Jul 15;22(14):1948-61.

[134] Rimbaud S, Garnier A, Ventura-Clapier R. Mitochondrial biogenesis in cardiac pathophysiology. Pharmacol Rep. 2009;61:131-138.

[135] Lee IH, Cao L, Mostoslavsky R, Lombard DB, Liu J, Bruns NE, Tsokos M, Alt FW, Finkel T: A role for the NAD-dependent deacetylase Sirt1 in the regulation of autophagy. Proc. Natl Acad. Sci. USA 105, 3374–3379 (2008).

[136] Schumer W, Das Gupta TK, Moss GS, Nyhus LM: Effect of endotoxemia on liver cell mitochondria in man. Ann Surg. 1970 ; 171:875-82.

[137] Mela L, Bacalzo LV Jr, Miller LD: Defective oxidative metabolism of rat liver mitochondria in hemorrhagic and endotoxin shock. Am J Physiol. 1971; 220:571-7.

[138] Exline MC, Crouser ED: Mitochondrial mechanisms of sepsis-induced organ failure. Mitochondria in Sepsis. Front Biosci. 2008 ;13:5030-41.

[139] Singer M: Mitochondrial function in sepsis: Acute phase versus multiple organ failure. Crit Care Med 2007; 35[Suppl.]:S441–S448.

[140] Smeding L, Plötz FB, Groeneveld AB, Kneyber MC: Structural changes of the heart during severe sepsis or septic shock. Shock. 2012 May;37(5):449-56.

[141] Suliman HB, Welty-Wolf KE, Carraway M, Tatro L, Piantadosi CA: Lipopolysaccharide induces oxidative cardiac mitochondrial damage and biogenesis. Cardiovasc Res 64:279Y288, 2004.

[142] Levy RJ, Piel DA, Acton PD, Zhou R, Ferrari VA, Karp JS, Deutschman CS: Evidence of myocardial hibernation in the septic heart. Crit Care Med 33:2752Y2756, 2005.

[143] Brealey D, Brand M, Hargreaves I, Heales S, Land J, Smolenski R, Davies NA, Cooper CE, Singer M: Association between mitochondrial dysfunction and severity and outcome of septic shock. Lancet. 2002 Jul 20;360(9328):219-23.

[144] Carré JE, Orban JC, Re L, Felsmann K, Iffert W, Bauer M, Suliman HB, Piantadosi CA, Mayhew TM, Breen P, Stotz M, Singer M: Survival in critical illness is associated with early activation of mitochondrial biogenesis. Am J Respir Crit Care Med. 2010 Sep 15;182(6):745-51.

[145] Singer M, De Santis V, Vitale D, Jeffcoate W: Multiorgan failure is an adaptive, endocrine-mediated, metabolic response to overwhelming systemic inflammation. Lancet 2004; 364:545-8.

[146] Levy RJ: Mitochondrial dysfunction, bioenergetic impairment and metabolic down-regulation in sepsis. Shock 2007; 28:24-28.

[147] Azevedo LC: Mitochondrial dysfunction during sepsis. Endocr Metab Immune Disord Drug Targets. 2010 Sep;10(3):214-23.

[148] Dyson A, Stidwill R, Taylor V, Singer M: Tissue oxygen monitoring in rodent models of shock. Am J Physiol Heart Circ Physiol. 2007 Jul;293(1):H526-33.

[149] Fink MP: Bench-to-bedside review: Cytopathic hypoxia. Critical Care 2002;6:491–499.

[150] Kato K, Giulivi C: Critical overview of mitochondrial nitric-oxide synthase. Front Biosci. 2006 ; 11:2725-38.

[151] Valdez LB, Boveris A: Mitochondrial nitric oxide synthase, a voltage-dependent enzyme, is responsible for nitric oxide diffusion to cytosol. Front Biosci 2007; 12:1210-9.

[152] Bateman RM, Sharpe MD, Goldman D, Lidington D, Ellis CG: Inhibiting nitric oxide overproduction during hypotensive sepsis increases local oxygen consumption in rat skeletal muscle. Crit Care Med 2008; 36:225-23.

[153] Brown GC: Nitric oxide and mitochondria. Front Biosci. 2007; 12:1024-33.

[154] Pun PB, Lu J, Kan EM, Moochhala S: Gases in the mitochondria. Mitochondrion: 2010 Mar;10(2):83-93.

[155] Cooper CE, Brown GC: The inhibition of mitochondrial cytochrome oxidase by the gases carbon monoxide, nitric oxide, hydrogen cyanide and hydrogen sulfide: chemical mechanism and physiological significance. J Bioenerg Biomembr. 2008 Oct;40(5):533-9.

[156] Blackstone E, Morrison M, Roth MB: H2S induces a suspended animation-like state in mice. Science 2005 Apr 22;308(5721):518.

[157] Nystul TG, Roth MB: Carbon monoxide-induced suspended animation protects against hypoxic damage in Caenorhabditis elegans. Proc Natl Acad Sci U S A. 2004 Jun 15;101(24):9133-6.

[158] Aslami H, Juffermans NP: Induction of a hypometabolic state during critical illness - a new concept in the ICU? Neth J Med. 2010 May;68(5):190-8.

[159] Baumgart K, Radermacher P, Wagner F: Applying gases for microcirculatory and cellular oxygenation in sepsis: effects of nitric oxide, carbon monoxide, and hydrogen sulfide. Curr Opin Anaesthesiol. 2009 Apr;22(2):168-76.

[160] Zegdi R, Perrin D, Burdin M, Boiteau R, Tenaillon A. Increased endogenous carbon monoxide production in severe sepsis. Intensive Care Med. 2002;28:793–796.

[161] Hoetzel A, Dolinay T, Schmidt R, Choi AM, Ryter SW: Carbon monoxide in sepsis. Antioxid Redox Signal. 2007 Nov;9(11):2013-26

[162] Hui Y, Du J, Tang C, Bin G, Jiang H: Changes in arterial hydrogen sulfide (H2S) content during septic shock and endotoxin shock in rats. J Infect. 2003 Aug;47(2):155-60.

[163] Schilling J, Lai L, Sambandam N, Dey CE, Leone TC, Kelly DP. Toll-like receptor-mediated inflammatory signaling reprograms cardiac energy metabolism by repressing peroxisome proliferator-activated receptor coactivator- 1 signaling. Circ Heart Fail. 2011;4:474–482.

[164] Smeding : Salutary effect of resveratrol on sepsis-induced myocardial depression. Crit Care Med. 2012

[165] Schrauwen P, Schrauwen-Hinderling V, Hoeks J, Hesselink MK. Mitochondrial dysfunction and lipotoxicity. Biochim Biophys Acta. 2010;1801:266–271.

[166] Zhang Z, Lowry SF, Guarente L, Haimovich B: Roles of SIRT1 in the acute and restorative phases following induction of inflammation. J Biol Chem. 2010 Dec 31;285(53):41391-401.

[167] Menconi MJ, Arany ZP, Alamdari N, Aversa Z, Gonnella P, O'Neal P, Smith IJ, Tizio S, Hasselgren PO: Sepsis and glucocorticoids downregulate the expression of the nuclear cofactor PGC-1beta in skeletal muscle. Am J Physiol Endocrinol Metab. 2010 Oct;299(4):E533-43.

[168] Soriano FG, Nogueira AC, Caldini EG, Lins MH, Teixeira AC, Cappi SB, Lotufo PA, Bernik MM, Zsengellér Z, Chen M, Szabó C: Potential role of poly(adenosine 5'-diphosphate-ribose) polymerase activation in the pathogenesis of myocardial contractile dysfunction associated with human septic shock. Crit Care Med. 2006 Apr;34(4):1073-9.

[169] Pacher P, Szabó C: Role of poly(ADP-ribose) polymerase 1 (PARP-1) in cardiovascular diseases: the therapeutic potential of PARP inhibitors. Cardiovasc Drug Rev. 2007 Fall;25(3):235-60.

[170] Melvin RG, Andrews MT: Torpor induction in mammals: recent discoveries fueling new ideas. Trends Endocrinol Metab. 2009 Dec;20(10):490-8.

[171] Liu TF, Brown CM, El Gazzar M, McPhail L, Millet P, Rao A, Vachharajani VT, Yoza BK, McCall CE: Fueling the flame: bioenergy couples metabolism and inflammation. J Leukoc Biol. 2012 May 9. [Epub ahead of print].

[172] Liu TF, Yoza BK, El Gazzar M, Vachharajani VT, McCall CE: NAD+-dependent SIRT1 deacetylase participates in epigenetic reprogramming during endotoxin tolerance. J Biol Chem. 2011 Mar 18;286(11):9856-64.

[173] Dare AJ, Phillips AR, Hickey AJ, Mittal A, Loveday B, Thompson N, Windsor JA: A systematic review of experimental treatments for mitochondrial dysfunction in sepsis and multiple organ dysfunction syndrome. Free Radic Biol Med. 2009 Dec 1;47(11):1517-25.

[174] Ruggieri AJ, Levy RJ, Deutschman CS: Mitochondrial dysfunction and resuscitation in sepsis. Crit Care Clin. 2010 Jul;26(3):567-75, x-xi.

[175] Protti A, Singer M: Bench-to-bedside review: potential strategies to protect or reverse mitochondrial dysfunction in sepsis-induced organ failure. Crit Care. 2006;10(5):228.

[176] Kozlov AV, Bahrami S, Calzia E, Dungel P, Gille L, Kuznetsov AV, Troppmair J: Mitochondrial dysfunction and biogenesis: do ICU patients die from mitochondrial failure? Ann Intensive Care. 2011 Sep 26;1(1):41.

[177] Lancel S, Joulin O, Favory R, Goossens JF, Kluza J, Chopin C, Formstecher P, Marchetti P, Neviere R: Ventricular myocyte caspases are directly responsible for endotoxin-induced cardiac dysfunction. Circulation. 2005 May 24;111(20):2596-604.

[178] Buerke U, Carter JM, Schlitt A, Russ M, Schmidt H, Sibelius U, Grandel U, Grimminger F, Seeger W, Mueller-Werdan U, Werdan K, Buerke M: Apoptosis contributes to septic cardiomyopathy and is improved by simvastatin therapy. Shock. 2008 Apr;29(4):497-503.

[179] Balija TM, Lowry SF: Lipopolysaccharide and sepsis-associated myocardial dysfunction. Curr Opin Infect Dis. 2011 Jun;24(3):248-53.

[180] Rossi MA, Celes MR, Prado CM: Myocardial structural changes in long term human severe sepsis\septic shock may be responsible for cardiac dysfunction. Shock 2007; 27:10-18.

[181] Celes MR, Torres-Duenas D, Prado CM, et al. Increased sarcolemmal permeability as an early event in experimental septic cardiomyopathy: a potential role for oxidative damage to lipids and proteins. Shock 2010; 33:322–331.

[182] Celes MR, Torres-Duenas D, Malvestio LM, et al. Disruption of sarcolemmal dystrophin and beta-dystroglycan may be a potential mechanism for myocardial dysfunction in severe sepsis. Lab Invest 2010; 90:531–542.

[183] Parker MM, Shelhamer JH, Bacharach SL, Green MV, Natanson C, Frederick TM, et al: Profound but reversible myocardial depression in patients with septic shock. Ann Intern Med 1984;/100:/483 90.

[184] G Redl , P Germann , H Plattner e Al: Right ventricular function in early septic shock states. Intensive Care Med 1993;19:3–7.

[185] Bouhemad B, Nicolas-Robin A, Arbelot C, Arthaud M, Féger F, Rouby JJ: Acute left ventricular dilatation and shock-induced myocardial dysfunction. Crit Care Med 2009, 37: 441-447.

[186] J Poelaert, C Declerck, D Vogelaers e Al: Left ventricular systolic and diastolic function in septic shock. Intensive Care Med 1997;23:553–60.

[187] Vieillard Baron A, Schmitt JM, Beauchet A et Al: Early preload adaptation in septic shock? A transesophageal echocardiographic study. Anesthesiology 2001;94:400–6.

[188] Vieillard-Baron A: Septic cardiomyopathy. Ann Intensive Care. 2011 Apr 13;1(1):6.

[189] Suffredini A, Fromm RE, Parker MM, Brenner M, Kovacs JA, Wesley RA,Parrillo JE: The cardiovascular response of normal humans to the administration of endotoxin. N Engl J Med 1989, 321: 280-287.

[190] Vieillard-Baron A, Caille V, Charron C, et al. Actual incidence of global left ventricular hypokinesia in adult septic shock. Crit Care Med 2008; 36:1701–1706.

[191] Vincent JL, Reuse C, Frank N, Contempré B, Kahn RJ: Right ventricular dysfunction in septic shock: assessment by measurements of right ventricular ejection fraction using thermodilution technique. Acta Anaesthesiol Scand 1989, 33: 34-38.

[192] Etchecopar-Chevreuil C, François B, Clavel M, Pichon N, Gastinne H, Vignon P: Cardiac morphological and functional changes during early septic shock: a transesophageal echocardiographic study. Intensive Care Med 2008, 34: 250-256.

[193] Jianhui L, Rosenblatt-Velin N, Loukili N, Pacher P, Feihl F, Waeber B, Liaudet L: Endotoxin impairs cardiac hemodynamics by affecting loading conditions but not by reducing cardiac inotropism. Am J Physiol Heart Circ Physiol. 2010 Aug;299(2):H492-501.192)Wiggers CJ. Myocardial depression in shock: a survey of cardiodynamic studies. Am Heart J. 1947;33:633– 650.

[194] Parrillo JE, Burch C, Shelhamer JH, Parker MM, Natanson C, Schuette W: A circulating myocardial depressant substance in humans with septic shock. Septic shock patients with a reduced ejection fraction have a circulating factor that depresses in vitro myocardial cell performance. J Clin Invest. 1985 Oct;76(4):1539-53.

[195] Kumar A, Thota V, Dee L, Olson J, Uretz E, Parrillo JE: Tumor necrosis factor alpha and interleukin 1beta are responsible for in vitro myocardial cell depression induced by human septic shock serum. J Exp Med 183(3):949Y958, 1996.

[196] Flynn A, Chokkalingam Mani B, Mather PJ: Sepsis-induced cardiomyopathy: a review of pathophysiologic mechanisms. Heart Fail Rev. 2010 Nov;15(6):605-11.

[197] Marchant DJ, Boyd JH, Lin DC, Granville DJ, Garmaroudi FS, McManus BM: Inflammation in myocardial diseases. Circ Res. 2012 Jan 6;110(1):126-44.

[198] Fallach R, Shainberg A, Avlas O, Fainblut M, Chepurko Y, Porat E, Hochhauser E: Cardiomyocyte Toll-like receptor 4 is involved in heart dysfunction following septic shock or myocardial ischemia. J Mol Cell Cardiol. 2010 Jun;48(6):1236-44.

[199] Zou L, Feng Y, Chen YJ, Si R, Shen S, Zhou Q, Ichinose F, Scherrer-Crosbie M, Chao W: Toll-like receptor 2 plays a critical role in cardiac dysfunction during polymicrobial sepsis. Crit Care Med. 2010 May;38(5):1335-42.

[200] Gao M, Ha T, Zhang X, Liu L, Wang X, Kelley J, Singh K, Kao R, Gao X, Williams D, Li C: Toll-like receptor 3 plays a central role in cardiac dysfunction during polymicrobial sepsis. Crit Care Med. 2012 May 24. [Epub ahead of print] J. [200] Rolli, N. Rosenblatt-Velin, J. Li et al: "Bacterial flagellin triggers cardiac innate immune responses and acute contractile dysfunction,". PLoS ONE, vol. 5, no. 9, Article ID e12687, 1–13, 2010.

[201] Boyd JH, Kan B, Roberts H, Wang Y, Walley KR. S100a8 and s100a9 mediate endotoxin-induced cardiomyocyte dysfunction via the receptor for advanced glycation end products. Circ Res. 2008;102:1239 –1246.

[202] Zhang Z, Schluesener HJ: Mammalian toll-like receptors: from endogenous ligands to tissue regeneration. Cell Mol Life Sci. 2006 Dec;63(24):2901-7.

[203] SP Jones, R Bolli: The ubiquitous role of nitric oxide in cardioprotection Journal of Molecular Cellul Cardiol 2006;40:16–23.

[204] De Backer D: Nitric oxide inhibition in septic shock. Reanimation 2006;15;145-149.

[205] LL Wu, C Tang, MS Liu: Altered phosphorylation and calcium sensitivity of cardiac myofibrillar proteins during sepsis . Am J Physiol Regul Integr Comp Physiol 281:408-416, 2001.

[206] Tavernier B, Li JM, El-Omar MM, Lanone S, Yang ZK, Trayer IP, Mebazaa A, Shah AM: Cardiac contractility impairment associated with increased phosphorylation of troponin I in endotoxemic rats. Faseb J 2001, 15:294-296.

[207] Hassoun SM, Marechal X, Montaigne D, et al. Prevention of endotoxin-induced sarcoplasmic reticulum calcium leak improves mitochondrial and myocardial dysfunction. Crit Care Med 2008; 36:2590–2596.

[208] Lehnart SE: Novel targets for treating heart and muscle disease: stabilizing ryanodine receptors and preventing intracellular calcium leak. Curr Opin Pharmacol. 2007 Apr;7(2):225-32.

[209] Huang J, Wang Y, Jiang D, Zhou J, Huang X: The sympathetic-vagal balance against endotoxemia. J Neural Transm. 2010 Jun;117(6):729-35.

[210] Slezak J, Tribulova N, Okruhlicova L, Dhingra R, Bajaj A, Freed D, Singal P: Hibernating myocardium: pathophysiology, diagnosis, and treatment. Can J Physiol Pharmacol. 2009;874:252-65.

[211] Hunter JD, Doddi M: Sepsis and the heart. Br J Anaesth. 2010;104: 3-11.

[212] Maeder M, Fehr T, Rickli H e Al: Sepsis-associated myocardial dysfunction: diagnostic and prognostic impact of cardiac troponins and natriuretic peptides. Chest. 2006 May;129:1349-66.

[213] McLean AS, Tang B, Nalos M, Huang SJ, Stewart DE: Increased B-type natriuretic peptide (BNP) level is a strong predictor for cardiac dysfunction in intensive care unit patients. Anaesth Intensive Care 2003, 31:21-27.

[214] de Bold AJ: Cardiac natriuretic peptides gene expression and secretion in inflammation. J Investig Med. 2009 Jan;57(1):29-32.

[215] Neubauer S: The failing heart--an engine out of fuel.N Engl J Med. 2007 Mar 15;356(11):1140-5.1.

[216] Neubauer S, Horn M, Cramer M, et al: Myocardial phosphocreatine-to-ATP ratio is a predictor of mortality in patients with dilated cardiomyopathy. Circulation 1997;96:2190-6.

[217] Neubauer S, Horn M, Pabst T, et al: Contributions of ^{31}P-magnetic resonance spectroscopy to the understanding of dilated heart muscle disease. Eur Heart J 1995;16:Suppl O:115-8.

[218] Sack MN, Rader TA, Park S, Bastin J, McCune SA, Kelly DP: Fatty acid oxidation enzyme gene expression is downregulated in the failing heart. Circulation. 1996 Dec 1;94(11):2837-42.

[219] Sihag S, Cresci S, Li AY, Sucharov CC, Lehman JJ. PGC-1alpha and ERRalpha target gene downregulation is a signature of the failing human heart. J Mol Cell Cardiol 46: 201–212, 2009.

[220] Abel ED, Doenst T: Mitochondrial adaptations to physiological vs. pathological cardiac hypertrophy. Cardiovasc Res. 2011 May 1;90(2):234-42.

[221] Lehman JJ, Barger PM, Kovacs A, Saffitz JE, Medeiros DM, Kelly DP: Peroxisome proliferator-activated receptor gamma coactivator-1 promotes cardiac mitochondrial biogenesis. J Clin Invest. 2000;106:847–856.

[222] L. K. Russell, C. M. Mansfield, J. J. Lehman, et al., "Cardiac specific induction of the transcriptional coactivator peroxisome proliferator-activated receptor γ coactivator-1α promotes mitochondrial biogenesis and reversible cardiomyopathy in a developmental stage-dependent manner," Circulation Research 2004; 94: 525–533.

[223] Leone TC, Lehman JJ, FinckBN et al: "PGC-1α deficiency causes multi-system energy metabolic derangements: muscle dysfunction, abnormal weight control and hepatic steatosis," PLoS Biology, vol. 3, no. 4, p. e101, 2005.

[224] Thum T, Galuppo P, Wolf C, Fiedler J, Kneitz S, van Laake LW, Doevendans PA, Mummery CL, Borlak J, Haverich A, Gross C, Engelhardt S, Ertl G, Bauersachs J: MicroRNAs in the human heart: a clue to fetal gene reprogramming in heart failure. Circulation. 2007 Jul 17;116(3):258-67.

[225] Sucharov C, Bristow MR, Port JD: miRNA expression in the failing human heart: functional correlates. J Mol Cell Cardiol. 2008 Aug;45(2):185-92.

[226] Divakaran V, Mann DL: The emerging role of microRNAs in cardiac remodeling and heart failure. Circ Res. 2008 Nov 7;103(10):1072-83.

[227] Molnár A, Tóth A, Bagi Z, Papp Z, Edes I, Vaszily M, Galajda Z, Papp JG, Varró A, Szüts V, Lacza Z, Gerö D, Szabó C: Activation of the poly(ADP-ribose) polymerase pathway in human heart failure. Mol Med. 2006 Jul-Aug;12(7-8):143-52.

[228] Sundaresan NR, Pillai VB, Gupta MP: Emerging roles of SIRT1 deacetylase in regulating cardiomyocyte survival and hypertrophy. J Mol Cell Cardiol. 2011 Oct;51(4):614-8.

[229] Rajamohan SB, Pillai VB, Gupta M, Sundaresan NR, Birukov KG, Samant S, Hottiger MO, Gupta MP: SIRT1 promotes cell survival under stress by deacetylation-dependent deactivation of poly(ADP-ribose) polymerase 1. Mol Cell Biol. 2009 Aug;29(15):4116-29.

[230] Virchow R. Cellular Pathology as Based Upon Physiological and Pathological Histology. London: John Churchill, 1860:325.

[231] Tontonoz P, Spiegelman BM. Fat and beyond: The diverse biology of PPARgamma. Annu Rev Biochem. 2008;77: 289-312.

[232] Medina-Gomez G, Gray S, Vidal-Puig A: Adipogenesis and lipotoxicity: role of peroxisome proliferator-activated receptor gamma (PPARgamma) and PPARgammacoactivator-1 (PGC1). Public Health Nutr. 2007 Oct;10(10A):1132-7.

[233] Bhayana S, Siu VM, Joubert GI, Clarson CL, Cao H, Hegele RA: Cardiomyopathy in congenital complete lipodystrophy. Clin Genet. 2002 Apr;61(4):283-7.

[234] Sharma S, Adrogue JV, Golfman L, Uray I, Lemm J, Youker K, Noon GP, Frazier OH, Taegtmeyer H: Intramyocardial lipid accumulation in the failing human heart resembles the lipotoxic rat heart. FASEB J. 2004 Nov;18(14):1692-700.

[235] Yagyu H, Chen G, Yokoyama M, Hirata K, Augustus A, Kako Y, Seo T, Hu Y, Lutz EP, Merkel M, Bensadoun A, Homma S, Goldberg IJ: Lipoprotein lipase (LpL) on the surface of cardiomyocytes increases lipid uptake and produces a cadiomyopathy. J Clin Invest. 2003 Feb;111(3):419-26.

[236] Unger RH, Clark GO, Scherer PE, Orci L. 2010. Lipid homeostasis, lipotoxicity and the metabolic syndrome. Biochim Biophys Acta 1801:209–214.

[237] Marfella R, Di Filippo C, Portoghese M, Barbieri M, Ferraraccio F, Siniscalchi M, Cacciapuoti F, Rossi F, D'Amico M, Paolisso G: Myocardial lipid accumulation in patients with pressure-overloaded heart and metabolic syndrome. J Lipid Res. 2009 Nov;50(11):2314-23.

[238] Finck BN, Han X, Courtois M, Aimond F, Nerbonne J, Kovacs A, Gross RW, Kelly DP: A critical role for PPARalpha-mediated lipotoxicity in the pathogenesis of diabetic cardiomyopathy: modulation by dietary fat content. Proc. Natl. Acad. Sci. USA 2003;100: 1226–1231.

[239] Son NH, Park TS, Yamashita H, Yokoyama M, Huggins LA, Okajima K, Homma S, Szabolcs MJ, Huang LS, Goldberg IJ: Cardiomyocyte expression of PPARgamma leads to cardiac dysfunction in mice. J Clin Invest. 2007 Oct;117(10):2791-801.

[240] Jozefowicz E, Brisson H, Rozenberg Mebazaa A, Gelé P, Callebert J, Lebuffe G, Vallet B, Bordet R, Tavernier B: Activation of peroxisome proliferatoractivated receptor-alpha by fenofibrate prevents myocardial dysfunction during endotoxemia in rats. Crit Care Med 2007; 35:856-63.

[241] Brindley DN, Kok BP, Kienesberger PC, Lehner R, Dyck JR: Shedding light on the enigma of myocardial lipotoxicity: the involvement of known and putative regulators of fatty acid storage and mobilization. Am J Physiol Endocrinol Metab. 2010 May;298(5):E897-908.

[242] Ilbäck NG, Mohammed A, Fohlman J, Friman G: 1990. Cardiovascular lipid accumulation with Coxsackie B virus infection in mice. Am. J. Pathol. 136: 159–167.

Chapter 15

Lipids as Markers of Induced Resistance in Wheat: A Biochemical and Molecular Approach

Christine Tayeh, Béatrice Randoux, Frédéric Laruelle,
Natacha Bourdon, Delphine Renard-Merlier and Philippe Reignault

Additional information is available at the end of the chapter

http://dx.doi.org/10.5772/51279

1. Introduction

Plant disease resistance can be defined as the ability of the plant to prevent or restrict pathogen growth and multiplication. All plants, whether they are resistant or susceptible, respond to pathogen attack by the induction of a coordinated resistance strategy. Acceleration and/or amplification of the plant responses by the application of resistance inducers could provide a biologically, environmentally and commercially viable alternative to existing pathogen control methods [1].

Among pathogenic fungi, the obligate parasite *Blumeria graminis* f. sp. *tritici* (*Bgt*) is responsible for wheat (*Triticum aestivum*) powdery mildew, one of the most damaging foliar diseases of this crop, especially in Northern Europe. Worldwide yield losses due to wheat powdery mildew would be about 30% without chemical treatments, so that an extensive use of conventional fungicides is undertaken. Moreover, populations of *Bgt* resistant to the main chemical fungicides (ergosterol biosynthesis inhibitors, EBIs and 2-aminopyridines) are rising, and these resistant strains emerged all over most European territories [2]. New disease management strategies based on the use of molecules that induce plant resistance *via* the elicitation of defence responses are therefore developed in order to reduce the use of conventional fungicides. These strategies match the growing concern about the consequences of the use of fungicides on both health and environment [3,4].

Induced partial resistance against *B. graminis* f.sp. *tritici* has been obtained in wheat with different elicitors and resistance inducers. Infection level was reduced to 57% and 58% relative to controls when nonacetylated and acetylated oligogalacturonides, respectively, were sprayed on wheat 48h before inoculation with *Bgt* [5]. Trehalose, a non-reducing disaccharide found in a wide variety of organisms, confers a 60% protection level against powdery mildew [6]. It has also been shown that a double spraying of wheat plantlets with salicylic acid (SA) confers a 65% protection level against powdery mildew [7]. Prophylactic efficacies of Iodus 40® and heptanoyl salicylic acid (HSA) against wheat powdery mildew have been tested [8]. Iodus 40®, a commercial product, is used to decrease wheat powdery mildew damage in the field. Its active ingredient is laminarin, a storage β-1,3-D-glucan (polysaccharide), extracted from the brown alga *Laminaria digitata*. It induces protection in grapevine against *Botrytis cinerea* and *Plasmopara viticola* [9] as well as in wheat against powdery mildew [8]. HSA is synthesized by esterification of 2-OH benzoic acid by heptanoic acid [7]. Plantlets treated twice exhibited 60% and 100% protection levels, respectively [8]. A long up-to-run-off spraying of wheat leaves with Milsana®, an ethanolic extract from leaves of the giant knotweed *Reynoutria sachaliensis*, 48h before inoculation led to a 97% protection level against powdery mildew [10]. No direct effect against the fungus has been noticed for any of these elicitors [8] except for Milsana® which exhibited a direct fungistatic effect on *B. graminis* conidia germination [10]. It is now necessary to understand the mode of action and the cascade of cellular and molecular events triggered by these wheat resistance inducers.

In the last fifteen years, SA itself has been described as playing a key role in the activation of defence systems against pathogens in plants. Despite several reports [11-14], works focusing on SA as a resistance inducer are far from being as extensive as those concerning BTH, a functional analogue of SA, and, as far as we know, a single one involved wheat [8].

Plant lipids and lipid metabolic pathways have been shown to be of crucial importance during a plant-pathogen interaction. Many changes in membrane lipids are known to occur in plants at the site of infection. Moreover, lipids and lipid metabolites, released from membranes, function and act as signal molecules in the activation of plant defence responses [15].

Over the past few years, it has become increasingly clear that phosphatidic acid (PA) is involved in stress signaling because it is rapidly and transiently formed in response to various environmental stimuli [16]. PA could be generated by 2 distinct pathways as shown in figure 1: a first one involves phospholipase D (PLD) acting hydrolytically on membrane phospholipids, particularly phosphatidylcholine (PC) and phosphatidylethanolamine (PE); a second one involves phospholipase C (PLC) acting sequentially with diacylglycerol kinase (DGK) *via* diacylglycerol (DAG) phosphorylation [17].

Phospholipid-signaling pathways are complex, interrelated, and involve numerous enzymes and substrates [18]. As an ubiquitous enzyme family, phospholipases play various roles in stress responses [19]. Beside PLC and PLD, a main class of phospholipases A (PLA) hydrolyze phospholipids (such as PC) into the corresponding free fatty acid and lysophospholipid (such as lysoPC). Such a fatty acid can be a precursor for oxylipin biosynthesis, and lysoPC may be involved in multiple cellular processes [20]. One important finding on functions of lysoPC is that it can activate H^+-ATPase in the tonoplast and cause cytoplasmic acidification, which is shown to activate defense responses and phytoalexin production [21]. The lipid messengers derived from hydrolysis of the plasma membrane are illustrated in figure 2.

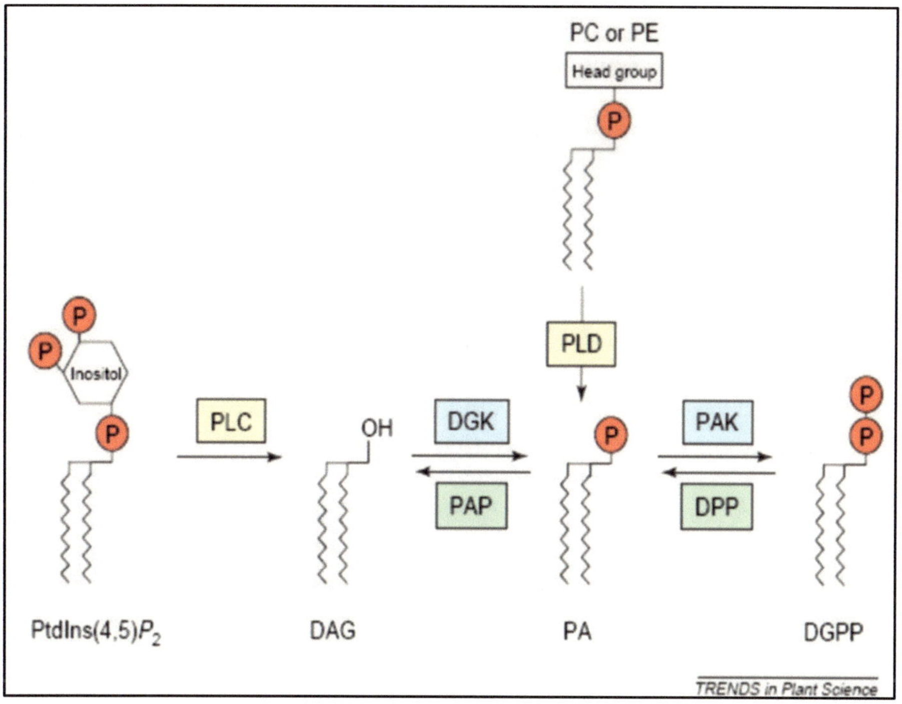

Figure 1. Formation and attenuation of phosphatidic acid (PA) [16]

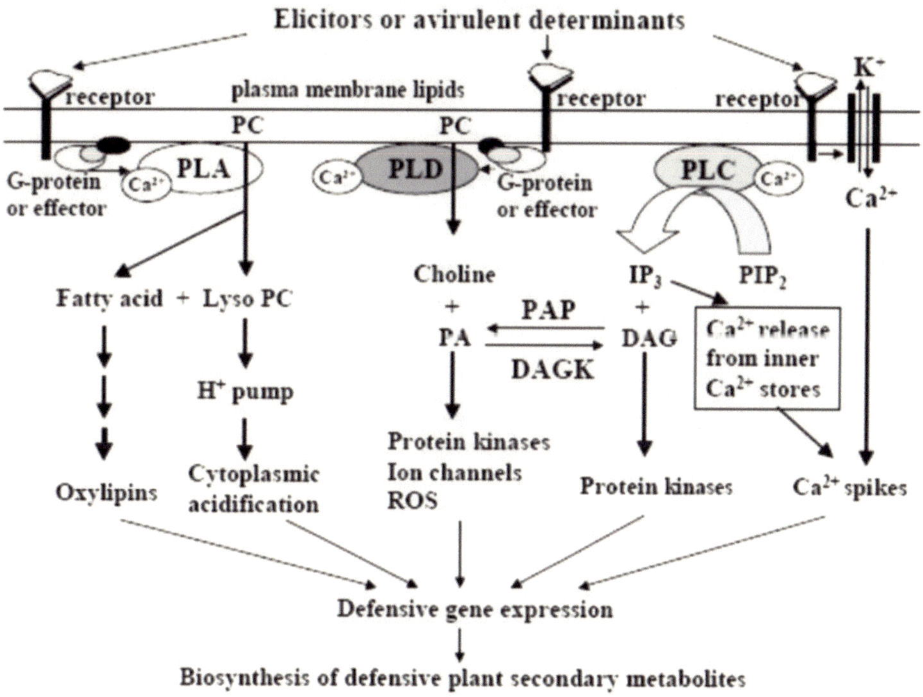

Figure 2. Lipid messengers derived from hydrolysis of plasma membrane [22]

Adaptation of higher plants to biotic and abiotic stress is often accompanied by the occurrence of lipid peroxidation and metabolites which derived therefrom are called oxylipins. Lipid peroxydation may be the result of a coordinated action of enzymes or the result of auto-oxidation (Figure 3). Oxylipins are potent signaling molecules in the defense response in plants [23]. The synthesis of oxylipins is first catalyzed by lipoxygenases (LOXs), which add molecular oxygen to polyunsaturated fatty acids (PUFAs) to yield the corresponding fatty acid hydroperoxides that are substrates for other enzymes (figure 4) [24]. Based on their regiospecificity, the dioxygenation occurs at C-9 or C-13 and LOXs have been thus classified as 9- and 13-LOX, which yield 9- or 13-hydroperoxides, respectively [25]. In the case of linolenic acid C18:3 and 13-LOX, the resulting product is 13-HPOT (hydroperoxy octadectrienoic acid) [15]. These LOX-derived hydroperoxides can be converted through different reactions of the LOX pathway, particularly by an allene oxide synthase (AOS) leading to jasmonic acid (JA). Most of the LOX-derived compounds are considered as acting in plant defense reactions: indeed, C6 volatiles induce defense-related genes expression [26], divinyl ethers are antifungal [27], and JA is an important signaling compound that is involved in plant response to biotic stress [28,29]. Jasmonates are primarily derived from the C18:3 FA, which is released from membrane lipids via the activity of phospholipase A1.

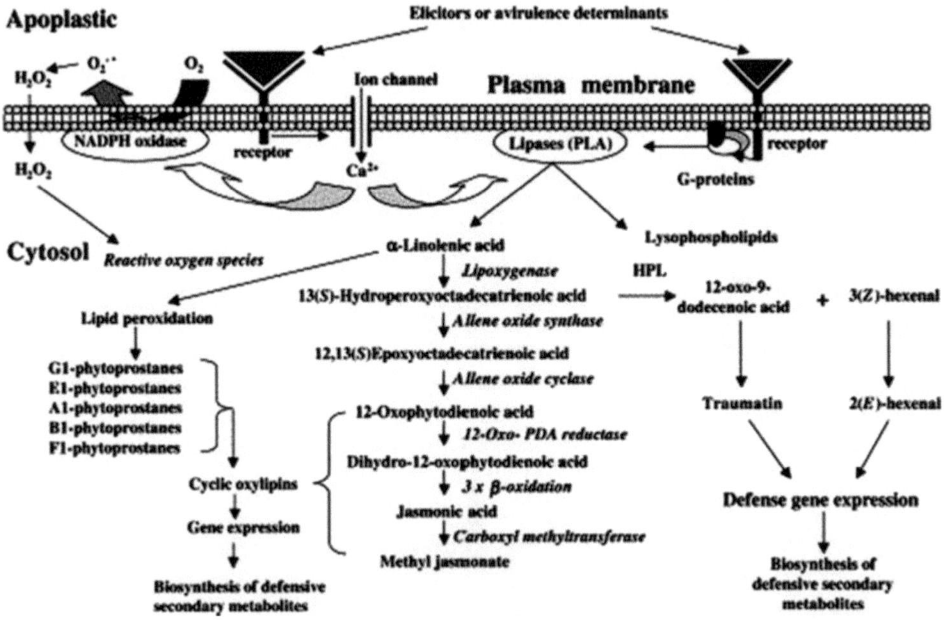

Figure 3. Schematic illustration of biosynthetic pathway of JA and other related oxylipins [22]

The phospholipase A (PLA) superfamily which catalyzes the hydrolysis of membrane phospholipids, acts up-stream the LOX to generate the corresponding PUFAs and lysophospholipids [30]. PLA may be involved in the release of free fatty acids for the biosynthesis of JA during the activation of plant defence responses. Indeed, three tobacco genes that encode putative members of the patatin family of PLAs, were identified [31].

Their expression is induced by microbial elicitors and upon exposure to pathogen. The high expression level of these PLA genes precedes the accumulation of JA in pathogen-inoculated or elicitor-treated tissues. Activation of PLA has also been reported in response to TMV infection in tobacco [32] and elicitor treatment of cultured parsley cells [33].

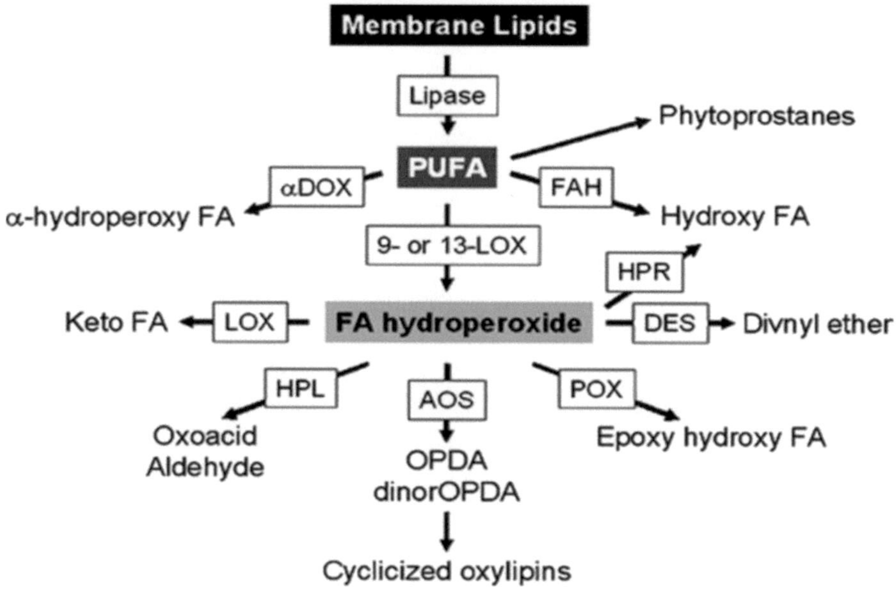

Figure 4. Enzymatic and non-enzymatic mechanisms leading to the synthesis of oxylipins in plants [15]

FAs not only serve as the major source of reserve energy but also consist of complex lipids, which are essential components of cellular membrane lipids. Increasing evidence also shows the involvement of FAs and their derivatives in signaling and altering normal and disease-related physiologies in microbes, insects, animals, and plants. In plants, FAs modulate a variety of responses to biotic and abiotic stresses. For instance, PUFAs levels in chloroplastic membranes affect membrane lipid fluidity and determine the plant's ability to acclimatize to temperature stress [34]. Linolenic acid (18:3) is involved in protein modifications in heat-stressed plants [35]. FAs also regulate salt, drought, and heavy metal tolerance as well as wound-induced responses and defense against insect and herbivore feeding in plants [36]. FA metabolic pathways play significant roles in defense against pathogens. Classically, only passive roles were assigned to FAs in plant defense such as providing biosynthetic precursors for cuticular components (studies of FA metabolic mutants also reveal an active signaling role for the cuticle in plant defense) or JA, well known for its role in wound responses and plant defense against insect pathogens. However, recent works demonstrate more direct roles for FAs and their breakdown products in inducing various modes of plant defenses. Both 16- and 18-carbon FAs participate in defense to modulate basal, effector-triggered, and systemic immunity in plants [37].

Furthermore, lipid transfer proteins (LTPs), located in the cell wall, participate in the *in vitro* transfer of phospholipids between membranes and can bind acyl chains. Based on these properties, LTPs are thought to be involved in membrane biogenesis and regulation of intracellular FA pools [38]. Many roles were suggested for LTPs: involvement in cutin formation, embryogenesis, symbiosis and adaptation of plants to various environmental conditions [39]. Among them, defensive role of LTPs has been proposed. Indeed, LTPs have been naturally classified as members of pathogenesis-related (PR) proteins belonging to the group PR-14 [40]. Some members of this family have the ability to inhibit the growth of fungal pathogens in barley and maize [41], in sunflower against *Fusarium solani* [42], in transgenic rice against *Magnaporthe grisea, Rhizoctonia solani* and *Xanthonomas oryzae* [43]. In transgenic wheat expressing *Ace-AMP,* the corresponding encoded LTP showed enhanced antifungal activity against *Bgt* [44]. *Ltp3F1,* a novel gene encoding an antifungal protein against *Alternaria sp., Curcularia lunata, Bipolaris oryzae* and *Sarocladium oryzae* was characterized from wheat [45].

In this review, we will discuss further and extend the study conducted by Renard-Merlier *et al.* [46], where a global investigation of total FA content in relation to treatment with four inducers of resistance and to powdery mildew infection was undertaken. Previous studies established that lipid metabolism is altered by Milsana®, Iodus 40®, HSA, SA and trehalose [8,10]; therefore, our work aimed to characterize their impact at the total FA level. During a time course experiment, content (quantitative analysis) and percentage (qualitative analysis) of FAs were compared in treated plants and in controls, as well as in non-inoculated (ni) plants and *Bgt*-challenged plants (i). Previous results will be considered and discussed relatively to new findings.

Moreover, the effect of one resistance inducer, namely SA, on lipid metabolism is evaluated by molecular and biochemical approaches.

Phospholipids being the major membrane components, we investigated PC, PE, DAG and PA content variation in wheat leaves infiltrated with salicylic acid (SA). SA can modulate the content variation of these compounds, reservoirs from which biologically active lipids and precursors of oxidized lipids are released.

At the transcriptional level, a PLC-encoding gene expression was investigated in an attempt to assign any participation of this pathway in the phospholipids equilibrium described above.

We also investigated free FAs and PLFAs content variations in SA-infiltrated wheat leaves; this pool of lipids is quite interesting since it ensures several functions, from being an energy source to acting as cellular messengers; the latter being highly related to resistance induction in plants. The lipoxygenase response to SA-infiltration, at the molecular and enzymatic level, was also evaluated; this enzyme activity is important for oxylipins biosynthesis in plants, because of its position upstream the cascade of enzymatic lipid peroxydation.

An LTP-encoding gene expression was also monitored, taking into account the possible antifungal activity of LTPs as well as their ability to bind and transport membrane lipids, thus participating in lipid-mediated signaling mechanisms.

2. Material and methods

2.1. Treatments application

Wheat (*Triticum aestivum*) cultivar Orvantis was used throughout the experiments. It was provided by Benoit C.C. (Orgerus, France). This cultivar is fully susceptible to the MPEBgt1 powdery mildew isolate. First leaf of ten-day-old wheat plantlets was infiltrated with salicylic acid (1g/L) solution using a hypodermic syringe without needle. Infiltrated area was delineated with a marker pen. Control plantlets were infiltrated with distillated water.

Ten-day-old wheat seedlings were treated with solutions of Iodus 40® (1g/L), HSA (1g/L), Milsana® (0.3% v/v) and trehalose (15g/L) as described by Renard-Merlier *et al.* [46]. Treatments consisted in "up-to-run-off" sprayings. Two days after inducer treatments, seedlings to be inoculated were sprayed with conidia of *Bgt* suspended in Fluorinert FC43 at a concentration of 5.10^6 spores.mL^{-1}.

2.2. RNA extraction and quantification of gene expression by real-time PCR

SA and water-infiltrated wheat leaves were sampled at 3, 6, 9, 12, 15, 18, 21, 24, 48, 72 and 96 hours after infiltration (hai) and stored at -80°C until use. Total RNA was extracted from 100 mg plant tissue using RNeasy Plant Mini Kit (Quiagen, The Netherlands) with some modifications of the protocol. cDNA synthesis was carried out using High Capacity cDNA Reverse Transcription Kit (Applied Biosystems, USA) according to the manufacturer's protocol. Real Time qPCR was performed using ABI Prism 7300 detection system (Applied Biosystems, USA). The *tub* and *ef1α* genes, encoding respectively for tubulin and elongation factor ef1alpha, were used as reference genes. The relative expression of the target genes was evaluated in SA-infiltrated wheat leaves compared with water-infiltrated leaves and normalized to the *tub* and *ef1a* expression level. The analyses were performed using the relative expression software tool REST® as described in [47]. The experiments were repeated twice with similar results and representative results are presented.

2.3. LOX assay

LOX was assayed as described in [10] according to [48] and [49] with slight modifications. The results are the mean of three biological repetitions.

2.4. Fatty acid extraction and analysis

Total cellular FAs extraction and purification were performed by the authors in [46] using adapted protocols from [50]. The results are means of three independent repetitions.

Free FAs, PLFA and PL extraction was carried out according to the method described in [51]. Data shown are the results of the first experiment, which need to be confirmed by a biological repetition.

3. Results and discussion

3.1. PA content increases after SA infiltration

Because of its central position in the pathways mentioned above, the first results presented here have been obtained for PA. Table 1 shows the variations in PA levels in SA-infiltrated leaves, compared to the control. No change in PA content was observed during the first 24 hours after infiltration (hai) of SA, compared to the water-infiltrated wheat leaves; even though a slight accumulation of PA was observed in water-infiltrated leaves in comparison to the untreated plants, probably due to the stress generated by the infiltration. However, SA induced increases in PA content from 24 h till 96 hai, with a maximum of 6.2-fold increase at 72 hai.

	Time after SA infiltration			
	24h	48h	72h	96h
PA content	2.2-fold increase	2.7-fold increase	6.2-fold increase	1.19-fold increase

Table 1. Variations in PA levels in SA-infiltrated wheat leaves compared to the water-infiltrated control

These results confirm some variations in PA content reported by several authors. Treatment of *A. thaliana* protoplasts with H_2O_2 increases PA content by 30% [52]. Furthermore, elicitors from plant pathogens activate the PLC-DGK pathway, which consisted of a rapid accumulation of PA within 2 minutes in transgenic tobacco cells treated with the race-specific elicitor Avr4 [53]. A transient accumulation of PA was also recorded in suspension-cultured tomato cells treated with the general elicitors N,N',N'',N'''-tetraacetyl-chitotetraose, xylanase, and the flagellin-derived peptide flg22 [54]. In rice cells, the PA amount increased rapidly after treatment with N-acetylchitooligosaccharide elicitor [55]. Moreover, the PA increase is likely to occur upstream of the oxidative burst [53,55]. Furthermore, method of PA assessment. Furthermore, all these studies point out the rapid accumulation of PA upon treatments, generally within minutes. According to [16], signaling lipids, unlike structural lipids, are present only in minute amounts, yet their levels increase rapidly in response to certain stimuli. Such an accumulation is transient because the signal is rapidly down regulated. However, none of these characteristics, namely the rapid and transient accumulation upon treatment, met our results. SA induces a PA accumulation that occurred not earlier than 24 h after SA infiltration and seemed to last for at least 4 days. This result, that does not match the general trend, may be explained by a late induction of one or both of the phospholipases pathways leading to PA formation. Since the magnitude of PA change varies upon the treatment, tissue and method of PA assessment [17], our findings could be attributed to the treatment and/or to the tissue nature - infiltration of SA and PA assessment *in planta* - whereas most of the studies are conducted on cellular cultures.

3.2. *PLC* gene expression is up-regulated and DAG content increases in SA-infiltrated leaves

In order to corroborate the PA formation with the PLC-DGK pathway activation, the expression of the *PLC* gene, encoding a phospholipase C, was measured over the time-course experiment, compared to the water-infiltrated wheat leaves, and normalized to two reference genes, *tub* and *ef1α*, encoding tubulin and elongation factor, respectively (Figure 5). The expression pattern of the *PLC* gene consisted of three up-regulations: 3.5 and 4.8-fold increases were induced at 9 and 21 hai, respectively. Furthermore, this gene expression was strongly increased from 48 till 96 hai, with an average of 9-fold increase over this period. This late high up-regulation of *PLC* gene correlates with the late PA detection in wheat leaves between 48 and 96 h after SA infiltration. The accumulation of PA is probably due to this pathway's stimulation after *PLC* gene's expression and synthesis of the corresponding enzyme.

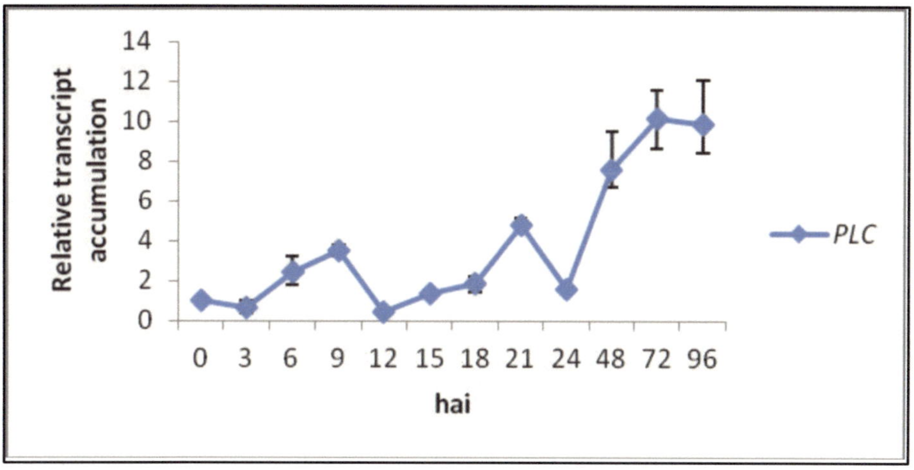

Figure 5. *PLC* gene expression in wheat leaves infiltrated with SA

PA formation through the phospholipase C pathway results from two enzymes acting sequentially: PLC hydrolyses phosphatidylinositol-4,5-bisphosphate [PtdIns(4,5)P2, also abbreviated as PIP2] into inositol-1,4,5-trisphosphate [Ins(1,4,5)P3] and DAG. DAG remains in the membrane and is rapidly phosphorylated to PA by DGK (Figure 1). The variation in DAG levels in SA-infiltrated wheat leaves is presented in table 2. During the first 24 h after SA infiltration, no clear variation pattern in DAG content was observed. However, SA induced the accumulation of DAG from 24 till 96 hai, with a maximum of 2.18-fold increase at 72hai. Interestingly, DAG accumulation, as well as *PLC* gene expression, was recorded in the same period of the time-course experiment, 24 till 96 h after SA infiltration. The DAG accumulation seems to be the consequence of the induction of *PLC* gene expression.

Twenty four hours after infiltration, SA induces the expression of PLC-encoding gene, simultaneously with an accumulation of DAG and PA. One could think that DAG content must decrease in order to fulfill PA formation; indeed, the contribution of DAG could only be confirmed by the investigation of DGK activity. Even if the subsequent enzymatic conversion of DAG doesn't lead to PA formation, one must keep in mind that the hydrolysis of PtdIns(4,5)P_2 into Ins(1,4,5)P_3 is of a great interest since the latter diffuses into the cytosol where it possibly triggers calcium flux/release from intracellular stores [20].

In addition, the simultaneous increase of these compounds could be due to the durable *PLC* gene expression, ensuring a continuous supply of DAG to be phosphorylated to PA.

	Time after SA infiltration						
	6h	12h	18h	24h	48h	72h	96h
DAG content	1.1-fold increase	1.1-fold decrease	Ø	1.26-fold increase	1.62-fold increase	2.18-fold increase	1.56-fold increase

Table 2. Variation in DAG level in SA-infiltrated wheat leaves compared to the control

3.3. PE and PC contents vary in SA-infiltrated leaves

PA could also be generated by the phospholipase D pathway which hydrolyzes structural membrane phospholipids such as PE and PC (Figure 1). The variations of PE and PC levels in SA-infiltrated leaves compared to the control are presented in table 3. While accumulation of PC was observed during the whole time-course experiment (except for 24 and 96 hai), PE accumulated the first 18h after treatment. Afterward, SA induced a decrease in the PE content between 24 and 96 hai, with a maximum decrease at 48 and 72 hai. These results match the increased PA level in SA-infiltrated wheat leaves in the same period, suggesting that this pathway is involved in PA formation. Since PC level was maintained and even increased, this phospholipid doesn't seem to be involved in PA production, under SA treatment. The PE/PC ratio is also reduced from 48 till 96 hai. Substantial alterations in the lipid composition of plasma membrane are a widely known process to stress adaptation, such as water deficit: the PC/PE ratio changed from 1.1 in plants non-acclimated to water stress to 0.69 in acclimated ones [56].

	Time after SA infiltration						
	6h	12h	18h	24h	48h	72h	96h
PE content	1.4-fold increase	1.3-fold increase	Ø	1.3-fold decrease	6.6-fold decrease	6.2-fold decrease	2.3-fold decrease
PC content	1.4-fold increase	2.9-fold increase	3.8-fold increase	Ø	1.8-fold increase	1.4-fold increase	Ø
PE/PC	2	1.2	1.2	2.2	0.2	0.5	0.6

Table 3. Variations in PE and PC levels (compared to the control) and PE/PC ratio induced in SA-infiltrated wheat leaves

In conclusion, SA seems to induce the formation of PA through the activation of phospholipases C and/or D pathways. In *Arabidopsis,* PLC signaling is involved in some responses mediated by ABA without any contribution of DGK activity or PA [57]. This signaling, *via* Ins(1,4,5)P3, is also reported as an early response to salinity and hyperosmotic stress [58,59]. The PLC-DGK pathway was sought in *Arabidopsis* after cold exposure [60], in transgenic tobacco cells upstream the oxidative burst as in [53] and after contact with pathogens. In suspension-cultured alfalfa cells, the nod factor activates this pathway [61].

Treatment of tomato cell cultures with the fungal elicitor xylanase resulted in a rapid and dose-dependent nitric oxide (NO) accumulation, required for PA production via the activation of PLC-DGK pathway. PA and, correspondingly, xylanase were shown to induce ROS production [62].

The PLD pathway is involved in every mentioned stress signaling, except cold-induced stress. Several *Arabidopsis* PLDs were found to be induced in response to *Pseudomonas* infection [63]. The PLD pathway contribution was also found in *Arabidopsis* upon drought [64], ethylene treatment [65], freezing [66] and wounding [67,68].

Moreover, signaling lipids can affect the activity of target enzymes. In [69], the authors showed an activation of a calcium-dependent protein kinase DcCPK1 by PA in *Daucus carota*. In *Arabidopsis,* the activation of AtPDK1, a protein kinase, target of PLD-generated PA, is involved in root hair growth [70]; the PLD-derived PA also interacts with ABI1 phosphatase and regulates ABA signaling [71].

All together, these results are the first evidence for SA as an inducer of PA formation in wheat leaves. Increases in PA levels in SA-treated wheat leaves seem to be highly related to the induction of plant genes encoding phospholipases that are involved in the synthesis or release of PA.

3.4. *LOX* gene expression and LOX activity are enhanced upon SA-infiltration

In the present experiments, the *lox* gene expression showed a 12 and 14-fold increase at 9 and 21 hai respectively, in SA-infiltrated leaves. This gene expression was also strongly induced later, with a 166 and 156-fold increase at 48 and 96 hai respectively (Figure 6).

In grapevine plantlets, rhamnolipids induced for *lox* gene expression a 7-fold increase 24 h after immersion in the rhamnolipids solution [72]. In wheat, transcripts of *WCI-2* (Wheat Chemically Induced gene) gene, which encodes a lipoxygenase, accumulated quickly in response to MeJA, SA and BTH treatments (from 2 h to 24h for MeJA, and from 4h and to 20 h for the other elicitors); however, SA induced this gene's expression to a lesser extent than the other two compounds [73]. The contribution of SA to early signaling events by the stimulation of lipoxygenase-encoding genes is therefore established. Nevertheless, the authors didn't record any accumulation of the transcripts of *WCI-2* gene the first 24 h after wheat seedlings inoculation with *Bgt* nor *Bgh* (incompatible interaction). However, accumulation of these transcripts was found in latter stages of wheat infection with powdery mildew. In infectious conditions, the *lox* gene seemed to be expressed quite late [74]. Infiltration with SA reproduced a similar lox-encoding transcripts profile with a late up-regulation of the *lox* gene to a 166 and 156-fold increase at 48 and 96 hai, respectively.

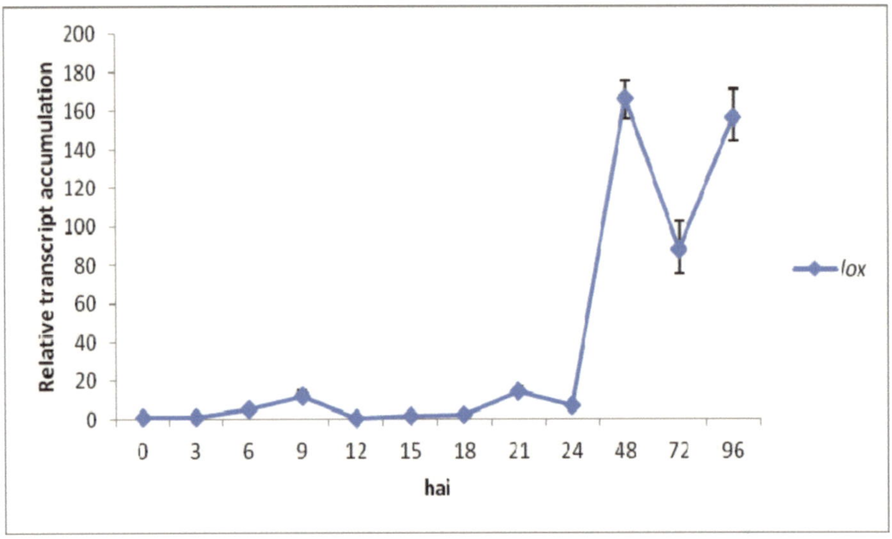

Figure 6. *lox* gene expression in wheat leaves treated with SA

Figure 7 shows the LOX activity in leaf extracts at 6, 12, 18, 24, 48, 72 and 96 h after SA infiltration in comparison to water-infiltrated leaves. During the first 48h, the LOX activity was decreased in SA-infiltrated leaves. However, SA induced significant 1.7 and 3.8-fold increases in LOX activity at 72h and 96hai, compared to the control.

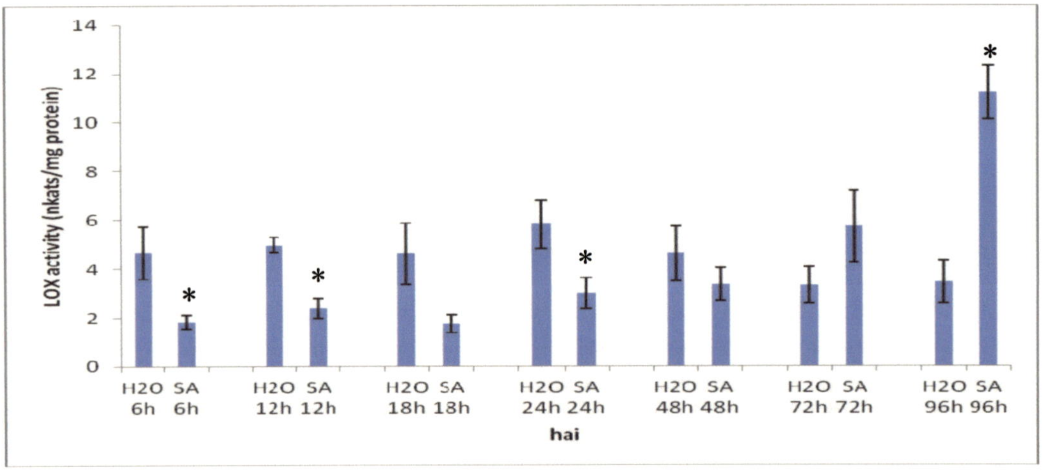

Figure 7. Time-course activity of LOX in water and SA-infiltrated wheat leaves. Data represent means of 3 independent experiments. Bars with an asterix are different from water control plantlets as determined by ANOVA followed by a multiple range test (LSD) ($P<0.05$).

When compared together, profiles of *lox* gene expression and LOX activity in SA-infiltrated leaves show interestingly that the first *lox* up-regulations, 24 h after SA infiltration, are not followed by the corresponding enzymatic activity. Induction of LOX activity by SA was only detectable after *lox* transcripts accumulation was the most important, between 48 and 96hai.

In non-infectious context, the induction of a LOX activity was also assessed in wheat by Renard-Merlier *et al.* [8]. Wheat sprayings with HSA enhanced a 1.5-fold increase in LOX activity, compared to corresponding ethanol control, only 96 h after treatment. Thus, infiltration of SA as well as HSA sprayings induced similar LOX enzymatic activity profile. However, these authors didn't report any significant difference in LOX activity between control and SA-sprayed leaves over the 4 days after treatment. This finding highlights the effect of SA functionalization, probably improving the penetration of HSA through the hydrophobic plant cuticle. Moreover, HSA, which increased the protection level against *Bgt* from 50% in SA-treated wheat leaves to 95%, induced an 8-fold increase of the LOX activity in inoculated conditions.

LOX-derived products such as hydroperoxy, hydroxyl and keto fatty acids accumulate in plants in response to attack by pathogens and treatment with inducers of plant defence responses [75]. For example, in *A. thaliana*, infection by *P. syringae* causes accumulation of ketodienoic fatty acids in *A.* leaves as well as the cell death and induces expression of the *GST1* gene, which encodes a glutathione-S-transferase [76]. In another study, SA treatment was shown to cause the accumulation of 13 (S)-hydroxyoctadecatrienoic acid (13-HOTrE) in barley leaves, and application of 13-HOTrE induces the expression of the PR1B gene, suggesting the involvement of 13-HOTrE in SA signaling in barley [77]. One must keep in mind that the primary products of PUFAs enzymatic oxidation are often converted to oxylipins such as JA. In barley leaves, 13-HOD and 13-HOT (hydroxyl PUFAs after reductase on HPOD and HPOT respectively) accumulated suggesting that the reductase branch of the LOX pathway is the object of preferential induction upon SA treatment, among the various metabolic transformations of the LOX-derived 13-HPOT or 13-HPOD. No accumulation of other LOX pathway-products was observed. SA as well as 13-HOT induced *PR1* gene expression, 48h after treatment. In barley leaves, at least one specific LOX is transcriptionnaly activated by SA and JA. This LOX-100 is a 13-LOX located in the chloroplast. However, this LOX-100 gene was not expressed upon infection with powdery mildew in susceptible and non-susceptible barley lines [78]. The co-induction of LOX and PR1 by SA suggests a role in plant defense reaction.

3.5. FAs content varies in resistance inducers-treated wheat plants

3.5.1. Total FAs content vary in trehalose, Iodus40, Milsana and HSA-treated wheat leaves

In wheat, Renard-Merlier *et al.* [46] conducted a global investigation of total FA content in relation to treatment with four inducers of resistance and to powdery mildew infection.

Table 4 presents a summary of the observed variations of several FAs content at the quantitative and qualitative levels induced by the four tested resistance inducers and these results are now discussed on the basis of the most recent literature as well as our results presented above.

	C12:0		C18:1		18:2		C20:2	
	quantitative	qualitative	quantitative	qualitative	quantitative	qualitative	quantitative	qualitative
Trehalose								
ni	Ø	Ø	Ø	Ø	Ø	Ø	Ø	Ø
i	4.0-fold increase	2.4-fold increase	Ø	Ø	Ø	Ø	Ø	1.3-fold decrease
Iodus 40								
ni	Ø	Ø	1.2-fold increase	2.2-fold increase	Ø	Ø	1.5-fold decrease	1.33-fold decrease
i	2.8-fold increase	1.5-fold increase	Ø	Ø	Ø	Ø	Ø	Ø
Milsana								
ni	Ø	Ø	Ø	Ø	Ø	Ø	2.3-fold decrease	Ø
i	4.8-fold increase	1.5-fold increase	Ø	Ø	Ø	Ø	1.8-fold decrease	2.0-fold decrease
HSA								
ni	Ø	Ø	Ø	Ø	Ø	1.15-fold increase	Ø	Ø
i	Ø	Ø	Ø	Ø	1.6-fold increase	1.15-fold increase	Ø	Ø

Table 4. Summary of variations observed in C12:0, C18:1, C18:2 and C20:2 content at the quantitative ($\mu g.mg^{-1}$ dry weight) and qualitative (percentage of total FAs) levels induced by inoculation, trehalose, Iodus 40®, Milsana® or HSA sprayings. These variations are observed 4 days after sprayings in non inoculated (ni) plants and 2 days post inoculation in inoculated (i) conditions

Lauric acid (C12:0) content quantitatively increased after Iodus 40® (2.8-fold), Milsana® (4.8-fold) and trehalose (4-fold) treatment in (i) plants (2 days after inoculation). In [79], the authors showed that *Vicia sativa* seedlings treated with MeJA exhibit an increase in lauric acid ω-hydroxylase activity, an enzyme that converts C12:0 into hydroxylated forms potentially involved in cutin monomer synthesis. Moreover, C12:0 itself has several relevant biological properties such as antifungal, antiviral, antiparasite and antibacterial activities [80,81]. However, none of the four compounds induced any variation in C12:0 level in non-infectious conditions. Since no elicitation was observed in this context, priming effect on C12:0 accumulations could be proposed for these resistance inducers in wheat against *Bgt*.

Contents of C20:2 (eicosadienoic acid) decreased in Iodus 40®- and Milsana®-treated (ni) plants compared to the corresponding controls (4 days after treatment). The decrease was confirmed at the qualitative level only for Iodus 40®. In (i) conditions, only Milsana® induced a significant decrease in C20:2 content at both levels whereas TR induced a decrease perceptible at the qualitative level only. In (i) plants, C20:2 increased (data not shown). C20:2 content seemed to be affected by fungal infection of the plant to a greater extent than by any of the resistance inducing treatments, since similar quantities were found in water-control (i) plants as well as in resistance inducers-treated plants. The link between C20:2 and infection was also reported in [82].Transgenic *A. thaliana* plants producing C20:2 exhibited enhanced resistance to the aphid *Myzus persicae*, the fungal pathogen *Botrytis cinerea* and to the oomycete pathogen *Phytophtora capsici*.

C18:1 (oleic acid) in Iodus 40®-treated (ni) plants showed a quantitative 1.2 fold-increase. C18:1, as well as other C18 and C16 FAs, are well known substrates for cutin monomer synthesis [83]. One could suggest that Iodus 40®, by stimulating the accumulation of this FA, contributes to the reinforcement of the plant cuticule prior to fungal contamination. In cultured parsley cells, a biphasic time-course for C18:1 increase was obtained upon treatment with peptidic or fungal elicitors [84]. In [85], the authors suggested that chloroplastic C18:1 level is critical for normal pathogen defense responses in *Arabidopsis*, including programmed cell death and systemic acquired resistance (SAR). In [86], it was shown that the oleic acid-mediated pathway induces constitutive defense signaling and enhances resistance to multiple pathogens in soybean. C18:1 and linoleic (18:2) acid levels, in part, regulate fungal development, seed colonization, and mycotoxin production by *Aspergillus* spp. [87]. Direct antifungal activity has also been reported for C18:1, since it inhibits, in a dose-dependent manner, the germination of *Erysiphe polygoni* spores [88].

The amount of C18:2 increased (1.6-fold) 4 days after HSA treatment in (i) plants. For C18:2, the accumulation in sorbitol-treated barley leaves was reported from 12 h till 72h after treatment [89]. Cold acclimating potato was found to accumulate linoleic acid (18:2) in the membrane glycerolipids of the leaves [90]. C18:2 is also a substrate for cutin monomer synthesis and can therefore contribute to cuticle reinforcement.

Among the four inducers tested, Iodus40® had the largest effects on FA levels, since it increased C12:0 and C18:1 and decreased C20:2. This product, which active ingredient is laminarin (polysaccharide), induced decreases in lipid peroxydation level all over the time-course experiment [8].

Trehalose and Milsana® had similar effects on FAs profile with induced increases in C12:0 and decreases in C20:2 contents. However, TR and Milsana® modes of action are quite different in the wheat-powdery mildew interaction. TR activates phenylalanine ammonia-lyase (PAL) and peroxydase activity and enhances papilla autofluorescence and H_2O_2 accumulation. However, it does not affect catalase (CAT), cinnamyl alcohol dehydrogenase (CAD), LOX or oxalate oxidase (OXO) activities, and does not alter lipid peroxide levels [8]. According to the authors in [10], treatments of wheat with Milsana® enhance H_2O_2 accumulation at the fungal penetration site without any possible correlation with the activation of enzymes involved in ROS metabolism. Only LOX, involved in both ROS regulation and lipid peroxidation, showed a 26 to 32% increase 48h postreatment in Milsana-infiltrated leaves. This weak effect of Milsana® on wheat lipid metabolism was confirmed at the lipid peroxydation level, which was shown to decrease in treated plants.

While HSA sprayings enhanced an increase in C18:2 levels only, HSA exhibited the most numerous and the highest effects in the wheat-powdery mildew interaction. HSA induced H_2O_2 accumulation, increases LOX activity in (i) conditions and decreases CAT activity in (ni) context [8].

While barley leaves treated with salicylate [77], sorbitol [89] or JA [91] accumulated C18:3, none of the 4 compounds tested induced any increase in C18:3 in wheat leaves according to our results.

3.5.2. Free FAs and PLFAs content vary in SA-infiltrated wheat leaves

The profile of free FAs and phospholipids FAs (PLFAs) in SA-infiltrated wheat leaves were also investigated and are presented in Table 5 and Table 6.

	C16:0	C18:0	C18:1	C18:2	C18:3
µg/mg dry weight	2.38-fold increase (48-96hai)	2.36-fold increase (48-96hai)	2-fold increase (48-96hai)	Ø	2.74-fold decrease (6-96hai)
%	1.4-fold increase (6-96hai)	1.47-fold increase (6-96hai)	Ø	Ø	2.3-fold decrease (6-96hai)

Table 5. Variations in free FAs content and % in SA-infiltrated leaves

	C16:0	C18:0	C18:1	C18:2	C18:3
µg/mg dry weight	1.5-fold increase (48-72hai)	1.9-fold increase (6-96hai)	Ø	2.7-fold decrease (72-96hai)	2.28-fold decrease (24-96hai)
%	1.6-fold increase (48-96hai)	2.5-fold increase (24-96hai)	Ø	Ø	1.27-fold decrease (24-96hai)

Table 6. Variations in PLFAs content and % in SA-infiltrated leaves

Upon treatment with SA, free palmitic acid (C16:0) accumulation was observed from 48 till 96 hai with an average of 2.38 fold-increase over this period and 1.4-fold increase at the qualitative level over the whole time-course experiment. Similar results were observed for the PLFAs C16:0, essentially the last 3 days of the experiment. Since monomers of cutin are synthesized C16:0, SA seems to induce the reinforcement of the plant cuticule. In *A. thaliana*, levels of the C16:3 (hexadecatrienoic acid) increase within a few hours of exposure to an avirulent strain of *P. syringae* [92].

Increases in both classes of stearic acid C18:0 content and percentage were observed in SA-infiltrated leaves. In soybean, increased levels of C18:0 likely inhibit soybean seed colonization by the seed-borne pathogen *Diaporthe phaseolorum* [93].

A transient 2-fold increase in free FAs C18:1 content was recorded. A sharp and rapid increase in C18:1 level was observed in parsley cells treated with a fungal elicitor [83]. Recent studies suggest that free oleic acid (18:1) levels in the chloroplast regulate the defense response of plants to pathogens including programmed cell death and SAR [94].

A 2,7-fold decrease in C18:2 PLFAs was observed 72 till 96 hai of SA. In sorbitol-treated barley leaves, the accumulation of C18:2 occurred from 12 h till 72h after treatment [89]. The development of asexual spores, and the formation of cleistothecia and sclerotia of *Aspergillus* spp are affected by C18:2 and light [95]. Avocado fruits infected with *Colletotrichum gleosporioides* spores accumulate C18:2 [96].

One of the most interesting results is the general decrease of C18:3 level after SA-infiltration. Most of the studies report increases in 18:3 levels such in suspension cells of California poppy (*Eschscholtzia californica*) treated with a yeast elicitor [97]. In *A. thaliana,* an increase of C18:3 occurred within a few hours of exposure to an avirulent strain of *P. syringae* [91]. The *Arabidopsis fad7 fad8* mutant defective in the generation of C18:3 in chloroplastic membranes is deficient in ROS production following infection with avirulent strains of *Pseudomonas syringae* and shows enhanced susceptibility to this pathogen [92]. C18:3 stimulates NADPH oxidase activity *in vitro,* which suggests that C18:3 modulates ROS production and the subsequent defense responses during *R* gene–mediated resistance in plants [92]. The *Arabidopsis fad3 fad7 fad8* triple mutant is unable to accumulate JA because of a deficiency in C18:3 and is highly susceptible to infection by insect larvae [98]. The *fad3 fad7 fad8* mutant plants are also highly susceptible to root rot by *Pythium jasmonium,* and this susceptibility can be alleviated by the exogenous application of MeJA [99]. Rhizobacteria-induced enhanced resistance to *Botrytis cinerea* is associated with the accumulation of C18:2 and C18:3 FAs in bean [100].

In barley leaves, 13-LOX are induced by SA and jasmonates. Upon SA treatment, free C18:3 and C18:2 accumulate in a 10:1 ratio reflecting their relative occurrence in leaf tissues [78]. The release of 18:3 from plant membrane lipids by stress-activated lipases is thought to provide the substrate for lipoxygenase and subsequent octadecanoid (oxylipin) pathway synthesis of JA and methyl jasmonate [101,102]. JA and methyl jasmonate participate in the signal regulation of a number of plant processes including wound and pathogen defense responses. Efforts have been successful to identify and characterize fatty acids esterifying lipases that are activated by pathogen attack and/or environmental stress. Results suggest that both A1 and A2 phospholipases are involved in 18:3 mobilization form membrane lipids [103]. In the C4 monocotyledon sorghum (*Sorghum bicolor L.),* SA induced genes of the octadecanoic acid pathway for JA synthesis which resulted in higher JA content [104].

However, in tobacco tissues expressing a hypersensitive response to TMV, an increase in the saturation of fatty acids contained in the microsomal phospholipids was observed while C18:3 content decreased by 9% [105]. Interestingly, the authors credited the change of FAs composition to a four-fold increase in LOX activity of the infected tobacco tissues.

The decreases in free FAs observed with our model could be explained by a rapid dioxygenation *via* LOX activity. Furthermore, accumulation of C16:0 and C18:0 coupled with no significant increase in C18:1 means that elongation of C16:0 into C18:0 is not followed by desaturation into C18:1, C18:2 and finally, C18:3. Such results could explain the reduced content level of C18:3.

3.6. *ltp* gene expression is induced by SA infiltration

The effect of SA on the expression of a lipid transfer protein-encoding gene *ltp* was also conducted according to the same time-course experiment (figure 8). SA induced a biphasic *ltp* expression pattern: a 1.7-fold increase at 9hai followed by an average of 4.6-fold increase between 48 and 96hai.

The LTPs extracellular distribution in the exposed surfaces in vascular tissue systems, high abundance and corresponding genes expression in response to infection by pathogens suggest that they are active plant-defense proteins [106]. A combined expression of chitinase and LTP-encoding genes in transgenic carrot plants enhances resistance to *Botrytis sp.* and *Alternaria sp.* [107]. A high global expression of an *ltp* gene in resistant wheat to *Tilletia tritici* was identified [108]. The nonspecific nsLTP-encoding gene expression profile was evaluated in grape cells suspension in response to various defense-realted signal molecules [109]. A rapid and strong accumulation of nsLTPs mRNAs was recorded upon treatment with ergosterol (5h after treatment with hybridation signal more than 300X A.U.) whereas JA, cholesterol and sitosterol promoted an accumulation but to a lesser extent (hybridation signal between 100 and 200X). However, SA had no effect on nsLTPs mRNAs accumulation.

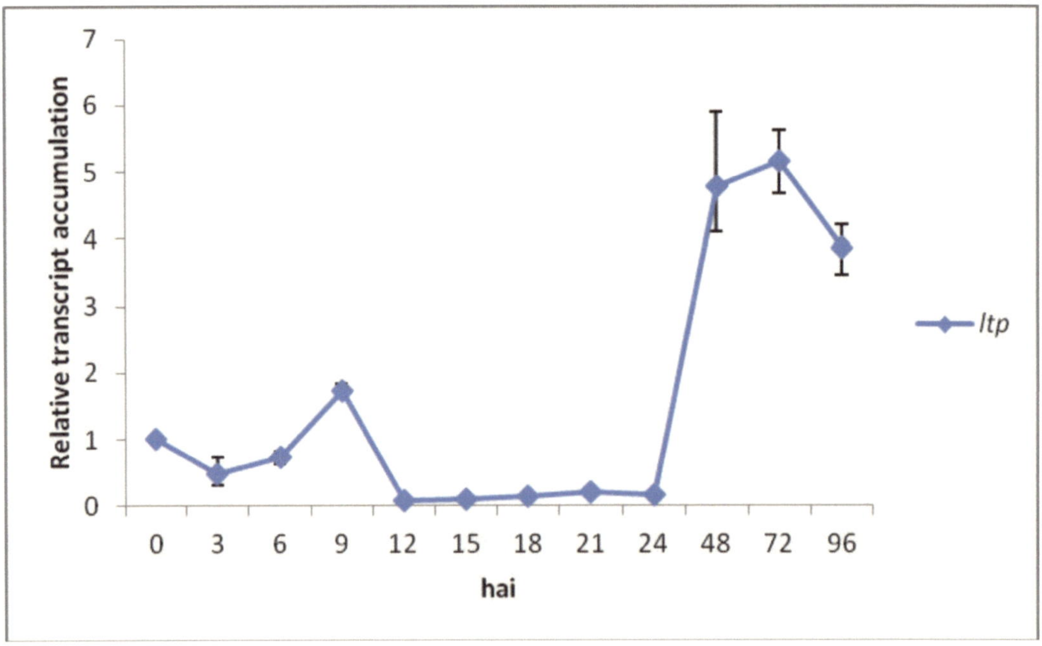

Figure 8. *ltp* gene expression in wheat leaves treated with SA

Moreover, LTPs are known to be differentially expressed during a pathogenic interaction because they are potentially good ligands to oleic C18:1, linoleic C18:2 and eicosadienoic acids C20:2 [110]. Among 28 identified wheat nsLTP, eight nsLTP expressed in yeast exhibited lipid binding activity [111]. These proteins could be involved in the intracellular traffic of phospholipids and in the transport of cutin monomers. Interestingly, SA induces the expression of the *ltp* gene in the same period when its impact on the lipid metabolism is the most important. One could think that the lipid transfer capacity of these binding proteins participate in the modulation of the lipid scenery upon resistance induction with SA.

4. Conclusion

The present chapter provides evidences for the effect of resistance inducers on wheat lipid metabolism and presents the strategy we used in order to characterize their mode of action at different levels: total FA content and relative proportion, PA, PE and DAG contents, expression of genes such as PLC and LTP-encoding ones. Lipid metabolism is therefore a marker of induced resistance in wheat. To our knowledge, such findings have never been presented before on *Triticum aestivum*.

Salicylic acid is very likely to induce the formation of PA through the activation of phospholipases C and/or D pathways: induction of *PLC* gene expression, together with DAG accumulation suggests that the PLC pathway is enhanced and leads to PA production. On the other hand, reduction of PE content suggests that PLD pathway is triggered upon SA infiltration in order to ensure PA synthesis. *lox* gene expression up-regulation and corresponding enzymatic activity, along with the decrease of linolenic acid content, suggests that SA modulates lipid enzymatic peroxidation. Moreover, the expression of *ltp* gene was induced by SA, showing the involvement of the corresponding protein in the lipid signaling metabolism.

The tested resistance inducers had some similarities in their mode of action, relatively to total FAs profiles. Trehalose and Milsana® seem to share similar modes of action via the increase of C12:0 and decrease of C20:2 contents. Iodus® exhibited the largest effects on FAs profiles, inducing increases in C12:0 and C18:1 and decreases in C20:2. HSA, however, was the only resistance inducer that modulated positively the content of C18:2.

Future investigations have to be extended to other genes expression and corresponding enzymatic activities acting downstream of lipoxygenase in order to figure out whether the LOX-derived hydroperoxides are metabolized during the JA synthesis. Furthermore, a global approach using microarrays based on wheat cDNA chips would be a useful tool for increasing our knowledge of the plant lipidome in our wheat-powdery pathosystem.

Author details

Christine Tayeh, Béatrice Randoux, Frédéric Laruelle,
Natacha Bourdon, Delphine Renard-Merlier and Philippe Reignault*
Université du Littoral Côte d'Opale, Unité de Chimie Environnementale et Interactions sur le Vivant (UCEIV), France

* Corresponding Author

Acknowledgement

Christine TAYEH is supported by the French Ministry of National Education and Research.

5. References

[1] Benhamou N. Elicitor-induced plant defense pathways. Trends in Plant Science 1996;1(7) 233-240.

[2] Walker AS, Leroux P, Bill L, Wilhelm E, Caron D. Oïdium du blé: quelles résistances aux fongicides en France? Phytoma 2004;577:49-54.

[3] Walters D, Walsh D, Newton A, Lyon G. Induced resistance for plant disease controls: maximizing the efficacy of resistance elicitors. Phytopathology 2005;95:1368-1373.

[4] Reignault P, Walters D. Topical application of inducers for disease control. In: Walters D (ed.). Induce resistance for plants defense. Oxford, Blackwell Publishing; 2007. p179-200.

[5] Randoux B, Renard-Merlier D, Mulard G, Rossard S, Duyme F, Sanssené J, Courtois J, Durand R, Reignault Ph. Distinct defenses induced in wheat against powdery mildew by acetylated and nonacteylated oligogalacturonides. Phytopathology 2010;100:1352-1363.

[6] Reignault Ph, Cogan A, Muchembled J, Lounes-Hadj Sahraoui A, Durand R, Sancholle M. Trehalose induces resistance to powdery mildew in wheat. New Phytologist 2001;149:519-529.

[7] Muchembled J, Lounes-Hadj Sahraoui A, Grandmoujin-Ferjani A, Sancholle M. Changes in lipid composition of *Blumeria graminis* f.sp. *tritici* conida produced on wheat leaves treated with heptanoyl salicylic acid. Phytochemistry, 2006;67(11) 1104-1109.

[8] Renard-Merlier D, Randoux B, Nowak E, Farcy F, Durand R, Reignault Ph. Iodus 40, salicylic acid, heptanoyl salicylic acid and trehalose exhibit different efficacies and defense targets during a wheat/powdery mildew interaction. Phytochemistry 2007;68:1156-1164.

[9] Aziz A, Poinssot B, Daire X, Adrian M, Bezier A, Lambert B, Joubert JM, Pugin A. Laminarin elicits defense responses in grapevine and induces protection against *Botrytis cinerea* and *Plasmopara viticola*. Molecular Plant-Microbe Interactions 2003;16:1118-1128.

[10] Randoux B, Renard D, Nowak E, Sanssené J, Courtois J, Durand R, Reignault P. Inhibition of *Blumeria graminis* f.sp. *tritici* germination and partial enhancement of wheat defenses by Milsana. Phytopathology 2006;96:1278-1286.

[11] Spletzer ME, Enyedi AJ. Salicylic acid induces resistance to *Alternaria solani* in hydroponically grown tomato. Phytopathology 1999;89:722-727

[12] Saika R, Singh T, Kumar R, Srivastava J, Srivastava AK, Signh K, Arora DK. Role of salicylic acid in systemic resistance induced by *Pseudomonas fluorescens* against *Fusarium oxysporum* f.sp. *ciceri* in chickpea. Microbiological Research 2003;158:203-213.
[13] Sparla F, Rotino L, Valgimigli MC, Pupillo P, Trost P. Systemic resistance induced by benzothiadiazole in pear inoculated with the agent of fire blight (*Erwinia amylovora*). *Scientia Horticulturae* 2004;101:269-279.
[14] Galis I, Smith JL, Jameson PE. Salicylic acid- , but not cytokinin-induced, resistance to WCIMV is associated with increased expression of SA-dependent resistance genes in *Phaseolus vulgaris.* Journal of Plant Pathology 2004;161:459-466.
[15] Shah J. Lipids, lipases and lipid-modifying enzymes in plant disease resistance. Annual Review of Phytopathology 2005;43:229-260.
[16] Testerink C, Munnik T. Phosphatidic acid: a multifunctional stress signaling lipid in plants. Trends in Plant Science 2005;10(8) 368-375.
[17] Wang X, Devaiah SP, Zhang W, Welti R. Signaling functions of phosphatidic acid. Progress in Lipid research 2006;45:250-278.
[18] Wang X. Lipid signaling. Current Opinion in Plant Biology 2004;7:329-336.
[19] Wang X. Phospholipase D in hormonal and stress signaling. Current Opinion in Plant Biology 2002;5:408–414.
[20] Meijer HJG, Munnik T. Phospholipid-based signaling in plants. Annual Review of Plant Biology 2003;54:265–306.
[21] Viehveger K, Dordschbal B, Roos W. Elicitor-activated phospholipase A2 generates lysophosphatidylcholines that mobilize the vacuolar H^+ pool for pH signaling via the activation of Na^+-dependent proton fluxes. Plant Cell 2002;14:1509-1525.
[22] Zhao J, Davis L, Verpoorte R. Elicitor signal transduction leading to production of plant secondary metabolites. Biotechnology Advances 2005;23:283-333.
[23] La Camera S, Gouzerh G, Dhondt S, Hoffmann L, Fritig B, Legrand M, Heitz T. Metabolic reprogramming in plant innate immunity: the contributions of phenylpropanoid and oxylipin pathways. Immunological Reviews 2004;198:267-284.
[24] Feussner I, Wasternack C. The lipoxygenase pathway. Annual Review of Plant Biology 2002;53:275-297.
[25] Christensen SA, Kolomiets MV. The lipid language of plant-fungal interactions. Fungal Genetics and Biology 2011;48:4-14.
[26] Bate NJ, Rothstein SJ. C6-volatiles derived from the lipoxygenase pathway induce a subset of defense-related genes. Plant Journal 1998;16:561-569.
[27] Weiler EW, Kutchan TM, Gorba T, Brodschelm W, Nieesel U, Bublitz F. The *Pseudomonas* phytotoxin coronatine mimics octadecanoid signalling molecules of higher plants. FEBS Letter 1994;345:9-13.
[28] Farmer EE, Almeras E, Krisnamurthy V. Jasmonates and related oxylipins in plant responses to pathogenesis and herbivory. Current Opinion in Plant Biology 2003;6:372-378.

[29] Browse J. Jasmonate passes muster: a receptor and targets for the defense hormone. Annual Review of Plant Biology 2008;60:183-205.
[30] Ryu SB. Phospholipid-derived signaling mediated by phospholipase A in plants. Trends in Plant Science 2004;9:229-235.
[31] Dhondt S, Gouzerh G, Muller A, Legrand M, Heitz T. Spatio-temporal expression of patatin-like lipid acyl hydrolases and accumulation of jasmonates in elicitor-treated tobacco leaves are not affected by endogeneous salicylic acid. Plant Journal 2002;32:749-762.
[32] Dhondt S, Geoffroy P, Stelmach BA, Legrand M, Heitz T. Soluble phospholipase A2 activity is induced before oxylipin accumulation in tobacco mosaic virus-infected tobacco leaves and is contributed by patatin-like enzymes. Plant Journal 2000;23:431-440.
[33] Scherer GFE, Paul RU, Holk A, Martinec J. Down-regulation by elicitors of hosphatidylcholine hydrolyzing phospholipase C and up-regulation of phospholipase A in plant cells. Biochemical and Biophysical Research Communications 2002;293:766-770.
[34] Routaboul JM, Fischer SF, Browse J. Trienoic fatty acids are required to maintain chloroplast function at low temperatures. Plant Physiology 2000;124:1697-1705.
[35] Yamauchi Y, Furutera A, Seki K, Toyoda Y, Tanaka K, Sugimoto Y. Malondialdehyde generated from peroxidized linolenic acid causes protein modification in heat-stressed plants. Plant Physiology and Biochemistry 2008;46:786-793.
[36] Tumlinson JH, Engelberth J. Fatty acid derived signals that induce or regulate plant defenses against herbivory. In: Schaller A. (ed.) Induced Plant Resistance to Herbivory. Amsterdam, The Netherlands, Springer; 2008. p389-407.
[37] Kachroo A, Kachroo P. Fatty acids-derived signals in plant defense. Annual Review of phytopathology 2009;47:153-176.
[38] Sossountzov L, Ruiz-Avila L, Vignols F, Jolliot A, Arondel V, Tchang F, Grosbois M, Guerbette F, Miginiac E, Delseny M. Spatial and temporal expression of a maize lipid transfer protein gene. Plant Cell 1991;3:923-933.
[39] Kader JC. Lipid-transfer proteins in plants. Annual Review of Plant Physiology and Plant Molecular Biology 1996;47:627-654.
[40] van Loon LC, van Strien EA. The families of pathogenesis-related proteins, their activities, and comparative analysis of PR-1 proteins. Physiological and Molecular Plant Pathology 1999;55:85-97.
[41] Molina A, Segura A, Garcia-Olmedo F. Lipid transfer proteins (ns-LTPs) from barley and maize leaves are potent inhibitors of bacterial and fungal plant pathogens. FEBS Letters 1993;316(2) 119-122.
[42] Regente MC, de La Canal L. Purification, characterization and antifungal properties of a lipid-transfer protein from sunflower (*Helianthus annuus*) seeds. Physiologia Plantarum 2001; 10:158-163.

[43] Patkar RN, Chattoo BB. Transgenic indica rice expressing ns-LTP-like protein shows enhanced resistance to both fungal and bacterial pathogens. Molecular Breeding 2006;17:159-171.

[44] Roy-Barman S, Sautter C, Chattoo BB. Expression of the lipid transfer protein Ace-AMP1 in transgenic wheat enhances antifungal activity and defense responses. Transgenic Research 2006;15:435-446.

[45] Kirubakaran IS, Mubarak Begum S, Ulaganathan K, Sakthivel N. Characterization of a new antifungal lipid transfer protein from wheat. Plant Physiology and Biochemistry 2008;46:918-927.

[46] Renard-Merlier D, Laruelle F, Nowak E, Durand R, Reignault Ph. Changes in C12:0, C18:1, C18:2 and C20:2 fatty acid content in wheat leaves treated with resistance inducers and infected by powdery mildew. Plant Biology 2009;11:75-82.

[47] Pfaffl MW, Horgan GW, Dempfle L. Relative expression software tool (REST©) for group-wise comparison and statistical analysis of relative expression results in real-time PCR. Nucleic Acids Research 2002;30(9) e36.

[48] Todd JF, Paliyath, G, Thompson, JE. Characteristics of a membrane-associated lipoxygenase in tomato fruit. Plant Physiology 1990;94:1225-1232.

[49] Avdiushko SA, Ye XS, Hildebrand DF, Kuc J. Induction of lipoxygenase activity in immunized cucumber plants. Physiological and Molecular Plant Pathology 1993;42:83-95.

[50] Morris K., editor Elsevier Science - Techniques of lipidology. Isolation, analysis and identification of lipids.Amsterdam, The Netherlands; 1986.

[51] Avalli A, Contarini G. Determination of phospholipids in dairy products by SPE/HPLC/ELSD. Journal Of Chromatography A 2005;1071:185-190.

[52] Zhang W, Wang C, Qin C, Wood T, Olafsdottir G, Wang X. The oleate-stimulated phospholipase D, PLDδ and phosphatidic acid decrease H_2O_2-induced cell death in *Arabidopsis*. Plant Cell 2003;15:2285-2295.

[53] de Jong CF, Laxalt AM, Bargmann BOR, de Wit PJGM, Joosten MHAJ, Munnik T. Phosphatidic acid accumulation is an early response in the Cf-4/Avr4 interaction. Plant Journal 2004;39:1-12.

[54] van der Luit AH, Piatti T, van Doorn A, Musqrave A, Felix G, Boller T, Munnik T. Elicitation of suspension-cultured tomato cells triggers formation of phopshatidic acid and diacylglycerol pyrophosphate. Plant Physiology 2000;123:1507-1515.

[55] Yamaguchi T, Minami E, Shibuya N. Activation of phospholipases by *N*-acetylchitooligosaccharide elicitor in suspension-cultured rice cells mediates reactive oxygen generation. Physiologia Plantarum, 2003 1189;3:361-370.

[56] Norberg P, Liljenberg C. Lipids of plasma membranes prepared from oat root cells. Plant Physiology 1991;96:1136-1141.

[57] Sanchez JP, Chua NH. Arabidopsis PLC1 is required for secondary responses to abscisic acid signals. Plant Cell 2001;13:1143-1154.

[58] Drøbak BK, Watkins PA. Inositol(1,4,5)trisphosphate production in plant cells: an early response to salinity and hyperosmotic stress. FEBS Letters 2000:481:240-244.

[59] Takahashi S, Katagiri T, Hirayama T, Yamaguchi-Shinozaki K, Shinozaki K. Hyperosmotic stress induces a rapid and transient increase inositol 1,4,5-trisphosphate independent of abscisic acid in *Arabidopsis* cell culture. Plant Cell Physiology 2001;42:214-222.

[60] Gomez-Merino FC, Brearley CA, Ornatowska M, Abdel-Haliem M, Zanor MI, Mueller-Roeber B. AtDGK2, a novel diacylglycerol kinase from Arabidopsis thaliana, phosphorylates 1-stearoyl-2-arachidonoyl-sn-glycerol and 1,2-dioleoyl-sn-glycerol and exhibits cold-inducible gene expression. Journal of Biological Chemistry 2004;279:8230-8241.

[61] Den Hartog M, Verhoef N, Munnik T. Nod factor and elicitors activate different phospholipid signaling pathways in suspension-cultured alfalfa cells. Plant Physiology 2003;132,311-317.

[62] Lazalt AM, Raho N, ten Have A, Lamattina L. Nitric oxide is critical for inducing phosphatidic acid accumulation in xylanase-elicited tomato cells. The Journal of Biological Chemistry 2007;282(29) 21160-21168.

[63] de Torres Zabela M, Fernandez-Delmond I, Niittyla T, Sanchez P, Grant M. Differential expression of genes encoding *Arabidopsis* phospholipases after challenge with virulent or avirulent *Pseudomonas* isolates. Molecular Plant-Microbe Interactions 2002;15:808-816.

[64] Katagiri T, Takahashi S, Shinozaki K. Involvement of a novel Arabidopsis phospholipase D, AtPLDδ in dehydration-inducible accumulation of phosphatidic acid in stress signaling. Plant Journal 2001;26:595-605.

[65] Fan L, Zheng S, Wang X. Antisense suppression of phospholipase Dδ retards abscisic acid- and ethylene-promoted senescence of postharvest Arabidopsis leaves. Plant Cell 1997;9:2183-2196.

[66] Li W, Li M, Zhang W, Welti R, Wang X. The plasma membrane-bound phospholipase Dδ enhances freezing tolerance in *Arabidopsis thaliana*. Nature Biotechnology 2004;22:427-433.

[67] Lee S, Suh S, Kim S, Crain, RC, Kwak JM, Nam HG, Lee Y. Systemic elevation of phosphatidic acid and lysophospholipid levels in wounded plants. Plant Journal 1997;12:547-556.

[68] Wang C, Zien CA, Afitlhile M, Weilt R, Hildebrand DF, Wang X. Involvement of phospholipase D in wound-induced accumulation of jasmonic acid in *Arabidopsis*. Plant Cell 2000;12:2237-2246.

[69] Farmer PK, Choi JH. Calcium and phospholipid activation of a recombinant calcium-dependent protein kinase (DcCPK1) from carrot (*Daucus carota* L.). Biochimica and Biophysica Acta 1999;1434(1) 6-17.

[70] Anthony RG, Henriques R, Helfer A, Mészáros t, Rios G, Testerink C, Munnik T, Deák M, Koncz C, Börge L. A protein kinase target of a PDK1 signalling pathway is involved in root hair growth in *Arabidopsis*. EMBO Journal 2004;23:572–581.

[71] Zhang W, Qin C, Zhao J, Wang X. Phospholipase Da1-derived phosphatidic acid interacts with ABI1 phosphatase 2C and regulates abscisic acid signaling. Proceedings of the National Academy of Science, USA 2004;101:9508-9513.

[72] Varnier AL, Sanchez L, Vatsa P, Boudesocque L, Garcia-Brugge A, Rabenoelina F, Sorokin A, Renault JH, Kauffman S, Pugin A, Clement C, Baillеul F, Dorey S. Bacterial rhamnolipids are novel MAMPs conferring resistance to *Botrytis cinerea* in grapevine. Plant, Cell and Environment 2009;32:178-193.

[73] Mauch F, Kmecl A, Schaffrath U, Volrath S, Gorlach J, Ward E, Ryals J, Dudler R. Mechanosensitive expression of a lipoxygenase gene in wheat. Plant Physiology 1997;114:1561-1566.

[74] Gorlach J, Volrath S, Knauf-Bieter G, Hengy G, Bechove U, Kogel KH, Oostendorp M, Staub T, Ward E, Kessman H, Ryals J. Benzothiadiazole, a novel class of inducers of systemic acquired resistance, activates gene expression and disease resistance in wheat. Plant Cell 1996;8:629-643.

[75] Weber H. Fatty acid-derived signals in plants. Trends in Plant Science 2002;7:217-224.

[76] Vollenweider S, Weber H, Stolz S, Chételat A, Farmer EE. Fatty acid ketodienes and fatty acid ketotrienes: Michael addition acceptors that accumulate in wounded and diseased *Arabidopsis* leaves. Plant Journal 2000;24:467-476.

[77] Weichert H, Stenzel I, Berndt E, Wasternack C, Feussner I. Metabolic profiling of oxylipins upon salicylate treatment in barley leaves – preferential induction of the reductase pathway by salicylate. FEBS Letters 1999;464:133-137.

[78] Hause B, Vörös K, Kogel KH, Besser K, Wasternack C. A jasmonate-responsive lipoxygenase of barley leaves is induced by plant activators but not by pathogens. Journal of Plant Physiology 1999;154:459-462.

[79] Pinot F, Benveniste I, Salaün JP, Durst F. Methyl jasmonate induces lauric acid ω-hydroxylase activity and accumulation of CYP94A1 transcripts but does not affect epoxide hydrolase activities in *Vicia sativa* seedlings. Plant Physiology 1998;118(4) 1481-1486.

[80] Zheng CJ, Yoo JS, Lee TG, Cho HY, Kim YH, Kim WG. Fatty acid synthesis is a target for antibacterial activity of unsaturated fatty acids. FEBS Letters 2005;579:5157-5162.

[81] Sado-Kamdem SL, Vannini L, Guerzoni ME. Effect of α-linolenic, capric and lauric acid on the fatty acid biosynthesis in *Staphylococcus aureus*. International Journal of Food Microbiology 2009;129:288-294.

[82] Savchenko T, Walley J, Chehab W, Xiao Y, Kaspi R, Pye M, Mohamed M, Lazarus C, Bostock R, Dehesh K. Arachidonic Acid: en evolutionary conserved signaling molecule modulates plant stress signaling networks. The Plant Cell 2010;22:3193-3205.

[83] Holloway PJ. The chemical constitution of plant cutins. In: Culter D. (ed). The plant cuticule. London: Linnaean Society Symposium Series; 1982. p45-85.

[84] Kirsh C, Takamiya-Wik M, Reinold S, Hahlbrock, Somssich IE. Rapid, transient, and highly localized induction of plastidial omega-3 fatty acid desaturase mRNA at fungal infection sites in *Petroselinum crispum*. Proceedings of the National Academy of Science, USA 1997;94:2079-2084.

[85] Kachroo P, Shanklin J, Shah J, Whittle EJ, Klessig DF. A fatty acid desaturase modulates the activation of defense signaling pathways in plants. Proceedings of the National Academy of Science, USA 2001;98 9448-9453.

[86] Kachroo A., Fu DQ, Havens W, Navarre D, Kachroo P, Ghabrial SA. An oleic acid-mediated pathway induces constitutive defense signaling and enhanced resistance to multiple pathogens in soybean. Molecular Plant-Microbe Interactions 2008;21(5) 564-575.

[87] Wilson RA, Calvo AM, Chang PK, Keller NP. Characterization of the *Aspergillus parasiticus* delta12-desaturase gene: a role for lipid metabolism in the *Aspergillus*-seed interaction. Microbiology 2004;150:2881-2888.

[88] Wang C, Xing J, Chin CK, Peters JS. Fatty acids with certain characteristics are potent inhibitors of germination and inducers of cell death of powdery mildew spores. Physiological and Molecular Plant Pathology 2002;61:151-161.

[89] Weichert H, Kohlmann M, Wasternack C, Freussner I. Metabolic profiling of oxylipins upon sorbitol treatment in barley leaves. Biochemical Society transactions 2000;28:861-862.

[90] Vega SE, del Rio AH, Bamberg JB, Palta JP. Evidence for the up-regulation of stearoyl-ACP (D9) desaturase gene expression during cold acclimation. American Journal of Potato Research 2004;81:125-135.

[91] Bachmann A, Hausse B, Maucher H, Garbe E, Vörös K, Weichert H, Wasternack C, Feussner I. Jasmonate induced lipid peroxidation in barley leaves initiated by distinct 13-LOX forms of choroplasts. Biological Chemistry 2002;383:1645-1657.

[92] Yaeno T, Matsuda O, Iba K. Role of cholorplast trienoic fatty acids in plant disease defense responses. Plant Journal 2004;40:931-941.

[93] Xue HQ, Upchurch RG, Kwanyuen P. Ergosterol as a quantifiable biomass marker for *Diaporthe phaseolorum* and *Cercospora kikuchii*. Plant Disease 2006;90:1395-1398.

[94] Upchurch RG. Fatty acid unsaturation, mobilization, and regulation in the response of plants to stress. Biotechnology Letters 2008;30:967-977.

[95] Calvo AM, Hinze LL, Gardner HW, Keller NP. Sporogenic effect of polyunsaturated fatty acids on development of *Aspergillus* spp. Applied and Environmental Microbiology 1999;65:3668-3673.

[96] Madi L,Wang X, Kobiler I, Lichter A, Prusky D. Stress on avocado fruits regulates Δ^9-stearoyl ACP desaturase expression, fatty acid composition, antifungal diene level and resistance to *Colletotrichum gleosporiodes* attack. Physiological and Molecular Plant Pathology 2009;62:277-283.

[97] Mueller MJ, Brodschelm W, Spannagl E, Zenk MH. Signaling in the elicitation process is mediated through the octadecanoid pathway leading to jasmonic acid. Proceedings of the National Academy of Science, USA 1993;90:7490-7494.

[98] McConn M, Creelman RA, Bell E, Mullet JE, Browse J. Jasmonate is essential for insect defense in *Arabidopsis*. Proc. Natl. Acad Sci. USA 1997;94:5473-5477.

[99] Vijayan P, Shockey J, Levesque CA, Cook RJ, Browse J. A role for jasmonate in pathogen defense of *Arabidopsis*. Proc. Natl. Acad. Sci. USA 1998;95:7209-7214.

[100] Ongena M, Duby F, Rossignol F, Fauconnier ML, Dommes J, Thonart P. Stimulation of the lipoxygenase pathway is associated with systemic resistance induced in bean by a nonpathogenic *Pseudomonas* strain. Molecular Plant-Microbe Interactions 2004;17:1009-1018.

[101] Padham AK, Hopkins MT, Wang TW, McNamara LM, Lo M, Richardson LG, Smith MD, Taylor CA, Thompson JE. Characterization of a plastid triacylglycerol lipase from *Arabidopsis*. Plant Physiology 2007;143:1372-1384.

[102] Wasternack C. Jasmonates: an update on biosynthesis, signal transduction and action in plant stress response, growth and development. Annals of Botany 2007;100:681-697.

[103] Grechkin A. Recent developments in biochemistry of the plant lipoxygenase pathway. Progress in Lipid Research 1998;37(5) 317-352.

[104] Salzman RA, Brady JA, Finlayson SA, Buchanan CD, Summer EJ, Sun F, Klein PE, Klein RR, Pratt LH, Cordonnier-Pratt MM, Mullet JE. Transcriptional profiling of sorghum induced by methyl jasmonate, salicylic acid, and aminocyclopropane carboxylic acid reveals cooperative regulation and novel gene responses. Plant Physiology 2005;138:352-368.

[105] Ruzicska P, Gombos Z, Farkas GL. Modification of the fatty acid composition of phospholipids during the hypersensitive reaction in tobacco. Virology 1983;128:60-64.

[106] Blein JP, Coutos-Thevenot P, Marion D, Ponchet M. From elicitins to lipid transfer proteins: a new insight in cell signaling involved in plant defense mechanism. Trends in Plant Science 2002;7:293-296.

[107] Jayaraj J, Punja ZK. Combined expression of chitinase and lipid transfer protein genes in transgenic carrot plants enhances resistance to foliar fungal pathogens. Plant Cell Reports 2007;26:1539-1546.

[108] Lu ZX, Gaudet DA, Frick Puchalski B, Genswein B, Laroche A. Identification and characterization of genes differentially expressed in the resistance reaction in wheat infected with *Tilletia tritici*, the common bunt pathogen. Journal of Biochemistry and Molecular Biology 2005;38(4) 420-431.

[109] Gomes E, Sagot E, Gaillard C, Laquitaine L, Poinssot B, Sanejouand YH, Delrot S, Coutos-Thévenot P. Nonspecific Lipid-Transfer Protein genes expression in grape (*Vitis* sp.) cells in response to fungal elicitor treatments. Molecular Plant-Microbe Interactions 2003;16(5) 456-464.

[110] Osman H, Mikes V, Milat ML, Ponchet M, Marion D, Prangé T, Maume BF, Vauthrin S, Blein JP. Fatty acids bind to fungal elicitor cryptogein and compete with sterols. FEBS Letters 2001;489:55-58.

[111] Sun JY, Gaudet D, Lu ZX, Frick M, Puchalski B, Laroche A. Characterization and antifungal properties of wheat nonspecific lipid transfer proteins. Molecular Plant-Microbe Interactions 2008;21(3) 346-360.

Section 4

Lipid Metabolism in Plants

Chapter 16

Jasmonate Biosynthesis, Perception and Function in Plant Development and Stress Responses

Yuanxin Yan, Eli Borrego and Michael V. Kolomiets

Additional information is available at the end of the chapter

http://dx.doi.org/10.5772/52675

1. Introduction

The oxidation products of unsaturated fatty acids are collectively known as oxylipins. These compounds represent a highly diverse group of substances that are involved in a number of developmental processes and various stress responses in plants (Andersson et al., 2006). Plant oxylipins can be formed enzymatically, by initial oxidation by lipoxygenases (LOXs) or α-dioxygenases (α-DOXs); however, non-enzymatic autoxidation of polyunsaturated fatty acids (PUFA) also contribute to oxylipin formation in plant (Göbel and Feussner, 2009). An array of these substances are known to exert protective activities either as signaling molecules in plants during development, wounding, and insect and pathogen attack, or direct anti-microbial substance that are toxic to the invader. Despite the recent progress in deciphering the function of some oxylipins, the role of the vast majority of plant oxylipins remains unclear. Particularly well studied examples of the plant oxylipins are jasmonates (JAs) including jasmonic acid (JA) and its derivatives such as methyl jasmonate (MeJA), *cis*-jasmone, jasmonoyl isoleucine (JA-Ile), jasmonoyl ACC (JA-ACC) and several other metabolites. Another important group of plant oxylipins is green leaf volatiles (GLV). Increasing evidence supports GLVs function in defense responses against herbivore. GLVs are C6 aldehydes, alcohols, and their esters formed through the hydroperoxide lyase (HPL) pathway downstream of LOXs. GLV can further trigger local and systemic volatile organic compounds (VOC) emissions upon insect feeding (Farag and Paré, 2002). A large number of VOC including monoterpenes, sesquiterpenes and carotenoid-type compounds can be biosynthesized in plants from the shikimic, lipidic and terpenic pathways (Fons et al., 2010). Most VOCs are not products of the LOX pathway but similar to LOX derivatives serve as signals for insects to choose a suitable host or to lay eggs (Müller and Hilker, 2001). The third better studied group of plant oxylipins is phytoprostanes, a category of non-enzymatically formed oxylipins, which play overlapped roles with OPDA in plant stress responses (Eckardt, 2008).

JA biosynthesis and signaling pathways have been extensively investigated in dicotyledonous plants such as *Arabidopsis*, tobacco and tomato. In monocotyledonous species, only a scant number of JA biosynthetic enzymes have been described (Tani et al., 2008; Yan et al., 2012). Jasmonates are formed from the LOX-catalyzed peroxidation of trienoic fatty acids at carbon atom 13 to form 13-hydroperoxide, which is modified to an allene oxide fatty acid and subsequently cyclized to the compound 12-oxo-phytodienoic acid (OPDA). Jasmonic acid (JA) is synthesized from OPDA by the reduction of a double bond and three consecutive rounds of β-oxidation. The pathway can accept C_{18}-PUFA (linolenic acid) as well as C_{16}-PUFA (hexadecatrienoic acid), in the latter case the intermediate is the so-called dinor-OPDA that may also be metabolized to JA. JA can be further enzymatically converted into numerous derivatives or conjugates, some of which have well-described biological activity such as free JA, MeJA, *cis*-jasmone and JA–Ile.

JA signaling pathway, the transition process of JA-Ile as a chemical signal to biological signal, was elucidated in recent years. JA initiates signaling process upon formation of a SCF^{COI1}-JA-Ile-JAZ ternary complex (JAZ: jasmonate ZIM-domain protein; Sheard et al., 2010), in which the JAZ repressors are ubiquitinated and subsequently degraded to release transcription factors, e.g., MYC2, causing downstream transcription activation of defense responses or developmental regulation (Chini et al., 2007; Thines et al., 2007). The only jasmonate receptor identified to date has been the COI1 protein (Katsir et al., 2008; Yan et al., 2009), but interestingly, only JA-Ile was found as a ligand of the SCF^{COI1} E3 ubiquitin ligase complex (Thines et al., 2007).

Since discovered in the 1960s as secondary metabolites from the oils of jasmine flowers (Demole *et al.*, 1962), the biological roles of JA have received increased attention of researchers in the past decades. Jasmonates have gradually become realized as a defense and fertility hormone, and as such modulate numerable processes relating to development and stress responses. In *Arabidopsis* and tomato, JAs are directly involved in stamen and trichome development, vegetative growth, cell cycle regulation, senescence, anthocyanin biosynthesis regulation, and responses to various biotic and abiotic stresses (Creelman and Mullet, 1997; Wasternack, 2007; Howe and Jander, 2008; Browse, 2009; Avanci et al., 2010; Pauwels and Goossens, 2011). In monocots, much less is known about the role of JAs, however, it has been shown they are required for sex determination, reproductive bud initiation and elongation, leaf senescence, pigmentation of tissues and responses to the attack by pathogens and insects (Engelberth et al., 2004; Tani et al., 2008; Acosta et al., 2009; Yan et al, 2012).

In plants, the JA signal acts co-operatively with other plant hormones. A number of studies have already attracted attention to plant hormone cross-talk as it relates to defense responses. In *Arabidopsis,* JA was shown to interact synergistically with ethylene (Xu et al 1994), and, depending on particular stress, both synergistically and antagonistically with salicylic acid (Beckers and Spoel, 2006) and abscisic acid (ABA) (Anderson et al 2004) in plant-pathogen or -insect interactions. Gibberellins (GA) interact with JA to control flower fertility in *Arabidopsis*. In maize, JA positively regulates ABA and ET biosynthesis in senescing leaves (Yan et al., 2012). In summary, it is clear that JA signaling exert its functions via interaction with multiple plant hormones; however the crossroads of these interactions still remain to be explored.

2. JA biosynthesis pathway and regulation

2.1. The scheme of JA biosynthesis pathway

In 1962, a floral scent compound, the methyl ester of jasmonic acid (MeJA) was isolated for the first time from the aromatic oil of *Jasminum grandiflorum* (Demole et al., 1962). However, the physiological effects of MeJA or its free acid (JA) were unknown until the 1980's when a senescence-promoting effect of JA (Ueda and Kato, 1980) and growth inhibition activity of MeJA to *Vicia faba* (Dathe, 1981) were observed. Now JA and derivatives (JAs) are the best characterized group of oxylipins in plants and are regarded as one of the the major hormones regulating both defense and development.

Biosynthesis of JAs originates from polyunsaturated fatty acids (PUFA) and is synthesized by one of the seven distinct branches of the lipoxygenase (LOX) pathway, the allene oxide synthase (AOS) branch (Feussner and Wasternack, 2002). The remaing six branches form other oxylipins including GLVs as well as epoxy-, hydroxy-, keto- or ether PUFA and epoxyhydroxy-PUFA (Feussner and Wasternack, 2002) (Figure 1). In the oxylipin biosynthesis (Figure 1), only 13-hydroperoxide from α-linolenic acid (18:3, α-LeA) can be utilized by the AOS branch for JA production. Other fatty acid hydroperoxides such as 9-13- and 2-hydroperoxide, oxygenated by 9-LOX, 13-LOX and α-dioxygenase (α-DOX), respectively, or those whose substrates originate from α-LeA, hexadecatrienoic acid (16:3, HTA) or linoleic acid (18:2, LA) may be channeled to form other oxylipin subgroups. Biological functions of the majority of estimated 400-500 oxylipins is mostly unknown.

The biosynthesis of JA and MeJA was elucidated by Vick and Zimmerman (1983), and Hamberg and Hughes (1988). The original precursors PUFA are released from chloroplast membranes by the action of lipid hydrolyzing enzymes. Upon α-LeA liberation, a molecular oxygen is incorporated by a 13-LOX at carbon atom 13 of the substrate leading to the formation of a fatty acid hydroperoxide, 13-HPOT (13*S*-hydroperoxy-(9*Z*,11*E*,15)-octadecatrienoic acid) (Figure 2). This intermediate compound can proceede to seven distinct enzymatic branches (Figure 1), one of which is dehydration by the allene oxide synthase (AOS) to an unstable allene oxide, 12,13-EOT ((9*Z*,13*S*,15*Z*)-12,13-oxido-9,11,15-octadecatrienoic acid) which can be cyclized to racemic 12-oxo-phytodienoic acid (OPDA). In the presence of an allene oxide cyclase (AOC), preferential product is the enantiomer, 9*S*,13*S*/*cis* (+)-OPDA (Figure 2). All the reactions from α-LeA to OPDA take place within a plastid. *cis* (+)-OPDA is subsequently transported into the peroxisome, where it is further converted into (+)-7-*iso*-JA by 12-oxo-phytodienoic acid reductase (OPR) and three beta oxidation steps involving three peroxisomal enzymatic functions (acyl-CoA oxidase, multi-functional protein, and l-3-ketoacyl-CoA thiolase) (Figure 2). (+)-7-*iso*-JA often epimerizes into a more stable *trans* configuration, (-)-JA or undergoes modifications to produce diverse JA derivatives including MeJA and (+)-7-*iso*-JA-Ile. The latter one is the bioactive form of JA produced by conjugation of JA to isoleucine by the enzyme encoded by the *JA resistant 1* (*JAR1*) gene (Staswick and Tiryaki, 2004).

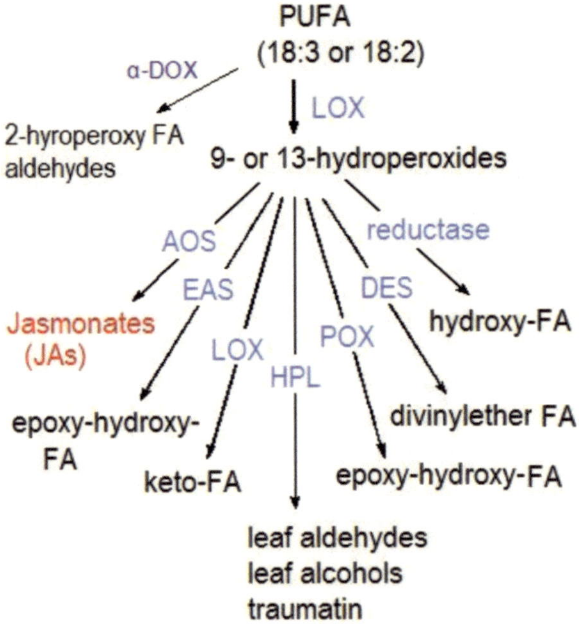

Figure 1. Overview of the oxylipin biosynthesis pathways in plants (Andreou et al., 2009)
In the first reaction, free fatty acids (18:3 or 18:2) are oxidized by the addition of molecular oxygen yielding hydroperoxides (HPOT, hydroperoxy-octadecatrienoic acid; HOPD, hydroperoxy-octadecadienoic acids) through activity of oxygenases, lipoxygenase (LOX) or α-dioxygenase (α-DOX). Hydroperoxide products formed by LOXs are further metabolized by other enzymes: allene oxide synthase (AOS), hydroperoxide lyase (HPL), divinyl ether synthase (DES), peroxygenase (POX) and epoxyalcohol synthases (EAS).

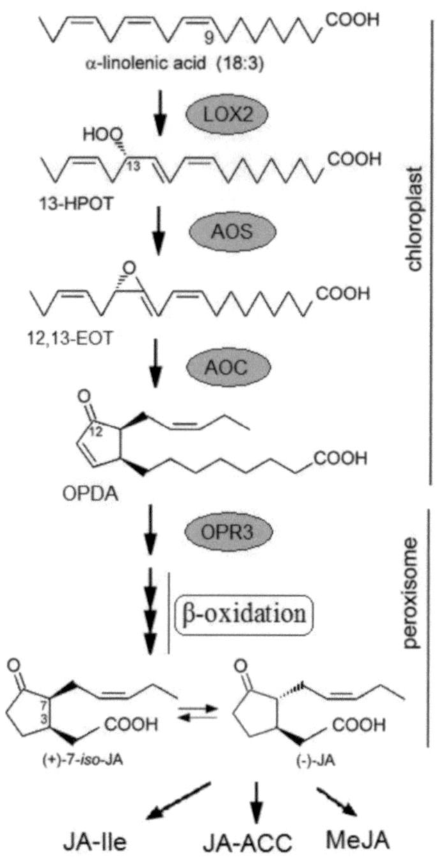

Figure 2. Scheme of JA biosynthesis pathway in *A. thaliana* (Delker et al., 2006)
The enzymes and the intermediates are indicated as LOX2 for lipoxygenase 2, AOS for allene oxide synthase, AOC for allene oxide cyclase, and OPR3 for 12-oxophytodienoate reductase 3; 13-HPOT for 13*S*-hydroperoxy-9*Z*,11*E*,15*Z*-octadecatrienoic acid, 12,13-EOT for 12,13-epoxyoctadecatrienoic acid, OPDA for 12-oxophytodienoic acid, JA for jasmonates, JA-Ile for jasmonoyl-isoleucine, JA-ACC for jasmonoyl-1-amino-1-cyclopropane carboxylic acid, and MeJA for methyl jasmonates.

2.2. The alternative routes of JA biosynthesis

JA biosynthesis beginning with free linolenic acid (18:3) as the substrate is referred to as the Vick and Zimmermann pathway (Schaller et al., 2004) which was considered the major source of JA production in plants. However, there are several variations of this pathway considered as the alternative routes of JA biosynthesis.

Linoleic acid (LA, 18:2) is a ubiquitous component of plant lipids. All seed oils of commercial importance including corn, sunflower and soybean oils usually contain over 50% of linoleate. Previously, LA was considered analogous to α-LeA for metabolism by the Vick and Zimmermann pathway (Schaller et al., 2004) yielding 9,10-dihydro-JA (DH-JA). This product was widely detected *in vivo* in some plant species (Miersch et al., 1999; Blechert et al., 1995; Gundlach and Zenk, 1998), but not others, suggesting DH-JA biosynthesis from LA through Vick and Zimmermann pathway is not conserved (Gundlach and Zenk, 1998). Investigation by Gundlach and Zenk (1998) revealed that allene oxide cyclase (AOC), unlike most of the other enzymes of the Vick and Zimmerman pathway, discriminates between 18:3 and 18:2-derived pathway intermediates. This implies that AOC is the bottleneck for DH-JA production or alternatively, DH-OPDA (precursor of DH-JA) may result from the spontaneous cyclization of the 18:2-derived allene oxide (Gundlach and Zenk, 1998).

Hexadecatrienoic acid (16:3) was proposed as an analog of linolenic acid for JA biosynthesis through the Vick and Zimmermann pathway (Weber et al., 1997), which is characterized by forming dinor-oxophytodienoic acid (dn-OPDA), a 16-carbon cyclopentanoic acid analog of *cis* (+)-OPDA. First identified in leaf extracts of *Arabidopsis* and potato plants (Weber et al., 1997), dn-OPDA dramatically accumulated upon wounding, suggesting an important role of this molecule in wounding response (Weber et al., 1997) (Figure 3). Although dn-OPDA forms after the first β-oxidation of *cis* (+)-OPDA (Figure 2), the detected dn-OPDA in wounded leaves believed to from 16:3 (Figure 3). Convincing genetic evidence for the role of 16:3 in JA biosynthesis came from the analysis ofthe *Arabidopsis* mutant *fad5* incapable of synthesizing 16:3 and JA (Weber et al., 1997).

OPDA and dn-OPDA are also constituents of arabidopsides (Figure 4), which are considered other alternative substrates for JA production in *Arabidopsis* (Gfeller et al., 2010). Arabidopsides are OPDA- and/or dn-OPDA-containing monogalactosyl-diacylglycerides

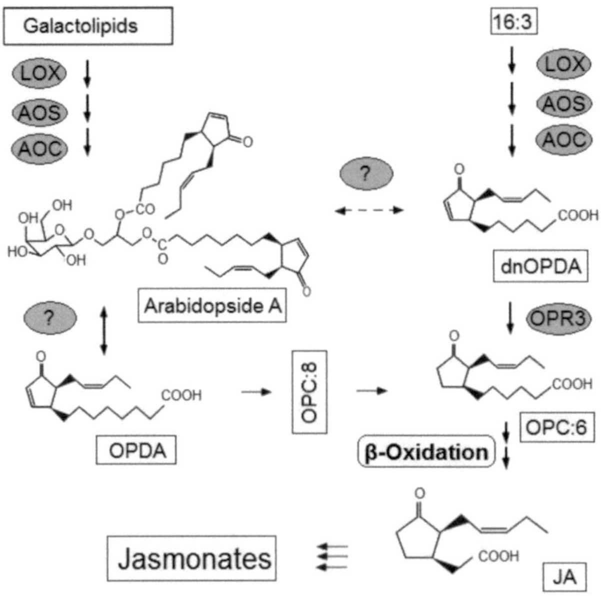

Figure 3. Alternative JA biosynthesis pathway (Schaller et al., 2004; Gfeller et al., 2010)
See the abbreviations of the enzymes in the Fig. 2. dnOPDA indicated the intermediate dinor-oxophytodienoic acid, OPC:8 is 3-oxo-2-(2'-[Z]-pentenyl)-cyclopentane-1-octanoicacid and OPC:6 is 3-oxo-2-(2'-pentenyl) cyclopentanehexanoic acid.

(MGDG) or digalactosyl-diacylglyceride (DGDG). Arabidopsides A, C, E and F have dino-OPDA at *sn2* position of glycerol backbone. Except for arabidopside F, all arabidopsides contain OPDA (Figure 4) (Hisamatsu et al., 2003; Hisamatsu 2005). At present, it is unclear whether the lipid-bound OPDA/dn-OPDA in the membranes is synthesized in situ from MGDG or DGDG or alternatively, OPDA/dn-OPDA is synthesized from free 18:3/16:3 and then incorporated into glycerol (Schaller et al., 2004). The latter possibility is supported by substantial amount of free 18:3 and 18:2 that were detected in tomato leaves after wounding (Conconi et al., 1996). However, Buseman et al. (2006) have shown that within the first 15 min after wounding, levels of OPDA-dnOPDA MGDG, OPDA-OPDA MGDG, and OPDA-OPDA DGDG increased 200 to 1000 folds. Yet in untreated leaves, the levels of these oxylipin-containing complex lipid species remained low, suggesting lipid-bound OPDA/dn-OPDA in wounding response synthesize on the esterified galactolipids rather than via the free fatty acids. Furthermore, OPDA and dn-OPDA sequestered in form of MGDG-O or DGDG-O may provide an abundant resource of OPDA/dn-OPDA, which may rapidly release under appropriate stress conditions for signaling or further metabolism (Schaller et al., 2004).

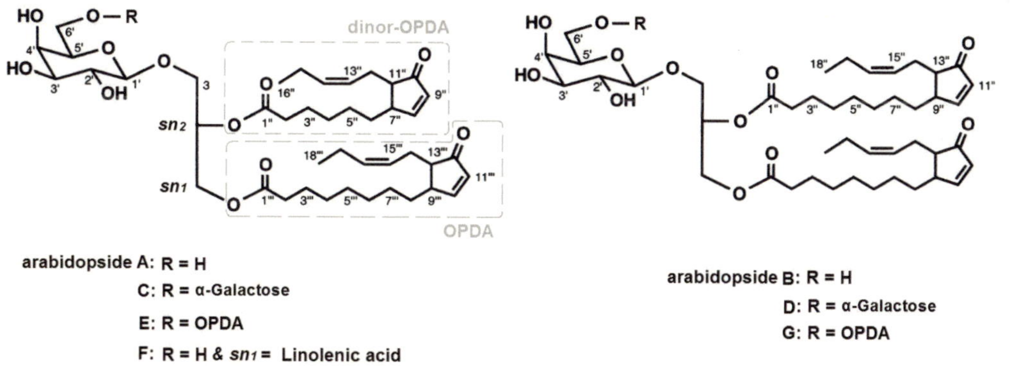

Figure 4. Arabidopsides of *Arabidopsis thaliana* (Hisamatsu et al., 2003, 2005)

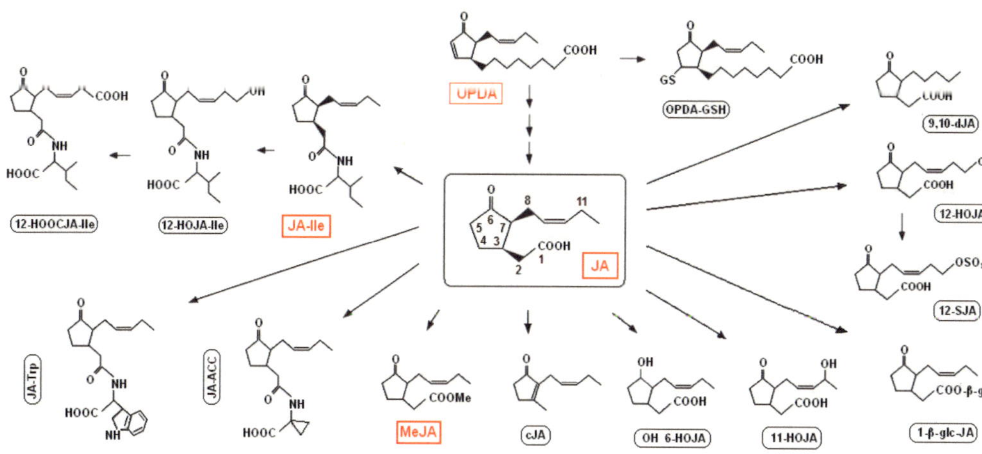

Figure 5. The metabolites produced from JA in plants (Gfeller et al., 2010)

2.3. Derivatives and Metabolites of JA

The JA biosynthetic pathway from linolenic acid yields (+)-7-*iso*-JA (3*R*,7*S*-JA) as the final product (Sembdner and Parthier, 1993). However, this molecule readily isomerizes to the thermodynamically favored stereoisomer (-)-JA (3*R*,7*R*-JA) (Figure 2) resulting in a molar equilibrium of about 9: 1 ((-)-JA : (+)-7-*iso*-JA) under normal conditions (Sembdner and Parthier, 1993). In addition to isomerization, JA undergoes a series of molecular modifications to form a variety of metabolites in plants (Figure 5).

1. C_1 carboxyl group can be methyl-esterified or conjugated with amino acids or with 1-Aminocyclopropane-1-carboxylic acid (ACC).
2. C_1 carboxyl group can be decarboxylated.
3. Glycosylation of C_1 carboxyl group.
4. Reduction of C_6 carbonyl group.
5. Reduction of $C_{9,10}$ double bond.
6. Hydroxylation of carbon at C_{11} or C_{12}.

With the above reactions, (+)-7-*iso*-JA can be converted into more than 30 distinct jasmonates which were found to be widespread in *Angiospermae, Gymnospermae, Pteridophyta, Algae* such as *Euglena, Spirulina,* and *Chiarella,* and the red alga *Gelidium* (Sembdner and Parthier, 1993). However, just several jasmonates *e.g.,* free JA, *cis*-jasmone, MeJA and JA-Ile, are considered to be the major bioactive JA forms in plants (Fonseca et al., 2009). Other jasmonate derivatives or conjugates have been viewed as clearance metabolites playing important roles in hormone homeostasis (Sembdner and Parthier, 1993), in which JA biosynthesis (and deconjugation) and JA degradation (or conjugation) are balanced to control the actual active JA level for fine-tuning developemental and defensive events.

2.4. The Enzymes for JA biosynthesis and derivation

The enzymes of JA biosynthesis and metabolism have been extensively investigated in *Arabidopsis* and several articles have reviewed structures, biochemical activities, and functional regulation (Schaller and Stintzi, 2009; Schaller, 2001; Delker et al., 2006). Here we focus on the genes encoding the enzymes for JA biosynthesis and metabolism.

2.5. Phosholipase A (PLA)

According to the classical Vick and Zimmerman pathway (Vick and Zimmerman, 1983), JA biosynthesis initiates by release of 18:3 from chloroplast membrane galactolipids by a lipase. The lipase belongs to one of the following five enzyme (Wasternack, 2007; Delker et al., 2006): (1) phospholipase A_1 (PLA1), which cleaves the acyl group of phospholipid and glycerolipids at the *sn*-1 position; (2) phospholipase A_2 (PLA2), which cleaves the acyl group in *sn*-2 position; (3) patatin-like acyl hydrolases, which has little *sn-1*/*sn-2* specificity and is homologous to animal Ca^{2+}-independent PLA_2; (4) DAD-like lipase with activity of phospholipid and galactolipid acyl hydrolase that may have *sn-1* or *sn-2* specificity; (5) SAG (senescence-associated gene) 101-like acyl hyrolase. The free hexadecatrienoic acid (16:3) liberated by a phospholipase A2 from the *sn-2* position of MGDG or DGDG can also become substrate for JA biosynthesis to form dn-OPDA (Figure 3). Alternatively, 13-LOX may oxygenate 18:3 and 16:3 esterified in galactolipids (Buseman et al., 2006; Kourtchenko et al., 2007). The resulting hydroperoxy galactolipids may then be substrates for AOS and AOC, yielding arabidopsides, which belong to galactolipid species containing esterified OPDA and dnOPDA in plastidic membranes. These lipid species may serve as storage lipids that may allow the rapid release of OPDA and dnOPDA, the JA biosynthetic intermediates. Conclusively, lipase activity is essential to supply the JA biosynthesis pathway with either free PUFA (18:3 and 16:3) or OPDA/dnOPDA as precursors.

The first reported lipase involved in JA biosynthesis was DEFECTIVE IN ANTHER DEHISCENCE1 (DAD1), a chloroplastic glycerolipid lipase. DAD1 belongs to phospholipase A_1 (PLA1) family. *Arabidopsis dad1* T-DNA insertion mutants are male sterile from decreased JA accumulation required for reproduction (Ishiguro et al., 2001), but remain capable of synthesizing JA, indicating that other lipases contribute to JA production.

A homolog of DAD1, the DONGLE protein was characterized as an essential lipase involved in the early wound response in *Arabidopsis* leaves. A DGL-overexpressing mutant *dgl-D* displayed dwarfism with small round leaves, extremely high basal JA accumulation, increased expression of JA-responsive genes, and increased resistance to the necrotrophic fungus *Alternaria brassicicola* (Hyun et al., 2008).

Arabidopsis PLA1 family comprises seven PLA1 with predicted plastidic transit signaling peptides: DGL (At1g05800; PLA-Iα1), DAD1 (At2g44810; PLA-Iβ1), At2g31690 (PLA-Iα2), At4g16820 (PLA-Iβ2), At1g06800 (PLA-Iγ1), At2g30550 (PLA-Iγ2), and At1g51440 (PLA-Iγ3) (Ryu, 2004). In addition to these seven PLA_1 lipases (DAD1-like lipases), Ellinger et al (2010), identified 14 additional putative lipases with predicted plastid transit peptides suggesting, up to 21 lipases may contribute to JA production in *Arabidopsis*. Mutant lines of 18 different lipases, including DGL and DAD1, have been assessed for wound-induced jasmonate levels. However, none of the single lipase mutants or the quadruple mutant line (*pla-Iβ2 / Iγ1 / Iγ2 / Iγ3*) were completely abolished in JA formation under basal and wound-induced conditions (Ellinger et al., 2010), indicating that multiple lipases with both *sn-1* and *sn-2* (or dual *sn-1/sn-2*) galactolipid substrate specificity participate in JA formation in plant.

2.6. Lipoxygenase (LOX)

Lipoxygenases (LOXs) are non-heme iron-containing dioxygenases widely distributed in yeast, algae, fungus, plant, and animal species (Shin et al, 2008). LOX is the first synthesis enzyme of Vick and Zimmermann pathway. LOX isozymes catalyze the incorporation of molecular oxygen at either position 9 or 13 of polyunsaturated fatty acids (PUFA) such as linoleic (LA,18:2) and α-linolenic (LeA,18:3) acid to produce PUFA hydroperoxides (HPOT and HPOD), which can be further converted to different oxidized fatty acids (oxylipins) through the action of enzymes participating in seven LOX-pathway branches (Figure 1).

Plant LOXs are classified with respect to their positional specificity of LA dioxygenation. LOXs adding O_2 to C-9 or C-13 of the hydrocarbon backbone of LA are designated as 9-LOX or 13-LOX (Feussner and Wasternack, 2002). However, in plants some LOXs have dual positional specificity to C-9 and C-13 of LA and produce both 9- and 13-hydroperoxides of linoleic acid (Hughes *et al*. 2001, Kim *et al*. 2002, Garbe *et al*. 2006). Plants LOXs were found in several subcellular compartments including chloroplast, vacuole and cytosol. According to their localization and sequence similarity, plant LOXs can be classified into type 1- and type 2-LOXs. Type 1-LOXs harbor no chloroplast-transit peptide but the members of this group share a high similarity (>75%) of amino acid sequence to one another. Type 2-LOXs carry a putative chloroplast transit peptide and show only a moderate overall similarity (~ 35%) of amino acid sequence to one another. To date, these LOX forms all belong to the subfamily of 13-LOXs (Feussner and Wasternack, 2002). After LOX activity and fluxing through the lipoxygenase pathway branches, PUFA (mainly LA and LeA) can be converted to hundreds of oxylipin species which physiological roles are largely unclear in plants. However, the jasmonates, a small group of oxylipins, whose members are well known signal molecules mediating defense responses against pathogens and insects. JA alone does not completely describe the effects of lipoxygenase activity, but the other hundreds of oxylipin compounds posses biochemical roles in determing a wide spectrum of responses. Plant LOXs have been correlated with seed germination, vegetative and reproductive growth, fruit maturation, plant senescence, and responses to pathogen attacks and insect wounding (Porta and Rocha-Sosa, 2002).

Every plant species harbors several LOX isozymes, encoded by a LOX gene family. For example, the *Arabidopsis* genome contains six LOX genes (Bannenberg et al., 2009), while rice and maize have 14 (Umate, 2011) and 13 LOX genes (Nemchenko et al. 2006), respectively. All LOX isoforms may contribute to oxylipin production, but only 13-LOXs with chloroplast-transit peptide participate in Vick and Zimmerman pathway for JA production. Additionally, several LOX genes may function for JA biosynthesis, e.g., LOX2, LOX3, LOX4 and LOX6 in *Arabidopsis* contain chloroplast signaling peptides and show 13S-lipoxygenase activity, both required for JA biosynthesis (Bannenberg et al., 2009). However, no LOX gene in *Arabidopsis* shows dual 9-/13-LOX activity (Bannenberg et al., 2009). Compelling evidence establishes LOXs involvment in JA biosynthesis in plants. LOX2 of *Arabidopsis* localizes to chloroplasts (Bell et al., 1995), and transgenic plants lacking LOX2 no longer produced JA as observed in control plants, indicating requirement of LOX2 for wound-induced accumulation of jasmonates in leaves (Bell et al., 1995). *lox3 lox4* double mutant is male sterilie, revealing redundant role of LOX3 and LOX4 in florescence JA biosynthesis (Caldelari et al., 2011). In maize strong evidence establishes *TS1* encoding ZmLOX8, as indispensible for JA biosynthesis in tassel (Acosta et al., 2009). In the *ts1* mutant, the male sex determination process – abortion of pistil primordia in bisexual floral meristem, fails from deficient lipoxygenase activity and subsequent low endogenous JA concentrations (Acosta et al., 2009). In addition to peroxidation of JA percurors, LOXs may indirectly regulate JA biosynthesis in plants. For example, the maize disruption mutant, *lox10,* is devoid of green leaf volatiles (GLV) and reduced JA production (Christensen et al., 2012).

2.7. Allene oxide synthase (AOS)

9-/13-HPOT, the product of LOXs can serve as substrate for several enzymes (Figure 1). Allene oxide synthase (AOS) catalyzes 9-/13-HPOT to the unstable epoxide, either 9,10-EOT (9,10-Epoxyoctadecatrienoic acid) or 12,13-EOT (12,13-Epoxyoctadecatrienoic acid). The unstable epoxide can be either hydrolysed non-enzymatically to α- and γ -ketols or cyclized to 12-oxo-phytodienoic acid (OPDA). Only 12, 13-EOT provides substrate for the following enzyme in JA biosynthesis, allene oxide cyclase (AOC) (Figure 1). AOS and other HPOT-utilizing enzymes such as HPL (hydroperoxide lyase) and DES (divinyl ether synthase) belong to the family of CYP74 enzymes, which are independent from molecular oxygen and NADPH, exhibit low affinity to CO, and use an acyl hydroperoxide as the substrate and the oxygen donor (Stumpe and Feussner, 2006). CYP74 enzymes have been phylogenetically classified into CYP74A, CYP74B, CYP74C, and CYP74D (Stumpe and Feussner, 2006). With some exceptions, plant AOS enzymes belong to CYP74A (Stumpe and Feussner, 2006). According to the specificity of AOS to the substrates, 9-/13-hydroperoxides, AOS enzymes specialize into 9- or 13-AOS, which use either 9- or 13-hydroperoxide, respectively, as substrate. AOS enzymes from barley and rice show no substrate specificity for either (9*S*)-hydroperoxides or (13*S*)-hydroperoxides, and designated 9/13-AOS (Stumpe and Feussner, 2006). Like LOXs, only 13-AOS functions in JA biosynthesis. All 13-AOS carry a plastid-transit peptide except AOS from guayule (Pan et al., 1995) and barley (Maucher at al., 2000), indicating that during JA biosynthesis, AOS localizes to chloroplast. Interestingly, barley AOS, which lacks plastid-transit peptide, was also found localized in plastid (Maucher at al., 2000). Plant species may contain one or multiple AOS genes. For example, *Arabidopsis* jus has a single copy of AOS gene while rice may have four AOS genes (Agrawal et al., 2004). AOS genes from plant species such as flax (Song *et al.*, 1993), guayule (Pan *et al.*, 1995), *Arabidopsis* (Laudert *et al.*, 1996), tomato (Howe *et al.*, 2000), barley (Maucher *et al.*, 2000), rice (Ha et al., 2002; Agrawal et al., 2004) and corn (Utsunomiya *et al.*, 2000) have been cloned or purified so far. The diagram of oxylipin biosynthesis (Figure 1) clearly showed AOS branch competes with other HPOT-using branches for substrate, indicating AOS activity is crucial to control influx of HPOT into JA biosynthesis (Figure 1 & 2). Overexpression of flax AOS in transgenic potato plants led to 6-12 folds increased of basal JA level (Harms et al., 1995). However, overexpression of *Arabidopsis* AOS in either *Arabidopsis* or tobacco did not alter the basal level of JA (Laudert et al., 2000), indicating that the basal expression level of AOS varied in plant species which may be the bottleneck or not for JA production in rest plants. One important property of *AOS* genes in plants is that they are strongly induced by wounding and JA- / MeJA-, and OPDA- treatment in many plant species (Harms et al., 1995; Laudert and weiler, 1998). Other plant hormones such and Ethylene and abscisic acid (ABA) can also induce AOS *Arabidopsis* (Laudert and weiler, 1998). *Arabidopsis* JA-deficient mutant *aos* (Park et al., 2002) or *dde2* (*delayed-dehiscence2*) (von Malek et al., 2002) showed male-sterile phenotype and no JA induction in wounding response, demonstrating AOS enzyme is essential for JA biosynthesis pathway in plants.

2.8. Allene oxide cyclase (AOC)

Allene oxide cyclase (AOC) catalyzes the stereospecific cyclization of the unstable allene oxide, the product of AOS into the cis-(+) enantiomer OPDA, the precursor of JA (Figure 2). The unstable allene oxide is either 9,10-EOT (9,10-Epoxyoctadecatrienoic acid) or 12,13-EOT (12,13-Epoxyoctadecatrienoic acid), corresponding to 9-/13-HPOT, the substrates of AOS. These unstable substrates of AOC, 9,10-EOT and 12,13-EOT can spontaneously and rapidly hydrolyze to a mixture of α- and γ- ketols ($t_{1/2}$ < 30 minutes in water) (Schaller et al., 2004). However, *in vivo* α- and γ- ketols are not detectable (Schaller et al., 2004), suggesting tight coupling of AOS and AOC reactions, which effectively convert HPOT into OPDA. AOC was firstly purified as a 47kDa dimer from maize kernals (Ziegler et al., 1997) and was found to accepted only 12,13-EOT (12,13(*S*)-epoxylinolenic acid) but not 12,13- EOD (12,13(*S*)-epoxylinoleic acid) as a substrate (Ziegler et al., 1999). This is in contrast to AOS, which produces both allene oxides using 13(*S*)-hydroperoxy 18:3 and 18:2. Thus, it appears AOC provides additional specificity to the octadecanoid pathway for JA production in plants (Schaller et al., 2004). To date, one *AOC* gene from tomato (Ziegler et al., 2000), one from barley (Maucher et al., 2004) and four from *Arabidopsis* (Stenzel et al., 2003) have been cloned. Monocot *AOC* genes are less stuied, but at least two exisist in the rice genome (Agrawal et al., 2004). *Arabidopsis* AOCs are enzymatically active and form *cis*-(+)-OPDA, with AOC2 having greatest activity. The N-terminal of cloned *AOC* genes revealed the presence of chloroplast-transit peptide and localization in chloroplast was confirmed immunohistochemically (Ziegler et al., 2000; Stenzel et al., 2003), supporting OPDA production of JA biosynthesis is localized in chloroplast. *Arabidopsis* and rice AOC genes, in particular AOC2 and AOC1, respectively are differentially regulated upon wounding, JA-treatment, and environmental stresses (Agrawal et al., 2004).

2.9. Oxo-phytodienoic acid reductase (OPR)

The second half of the JA biosynthesis pathway, beginning with *cis*-(+)-OPDA, occurs in the peroxisome, requiring OPDA or its CoA ester to transport from the chloroplast into the peroxisome. An OPDA-specific transporter is not yet known, however a peroxisomal ABC transporter protein COMATOSE (CTS, Footitt et al., 2002), also known as PXA1 (Zolman et al., 2001) or PED3 (Hayashi et al., 2002), may mediate transportation of OPDA into peroxisome. While *cts* mutants are JA-deficient, suggesting involvement of CTS with JA-production, substantial residual JA implicates CTS-independent OPDA transport, possiblely by ion trapping of OPDA (Theodoulou et al., 2005).

The first step of peroxisomal JA biosynthesis is the conversion of OPDA, a cyclopentenone to cyclopentanone (3-oxo-2-(2′(Z)-pentenyl)-cyclopentane-1-octanoic acid, OPC-8:0) catalyzed by OPDA reductase (OPR). OPR enzymes belong to Old Yellow Enzyme (OYE) (EC 1.6.99.1), initially isolated from brewer's bottom yeast and shown to possess a flavin cofactor. Despite extensive biochemical and spectroscopic characterization, the physiological role of the enzyme remained obscure. OYE has been described as a diaphorase catalyzing the oxidation of NADPH in presence of molecular oxygen, but the physiological oxidant remains unknown (Schaller, 2001). A number of compounds containing an olefinic bond of α,β-unsaturated ketones and aldehydes may be substrates of OYE (Schaller, 2001). Several OYE homologues have been identified in prokaryotic and eukaryotic organisms (Vaz et al., 1995; Kohli and Massey, 1998; Xu et al., 1999). The first identified OYE in higher plant is OPR1 of *Arabidopsis* (Schaller and Weiler, 1997). Plant OPR isomers are encoded by small gene families identified in across broad plant genre, (Schaller et al., 2004). Better-studied OPR families include five *OPRs* (three of which are characterized) in *Arabidopsis* (Sanders et

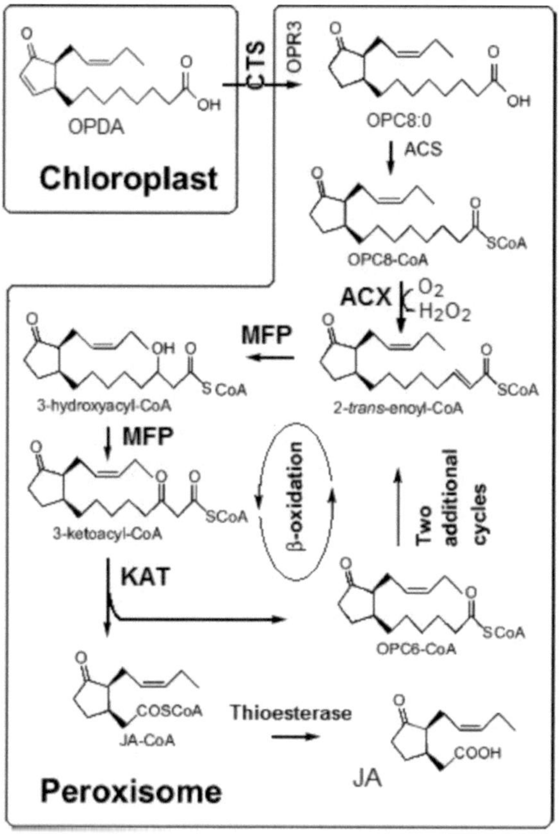

Figure 6. β-Oxidation Scheme of JA Biosynthesis (Li et al., 2005)
Abbreviations: ACS (acyl-CoA synthetase), ACX (acyl-CoA oxidase), MFP (multifunctional protein), KAT (3-ketoacyl-CoA thiolase), and OPC8:0 (3-oxo-2(2'[Z]-pentenyl)-cyclopentane-1-octanoic acid)

al., 2000), six in pea (Matsui et al., 2004), three in tomato (Strassner et al., 2002), 13 in rice (Agrawal et al., 2004), and eight in maize (Zhang et al., 2005). All theses OPRs can catalyze the reduction of α,β-unsaturated carbonyls (conjugated enones) in a wide spectrum of substrates in including four stereoisomers of OPDA(Sanders et al., 2000). Earlier studies on the enzymatic activity of OPRs in *Arabidopsis* and tomato revealed that different OPR isomers have distinct substrate preferences to warrant classification into separate groups, group I and II, depending on their substrate specificity to OPDA stereoisomers (Schaller et al., 1998). OPR group I enzymes preferentially catalyze the reduction of (9*R*,13*R*)-12-oxo-

10,15(*Z*)-octadecatrienoic acid (9*R*,13*R*-OPDA), while OPR group II enzymes preferentially catalyze (9*S*,13*S*)-12-oxo-10,15(*Z*)-octadecatrienoic acid (9*S*,13*S*-OPDA), a intermediate biosynthetic precursor in JA biosynthesis (Schaller et al., 1998). OPR3 of *Arabidopsis* and tomato, belonging to group II, have been shown to efficiently reduce the natural isomer 9*S*,13*S*-OPDA to OPC 8:0, the precursor of JA (Schaller et al., 1998). In contrast, OPR group I enzymes such as OPR1/2 of *Arabidopsis* and tomato have very low affinity for 9*S*,13*S*-OPDA (Schaller et al., 1998) and unlikely to be involved in JA biosynthesis but instead function in other yet unknown biochemical processes. In addition, to uncover the molecular determinants of substrate specificity between OPR group I and II, crystal structural comparison and mutational analysis of tomato OPR1/3 in complex with OPDA enantiomers revealed that two active-site residues, i.e., Tyr78 and Tyr246 in OPR1 and Phe74 and His244 in OPR3 of tomato, are critical for substrate specificity (Breithaupt et al. 2009). Thus, the biochemical studies conclude OPR3 rather than OPR1 and OPR2, is responsible for JA production in *Arabidopsis* and tomato.

Numerous genetic studies identifed JA biosynthetic OPR enzymes across several plant species. A knockout *Arabidopsis* mutant, *dde1/opr3,* displayed male sterilility and compromised defense responses resulting from JA deficiency, indicating OPR3 is essential for the JA biosynthesis pathway and other OPR isomers such as OPR1/2 can not substitute for OPR3 in JA production (Sanders et al., 2000; Stintzi and Browse, 2000). One orthologue of OPR3, i.e., OsOPR7, was identified as a JA biosynthetic OPR in rice (Tani et al., 2008). *OPR7* and *OPR8* in maize, orthologous to *OPR3* of *Arabidopsis,* are segmentally duplicated genes, sharing 94.5% identity in amino acid sequence to each other and responsible for JA biosynthesis in maize (Yan et al., 2012). *opr7 opr8* double mutant showed a number of genetic phenotypes such as tasselseed and susceptibility to insect and pathogen, reflecting JA essential functions in monocotyledonous plants (Yan et al., 2012). Thus in plants, the physiological role of OPR group II enzymes in plants is primarily for production of the jasmonates, which mediate many development and defense-related processes (Yan et al., 2012). However, the biological significance of plants with multiple OPR group I enzymes is not clearly understood so far.

2.10. β-Oxidation enzymes

β-oxidation in lipid metabolism was believed to be located in the peroxisomes of all higher plants (Masterson and Wood, 2001) but also detected in mitochondria in a non-oilseed plant (Masterson and Wood, 2001). The terminal steps of peroxisomal JA biosynthesis are three β-oxidation reactions, which shorten the carboxyl side chain from the intermediates OPC-8:0 or OPC-6:0 produced from OPDA or dn-OPDA (Vick and Zimmernan, 1983). Prior to entry into the β-oxidation reactions, the carboxylic group of OPC-8:0 or OPC-6:0 must activate as a CoA ester. *Arabidopsis* possesses an acyl-activating superfamily containing 63 different genes, whose proteins are potential acyl-activating enzymes (AAEs) (Shockey et al., 2003). Within this superfamily, a subgroup, called the 4-coumarate:CoA ligase (4CL)-like family, contains 13 members shown to possess peroxisomal acyl-activating activity involved in the biosynthesis of jasmonic acid (Koo et al., 2006). One of these 13 genes, At1g20510 was confirmed as an OPC-activating enzyme, designated OPCL1 (OPC-8:CoA ligase 1) (Koo et al., 2006). Loss-of-function mutants for *OPCL1* hyper-accumulate OPC-8:0, OPC-6:0, and OPC-4:0, suggesting a metabolic block in OPC-CoA ester formation. The mutants are also compromised in wound-induced JA accumulation. However, about 50% of wild-type levels remain in the mutants indicating that OPCL1 is responsible for only part of the wound-induced JA production, and that additional acyl-CoA synthetases may be involved in OPC-8:0-activation (Koo et al., 2006). Another two 4CL-like proteins At4g05160 and At5g63380, were selected as acyl-CoA synthetases for JA biosynthesis. The recombinant At4g05160 protein showed, *in vitro,* a distinct activity with broad substrate specificity including, medium-chain fatty acids, long-chain fatty acids, as well as, OPDA and OPC-8:0. The closest paralogue of At4g05160, At5g63380, showed high activity with long-chain fatty acids and OPDA (Schneider et al., 2005), suggesting OPDA-CoA could function as substrate for OPR3 to form OPC-CoA, the substrate of β-oxidation.

Peroxisomal β-oxidation (Figure 6) of JA biosynthesis is catalyzed by three proteins (1) acyl-CoA oxidase (ACX), (2) the multifunctional protein (MFP) which exhibits 2-*trans*-enoyl-CoA hydratase, L-3-hydroxyacyl-CoA dehydrogenase, D-3-hydroxyacyl-CoA epimerase and Δ^3, Δ^2-enoyl-CoA isomerase activities, and (3) L-3-ketoacyl-CoA thiolase (KAT) (Schaller et al., 2004). The first *ACX* gene, named *ACX1A* was isolated from tomato. ACX1A was shown to catalyze the first step in the peroxisomal beta-oxidation stage of JA biosynthesis (Li et al., 2005). Recombinant ACX1A exhibited a preference for C12 and C14 straight-chain acyl-CoAs and also was active in the metabolism of cyclopentanoid-CoA precursors of JA (Li et al., 2005). *acx1* tomato mutant produced very little JA in wounded leaves (for 1-hour wound, 5% of wild type) and impaired in wound-induced defense gene activation and insect resistance (Li et al., 2005). *Arabidopsis* genome contains six *ACX* genes, designated *ACX1 to ACX6* (Rylott et al., 2003). *acx1* mutant of Arabidopsis produced 20% of JA production in wild type while *acx1/5* double mutant showed severe JA deficiency symptoms including impaired male fertility and susceptible to leaf-chewing insect (Schilmiller et al., 2007). For MFP roles in JA biosynthesis Arabidopsis *aim1* mutant, in which one of two MFP i.e. MFP2 is disrupted, showed impairment in wound-induced JA accumulation and defensive gene expression (Delker et al., 2007). In tobacco a similar result was obtained, that is, a stress-responsive MFP orthologous to *Arabidopsis* AIM1 are involved in β-oxidation (Ohya et al., 2008). Among five *KAT* genes in *Arabidopsis*, *KAT2* was shown to play a major role in driving wound-activated responses by participating in the biosynthesis of JA in wounded leaves (Castillo et al., 2004). The final step of JA biosynthesis is that jasmonyl-CoA releases free acid by jasmonyl-thioesterase. There is no report of cloning of jasmonyl-thioesterase in plant so far except that in *Arabidopsis* two peroxyisomal acyl-thioesterases, ACH1 and ACH2 have showed thioesterase activity of hydrolyzing both medium and long-chain fatty acyl-CoAs but not jasmonyl-CoA (Tilton et al., 2004).

2.11. Carboxyl methyltransferase (JMT)

The floral scent methyl jasmonate (MeJA) has been identified as a vital cellular regulator that mediates diverse developmental processes and defense responses against biotic and abiotic stresses (Cheong and Choi, 2003). The enzyme converting JA to methyl jasmonates (MeJA) is JA carboxyl methyltransferase (JMT), which was first cloned and characterized from *Arabidopsis* (Seo et al., 2001). As JMT does not carry any transit signal peptides, it is presumably a cytoplasmic enzyme (Seo et al., 2001). JMT is constitutively expressed in almost all the organs of mature plants, but not in young seedling (Seo et al., 2001), indicating young plant avoids to produce MeJA. However, JMT can be induced by both wounding and MeJA treatment (Seo et al., 2001). Transgenic *Arabidopsis* overexpressing *JMT* exhibited constitutive expression of jasmonate-responsive genes, including *VSP* and *PDF1.2,* and enhanced level of resistance against the virulent fungus *Botrytis cinerea* (Seo et al., 2001), indicating JMT is a key enzyme for airborne-jasmonate-regulated plant responses.

2.12. JA-amino acid synthetase (JAR1)

Since jasmonoyl-L-isoleucine (JA-Ile) is the only one bioactive ligand, known so far, involving in JA signaling, JAR1 (JASMONATE RESISTANT 1), a JA amino acid synthetase that conjugates isoleucine to JA (Staswick and Tiryaki, 2004), was assumed a most important JA derivation enzyme in plants. Recent studies indicate JA-Ile promotes binding of the JAZ proteins to SCF^{COI1} complexes and results in subsequent degradation of JAZ by the ubiquitination/26S-proteasomes (Thines et al., 2007). *JAR1* is one of 19 closely related *Arabidopsis* genes that are similar to the auxin-induced soybean *GH3* gene family (Staswick et al., 2002). Analysis of fold-predictions for this protein family suggested that JAR1 might belong to the acyl adenylate-forming firefly luciferase superfamily. These enzymes activate the carboxyl groups of a variety of substrates including JA, indole-3-acetic acid (IAA) and salicylic acid (SA) for their subsequent biochemical modification (Staswick et al., 2002), thereby regulating hormone activity. The first *jar1* mutant was identified that affected signaling in the jasmonate pathway. *jar1* plants have reduced sensitivity to root growth inhibition in the presence of exogenous JA (Staswick *et al.*, 2002). *jar1* was shown to be susceptible to soil oomycete (Staswick et al., 1998) and necrotrophic pathogens (Antico et al., 2012). In wounding *JAR1* transcript was found increased dramatically in wounded tissue and JA–Ile accumulated mostly near the wound site with a minor increase in unwounded tissue (Suza and Staswick, 2008). However, the reduced accumulation of JA–Ile had little or no effect on several jasmonate-dependent wound-induced genes such as *VSP2,* for *LOX2, PDF1.2, WRKY33, TAT3* and *CORI3*. Morphologically, *jar1* mutation is male fertile while JA biosynthesis and signaling mutants are male sterile (Suza and Staswick, 2008).

2.13. JA Biosynthesis Regulation

The levels of jasmonic acid in plants vary with developmental stage, organs, and are variable in response to different environmental stimuli (Creelman and Mullet, 1995). High levels of jasmonates are found in flowers, pericarp tissues of developing fruit, and in the chloroplasts of illuminated plants; Jasmonate levels increase rapidly in response to mechanical perturbations such as tendril coiling and when plants suffer wounding (Creelman and Mullet, 1995). There are several strategies applicable for plants to regulate generation or activities of jasmontes. The first strategy is to regulate the expression of the enzymes in JA biosynthesis pathway. Many studies show that most enzyme genes for JA biosynthesis such as *LOX, AOS, AOC, OPR3, JMT* and *JRA1* are induced by JA treatment (Wasternack, 2007) or wounding (Schaller, 2001), implying that JA biosynthesis is a JA-dependent process in plants. Monitoring of MeJA-responsive genes in *Arabidopsis* by cDNA microarrays also concluded that JA biosynthesis is regulated by a positive feedback loop (Sasaki et al., 2001). Further evidence for this conclusion has come from mutants with constitutively up-regulated JA levels such as *cev1* and *fou2*. These mutants showed typical phenotypes associated with exogenous JA treatment such as roots/shoots growth inhibition, anthocyanin accumulation in the leaves, and over-expression of JA-dependent genes (Ellis and Turner, 2001; Bonaventure et al., 2007). However, the expression levels of JA biosynthetic enzymes do not determine the actual output of JA biosynthesis in limited substrate conditions. The second strategy for JA biosynthesis regulation is controlling the substrate availability. For example, the fully expanded leaves of *Arabidopsis* carry LOX, AOS, and AOC proteins abundantly; however, JA formation is at a substantially low level. JA production rapidly occurs only upon strong external stimuli such as wounding, which largely induces JA biosynthesis enzymes and releases the substrate LA from the membranes (Stenzel et al., 2003). Furthermore, wound induction of JA is transient and appears before the expression induction of *LOX, AOS,* and *AOC* genes (Howe et al., 2000). These data clearly show that JA biosynthesis is regulated by enzyme activities and substrate availability. The third strategy of JA biosynthesis regulation is to store or reuse intermediates or conjugates of jasmonate in case of over-produced or quick release release is required for healing in situation of insect or pathogen attacks. Recently, esterified OPDA was found in galactolipids (monogalactosyldiacylglycerol, MGDG and digalactosyldiacylglycerol, DGDG) (Stelmach et al., 2001). A novel oxylipin category, so-called arabidopsides A, B, C, D, E, F, G and F (Figure 4) were found containing OPDA and/or dino-OPDA (Hisamatsu et al., 2003; Hisamatsu, 2005). These compounds could accumulate to 7-8% of total lipids in plants if challenged by pathogens (Anderson et al., 2006). In addition, JA derivatives including jasmonyl-amino acids such as JA-Ile (jasmonoyl-isoleucine), JA-Leu (jasmonoyl-leucine), and JA-Val (jasmonoyl-valine) and jasmonyl-ACC (1-amino- cyclopropane-1-carboxylic acid) conjugates are present and all, except JA-Ile, are considered storage forms of jasmonates in plants (Staswick et al., 2002).

3. JA perception and signaling pathway

3.1. Bioactive JA forms and JA signaling ligand

The initial product (+)-7-*iso*-JA, synthesized in peroxisomes epimerizes simultaneously to a more thermo-stable *trans* configuration, (-)-JA, which is generally known as jasmonic acid (JA) (Wasternack, 2007; Creelman and Mullet, 1997). Both (-)-JA and (+)-7-iso-JA are bioactive but the former is more active (Wasternack, 2007). JA can convert into a number of derivatives and conjugates (Figure 5). The JA precursor OPDA, the free acid and methyl ester of JA, i.e., JA and MeJA, and conjugates JA-Ile and JA-trp (jasmonyl-L-tryptophan) are assumed the most active JA forms in plants (Fonseca ea al., 2009). However, in COI1-JAZ (Coronatine Insensitive 1 and Jasmonate ZIM-domain-containing protein, respectively) binding experiments JA-Ile rather than OPDA, JA, and MeJA can promote COI1-JAZ binding, indicating only JA-Ile is the direct JA signaling ligand in plants (Thines et al, 2007). The trans configuration, (-)-JA-L-isoleucine was demonstrated to be the active molecule form of JA for COI1-JAZ binding (Thines et al, 2007). However, the recent study showed that (+)-7-iso-JA-L-Ile, which is also structurally more similar to coronatine, is highly active. The previously proposed active form (-)-JA-L-Ile, which contains a small amount of the C7 epimer (+)-7-iso-JA-L-Ile, if purified, is inactive (Fonseca ea al., 2009). In summary, currently (+)-7-iso-JA-L-Ile is the only proven ligand for JA signaling in plants.

3.2. Ubiquitination-based JA receptor: COI1-JAZ complex

Critical to comprehending hormonal control of development and defense events is the understanding of hormone perception. In the past decades, several mechanisms of plant hormone perception have been elucidated (Spartz and Gray, 2008; Chow and MeCourt, 2006). Cytokinins (CK) and ethylene were found to be perceived by two-component-based hormone receptors while brassinosteroids (BR) by leucine-rich repeat (LRR)-based hormone receptors (Chow and MeCourt, 2006) and ABA (abscisic acid) by nuclear RCAR/PYR1/PYL–PP2C complexes (Raghavendra et al, 2010). More recently, auxin, JA, GA (gibberellic acid), and SA (salicylic acid) are found to be perceived by nuclear SCF^{TIR1}, SCF^{COI1}, SCF^{DELLA}, and SCF^{NPR} complexes respectively (Chow and MeCourt, 2006; Lumba et al., 2010; Fu et al. 2012).

Early researchers believed that screening for Arabidopsis mutants insensitive to growth inhibition by bacterial coronatine, which is structurally analogous to JA and MeJA, would result in discovering JA receptor protein(s) in plants. Exhaustive screens identified only the alleles of *coronatine insensitive 1 (coi1)* and *jasmonates resistant 1 (jar1),* suggesting COI1 and JAR1 function in JA perception in plant. However, cloning of COI1 and JAR1 showed that COI1 encodes an F-box protein (Xie et al., 1998) and JAR1 an auxin-induced GH3 protein (Staswick and Tiryaki, 2004), and neither protein shows homology to known plant receptor proteins. The investigators reasoned that COI1, rather than JAR1, is a potential JA-receptor or a component of a receptor complex from two lines of evidence. First, *coi1* mutant displays severe JA signal-phenotypes such as male sterility, defective responses to JA-treatment and wounding, and high susceptiblity to insect and necrotrophic pathogens whereas *jar1* is fertile and only partially defective to JA-treatment and wounding. Secondly, *COI1* locus encodes an F-box protein which is known to associate with SKP1, Cullin, and Rbx proteins to form an E3 ubiquitin ligase, known as the SCF complex. Several SCF complexes in plant have been implicated in a number of important processes, for example, SCF^{TIR1} complex is an auxin receptor, implying SCF^{COI1} may function as analog of SCF^{TIR1} for JA signaling. The components of SCF^{COI1} complex were demonstrated to exist in Arabidopsis and mutations in the components of SCF resulted in reduced JA-dependent responses (Xu et al., 2002). Now the question becomes: what is the substrate(s) of SCF^{COI1} E3 ubiquitin ligase complex? This substrate was anticipated to function as a key negative regulator in JA signaling (Turner et al., 2002; Browse, 2005). Later, three laboratories simultaneously found the substrates of SCF^{COI1} complex, which were called JAZ proteins consisting of 12 members in Arabidopsis (Chini et al., 2007; Thines et al., 2007; Yan et al., 2007). Bioactive JA forms JA, OPDA, MeJA, and JA-Ile were tested for affinity in COI1-JAZ1 binding. Surprisingly, only JA-Ile functioned as ligand for COI1-JAZ interaction (Thines et al., 2007). JA-Ile is a conjugate product of JA with isoluecine by JAR1, a JA-amino acid conjugation enzyme similar to auxin-responsive GH3 family proteins of soybean (Staswick and Tiryaki, 2004). This provided biochemical explination as to why *jar1* mutant showed the phenotype 'JA-RESISTANT' and demonstrating JAR1 as a provider of a JA signal rather than a component of JA perception machinery in plant. More recently, inositol pentakisphosphate (IP5) was found as an existing cofactor of COI1 crystal structure and COI1 protein lacking IP5 lost ligand-binding acivity (Sheard et al., 2010). Based on the information available so far, the true jasmonates receptor is a co-repressor complex, consisting of the SCF^{COI1} E3 ubiquitin ligase complex, JAZ degrons (JAZ1 to JAZ12), and a newly discovered third component, inositol pentakisphosphate (IP5) (Sheard et al., 2010).

3.3. JA Signaling Model: SCF^{COI1}/JAZ Proteins Imitates SCF^{TIR1}/AUX/IAA Proteins

coi1 is a completely insensitive mutant to JA/coronatine. COI1 was map-cloned and revealed as an F-box protein that functions as the substrate-recruiting element of the Skp1–Cul1–F-box protein (SCF) ubiquitin E3 ligase complex. As described above, JAZ family proteins are transcriptional repressors and SCF^{COI1} substrate targets, which associate with COI1 in a hormone-dependent manner. Recent research established JA signaling model (Figure 7) (Chini et al, 2007; Thines et al., 2007; Sheard et al., 2010). In the absence or low level of hormone signal, JAZ repressor complex, including JAZ proteins, adaptor protein NINJA, and co-repressor TPL, actively repress the activity of JA-responsive transcription factors

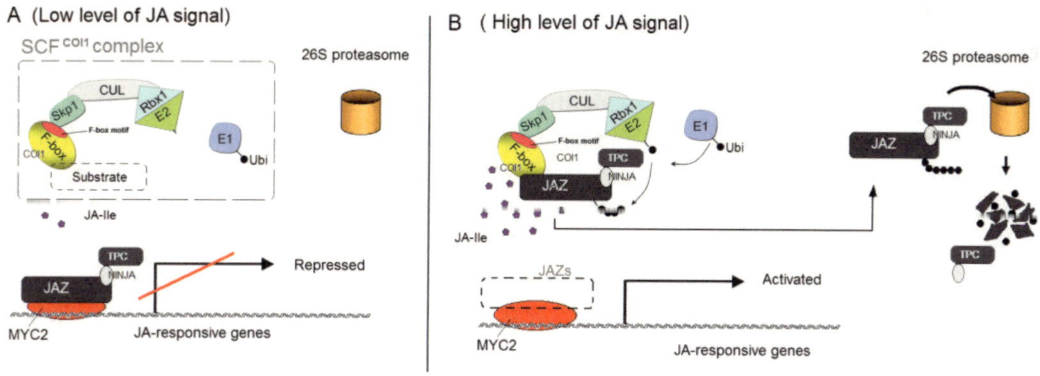

Figure 7. Model of JA signaling in *Arabidopsis* (Browse and Howe, 2008). (A) At low intracellular levels of JA signal (JA-Ile), SCF^{COI1} complex has no essential activity of E3 ubiquitin ligase, resulting in accumulation of JAZ proteins which repress the activity of transcription factors such as MYC2 that positively regulate JA-responsive genes. (B) At high level of JA signal such as upon wounding, rapid accumulation of bioactive JA-Ile promotes SCF^{COI1}-mediated ubiquitination and subsequent degradation of JAZ proteins via the 26S proteasome. JA-induced removal of JAZ proteins causes derepression of transcription factors and the activation of JA-responsive genes.

(e.g., MYC2), which bind to *cis*-acting elements of jasmonate-response genes, preventing transcription activity. In response to stimuli such as wounding JA-Ile stimulates the specific binding of JAZ proteins to COI1, leading to poly-ubiquitination and subsequent degradation of JAZs by the 26S proteasome. JAZ degradation relieves repression of MYC2 and other transcription factors, permitting the expression of jasmonate-responsive genes such as *PDF1.2*. The role of COI1-mediated JAZ degradation in jasmonate signaling is analogous to auxin signaling through the receptor SCF^{TIR1} complex, which degrades the AUX/IAA transcriptional repressors in hormone-dependent manner (Gray et al., 2001; Kepinski and Leyser, 2005). Supported by its sequence homology and functional similarity to TIR1, COI1 is recognized for a critical role in the direct perception of the jasmonate signal (Xie et al., 1998; Katsir et al., 2008; Sheard et al., 2010). Mimicking AUX/IAA proteins which are induced specifically in response to auxin (Gray et al., 2001), JAZ proteins are highly inducible by JA/MeJA treatment or wounding (Thines et al., 2007; Chung et al., 2008).

3.4. Characterization of JA Signaling Repressors: JAZs, NINJA, and TPL

JAZs proteins were designated as JAZs because they were annotated as ZIM-domain containing proteins (ZIM: Zinc-finger protein expressed in Inflorescence Meristem) and their expression depends on jasmonates (Chini et al, 2007; Thines et al., 2007). Thines et al., (2007) in their study found that eight ZIM-domain containing unknown proteins (JAZs) were significantly induced in stamens and seedlings of *opr3* mutant after JA application. JAZ1 protein, one out of the eight JAZs that were tested for activity as a substrate of SCF^{COI1} complex, acts to repress transcription of jasmonate-responsive genes. Jasmonate treatment causes JAZ1 degradation and JA–Ile promotes physical interaction between COI1 and JAZ1 proteins in the absence of other plant proteins (Thines et al., 2007). Additionally, *JAZ1Δ3A*, a mutant with distruption of conserved domain 3A (i.e., Jas domain in Yan et al., 2007) shows typical JA-signaling phenotypes such as male sterility and root growth insensitivity to JA (Thines et al., 2007). In a separate study, Chini et al., (2007) characterized the mutant *jasmonate-insensitive3-1* (*jai3-1*) they identified in a genetic screen for JA-insensitivity. Positional cloning of the *jai3-1* mutation revealed that a base substitution in JAI3 results in a truncated protein that causes a jasmonate-insensitive phenotype and impaired transcriptional responses to jasmonate (Chini et al., 2007). *jai3-1* is a dominant mutant with a missing conserved CT/Jas domain of JAI3, which encodes JAZ3.,This mutant showed some JA-deficiency phenotypes such as root growth insensitivity to JA treatment (Chini et al., 2007). In the third independent study, Yan et al. (2007) profiled the transriptome depletion of *aos* mutant compared to wild type and identified 35 JA-dependent genes responsible for JA signaling depletion in *aos* mutant. Three of these genes encode ZIM-domain containing proteins. Overexpression of a predicted alternatively spliced transcript At5g13220.3, called *Jasmonate-Associated 1* (*JAS1*, identical to *JAZ10*), resulted in reduced sensitivity to MeJA and elevated growth of roots and shoots under MeJA treatment (Yan et al., 2007). In total, 12 *JAZ* genes (Figure 8) have been identified so far in *Arabidopsis* (Chini et al., 2007; Yan et al., 2007; Browse, 2009). All are believed to have redundant function in JA signaling pathway as transcription repressors (Chini et al., 2007). The gene family of ZIM-domain containing proteins is also known as TIFY family (Vanholme et al., 2007). 12 of 18 TIFY proteins are JAZs. The functions of the remaining TIFYs are unknown, except PPD1 and PPD2, which showed, to additively repress the proliferation of dispersed meristematic cells (DMCs) in leaves (Pauwels and Goossens, 2011).

The first prominent characteristic of JAZ proteins is that they possess two domains, ZIM and Jas domains, and both are important for JAZs function (Thines et al., 2007). The former may have two biochemical roles *in vivo*. 1) JAZ1ΔJas and JAZ3ΔJas can not be degraded by SCF^{COI1} complex plus 26S proteasome but still can suppress JA signaling, indicating JAZ may interact with MYC2 via the first conserved domain ZIM (Chini et al., 2007; Thines et al., 2007). 2) ZIM domains are responsible for homo- and hetero dimerization (Chini et al., 2009; Chung and Howe, 2009). All JAZs except JAZ7 are prone to form homo-/hetero-dimers (Pauwels and Goossens, 2011). The biological meaning of JAZ dimerization *in vivo* remains elusive but extensive dimerization of JAZs or JAZ with other proteins such as MYC2 and NINJA may help to establish insensitivity to SCF^{COI1} E3 ubiquitin ligase in the situation of low JA signal. The second prominent feature of JAZs is "logically-paradoxical"; most *JAZ* genes are highly induced upon JA treatment or by wounding in JA-dependent manner (Chini et al., 2007; Thines et al., 2007; Yan et al., 2007) but, on the other hand, JAZ proteins are degraded during activated signaling (Chini et al., 2007; Thines et al., 2007). Similarly, AUX/IAA proteins have the same paradoxical feature, that is, AUX/IAA genes are induced by auxin but the proteins disappear rapidly (Abel et al., 1994). The third important feature of JAZ genes is that several splice-variant transcripts of single *JAZ* gene exist naturally in plants (Figure 9). For example, *JAZ10* has four alternative splice variants and three of them, *At5g13220.2, At5g13220.3,* and *At5g13220.4* encode stable JAZΔJas isomers, which attenuate JA signal output (Yan et al., 2007 Chung and Howe, 2009).

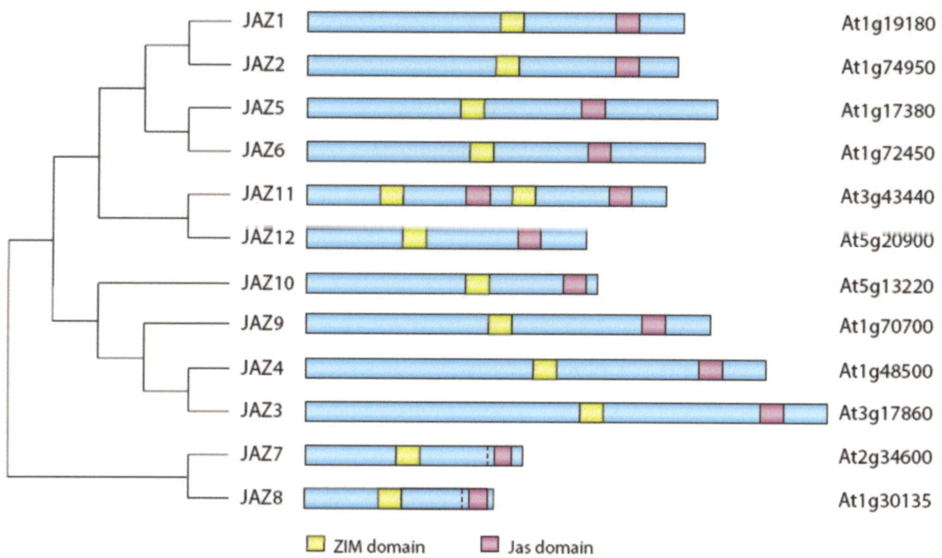

Figure 8. The structures and phylogeny of *Arabidopsis* ZIM-Domain containing proteins JAZs. ZIM domain and Jas domain are shown in yellow and pink bars, respectively (Browse, 2009).

The molecular mechanism by which JAZ proteins repress downstream gene expression is unknown. Pauwels et al. (2010) reported a mechanism that JAZ proteins co-repress JA signal by recruiting the Groucho/Tup1-type co-repressor TOPLESS (TPL) and TPL-related proteins (TPRs) through a newly characterized adaptor protein, designated Novel Interactor of JAZ (NINJA). NINJA acts as a transcriptional repressor whose activity is mediated by a functional TPL-binding motif EAR (ERF-associated amphiphilic repression). Accordingly, both NINJA and TPL proteins function as negative regulators of JA response (Pauwels et al., 2010).

Protein Name	Protein #	Sequence of ZIM domain	Sequence of Jas domain
JAZ1	At1g19180.1	PLTIFYAGQVIVFNDFSAEKAKEVINLA	PIARRASLHRFLEKRKDRVTSKAPY
	At1g19180.2	PLTIFYAGQVIVFNDFSAEKAKEVINLA	PIARRASLHRFLEKRKDRVTSKAPY
JAZ2	At1g74950.1	PLTIFYGGRVMVFDDFSAEKAKEVIDLA	PIARRASLHRFLEKRKDRITSKAPY
JAZ3	At3g17860.1	QLTIFYAGSVCVYDDISPEKAKAIMLLA	PLARKASLARFLEKRKERVTSVSPY
	At3g17860.2	QLTIFYAGSVCVYDDISPEKAKAIMLLA	PLARKASLARFLEKRKERVTSVSPY
	At3g17860.3	QLTIFYAGSVCVYDDISPEKAKAIMLLA	PLARKASLARFLEKRKERVTSVSPY
JAZ4	At1g48500.1	QLTIFYAGSVLVYQDIAPEKAQAIMLLA	PQTRKASLARFLEKRKERVINVSPY
	At1g48500.2	QLTIFYAGSVLVYQDIAPEKAQAIMLLA	PQTRKASLARFLEKRKERY*
	At1g48500.3	QLTIFYAGSVLVYQDIAPEKAQAIMLLA	PQTRKASLARFLEKRKERY*
JAZ5	At1g17380.1	LTIFFGGKVLVYNEFPVDKAKEIMEVA	RIARRASLHRFFAKRKDRAVARAPY
JAZ6	At1g72450.1	QLTIFFGGKVMVFNEFPEDKAKEIMEVA	RIARRASLHRFFAKRKDRAVARAPY
JAZ7	At2g34600.1	ILTIFYNGHMCVSSDLTHLEANAILSLA	KASMKRSLHSFLQKRSLRIQATSPY
JAZ8	At1g30135.1	RITIFYNGKMCFSSDVTHLQARSIISIA	KASMKKSLQSFLQKRKIRIQATSPY
JAZ9	At1g70700.1	QLTIFYGGTISVFNDISPDKAQAIMLCA	PQARKASLARFLEKRKERLMSAMPY
	At1g70700.2	QLTIFYGGTISVFNDISPDKAQAIMLCA	PQARKASLARFLEKRKERLMSAMPY
JAZ10	At5g13220.1	MTIFYNGSVSVFQVSRNKAGEIMKVA	PIARRKSLQRFLEKRKERLVSTSPY
	At5g13220.2	MTIFYNGSVSVFQVSRNKAGEIMKVA	PIARRKSLQRFLEKRKER*
	At5g13220.3	MTIFYNGSVSVFQVSRNKAGEIMKVA	PIARRKSLQRFLEKRKER*
	At5g13220.4	MTIFYNGSVSVFQVSRNKAGEIMKVA	*
JAZ11	At3g43440.1	QLTIIFGGSFSVFDGIPAEKVQEILHIA	PIARRRSLQRFFEKRRHRFVHTKPY
	At3g43440.2	-------------------GVPAQKVQEILHIA	PIARRRSLQRFFEKRRHRFVHTKPY
JAZ12	At5g20900.1	QLTIFFGGSVTVFDGLPSEKVQEILRIA	PIARRHSLQRFLEKRRDRLVNKNPY
	At5g20900.2	QLTIIFGGSCRVFNGVPAQKVQEILHIA	PIARRRSLQRFFEKRRHRFVHTKPY

Figure 9. The sequences of ZIM and Jas domains in the transcripts of JAZs (Yan et al., 2007)

3.5. JAZ proteins control the MYC-type transcription factors activity

Transcription factors dependent on JA signal are supposed to be the key components for JA signaling pathway. Up to date, MYC2 is the only transcription factor known to interact directly with JAZ proteins. According to the current model of JA signaling (Figure 7), MYC2 is the most important transcription factor to activate transcription of the early JA-responsive genes including downstream transcription factors (such as WRKYs, MYBs, and AP2/ERFs), JA biosynthesis genes, and JAZ proteins (Lorenzo et al., 2004; Chini et al.,

2007; Chung and Howe, 2009). MYC2 was identified as a key regulator of JA signaling, acting as a basic helix-loop-helix (bHLH, also called MYC) transcription factor for JA signal transduction. MYC2 was map-cloned from *jai1* (*jasmonate-insensitive 1*) mutant mutant (Lorenzo et al., 2004), which is allelic to the previously characterized mutant *jin1* (*methyl jasmonate-insensitive 1*) (Berger et al., 1996). MYC2 differentially regulates two branches of JA-mediated responses. That is, it positively regulates a wound-responsive gene set, including *VSP2, LOX3,* and *TAT,* but represses the expression of a pathogen-responsive gene set such as *PR4, PR1,* and *PDF1.2* (Lorenzo et al., 2004). Interestingly, the ethylene-responsive transcription factor ERF1 also co-regulated these two gene sets, but in opposite direction, i.e., ERF1 activated pathogen-responsive genes but represses wound-responsive genes (Lorenzo et al., 2004).

In Arabidopsis, there are 133 bHLH genes, constituting one of the largest families of transcription factors (Heim et al., 2003). Based on the amino acid sequence similarity of both the entire protein and of the bHLH domain, Arabidopsis bHLH proteins are divided into 12 major groups and 25 subgroups (Heim et al., 2003). MYC2 is a member of the subgroup IIIe, along with MYC3 (At5g46760), MYC4 (At4g17880), and MYC5 (At5g46830) (Heim et al., 2003). In contrast to severe JA-synthesis and JA-perception mutants such as *aos* and *coi1, myc2* plants are male-fertile and only partially defense-compromised (Lorenzo et al., 2004). This indicates that other JAZ-interacting transcription factors activate the expression of early JA-responsive genes following JA-mediated ubiquitination-proteasomal removal of JAZ repressors. The close paralogues MYC3 and MYC4, but not MYC5, showed to interact with JAZ1, JAZ3, and JAZ9 proteins in both pull-down and yeast two-hybrid assays. Although *myc3* and *myc4* loss-of-function mutants did not show an evident JA-related phenotype, the triple mutant *myc2 myc3 myc4* is as impaired *as coi1-1* in the activation of several, but not all, JA-mediated responses such as the defense against bacterial pathogens and insect herbivory. Moreover, overexpression of cDNAs encoding MYC3 and MYC4 proteins resulted in anthocyanin accumulation and higher transcript levels of JA-responsive genes compared to wild type. In addition, similar to plants overexpressing MYC2, MYC3 overexpression plants were hypersensitive to JA-mediated root growth inhibition. Based on these results, it is concluded that in addition to previously characterized MYC2, MYC3 and MYC4 are also JAZ-interacting transcription factors that activate JA-responses through SCF^{COI1} complex plus 26S proteasome (Niu et al., 2011; Brown et al., 2003; Cheng et al., 2011; Fernández-Calvo et al., 2011).

3.6. AP2/ERF Transcription Factors Involve in JA Signaling Network

AP2/ERF transcription factors are considered the second important group of transcription factors that belong to a large plant-specific APETALA2/ETHYLENE RESPONSE FACTOR (AP2/ERF) superfamily, containing at least 122 members in *Arabidopsis* (Nakano et al., 2006). Many ERF genes have been shown to be regulated by a variety of stress related stimuli, such as wounding, JA, ethylene, salicylic acid, or infection by different types of pathogens (Pré et al., 2008). Four transcription factors, ERF1, AtERF2, AtERF14, and ORA59, were suggested to function as positive regulators involving in JA signing pathway while AtERF4 was identified as a negative regulator for this process (Lorenzo et al., 2003; Oñate-Sánchez et al., 2007; Pré et al., 2008; McGrath et al., 2005).

The expression of *ERF1* can be activated rapidly by ethylene or jasmonate in wild-type plant but not in JA or ethylene (ET) signaling mutants *coi1* or *ein2* (*ethylene insensitive2*), suggesting *ERF1* expression depends on JA and/or ethylene signal. Constitutive overexpression of *ERF1* activates the expression of several defense-related genes, including *PLANT DEFENSIN1.2* (*PDF1.2*) and *BASIC CHITINASE* (*ChiB*) (Lorenzo et al., 2003), and was shown to confer resistance to necrotrophic fungi such as *Botrytis cinerea* and *Plectosphaerella cucumerina* (Lorenzo et al., 2003). All these results suggest that ERF1 acts downstream of the intersection between ethylene and jasmonate pathways and suggest that this transcription factor is a key element in the integration of both signals for the regulation of defense response genes (Lorenzo et al., 2003). *ORA59,* a close paralogue of *ERF1* in *Arabidopsis*, has also been shown to integrate JA and ET signals in defense responses against *B. cinerea*. Overexpression line of ORA59 showed a severe dwarf phenotype under normal growth conditions, similar to plant overexpressing *ERF1* (Pré et al., 2008). RNAi-silencing of *ORA59* compromises JA- and ET-induced expression of several defense-related genes such as *PDF1.2, HEL,* and *ChiB* (Pré et al., 2008). Two more *ERF1*-like genes, *AtERF2* and *AtERF14* have shown to behave similarly as *ERF1* and *ORA59*. Constitutive overexpression of *AtERF2* or AtERF14 causes high levels of *PDF1.2* and *ChiB* gene expression in transgenic *Arabidopsis* plants (Brown et al., 2003; Oñate-Sánchez et al., 2007). In contrast to *ERF1, ORA59, AtERF2,* and *AtERF14,* AtERF4 (At3g15210) negatively regulates the expression of *PDF1.2* (McGrath et al., 2005). Loss-of-function mutants of *AtERF4* showed impaired induction of defense genes following exogenous ET treatment and increased susceptibility to *Fusarium oxysporum*. Moreover, the expression of other *ERF* genes such as *ERF1* and *AtERF2* depends on *AtERF14* expression (McGrath et al., 2005). Collectively, several of members of the ERF family negatively and positively control the expression of a number of defense genes mediated by jasmonates.

3.7. JA-signaling controlling anthocyanin accumulation and trichome development via transcription factors WD40/bHLH/R2R3-MYB complex

Current genetic and physiological evidence shows that JA regulates the activity of "WD-repeat/bHLH/MYB complex", which mediates anthocyanin accumulation and trichome initiation in a *COI1*-dependent manner. Overexpression of the MYB transcription factor MYB75 and bHLH factors such as GL3 (GLABRA 3) and EGL3 (ENHANCER OF GLABRA 3) restored anthocyanin accumulation and trichome initiation in the *coi1* mutant, respectively (Qi et al., 2011). Anthocyanin biosynthesis and trichome initiation are both inducible by JA (Maes et al., 2008; Qi et al., 2011). This induction requires both the JA receptor component COI1 and the GL3/EGL3/TT8-type bHLH proteins (Maes et al., 2008; Qi et al., 2011). Interestingly, the major JA signaling players, MYC2/MYC3/MYC4 are also involved in the JA-mediated anthocyanin accumulation (Lorenzo et al., 2004; Niu et al., 2011), but may not be required for trichome induction. bHLH factors GL3, EGL3 and TT8 (TRANSPARENT TESTA 8) function in complexes in which they interact directly with the

WD40 protein TTG1 (TRANSPARENT TEXTA GLABRA 1) and R2R3-MYB proteins such as MYB75 and GL1 (GLABRA 1). Apart from anthocyanin biosynthesis and trichome formation, GL3/EGL3/TT8 complex may be involved in many other processes including root hair formation, flavonoid biosynthesis, stomata patterning, and seed coat mucilage production (Pauwels and Goossens, 2011). JAZ-interacting domain (JID) was found in a number of bHLH transcription factors including MYC2/MYC3/MYC4, indicating that JAZs may have much wider function spectrum than currently known. Indeed, JID domain is present in GL3, EGL3 and TT8, and interaction of these proteins with eight different JAZs has been detected (Qi et al., 2011).

3.8. JA-Signaling regulates Male Fertility via Transcription Factors MYB21 and MYB24

JA was repeatedly shown to be essential for male fertility in *Arabidopsis*. Many JA biosynthesis and signaling mutants such as *dad1, fad3/7/8, lox3/4, aos, opr3,* and *coi1* are male sterile because of a combination of defective anther dehiscence, insufficient filament elongation, and severely reduced pollen viability (Browse, 2009). Transcriptome analysis of JA-treated stamens in *opr3* and wild type identified two R2R3 MYB proteins, MYB21 and MYB24, as key regulators of the stamen maturation processes triggered by JA (Mandaokar et al., 2006). Overexpression of *MYB21* in the *coi1-1* or *opr3* mutants could partially restore male fertility (Cheng et al., 2009), whereas the *myb21-1* knockout mutant had strong reduction of fertility that could not be rescued by exogenous JA (Mandaokar et al., 2006).

On the other hand, as the major JA-signaling components, JAZ proteins were found directly involved in stamen development. Overexpression of JAZ1ΔJas (Thines et al., 2007) and JAZ10.4 (Chung and Howe, 2009), both of which lack the full Jas domain and are resistant to degradation by SCFCOI1/26S proteasome, results in male sterility. However, the JAZ3 splice acceptor mutant *jai3-1,* which expresses *JAZ3* without the Jas domain (Chini et al., 2007) and JAZ10.3 (Yan et al., 2007), which lost a portion of Jas domain, are still fertile. This suggests a threshold level of JA signaling determines fertility. This notion was also strongly supported by the findings that COI1 leaky mutant allele coi1-16 is only partially male-sterile (Xiao et al., 2004). Interestingly, JAZ proteins were shown to regulate MYB21/MYB24, the transcription factors responsible for stamen and pollen maturation. A select set of JAZ proteins (JAZ1, JAZ8, and JAZ11) interact directly with MYB21 and MYB24, revealing a mechanism in which JA triggers COI1-dependent JAZ degradation to control MYB21 and MYB24 levels and thereby stamen development (Song et al., 2011). In addition, GA was found to promote JA biosynthesis in flower to control the expression of MYB21, MYB24, and MYB57 in the filament of the flower (Cheng et al., 2009).

3.9. JA Signal Interaction with GA, SA, Ethylene and ABA

As an important signal for plant development and defense, JA does not act independently but cooperatively with other phytohormonal signaling pathways including GA (gibberellin), SA (salicylic acid), Ethylene, and ABA (abscisic acid). For JA-GA interaction, a "relief of repression" model has been proposed; in which DELLAs compete with MYC2 for binding to JAZ1 in *Arabidopsis*. Without GA, stabilized DELLA proteins bind to JAZ1 and release MYC2 to promote JA signaling. GA triggers degradation of DELLAs, which releases free JAZ1 to bind to MYC2 and, thus, attenuates JA signaling (Hou et al., 2010). Furthermore, GA significantly suppresses JA-activation of JA-responsive genes, whereas, GA alone does not significantly affect the expression of JA-responsive genes (Hou et al., 2010). This study suggested GA negatively regulates JA signaling. However, GA was found to mobilize the expression of DAD1, a key enzyme of JA biosynthesis in flowers. This is consistent with the observation that the JA content in the young flower buds of the GA-deficient quadruple mutant *ga1-3 gai-t6 rga-t2 rgl1-1* is much lower than that in the WT. The conclusion of these observervations suggests that GA promotes JA biosynthesis to control the expression of MYB21, MYB24, and MYB57, which are essential for male anther development (Cheng et al., 2009).

The mutually antagonistic interactions between SA and JA pathways were shown by analysis of SA- and JA-marker gene expression in SA and JA signaling mutants of *Arabidopsis*. JA-signaling mutant *coi1* displayed enhanced basal and inducible expression of SA marker gene *PR1*, while SA signaling mutant *npr1* (*non-repressor of pr genes 1*) showed concomitant increases in basal or induced levels of JA marker gene *PDF1.2* (Mur et al., 2006). Interestingly, exogenous SA promotes JA-dependent induction of defense gene *PDF1.2* when applied at low concentrations. However, at higher SA concentrations, JA-induced induction of *PDF1.2* is suppressed, suggesting the interaction between these pathways may be dose dependent (Mur et al., 2006). The antagonistic interaction between SA and JA is mediated by NPR1, the centrral regulator of SA signaling (Spoel et al., 2003). WRKY70 is a versatile transcription factor with roles in multiple signaling pathways and physiological processes. It regulates the antagonistic interactions between SA and JA pathways. Overexpression of WRKY70 leads to the constitutive expression of the SA-responsive *PR* genes and increased resistance to SA-sensitive pathogens but reduces resistance to JA-sensitive pathogens. In contrast, suppression of WRKY70 leads to increased expression of JA-responsive genes and increased resistance to a pathogen sensitive to JA-dependent defenses (Li et al., 2004). Another important negative regulator of SA signaling is MPK4. The *Arabidopsis mpk4* mutant exhibits increased SA levels, constitutive expression of *PR1*, and increased resistance to *P. syringae* in the absence of pathogen attack. In contrast, the JA-dependent induction of the *PDF1.2* gene was abolished in the *mpk4* mutant (Petersen et al., 2000).

A number of studies provide evidence for positive interactions between the JA and ET signaling pathways. For example, both JA and ET signaling are required for the expression of the defense-related gene *PDF1.2* in response to infection by *Alternaria brassicicola* (Penninckx et al., 1998). Evidence that JA and ET coordinatively regulate many other defense-related genes was obtained in an *A. thaliana* microarray experiment, which showed nearly half of the genes that were induced by ET were also induced by JA treatment (Schenk et al., 2000). Some evidence suggest also antagonistic interactions between the JA and ET defense pathways although a number of JA-specific or ET-specific genes were found in wounding and defense responses (Lorenzo et al., 2003). Crosstalk between JA and ET was found mediated through the physical interaction of JAZ proteins with ETHYLENE

INSENSITIVE3 (EIN3) and EIN3-LIKE1 (EIL1), two central positive transcription factors for the ET responses (Zhu et al., 2011). At least JAZ1, JAZ3, and JAZ9 can bind EIN3 and EIL1. Therefore, the JAZ proteins can repress the function of EIN3/EIL1, possibly by suppressing the DNA binding of EIN3 (Zhu et al., 2011). In the current model, ET is needed for EIN3/EIL1 stabilization and JA for EIN3/EIL1 release from the JAZ protein repression due to ubiquitin-mediated proteolysis, providing a reasonable explanation for the synergy in many ET/JA-regulated processes (Zhu et al., 2011). As we described above, MYC2, MYC3, and MYC4 are the key signaling players for JA signaling downstream JAZs are also required for ET signaling (Lorenzo et al., 2004). On the other hand, Overexpression of ET-responsive transcription factors ERF1 and ORA59 significantly activates JA responses (Lorenzo et al., 2003; Pré et al., 2008).

Very limited information for the interaction between JA and ABA is available so far. ABA and MeJA were reported to induce stomatal closure, most likely by triggering the production of reactive oxygen species (ROS) in stomatal guard cells (Munemasa et al., 2007). The *coi1* mutation suppresses only MeJA-mediated ROS production without influencing ABA-mediated ROS production, suggesting that *COI1*-dependent JA signaling acts through ABA pathway for stomatal closure (Munemasa et al., 2007). Anderson et al. (2004) showed that interaction between ABA and ethylene signaling is mutually antagonistic in vegetative tissues. Exogenous ABA suppressed both basal and JA/ethylene–activated transcription of defense genes. By contrast, ABA deficiency as conditioned by mutations in the *ABA1* and *ABA2* genes, which encode enzymes involved in ABA biosynthesis, resulted in up-regulation of basal and induced transcription from JA-ethylene responsive defense genes (Anderson et al., 2004).

4. THE physiological roles of JA in plant development and defense

4.1. JA is an essential signal for plant defense against insect herbivory

JA is one of the major defense hormones in plants (Browse, 2009), and it provides a major mechanism of induced defenses against insects herbivores and a wide spectrum of pathogen species, especially necrotrophic fungi. The defense property of jasmonates to various insect herbivores has been extensively studied in the past decades. To the best of our knowledge, there is no report supporting a negative role of jasmonates in defense against insect species This topic has been covered by a number of excellent reviews (Farmer et al., 2003; Felton and Tumlinson, 2008; Browse, 2009; Howe and Jander, 2008). Here, we describe the major lines of evidence that point to the evolution, action and significance of JA as a defense hormone *in planta*. (1) Mechanical wounding or damage caused by herbivore feeding results in rapid accumulation of JAs at the site of wounding (Glauser et al., 2008). Successive feeding on the leaves causes steady increase of JA content throughout the entire plant (Reymond et al., 2004). (2) Wounding or exogenous application of JA/MeJA generally up-regulates the genes involved in JA biosynthesis (Mueller, 1997; Leon and Sanchez-Serrano, 1999). Most JA biosynthesis genes such as *LOX2*, *LOX3*, *LOX4*, *AOS*, *OPR3*, and *AOC3* and signaling genes such as *MYC2*, *JAZ1*, *JAZ2*, *JAZ5*, *JAZ6*, *JAZ7*, *JAZ8*, *JAZ9*, and *JAZ10* were found highly inducible in response to wounding, MeJA treatment, and herbivore feeding (Chung et al.,

2008). (3) Insect feeding or wounding induces hundreds of defense-related genes in JA-dependent manner, including genes involved in pathogenesis, indole glucosinolate metabolism, and detoxification (Reymond et al., 2004). (4) Insect feeding, wounding, or MeJA treatment activates synthesis of anti-insect substance, e.g., proteinase inhibitors (PIs) in *Arabidopsis* (Farmer et al., 1992), nicotine in tobacco, papain inhibitor(s) in tomato (Bolter, 1993), vinblastine in rose periwinkle (*Catharanthus roseus*), artemisinin in annual wormwood (*Artemisia annua*) (De Geyter et al., 2012), and poisonous secondary metabolites such as glucosinates and camalexin in *Arabidopsis*. (5) JA biosynthesis or perception mutants of *Arabidopsis* such as, *fad3-2 fad7-2 fad8*, *aos*, *opr3*, *jar1*, and *coi1*, as well as those from other species such as tomato *jar1*, and maize *opr7 opr8* are highly susceptible to insect attack (McConn et al. 1997; Laudert and Weiler, 1998; Stintzi et al., 2001; Staswick et al., 1998; Xie et al., 1998; Li et al., 2004; Yan et al., 2012). These JA mutants are shown to be compromised in resistance to a wide range of arthropod herbivores including caterpillars (*Lepidoptera*), beetles (*Coleoptera*), thrips (*Thysanoptera*), leafhoppers (*Homoptera*), spider mites (*Acari*), fungal gnats (*Diptera*), and mirid bugs (*Heteroptera*) (Howe and Jander, 2008). On the other hand, JA-pathway overexpression mutants such as *cev1*, cex1, and *fou2* are highly resistant to insect and pathogen attacks (Ellis and Turner, 2001; Xu et al., 2001; Bonaventure et al., 2007). (6) Exogenous application of JA or MeJA can elevate resistance of a number of plant species to insects attack (Avdiushko et al., 1997). The JA precursor OPDA also contributes to plant defense against insect attacks (Stintzi et al., 2001). (7) When attacted by herbivores, plants can rapidly release volatile organic compounds (VOC, consisting mainly of fatty acid-derived products and terpenes) and green leafy volatiles (GLV, including mainly of (Z)-3-hexenal, (Z)-3-hexenol, and (Z)-3-hexenyl acetate). These can effectively induce direct defense response — activation of JA biosynthesis pathway in the attacked and neighboring plants, and indirect defense response — attraction of insect enemies that parasitize or prey on feeding insects (Paré and Tumlinson, 1999; Engelberth et al., 2004).

4.2. The roles of JA in induced systemic resistance (ISR) against microbial pathogens

JA is an essential phytohormone for defense response against a wide spectrum of pathogens, alone or in combination with other hormones, such as ET, SA, and ABA (Browse, 2009; Adie et al., 2007). Although all plant hormones including GA, auxin (IAA), and brassinosteroids (BR) may be involved in plant defense responses against pathogens (Smith et al., 2009), numerous studies have shown that SA, JA, and ET are the major players in induced resistance of plants (Dong, 1998; Kunkel and Brooks, 2002). The SA-mediated pathway is typically activated in response to pathogens and mediates the initiation of a hypersensitive response (HR) and induction of pathogenesis-related proteins (PRs) that confer systemic acquired resistance (SAR) against a broad array of pathogens (Smith et al., 2009). Rhizobacteria-mediated induced systemic resistance (ISR) in plants primarily depends on JA and ET (Pieterse et al., 1998). Regarding the relationship of JA with ET, the widely held belief is that ET acts synergistically with JA in the activation of responses to pathogens (Lorenzo and Solano, 2005). Several defense-related genes including *PR1*, *PR3*, *PR4*, *PR5*, and *PDF1.2* are synergistically induced by JA and ET (Lorenzo et al., 2003). Exogenous application of JA and ET can activate expression of genes in both JA biosynthesis and signaling pathway (Chung et al., 2008; Pré et al., 2008). As to SA interaction with JA/ET, either to biotrophic or necrotrophic pathogens, SA was suggested to act mutually antagonistically with JA/ET pathways (Lorenzo and Solano, 2005).

Considering only the role of JA, it has been frequently demonstrated to be an indispensible phytohormone signal for resistance/susceptibility to several diseases caused by fungal, bacterial, and viral pathogens.

1. **JA mediates resistance of plant to necrotrophic pathogens such as *Botrytis cenerea* and *Alternaria brassicicola*.** JA perception mutant *coi1* display enhanced susceptibility to *B. cenerea* and *A. brassicicola* (Thomma et al., 1998) and JA biosynthesis mutant *aos* as well as signaling mutant *coi1* is also highly susceptible to *B. cenerea* (Rowe et al., 2010). Interestingly, there are exceptions that JA negatively regulates resistance to necrotrophic fungi. For example, JA signaling mutant *jin1/jai1*, which acts downstream of *COI1* in JA signaling pathway, showed higher resistance to necrotrophic fungi such as *B. cinerea* and *Plectosphaerella cucumerina* (Lorenzo et al., 2004). JA signaling mutant *coi1* displayed enhanced resistance to necrotrophic fungus *Fusarium oxysporium* (Thatcher et al., 2009).
2. **JA biosynthesis mutants show extremely high susceptibility to soil-borne oomycete *Pythium* spp.** *Arabidopsis* fatty acid desaturase triple mutant *fad3-2 fad7-2 fad8*, deficient in biosynthesis of the JA precursor linolenic acid, is more susceptible to the root pathogen *Pythium mastophorum*; 90% of the triple mutant plants did not survive the infection as compared to only 10% of wild-type plants (Vijayan et al., 1998). Exogenously applied MeJA reduced death rate of *fad3-2 fad7-2 fad8*. Another *Arabidopsis* JA mutany *jar1* (*jasmonic-acid resistant 1*), shows reduced sensitivity to jasmonates and deficient JA signaling (Staswick et al., 1998). Both *fad3-2 fad7-2 fad8* and *jar1* plants exhibit enhanced susceptibility to *Pythium irregulare* (Staswick et al., 1998). In maize, the double mutant *opr7 opr8*, deficient in JA biosynthesis, showed extreme susceptibility to *Pythium aristosporium* (Yan et al., 2012). When tarnsfered to a field from sterile soil *opr7 opr8* plants displayed "wilting" phenotype due to root rots 6 d after the transfer (Figure 10H and 10I), and 11 days after transplanting, all the *opr7 opr8* plants died, while wild-type plants continued to display normal growth (Yan et al., 2012).
3. **JA signaling promotes pathogenesis of biotrophic pathogens.** Resistance of host plants against fungal and bacterial biotrophic pathogens is associated with activation of SA-dependent signaling and SAR. As SA and JA/ET signaling tend to be mutually inhibitory, JA/ET signaling is expected to have negative effects on resistance to these pathogens. Results from studies of *Peronospora parasitica, Erysiphe* spp., and *Pseudomonas syringae* support the idea that SA signaling is important for resistance against biotrophs. In the cases of *P. parasitica* and *Erisyphe* spp., JA/ET-dependent responses do no seem to play a major role because infection does not induce JA/ET pathways. However, JA/ET signaling may also be effective if activated artificially (Glazebrook, 2005). In the case of *bacterial biotroph P.syringae,* SA-dependent defense responses clearly play an important role in limiting *P.syringae* growth. Mutants with defects in SA signaling, including *eds1, pad4, eds5, sid2,* and *npr1,* show enhanced susceptibility to virulent strains and in some

cases, avirulent strains. *P. syringae* DC3000 inhibits SA signaling by producing a toxin called coronatine, which imitates JA-Ile (a bioactive JA-amino acid conjugate). The coronamic acid moiety of coronatine structurally resembles ACC (the ET precursor, aminocyclopropane carboxylic acid). Resistance of JA insensitive mutant *coi1* to *P. syringae* DC3000 is associated with elevated levels of SA and enhanced expression of SA-regulated genes, suggesting that coronatine contributes to virulence by activating JA signaling, thereby repressing SA-dependent defense mechanisms that limit *P. syringae* growth (Glazebrook, 2005).

4. **JAs may have positive roles in plant resistance against viruses.** Members of the geminivirus family are plant viruses with circular, single-stranded DNA genomes that infect a wide range of plant species and cause extensive yield losses in important crops such as tomato, maize, and cotton. In *Arabidopsis*, exogenous application of jasmonates reduces susceptibility to geminivirus infection (Lozano-Durán et al., 2011). In a case of turnip crinkle virus (TCV), SA, but not JA/ET, is required for the development of hypersensitive reaction (HR) and systemic resistance in *Arabidopsis* (Kachroo et al., 2000). However, applying 60 μM JA and then 100 μM SA 24 h later, enhanced resistance to *Cucumber mosaic virus* (CMV), *Tobacco mosaic virus* (TMV), and TCV in *Arabidopsis*, tobacco, tomato, and hot pepper (Shang et al., 2011), indicating JA and SA have additive positive effects to resistance against RNA viruses.
5. **JA positively regulates resistance against parasitic plants.** In plant-parasitic plants interaction, both JA and SA were found to positively regulate host-plant defense responses to parasitic plants (Bar-Nun et al., 2008; Runyon et al., 2010). The holoparasitic plant, *Orobanche aegyptiaca*, is capable of infecting many host plants, including *Arabidopsis thaliana*. Low dose exposure to MeJA or methyl salicylic acid (MeSA) effectively induced resistance of *Arabidopsis* seedlings to *O. aegyptiaca* (Bar-Nun et al., 2008). Runyon et al. (2010) reported that the parasitic plant *Cuscuta pentagona* grew larger on mutant tomato plants, in which the SA (*NahG*) or JA (*jin1*) pathways were disrupted, suggesting that these hormones can act independently to reduce parasite growth. Large increases of both JA and SA were detected in host plant tomato after parasitism was established (*i.e.*, haustoria formation) (Runyon et al., 2010). Host production of JA was transitory and reached a maximum at 36 hr, whereas SA peaked 12 hr later and remained elevated 5 d later (Runyon et al., 2010).
6. **JA is a key player in induced systemic resistance against root knot nematodes (RKN).** Foliar application of JA induces a systemic defense response that reduces avirulent nematode reproduction on susceptible tomato plants. JA enhances *Mi*-mediated resistance (*Mi* is a resistant gene in tomato) of resistant lines at high temperature (Cooper et al., 2005). However, using JA-signaling mutant *jar1* (equal to *coi1* of *Arabidopsis*) and JA biosynthesis mutant *def1*, it was found that endogenous JA signaling pathway is required for tomato susceptibility to RKNs (Bhattarai et al., 2008).

4.3. JAs serve an important role against abiotic stresses

Salinity is one better studied abiotic stress in plants. Foliar application of MeJA can effectively alleviate salinity stress symptoms in soybean seedlings (Yoon et al., 2009). In grapevine, exogenous jasmonate can rescue growth in the salt-sensitive cell line and salt stress response is modulated by JA-signaling components such as JAZ proteins (Ismail et al., 2012).

JA plays import role of plant resistance against ozone (O_3) stress. JA biosynthesis mutant *fad3/7/8* and JA-signaling mutant *jar1* have greater sensitivity to O_3 (Rao et al., 2000). Furthermore, MeJA pretreatment decreased O_3-induced H_2O_2 content and SA concentrations and completely abolished O_3-induced cell death (Rao et al., 2000).

4.4. JAs are required signals for pollen development in dicots and for sex determination in monocots

In addition to defense function, jasmonate was frequently shown to serve essential roles in reproductive processes of plants. In *Arabidopsis*, JA biosynthesis mutants such as *fad3/7/8, aos, opr3,* and JA signaling mutant *coi1* are male sterile, strongly supporting JA as an essential signal for development of male organ of bisexual flowers (Browse, 2009). This JA-dependent male sterility phenotype consists of three characteristics: 1) the anthers of mutants lost dehiscence to shed pollen at flowering time; 2) the pollen grains in the anthers are predominantly (>97%) inviable; 3) the stamen filaments are substantially shorter in mutant, that is, the anthers do not elongate sufficiently to the stigma level (Browse, 2009). The fertility defective phenotype of JA biosynthetic mutants is rescued by exogenous JA treatment; however, the signaling mutant *coi1* cannot be rescued by JA application (Browse, 2009). Some JA signaling components have also been implicated in stamen development. *MYB21* and *MYB24* are JA-responsive transcription factors in *opr3* stamens and were isolated as JA-dependent transcription factors for flower development (Mandaokar et al., 2006). A *myb21* mutants exhibited shorter anther filaments, delayed anther dehiscence, and greatly reduced male fertility. A *myb24* mutants was phenotypically wild type, but creation of a *myb21myb24* double mutant indicated that introduction of the *myb21* mutation exacerbated all three aspects of the *myb24* phenotype. Exogenous jasmonate could not restore fertility to *myb21* or *myb21myb24* mutant plants. All these results indicate that *MYB21* and *MYB24* are JA signaling components mediating JA response during stamen development (Mandaokar et al., 2006).

In addition, overexpression of Jas domain defective JAZ proteins such as JAZ1-ΔJas and JAZ10.4 which are resistant to SCF^{COI1}/26S proteolysis complex resultes male sterile phenotypes, further demonstrating that JA is essential for male fertility in *Arabidopsis* (Thines et al., 2007; Chung and Howe, 2009). However, some JA signaling mutants are male fertile instead of sterile. For example, *myc2* mutant does not show a male-sterile phenotype (Lorenzo et al., 2004); *jar1* mutant is male fertile (Staswick and Tiryaki, 2004). In these mutants, it may be possible that an alternative component or ligand for JA signaling exists. Surprisingly, in contrast to *Arabidopsis*, JA perception mutant *jar1* of tomato (*Solanum lycopersicum*) are male-fertile but female-sterile (Li et al., 2004), suggesting that JA roles in reproductive differentiation of plants largely depend on the species.

Like *Arabidopsis*, the monocotyledonous plant rice bears bisexual flowers. The JA-deficient mutant of rice *hebiba* showed male sterility (Riemann et al., 2003), supporting that JA is required for male organ formation of bisexual flower plants. Maize is another monocot and belongs to monoecious plants, which bears distinct male inflorescence (called tassel) and female inflorescence (called ear) on the same plant. The monosexual florets in the tassel or the ears develop from bisexual floret primordia of top or axillary meristems though a sex determination program mediated by a number of sex-determining genes (Bortiri and Hake, 2007). Recent study on *ts1* (*tasselseed1*), a mutant in which male inflorescence (tassel) becomes female-fertile structure that can be pollinated to bear seeds, showed that jasmonates is an essential phytohormone that initiates sex determination program of tassel (Acosta et al., 2009). In our recent study, the JA-deficient mutant *opr7 opr8* showed 100%-feminized tassel, strongly supporting the JA signal requirement for tassel formation in maize (Figure 10A and 10B) (Yan et al., 2012). *TS1* encodes a 13-lipoxygenase (i.e. *LOX8*), disruption of which causes JA-deficiency locally in the tassel meristem. *opr7 opr8* is a double mutant of OPR isoforms required for JA biosynthesis, mutation of which results in JA depletion systemically in the plant. Several studies have showed that gibberellin (GA) is involved in ear formation. GA biosynthesis mutants such as *an1*, *d1*, *d2*, *d3,* and *d5* and GA perception mutants *D8* and *D9*, all showed dwarfism and masculinized ears (i.e. male florets are produced in ears), indicating GA is another important phytohormone for sex determination in maize (Chuck, 2010). Putting the studies of JA and GA together, we may hypothesize that JA and GA act antagonistically in male and female flowers, respectively, in maize sex determination process.

4.5. JAs has a role in female organgenesis in some plant species

In tomato, JA signaling mutant *jar1* (the ortholog of *coi1*) showed seed-bearing sterility: 1) the size and mass of mature ripened *jai1-1* fruit were significantly less than those of mature wild-type fruit; 2) vast majority (>99%) of fertilize ova of the mutant fruit were not viable during the fruit development and only a few viable seeds were recovered from the fruit. It is estimated that the number of viable seeds produced by *jai1-1* plants was <0.1% of the viable seed yield from wild-type plants grown under identical conditions (Li et al., 2004). In maize, JA-deficient mutant *opr7 opr8* showed outgrowth of multiple female reproductive buds and extreme elongation of ear shanks, indicating JA is a crucial signal for female organ growth (Figure 10C and 10D) (Yan et al., 2012).

4.6. JAs regulate vegetative growth

Activation of JA defense signaling against biotic and abiotic stresses depletes available resources and severely restricts plant growth. It is well known that JAs act in plant as growth inhibitors in root and shoots (Staswick et al., 1992). Wound-induced accumulation of endogenous JAs strongly suppresses plant growth of roots and shoots by inhibiting cell mitosis (Zhang and Turner, 2008). The inhibition role of JAs depends on JA signaling pathway. JA perception mutant *coi1* relieved JA inhibition to roots and shoots (Xie et al., 1998). JA-signaling mutants such as *jin1/myc2, jin4/jar1,* and *jai3* have largely reduced growth inhibition to roots and leaves by JA application (Lorenzo et al., 2004). JA signal integrates other plant hormones including CK (cytokinins), GA, IAA, ABA, and ET to regulate growth processes and defense responses (Sano et al., 1996; Cheng et al., 2009; Nagpal et al., 2005; Anderson et al., 2004; Lorenzo et al., 2003).

4.7. JA involved in trichome development

Trichomes are branching structures or hair-like appendages differentiated from epidermal cells in the aerial part of plant, which function as barriers to protect plants against herbivores, insects, abiotic damage, UV irradiation, and excessive transpiration (Ishida et al., 2008). Trichome formation is initiated by various environmental cues, such as wounding and insect attack (Yoshida et al., 2009), and by different endogenous developmental signals, including phytohormones, such as jasmonate (Traw and Bergelson, 2003; Li et al., 2004; Yoshida et al., 2009), gibberellin (Perazza et al., 1998), ethylene (Plett et al., 2009), and salicylic acid (Traw and Bergelson, 2003). Tomato JA perception mutant *jar1* has no trichomes on the surface of young fruit and significantly less on the leaf and stem surfaces (Li et al., 2004). JA biosynthesis mutant *aos* and perception mutant *coi1* produced fewer trichomes than the wild type and MeJA treatment increases trichome density in *aos* but not *coi1*, indicating JA signal is a positive regulator of trichome development in *Arabidopsis* (Yoshida et al., 2009). JA signal controls trichome patterning in *Arabidopsis* via a key transcription factor GRABRA3 of which JA treatment enhanced expression prior to trichome initiation (Yoshida et al., 2009). GRABRA3 interacts with other transcription factors such as TRANSPARENT TESTA GLABRA1 (TTG1) and GLABRA1 (GL1) to control trichome initiation (Yoshida et al., 2009). Furthermore, a recent study showed that JAZ proteins interact with these transcription factors to regulate trichome development (Qi et al., 2011).

4.8. JAs promote fruit/seed ripening

JA perception mutant *jar1* of tomato bears much smaller fruits compared with wild type, and the young seeds of the mutant fruits suffer from high rate of seed abortion (>99%), indicating that JA signal is an essential signal during the early stage of fruit development and seed maturation in tomato (Li et al., 2004). In apples (*Malus sylvestris*) and sweet cherries (*Prunus avium*), endogenous JA accumulated in the early ripening stage of the fruit and seeds, also indicating that JA plays an important role in fruit/seed development (Kondo et al., 2000).

4.9. JAs act as an internal signal facilitating leaf senescence

Leaf senescence involves senescence-associated cell death (PCD), which is controlled by age under the influence of endogenous and environmental factors (Lim et al., 2007). Several phytohormones including JA, cytokinins, ethylene, ABA, and SA were implicated in leaf senescence program (Lim et al., 2007). Regarding the role of JA in leaf senescence, most studies support that JA positively regulates leaf senescence process (Ueda and Kato, 1980; He et al., 2002; Schenk et al., 2000; Castillo and León, 2008). Senescence-like phenotypes are induced by exogenous application of MeJA or JA in *Artemisia absinthium* or *Arabidopsis* (Ueda and Kato, 1980; He et al., 2002); and some senescence-up-regulated genes such as

SEN1, *SEN4*, *SEN5*, *SAG12*, *SAG14*, and *SAG15* are responsive to JA treatment (He et al., 2002; Schenk et al., 2000). Delayed yellowing phenotype during natural senescence and upon dark incubation of detached leaves was observed in JA biosynthesis mutant *kat2* and signaling mutant *coi1* (Castillo and León, 2008). Casting doubt about the role of JA in senescence, JA-defective mutants *aos* and *opr3* senesced similar ro wild type under natural senescence conditions or upon dark treatment (He et al., 2002; Schommer et al., 2008). In maize, strong genetic evidence was obtained for JA involvement in the leaf senescence (Yan et al., 2012). The leaves of JA-deficient mutant *opr7 opr8* displayed senesced substantially later than wild type (Figure 10G).

4.10. JAs activate secondary metabolism beneficial to development and defense

Secondary metabolites play diverse roles in plants. For example, flowers synthesize and accumulate anthocyanin pigments in petals to attract pollinating insects. In addition, anthocyanins absorb visible as well as UV radiation and are effective antioxidants and scavengers of reactive oxygen species, protecting plant tissues from the effects of excess incidental visible or UV-B radiation and oxidative stress (Quina et al., 2009). Other secondary metabolites such as polyamines, quinones, terpenoids, alkaloids, phenylpropanoids, and glucosinolates act as phytoalexins to protect plants against microorganisms or herbivores (Chen et al., 2006).

Gaseous MeJA enhance production of anthocyanins in soybean seedlings (Franceschi and Grimes, 1991). Wounding or MeJA treatment activates rapidly the expression of anthocyanin biosynthesis genes and increase anthocyanin level in the detached corolla of *Petunia hybrida* (Moalem-Beno *et al.*, 1997). In *Arabidopsis*, JA or MeJA treatment strongly enhances anthocyanin accumulation in the shoots, especially in the petiole of the seedling (Lorenzo et al., 2004) and this JAs-activating anthocyanin accumulation depends on COI1-mediated JA signaling pathway (Shan et al., 2009). JA induces anthocyanin biosynthesis via up-regulation of the 'late' anthocyanin biosynthetic genes *DFR*, *LDOX*, and *UF3GT* (Shan et al., 2009). JA coincidently activates anthocyanin biosynthetic regulators such as transcription factors *PAP1*, *PAP2*, and *GL3* (Shan et al., 2009). Either these biosynthetic genes or transcription factors are *COI1*-dependent (Shan et al., 2009). In the monocot plant maize, *opr7opr8* double mutant lack anthocyanin pigmentation in brace roots and auricles (Figure 10E and 10F), but not in leaf blade or sheath, indicating that endogenous JA controls anthocyanins pigmentation in specific tissues of maize (Yan et al., 2012).

JAs also effectively activate defensive metabolites against insects or pathogens. Early studies concluded that MeJA application strongly induced anti-insect protein accumulation such as proteinase inhibitors I and II (PI-I, II) (Farmer et al., 1992) and vegetative storage protein (VSP) (Liu et al., 2005). Nicotine, an alkaloid toxic to most insects by interfering with the transmitter substance between nerves and muscles, widely exists in tobacco (*Nicotiana tabacum*) and related species. Exogenous application of JA or wounding of leaves activate nicotine biosynthesis in a *COI1*- and *MYC2*-dependent manner, indicating JA signal is required in tobacco to control nicotine metabolism (Shoji et al., 2008; Shoji and Hashimoto,

2011). In *Arabidopsis*, camalexin (3-thiazol-2'yl-indole) is the main phytoalexin induced by a variety of microorganisms including bacteria, fungi, and oomycetes. JA signaling is required for the activation of camalexin synthesis in response to infection by *P. syringae* pv. *maculicola* ES4326 (Zhou et al., 1999). Glucosinolates are a group of thioglucosides found in all cruciferous plants such as *Arabidopsis* and *Brassica napus*. The hydrolysed products of glucosinolates contribute to plant defense against microorganisms. MeJA treatment increases total glucosinolate content in leaves of *B. napus* up to 20 fold (Doughty et al., 1995). In *Arabidopsis*, accumulation of camalexin and indole glucosinolates can be trigged by elicitors from the plant pathogen *Erwinia carotovora,* and this induction effect is *COI1*-dependent (Brader et al., 2001). There are also a number of examples that jasmonates effectively activate secondary metabolites in medicinal plant species such as artemisinin synthesis in *Artemisia annua* and vinblastine (an alkaloid) in *Catharanthus roseus* (De Geyter et al., 2012). All pathways of the above metabolites, including nicotine, camalexin, glucosinolates, artemisinin, and vinblastine belong to JA-elicited plant secondary metabolism, which is regulated by JA-signaling components such as *COI1, MYC2, ERF1* and *JAZs* (De Geyter et al., 2012).

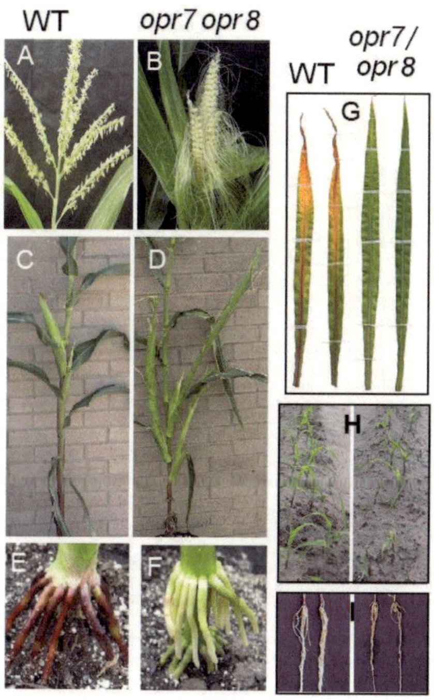

Figure 10. Genetic morphological phenotypes of JA-deficient mutant in maize
(A) Tassel of wild type. (B) Feminized tassel structure of JA deficient mutant *opr7 opr8*. (C) The ear of wild type. (D) Multiple elongated ears of *opr7 opr8*.(E) Anthocyanins accumulation in the brace roots of wildtype. (F) Lack anthocyanins pigmentation of *opr7 opr8* brace roots. (G) The senescence phenotype of third leaves of wild type (left) and *opr7 opr8* (right). (H) & (I) *opr7 opr8* (right) is highly susceptible to *Pythium aristosporum* compared with wild type (left).

5. Conclusion

Our understanding of the biosynthesis, regulation, and signaling mechanisms of jasmonates has increased substantially in the last few years. JA biosynthesis enzymes showed 'self-activation', in which the final product, JA, positively regulate the enzyme activity of this pathway. Currently, only (+)-7-iso-jasmonoyl-L-Ile has been conclusively shown to function as the bioactive ligand to JA signaling machinery SCF^{COI1}/JAZs complex. The molecular mechanism of JA signal perception and transduction was found to mimic many aspects of the auxin signaling process. In the presence of low levels of JA, JAZ proteins repress the expression of JA-responsive genes by interacting directly with the bHLH (basic helix-loop-helix) transcription factors MYC2, MYC3, and MYC4, which are positive regulators of JA responses. When JA levels increased, the bioactive form of ligand JA-Ile promotes binding of JAZs to SCF^{COI1} to form SCF^{COI1}-JAZ-JA-Ile reception complex and subsequent degradation of JAZ repressors via the ubiquitin/26S proteasome pathway, resulting in derepression of primary response genes. A number of recent studies found a wide spectrum of JA functions in plant including the regulation of developmental and defense processes, such as, resistance against insects and pathogens, root growth, fruit/seed maturation, leaf senescence, anthocyanin pigmentation, sex determination (of monoecious plant), female or reproductive organ formation.

Author details

Yuanxin Yan, Eli Borrego and Michael V. Kolomiets
Department of Plant Pathology and Microbiology, Texas A&M University, College Station, Texas, USA

Acknowledgement

This work was supported by the NSF grants IOS-0925561 and IOS-0951272 to Dr. Michael Kolomiets.

6. References

Abel S, Oeller PW, and Theologis A (1994) Early auxin-induced genes encode short-lived nuclear proteins. Proc Natl Acad Sci U S A 91:326–330.

Acosta IF, Laparra H, Romero SP, Schmelz E, Hamberg M, Mottinger JP, Moreno MA, and Dellaporta SL (2009) tasselseed1 is a lipoxygenase affecting jasmonic acid signaling in sex determination of maize. Science 323:262-265.

Adie BA, Perez-Perez J, Perez-Perez MM, Godoy M, Sanchez-Serrano JJ, Schmelz EA, and Solano R (2007) ABA is an essential signal for plant resistance to pathogens affecting JA biosynthesis and the activation of defenses in Arabidopsis. Plant Cell 19:1665-1681.

Agrawal GK, Tamogami S, Han O, Iwahashi H, and Rakwal R (2004) Rice octadecanoid pathway. Biochem Biophys Res Commun 317:1-15.

Anderson JP, Badruzsaufari E, Schenk PM, Manners JM, Desmond OJ, Ehlert C, Maclean DJ, Ebert PR, and Kazan K (2004) Antagonistic interaction between abscisic acid and jasmonate-ethylene signaling pathways modulates defense gene expression and disease resistance in Arabidopsis. Plant Cell 16:3460-3479.

Andersson MX, Hamberg M, Kourtchenko O, Brunnstrom A, McPhail KL, Gerwick WH, Gobel C, Feussner I, and Ellerstrom M (2006) Oxylipin profiling of the hypersensitive response in Arabidopsis thaliana. Formation of a novel oxo-phytodienoic acid-containing galactolipid, arabidopside E. J Biol Chem 281:31528-31537.

Andreou A, Brodhun F, and Feussner I (2009) Biosynthesis of oxylipins in non-mammals. Prog Lipid Res 48:148-170.

Antico CJ (2012) Insights into the role of jasmonic acid-mediated defenses against necrotrophic and biotrophic fungal pathogens. Frontiers in Biology 7:48.

Avanci NC, Luche DD, Goldman GH, and Goldman MH (2010) Jasmonates are phytohormones with multiple functions, including plant defense and reproduction. Genet Mol Res 9:484-505.

Avdiushko SA, Brown GC, Dahlman DL, and Hildebrand DF (1997) Methyl jasmonate exposure induces insect resistance in cabbage and tobacco. Environmental Entomology 26:642-654.

Bannenberg G, Martinez M, Hamberg M, and Castresana C (2009) Diversity of the enzymatic activity in the lipoxygenase gene family of Arabidopsis thaliana. Lipids 44:85-95.

Bar-Nun N, Sachs T, andMayer AM (2008) A role for IAA in the infection of Arabidopsis thaliana by Orobanche aegyptiaca Ann Bot 101:261-265.

Beckers GJ, and Spoel SH (2006) Fine-tuning plant defence signalling: salicylate versus jasmonate. Plant Biol (Stuttg) 8:1-10.

Bell E, Creelman RA, and Mullet JE (1995) A chloroplast lipoxygenase is required for wound-induced jasmonic acid accumulation in Arabidopsis. Proc Natl Acad Sci U S A 92:8675-8679.

Berger S, Bell E, and Mullet JE (1996) Two methyl jasmonate-insensitive mutants show altered expression of AtVsp in response to methyl jasmonate and wounding. Plant Physiology 111:525-531.

Bhattarai KK, Xie QG, Mantelin S, Bishnoi U, Girke T, Navarre DA, and Kaloshian I (2008) Tomato susceptibility to root-knot nematodes requires an intact jasmonic acid signaling pathway. Mol Plant Microbe Interact 21:1205-1214.

Blechert S, Brodschelm W, Holder S, Kammerer L, Kutchan TM, Mueller MJ, Xia ZQ, and Zenk MH (1995) The octadecanoic pathway: signal molecules for the regulation of secondary pathways. Proc Natl Acad Sci U S A 92:4099-4105.

Bolter CJ (1993) Methyl Jasmonate Induces Papain Inhibitor(s) in Tomato Leaves. Plant Physiol 103:1347-1353.

Bonaventure G, Gfeller A, Proebsting WM, Hortensteiner S, Chetelat A, Martinoia E, and Farmer EE (2007) A gain-of-function allele of TPC1 activates oxylipin biogenesis after leaf wounding in Arabidopsis. Plant J 49:889-898.

Bortiri E, and Hake S (2007) Flowering and determinacy in maize. J Exp Bot 58:909-916.

Brader G, Tas E, Palva ET (2001) Jasmonate-dependent induction of indole glucosinolates in arabidopsis by culture filtrates of the nonspecific pathogenerwinia carotovora. Plant Physiology 126:849-860.

Breithaupt C, Kurzbauer R, Schaller F, Stintzi A, Schaller A, Huber R, Macheroux P, and Clausen T (2009) Structural basis of substrate specificity of plant 12-oxophytodienoate reductases. J Mol Biol 392:1266-1277.

Brown RL, Kazan K, McGrath KC, Maclean DJ, and Manners JM (2003) A role for the GCC-box in jasmonate-mediated activation of the *PDF1.2* gene of Arabidopsis. Plant Physiol 132:1020-1032.

Browse J (2005) Jasmonate: an oxylipin signal with many roles in plants. Vitam Horm 72: 431-456.

Browse J (2009) Jasmonate passes muster: a receptor and targets for the defense hormone. Annu Rev Plant Biol 60:183-205.

Browse J (2009) The power of mutants for investigating jasmonate biosynthesis and signaling. Phytochemistry 70:1539-1546.

Browse J, and Howe GA (2008) New weapons and a rapid response against insect attack. Plant Physiol 146:832-838.

Buseman CM, Tamura P, Sparks AA, Baughman EJ, Maatta S, Zhao J, Roth MR, Esch SW, Shah J, Williams TD, and Welti R (2006) Wounding stimulates the accumulation of glycerolipids containing oxophytodienoic acid and dinor-oxophytodienoic acid in Arabidopsis leaves. Plant Physiol 142:28-39.

Caldelari D, Wang G, Farmer EE, and Dong X (2011) Arabidopsis lox3 lox4 double mutants are male sterile and defective in global proliferative arrest. Plant Mol Biol 75:25-33.

Castillo MC, Martínez C, Buchala A, Métraux JP, León J (2004) Gene-specific involvement of β-oxidation in wound-activated responses in Arabidopsis. Plant physiology 135:85-94.

Castillo MC, León J (2008) Expression of the β-oxidation gene 3-ketoacyl-CoA thiolase 2 (KAT2) is required for the timely onset of natural and dark-induced leaf senescence in Arabidopsis. Journal of Experimental Botany 59:2171-2179.

Chen H, Jones AD, and Howe GA (2006) Constitutive activation of the jasmonate signaling pathway enhances the production of secondary metabolites in tomato. FEBS Lett 580:2540-2546.

Cheng H, Song S, Xiao L, Soo HM, Cheng Z, Xie D, and Peng J (2009) Gibberellin acts through jasmonate to control the expression of *MYB21*, *MYB24*, and *MYB57* to promote stamen filament growth in Arabidopsis. PLoS Genet 5:e1000440.

Cheng Z, Sun L, Qi T, Zhang B, Peng W, Liu Y, and Xie D (2011) The bHLH transcription factor MYC3 interacts with the Jasmonate ZIM-domain proteins to mediate jasmonate response in Arabidopsis. Mol Plant 4:279-288.

Cheong JJ, and Choi YD (2003) Methyl jasmonate as a vital substance in plants. Trends in genetics 19:409-413.

Chini A, Fonseca S, Chico JM, Fernández-Calvo P, and Solano R (2009) The ZIM domain mediates homo - and heteromeric interactions between Arabidopsis JAZ proteins. Plant J 59:77.

Chini A, Fonseca S, Fernandez G, Adie B, Chico JM, Lorenzo O, Garcia-Casado G, Lopez-Vidriero I, Lozano FM, Ponce MR, Micol JL, and Solano R (2007) The JAZ family of repressors is the missing link in jasmonate signalling. Nature 448:666-671.

Christensen, SA (2009) The function of the lipoxygenase ZmLOX10 in maize interactions with insects and pathogens. Doctoral dissertation, Texas A&M University. Available electronically from http : / /hdl .handle .net /1969 .1 /ETD -TAMU -2009 -12 -7459

Chow B, and McCourt P (2006) Plant hormone receptors: perception is everything. Genes Dev 20:1998-2008.

Chuck G (2010) Molecular mechanisms of sex determination in monoecious and dioecious plants. Advances in Botanical Research. K. Jean-Claude and D. Michel. Academic Press. Volume 54: 53-83.

Chung HS, and Howe GA (2009) A critical role for the TIFY motif in repression of jasmonate signaling by a stabilized splice variant of the JASMONATE ZIM-domain protein JAZ10 in Arabidopsis. Plant Cell 21:131-145.

Chung HS, Koo AJ, Gao X, Jayanty S, Thines B, Jones AD, and Howe GA (2008) Regulation and function of Arabidopsis JASMONATE ZIM-domain genes in response to wounding and herbivory. Plant Physiol 146:952-964.

Conconi A, Miquel M, Browse JA, and Ryan CA (1996) Intracellular levels of free linolenic and linoleic acids increase in tomato leaves in response to wounding. Plant Physiol 111:797-803.

Cooper WR, Jia L, and Goggin L (2005)Effects of jasmonate-induced defenses on root-knot nematode infection of resistant and susceptible tomato cultivars. J Chem Ecol 31:1953-1967.

Creelman RA, and Mullet JE (1995) Jasmonic acid distribution and action in plants: regulation during development and response to biotic and abiotic stress. Proc Natl Acad Sci U S A 92:4114-4119.

Creelman RA, and Mullet JE (1997) Biosynthesis and Action of Jasmonates in Plants. Annu Rev Plant Physiol Plant Mol Biol 48:355-381.

Dathe W (1981) Endogenous plant hormones of the broad bean, Vicia faba L.(-)-jasmonic acid, a plant growth inhibitor in pericarp. Planta 153:530.

De Geyter N, Gholami A, Goormachtig S, and Goossens A (2012) Transcriptional machineries in jasmonate-elicited plant secondary metabolism. Trends Plant Sci 17:349-359.

Delker C, Stenzel I, Hause B, Miersch O, Feussner I, and Wasternack C (2006) Jasmonate biosynthesis in Arabidopsis thaliana--enzymes, products, regulation. Plant Biol (Stuttg) 8:297-306.

Delker C, Zolman BK, Miersch O, and Wasternack C (2007) Jasmonate biosynthesis in Arabidopsis thaliana requires peroxisomal beta-oxidation enzymes--additional proof by properties of pex6 and aim1. Phytochemistry 68:1642-1650.

Demole E, Lederer E, and Mercier D (1962) Isolement et détermination de la structure du jasmonate de méthyle, constituant odorant charactéristique de l'essence de jasmin. Helvetica Chimica Acta 45:675-685.

Dong X (1998) SA, JA, ethylene, and disease resistance in plants. Curr Opin Plant Biol 1:316-323.

Doughty KJ, Kiddle GA, Pye BJ, Wallsgrove RM, and Pickett JA (1995) Selective induction of glucosinolates in oilseed rape leaves by methyl jasmonate Phytochem 38:347-350.

Eckardt NA (2008) Oxylipin signaling in plant stress responses. Plant Cell 20:495-497.

Ellinger D, Stingl N, Kubigsteltig II, Bals T, Juenger M, Pollmann S, Berger S, Schuenemann D, and Mueller MJ (2010) DONGLE and DEFECTIVE IN ANTHER DEHISCENCE1 lipases are not essential for wound-and pathogen-induced jasmonate biosynthesis: redundant lipases contribute to jasmonate formation. Plant Physiol 153:114.

Ellis C, and Turner JG (2001) The Arabidopsis mutant cev1 has constitutively active jasmonate and ethylene signal pathways and enhanced resistance to pathogens. Plant Cell 13:1025-1033.

Engelberth J, Alborn HT, Schmelz EA, and Tumlinson JH (2004) Airborne signals prime plants against insect herbivore attack. Proc Natl Acad Sci U S A 101:1781-1785.

Farag MA, and Paré PW (2002) C-6 Green leaf volatiles trigger local and systemic VOC emissions in tomato. Phytochemistry 61:545-554.

Farmer EE, Almeras E, and Krishnamurthy V (2003) Jasmonates and related oxylipins in plant responses to pathogenesis and herbivory. Curr Opin Plant Biol 6:372-378.

Farmer EE, Johnson RR, and Ryan CA (1992) Regulation of expression of proteinase inhibitor genes by methyl jasmonate and jasmonic Acid. Plant Physiol 98:995-1002.

Felton GW, Tumlinson JH (2008) Plant–insect dialogs: complex interactions at the plant–insect interface. Curr Opin Plant Biol 11:457-463.

Fernandez-Calvo P, Chini A, Fernandez-Barbero G, Chico JM, Gimenez-Ibanez S, Geerinck J, Eeckhout D, Schweizer F, Godoy M, Franco-Zorrilla JM, Pauwels L, Witters E, Puga MI, Paz-Ares J, Goossens A, Reymond P, De Jaeger G, and Solano R (2011) The Arabidopsis bHLH transcription factors MYC3 and MYC4 are targets of JAZ repressors and act additively with MYC2 in the activation of jasmonate responses. Plant Cell 23:701-715.

Feussner I, and Wasternack C (2002) The lipoxygenase pathway. Annu Rev Plant Biol 53:275-297.

Fons F, Froissard D, Bessière JM, Buatois B, and Rapior S (2010) Biodiversity of volatile organic compounds from five French ferns. Nat Prod Commun 5:1655-1658.

Fonseca S, Chini A, Hamberg M, Adie B, Porzel A, Kramell R, Miersch O, Wasternack C, Solano R (2009) (+)-7-iso-Jasmonoyl-L-isoleucine is the endogenous bioactive jasmonate. Nat Chem Biol 5: 344-350.

Footitt S, Slocombe SP, Larner V, Kurup S, Wu Y, Larson T, Graham I, Baker A, and Holdsworth M (2002) Control of germination and lipid mobilization by COMATOSE, the Arabidopsis homologue of human ALDP. EMBO J 21:2912-2922.

Franceschi VR, and Grimes HD (1991) induction of soybean vegetative storage proteins and anthocyanins by low-level atmospheric methyl jasmonate. Proc Natl Acad Sci U S A 88:6745-6749.

Fu ZQ, Yan S, Saleh A, Wang W, Ruble J, Oka N, Mohan R, Spoel SH, Tada Y, Zheng N, and Dong X (2012) NPR3 and NPR4 are receptors for the immune signal salicylic acid in plants. Nature 486:228-232.

Garbe LA, Barbosa de Almeida R, Nagel R, Wackerbauer K, and Tressl R (2006) Dual positional and stereospecificity of lipoxygenase isoenzymes from germinating barley (green malt): biotransformation of free and esterified linoleic acid. J Agric Food Chem 54:946-955.

Gfeller A, Dubugnon L, Liechti R, and Farmer EE (2010) Jasmonate Biochemical Pathway. Sci Signal 3:cm3.

Glauser G, Grata E, Dubugnon L, Rudaz S, Farmer EE, and Wolfender JL (2008) Spatial and temporal dynamics of jasmonate synthesis and accumulation in Arabidopsis in response to wounding. J Biol Chem 283:16400-16407.

Glazebrook J (2005) Contrasting mechanisms of defense against biotrophic and necrotrophic pathogens. Annu Rev Phytopathol 43:205-227.

Göbel C, and Feussner I (2009) Methods for the analysis of oxylipins in plants. Phytochemistry 70:1485-1503.

Gray WM, Kepinski S, Rouse D, Leyser O, and Estelle M (2001) Auxin regulates SCF^{TIR1}-dependent degradation of AUX/IAA proteins. Nature 414:271-276.

Gundlach H, and Zenk MH (1998) Biological activity and biosynthesis of pentacyclic oxylipins: The linoleic acid pathway. Phytochemistry 47:527-537.

Ha SB, Lee BC, Lee DE, Kuk YI, Lee AY, Han O, and Back K (2002) Molecular characterization of the gene encoding rice allene oxide synthase and its expression. Biosci Biotechnol Biochem 66:2719-2722.

Hamberg M, and Hughes MA (1988) Fatty acid allene oxides. III. Albumin-induced cyclization of 12,13(S)-epoxy-9(Z), 11-octadecadienoic acid. Lipids 23:469-475.

Harms K, Atzorn R, Brash A, Kuhn H, Wasternack C, Willmitzer L, Pena-Cortes H (1995) Expression of a flax allene oxide synthase cDNA leads to increased endogenous jasmonic acid (JA) levels in transgenic potato plants but not to a corresponding activation of JA-responding genes. Plant Cell 7:1645-1654.

Hayashi M, Nito K, Takei-Hoshi R, Yagi M, Kondo M, Suenaga A, Yamaya T, and Nishimura M (2002) Ped3p is a peroxisomal ATP-binding cassette transporter that might supply substrates for fatty acid beta-oxidation. Plant Cell Physiol 43: 1-11.

He Y, Fukushige H, Hildebrand DF, and Gan S (2002) Evidence supporting a role of jasmonic acid in Arabidopsis leaf senescence. Plant Physiol 128:876-884.

Heim MA, Jakoby M, Werber M, Martin C, Weisshaar B, and Bailey PC (2003) The basic helix-loop-helix transcription factor family in plants: a genome-wide study of protein structure and functional diversity. Mol Biol Evol. 20:735-747.

Hisamatsu Y (2005) Oxylipin arabidopsides C and D from *Arabidopsis t haliana*. Journal of Natural Products 68:600.

Hisamatsu Y, Goto N, Hasegawa K, and Shigemori H (2003) Arabidopsides A and B, two new oxylipins from Arabidopsis thaliana. Tetrahedron letters 44:5553-5556.

Hou X, Lee LY, Xia K, Yan Y, and Yu H (2010) DELLAs modulate jasmonate signaling via competitive binding to JAZs. Dev Cell 19:884-894.

Howe GA, and Jander G (2008) Plant immunity to insect herbivores. Annu Rev Plant Biol 59:41-66.

Howe GA, Lee GI, Itoh A, Li L, and DeRocher AE (2000) Cytochrome P450-dependent metabolism of oxylipins in tomato. Cloning and expression of allene oxide synthase and fatty acid hydroperoxide lyase. Plant Physiol 123:711-724.

Hughes RK, Lawson DM, Hornostaj AR, Fairhurst SA, and Casey R (2001) Mutagenesis and modelling of linoleate-binding to pea seed lipoxygenase. Eur J Biochem 268:1030-1040.

Hyun Y, Choi S, Hwang HJ, Yu J, Nam SJ, Ko J, Park JY, Seo YS, Kim EY, Ryu SB, Kim WT, Lee YH, Kang H, and Lee I (2008) Cooperation and functional diversification of two closely related galactolipase genes for jasmonate biosynthesis. Dev Cell 14:183-192.

Ishida T, Kurata T, Okada K, and Wada T (2008) A genetic regulatory network in the development of trichomes and root hairs. Annu Rev Plant Biol 59:365-386.

Ishiguro S, Kawai-Oda A, Ueda J, Nishida I, and Okada K (2001) The *DEFECTIVE IN ANTHER DEHISCENCE1* gene encodes a novel phospholipase A1 catalyzing the initial step of jasmonic acid biosynthesis, which synchronizes pollen maturation, anther dehiscence, and flower opening in Arabidopsis. Plant Cell 13:2191-2209.

Ismail A, Riemann M, and Nick P (2012) The jasmonate pathway mediates salt tolerance in grapevines. J Exp Bot 63:2127-2139.

Katsir L, Schilmiller AL, Staswick PE, He SY, and Howe GA (2008) COI1 is a critical component of a receptor for jasmonate and the bacterial virulence factor coronatine. Proc Natl Acad Sci U S A 105:7100-7105.

Kepinski S, and Leyser O (2005) The Arabidopsis F-box protein TIR1 is an auxin receptor. Nature 435:446-451.

Kim ES, Kim H, Park RD, Lee Y, and Han O (2002) Dual positional specificity of wound-responsive lipoxygenase from maize seedlings. Journal of Plant Physiology 159:1263-1265.

Kohli RM, and Massey V (1998) The oxidative half-reaction of Old Yellow Enzyme. The role of tyrosine 196. J Biol Chem 273:32763-32770.

Kondo S, Tomiyama A, and Seto H (2000) Changes of endogenous jasmonic acid and methyl jasmonate in apples and sweet cherries during fruit development. Journal of the American Society for Horticultural Science 125:282-287.

Koo AJ, Chung HS, Kobayashi Y, and Howe GA (2006) Identification of a peroxisomal acyl-activating enzyme involved in the biosynthesis of jasmonic acid in Arabidopsis. J Biol Chem 281:33511-33520.

Kourtchenko O, Andersson MX, Hamberg M, Brunnstrom A, Gobel C, McPhail KL, Gerwick WH, Feussner I, and Ellerstrom M (2007) Oxo-phytodienoic acid-containing galactolipids in Arabidopsis: jasmonate signaling dependence. Plant Physiol 145:1658-1669.

Kunkel BN, and Brooks DM (2002) Cross talk between signaling pathways in pathogen defense. Curr Opin Plant Biol 5:325-331.

Laudert D, Pfannschmidt U, Lottspeich F, Hollander-Czytko H, and Weiler EW (1996) Cloning, molecular and functional characterization of Arabidopsis thaliana allene oxide synthase (CYP 74), the first enzyme of the octadecanoid pathway to jasmonates. Plant Mol Biol 31:323-335.

Laudert D, Schaller F, and Weiler EW (2000) Transgenic Nicotiana tabacum and Arabidopsis thaliana plants overexpressing allene oxide synthase. Planta 211:163-165.

Laudert D, and Weiler EW (1998) Allene oxide synthase: a major control point in Arabidopsis thaliana octadecanoid signalling. Plant J 15:675-684.

Leon J, and Sanchez-Serrano JJ (1999) Molecular biology of jasmonic acid biosynthesis in plants. Plant Physiol and Biochem 37:373-380.

Li C, Schilmiller AL, Liu G, Lee GI, Jayanty S, Sageman C, Vrebalov J, Giovannoni JJ, Yagi K, Kobayashi Y, and Howe GA (2005) Role of ß-oxidation in jasmonate biosynthesis and systemic wound signaling in tomato. Plant Cell 17:971.

Li J, Brader G, and Palva ET (2004) The WRKY70 transcription factor: a node of convergence for jasmonate-mediated and salicylate-mediated signals in plant defense. Plant Cell 16:319-331.

Li L, Zhao Y, McCaig BC, Wingerd BA, Wang J, Whalon ME, Pichersky E, Howe GA (2004) The tomato homolog of CORONATINE-INSENSITIVE1 is required for the maternal control of seed maturation, jasmonate-signaled defense responses, and glandular trichome development. Plant Cell 16:126-143.

Lim PO, Kim HJ, and Nam HG (2007) Leaf senescence. Annu Rev Plant Biol 58:115-136.

Liu YL, Ahn JE, Datta S, Salzman RA, Moon J, Huyghues-Despointes B, Pittendrigh B, Murdock LL, Koiwa H, and Zhu-Salzman K (2005) Arabidopsis vegetative storage protein is an anti-insect acid phosphatase. Plant Physiol 139:1545-1556.

Lorenzo O, Chico JM, Sanchez-Serrano JJ, and Solano R (2004) JASMONATE-INSENSITIVE1 encodes a MYC transcription factor essential to discriminate between different jasmonate-regulated defense responses in Arabidopsis. Plant Cell 16:1938-1950.

Lorenzo O, Piqueras R, Sanchez-Serrano JJ, and Solano R (2003) ETHYLENE RESPONSE FACTOR1 integrates signals from ethylene and jasmonate pathways in plant defense. Plant Cell 15:165-178.

Lorenzo O, and Solano R (2005) Molecular players regulating the jasmonate signalling network. Curr Opin Plant Biol 8:532-540.

Lozano-Duran R, Rosas-Diaz T, Gusmaroli G, Luna AP, Taconnat L, Deng XW, and Bejarano ER (2011) Geminiviruses subvert ubiquitination by altering CSN-mediated derubylation of SCF E3 ligase complexes and inhibit jasmonate signaling in Arabidopsis thaliana. Plant Cell 23:1014-1032.

Lumba S, Cutler S, and McCourt P (2010) Plant nuclear hormone receptors: a role for small molecules in protein-protein interactions. Annu Rev Cell Dev Biol 26:445-469.

Maes L, Inze D, and Goossens A (2008) Functional specialization of the TRANSPARENT TESTA GLABRA1 network allows differential hormonal control of laminal and marginal trichome initiation in Arabidopsis rosette leaves. Plant Physiol 148:1453-1464.

Mandaokar A, Thines B, Shin B, Lange BM, Choi G, Koo YJ, Yoo YJ, Choi YD, Choi G, and Browse J (2006) Transcriptional regulators of stamen development in Arabidopsis identified by transcriptional profiling. Plant J 46:984-1008.

Masterson C, and Wood C (2001) Mitochondrial and peroxisomal beta-oxidation capacities of organs from a non-oilseed plant. Proc Biol Sci 268:1949-1953.

Matsui H, Nakamura G, Ishiga Y, Toshima H, Inagaki Y, Toyoda K, Shiraishi T, and Ichinose Y (2004) Structure and expression of 12-oxophytodienoate reductase (subgroup I) genes in pea, and characterization of the oxidoreductase activities of their recombinant products. Molecular Genetics and Genomics 271:1-10.

Maucher H, Hause B, Feussner I, Ziegler J, and Wasternack C (2000) Allene oxide synthases of barley (Hordeum vulgare cv. Salome): tissue specific regulation in seedling development. Plant J 21:199-213.

Maucher H, Stenzel I, Miersch O, Stein N, Prasad M, Zierold U, Schweizer P, Dorer C, Hause B, and Wasternack C (2004) The allene oxide cyclase of barley (Hordeum vulgare L.)--cloning and organ-specific expression. Phytochemistry 65:801-811.

McConn M, Creelman RA, Bell E, Mullet JE, Browse J (1997) Jasmonate is essential for insect defense in Arabidopsis. Proc Natl Acad Sci U S A 94:5473-5477.

McGrath KC, Dombrecht B, Manners JM, Schenk PM, Edgar CI, Maclean DJ, Scheible WR, Udvardi MK, and Kazan K (2005) Repressor- and activator-type ethylene response factors functioning in jasmonate signaling and disease resistance identified via a genome-wide screen of Arabidopsis transcription factor gene expression. Plant Physiol 139:949-959.

Miersch O, Porzel A, and Wasternack C (1999) Microbial conversion of jasmonates-hydroxylations by Aspergillus niger. Phytochemistry 50:1147-1152.

Moalem-Beno D, Tamari G, Leitner-Dagan Y, Borochov A, and Weiss D (1997) Sugar-dependent gibberellin-induced chalcone synthase gene expression in Petunia corollas. Plant Physiol 113:419-424.

Mueller MJ (1997) Enzymes involved in jasmonic acid biosynthesis. Physiologia Plantarum 100:653-663.

Müller C (2001) Host Finding and Oviposition Behavior in a Chrysomelid Specialist--the Importance of Host Plant Surface Waxes. Journal of Chemical Ecology 27:985.

Munemasa S, Oda K, Watanabe-Sugimoto M, Nakamura Y, Shimoishi Y, and Murata Y (2007) The coronatine-insensitive 1 mutation reveals the hormonal signaling interaction between abscisic acid and methyl jasmonate in arabidopsis guard cells. Specific impairment of ion channel activation and second messenger production. Plant Physiol 143:1398-1407.

Mur LAJ, Kenton P, Atzorn R, Miersch O, and Wasternack C (2006) The outcomes of concentration-specific interactions between salicylate and jasmonate signaling include synergy, antagonism, and oxidative stress leading to cell death. Plant Physiol 140:249-262.

Nagpal P, Ellis CM, Weber H, Ploense SE, Barkawi LS, Guilfoyle TJ, Hagen G, Alonso JM, Cohen JD, Farmer EE, Ecker JR, and Reed JW (2005) Auxin response factors ARF6 and ARF8 promote jasmonic acid production and flower maturation. Development 132:4107-4118.

Nakano T, Suzuki K, Fujimura T, and Shinshi H (2006) Genome-wide analysis of the ERF gene family in Arabidopsis and rice. Plant Physiol 140:411-432.

Nemchenko A, Kunze S, Feussner I, and Kolomiets M (2006) Duplicate maize 13-lipoxygenase genes are differentially regulated by circadian rhythm, cold stress, wounding, pathogen infection, and hormonal treatments. J Exp Bot 57: 3767–3779.

Niu YJ, Figueroa P, and Browse J (2011) Characterization of JAZ-interacting bHLH transcription factors that regulate jasmonate responses in Arabidopsis. Journal of Experimental Botany 62:2143-2154.

Ohya H, Ogata A, Nakamura K, Chung KM, and Sano H (2008) A stress-responsive multifunctional protein involved in beta-oxidation in tobacco plants. Plant Biotechnology 25:503-508.

Oñate-Sánchez L, Anderson JP, Young J, Singh KB (2007) AtERF14, a member of the ERF family of transcription factors, plays a nonredundant role in plant defense. Plant Physiol 143:400-409.

Pan ZQ, Durst F, Werckreichhart D, Gardner HW, Camara B, Cornish K, and Backhaus RA (1995) The major protein of guayule rubber particles is a cytochrome-p450 - characterization based on cdna cloning and spectroscopic analysis of the solubilized enzyme and its reaction-products. Journal of Biological Chemistry 270:8487-8494.

Paré PW, and Tumlinson JH (1999) Plant volatiles as a defense against insect herbivores. Plant physiology 121:325-331.

Park JH, Halitschke R, Kim HB, Baldwin IT, Feldmann KA, and Feyereisen R (2002) A knock-out mutation in allene oxide synthase results in male sterility and defective wound signal transduction in Arabidopsis due to a block in jasmonic acid biosynthesis. Plant J 31:1-12.

Pauwels L, Barbero GF, Geerinck J, Tilleman S, Grunewald W, Pérez AC, Chico JM, Bossche RV, Sewell J, Gil E, García-Casado G, Witters E, Inzé D, Long JA, De Jaeger G, Solano R, and Goossens A (2010) NINJA connects the co-repressor TOPLESS to jasmonate signalling. Nature 464:788-791.

Pauwels L, and Goossens A (2011) The JAZ proteins: a crucial interface in the jasmonate signaling cascade. Plant Cell 23:3089-3100.

Penninckx IAMA, Thomma BPHJ, Buchala A, Metraux JP, and Broekaert WF (1998) Concomitant activation of jasmonate and ethylene response pathways is required for induction of a plant defensin gene in Arabidopsis. Plant Cell 10:2103-2113.

Perazza D, Vachon G, and Herzog M (1998) Gibberellins promote trichome formation by up-regulating *GLABROUS1* in Arabidopsis. Plant Physiol 117:375-383.

Petersen M, Brodersen P, Naested H, Andreasson E, Lindhart U, Johansen B, Nielsen HB, Lacy M, Austin MJ, Parker JE, Sharma SB, Klessig DF, Martienssen R, Mattsson O, Jensen AB, and Mundy J (2000) Arabidopsis MAP Kinase 4 negatively regulates systemic acquired resistance. Cell 103:1111-1120.

Pieterse CM, van Wees SC, van Pelt JA, Knoester M, Laan R, Gerrits H, Weisbeek PJ, and van Loon LC (1998) A novel signaling pathway controlling induced systemic resistance in Arabidopsis. Plant Cell 10:1571-1580.

Plett JM, Mathur J, and Regan S (2009) Ethylene receptor ETR2 controls trichome branching by regulating microtubule assembly in Arabidopsis thaliana. J Exp Bot 60:3923-3933.

Porta H, and Rocha-Sosa M (2002) Plant lipoxygenases. Physiological and molecular features. Plant Physiol 130:15-21.

Pré M, Atallah M, Champion A, De Vos M, Pieterse CM, and Memelink J (2008) The AP2/ERF domain transcription factor ORA59 integrates jasmonic acid and ethylene signals in plant defense. Plant Physiol 147:1347-1357.

Qi T, Song S, Ren Q, Wu D, Huang H, Chen Y, Fan M, Peng W, Ren C, and Xie D (2011) The Jasmonate-ZIM-domain proteins interact with the WD-Repeat/bHLH/MYB complexes to regulate Jasmonate-mediated anthocyanin accumulation and trichome initiation in Arabidopsis thaliana. Plant Cell 23:1795-1814

Quina FH, Moreira PF, Vautier-Giongo C, Rettori D, Rodrigues RF, Freitas AA, Silva PF, and Macanita AL (2009) Photochemistry of anthocyanins and their biological role in plant tissues. Pure and Applied Chemistry 81:1687-1694.

Raghavendra AS, Gonugunta VK, Christmann A, and Grill E (2010) ABA perception and signalling. Trends Plant Sci 15:395-401.

Rao MV, Lee H, Creelman RA, Mullet JE, and Davis KR (2000) Jasmonic acid signaling modulates ozone-induced hypersensitive cell death. Plant Cell 12:1633-1646.

Reymond P, Bodenhausen N, Van Poecke RM, Krishnamurthy V, Dicke M, and Farmer EE (2004) A conserved transcript pattern in response to a specialist and a generalist herbivore. Plant Cell 16:3132-3147.

Riemann M, Muller A, Korte A, Furuya M, Weiler EW, and Nick P (2003) Impaired induction of the jasmonate pathway in the rice mutant hebiba. Plant Physiol 133:1820-1830.

Rowe HC, Walley JW, Corwin J, Chan EK, Dehesh K, and Kliebenstein DJ (2010) Deficiencies in jasmonate-mediated plant defense reveal quantitative variation in Botrytis cinerea pathogenesis. PLoS Pathog 6:e1000861.

Runyon JB, Mescher MC, and De Moraes CM (2010) Plant defenses against parasitic plants show similarities to those induced by herbivores and pathogens. Plant signaling & behavior 5:929.

Rylott EL, Rogers CA, Gilday AD, Edgell T, Larson TR, and Graham IA (2003) Arabidopsis mutants in short- and medium-chain acyl-CoA oxidase activities accumulate acyl-CoAs and reveal that fatty acid beta-oxidation is essential for embryo development. J Biol Chem 278:21370-21377.

Ryu SB (2004) Phospholipid-derived signaling mediated by phospholipase A in plants. Trends Plant Sci 9:229-235.

Sanders PM, Lee PY, Biesgen C, Boone JD, Beals TP, Weiler EW, and Goldberg RB (2000) The arabidopsis *DELAYED DEHISCENCE1* gene encodes an enzyme in the jasmonic acid synthesis pathway. Plant Cell 12:1041-1061.

Sano H, Seo S, Koizumi N, Niki T, Iwamura H, and Ohashi Y (1996) Regulation by cytokinins of endogenous levels of jasmonic and salicylic acids in mechanically wounded tobacco plants. Plant and Cell Physiology 37:762-769.

Sasaki Y, Asamizu E, Shibata D, Nakamura Y, Kaneko T, Awai K, Amagai M, Kuwata C, Tsugane T, Masuda T, Shimada H, Takamiya K, Ohta H, and Tabata S (2001) Monitoring of methyl jasmonate-responsive genes in Arabidopsis by cDNA macroarray: self-activation of jasmonic acid biosynthesis and crosstalk with other phytohormone signaling pathways. DNA Res 8:153-161.

Schaller A, and Stintzi A (2009) Enzymes in jasmonate biosynthesis - structure, function, regulation. Phytochemistry 70:1532-1538.

Schaller F (2001) Enzymes of the biosynthesis of octadecanoid-derived signalling molecules. J Exp Bot 52:11-23.

Schaller F, Hennig P, and Weiler EW (1998) 12-Oxophytodienoate-10,11-reductase: occurrence of two isoenzymes of different specificity against stereoisomers of 12-oxophytodienoic acid. Plant Physiol 118:1345-1351.

Schaller F, Schaller A, and Stintzi A (2004) Biosynthesis and metabolism of jasmonates. J Plant Growth Regul 23:179-199.

Schaller F, and Weiler EW (1997) Molecular cloning and characterization of 12-oxophytodienoate reductase, an enzyme of the octadecanoid signaling pathway from Arabidopsis thaliana. Structural and functional relationship to yeast old yellow enzyme. J Biol Chem 272:28066-28072.

Schenk PM, Kazan K, Wilson I, Anderson JP, Richmond T, Somerville SC, and Manners JM (2000) Coordinated plant defense responses in Arabidopsis revealed by microarray analysis. Proc Natl Acad Sci U S A 97:11655-11660.

Schilmiller AL, Koo AJ, and Howe GA (2007) Functional diversification of acyl-coenzyme A oxidases in jasmonic acid biosynthesis and action. Plant Physiol 143:812-824.

Schneider K, Kienow L, Schmelzer E, Colby T, Bartsch M, Miersch O, Wasternack C, Kombrink E, and Stuible HP (2005) A new type of peroxisomal acyl-coenzyme A synthetase from Arabidopsis thaliana has the catalytic capacity to activate biosynthetic precursors of jasmonic acid. J Biol Chem 280:13962-13972.

Schommer C, Palatnik JF, Aggarwal P, Chetelat A, Cubas P, Farmer EE, Nath U, and Weigel D (2008) Control of jasmonate biosynthesis and senescence by miR319 targets. PLoS Biol 6:e230.

Sembdner G, and Parthier B (1993) The Biochemistry and the Physiological and Molecular Actions of Jasmonates. Annu Rev Plant Physiol and Plant Mol Biol 44:569-589.

Seo HS, Song JT, Cheong JJ, Lee YH, Lee YW, Hwang I, Lee JS, and Choi YD (2001) Jasmonic acid carboxyl methyltransferase: a key enzyme for jasmonate-regulated plant responses. Proc Natl Acad Sci U S A 98:4788-4793.

Shan X, Zhang Y, Peng W, Wang Z, and Xie D (2009) Molecular mechanism for jasmonate-induction of anthocyanin accumulation in Arabidopsis. J Exp Bot 60:3849-3860.

Shang J, Xi DH, Xu F, Wang SD, Cao S, Xu MY, Zhao PP, Wang JH, Jia SD, Zhang ZW, Yuan S, and Lin HH (2011) A broad-spectrum, efficient and nontransgenic approach to control plant viruses by application of salicylic acid and jasmonic acid. Planta 233:299-308.

Sheard LB, Tan X, Mao H, Withers J, Ben-Nissan G, Hinds TR, Kobayashi Y, Hsu FF, Sharon M, Browse J, He SY, Rizo J, Howe GA, and Zheng N (2010) Jasmonate perception by inositol-phosphate-potentiated COI1-JAZ co-receptor. Nature 468:400-405.

Shin JH, Van K, Kim DH, Kim KD, Jang YE, Choi BS, Kim MY, and Lee SH (2008) The lipoxygenase gene family: a genomic fossil of shared polyploidy between Glycine max and Medicago truncatula. BMC Plant Biol 8:133.

Shockey JM, Fulda MS, and Browse J (2003) Arabidopsis contains a large superfamily of acyl-activating enzymes. Phylogenetic and biochemical analysis reveals a new class of acyl-coenzyme a synthetases. Plant Physiol 132:1065-1076.

Shoji T, and Hashimoto T (2011) Tobacco MYC2 regulates jasmonate-inducible nicotine biosynthesis genes directly and by way of the NIC2-locus ERF genes. Plant Cell Physiol 52:1117-1130.

Shoji T, Ogawa T, and Hashimoto T (2008) Jasmonate-induced nicotine formation in tobacco is mediated by tobacco COI1 and JAZ genes. Plant Cell Physiol 49:1003-1012.

Smith JL, De Moraes CM, and Mescher MC (2009) Jasmonate- and salicylate-mediated plant defense responses to insect herbivores, pathogens and parasitic plants. Pest Manag Sci 65:497-503.

Song S, Qi T, Huang H, Ren Q, Wu D, Chang C, Peng W, Liu Y, Peng J, and Xie D (2011) The Jasmonate-ZIM domain proteins interact with the R2R3-MYB transcription factors MYB21 and MYB24 to affect Jasmonate-regulated stamen development in Arabidopsis. Plant Cell 23:1000-1013.

Song WC, Funk CD, and Brash AR (1993) Molecular cloning of an allene oxide synthase: a cytochrome P450 specialized for the metabolism of fatty acid hydroperoxides. Proc Natl Acad Sci U S A 90:8519-8523.

Spartz AK, and Gray WM (2008) Plant hormone receptors: new perceptions. Genes Dev 22:2139-2148.

Spoel SH, Koornneef A, Claessens SMC, Korzelius JP, Van Pelt JA, Mueller MJ, Buchala AJ, Metraux JP, Brown R, Kazan K, Van Loon LC, Dong XN, and Pieterse CMJ (2003) NPR1 modulates cross-talk between salicylate- and jasmonate-dependent defense pathways through a novel function in the cytosol. Plant Cell 15:760-770.

Staswick PE, Su W, and Howell SH (1992) Methyl jasmonate inhibition of root growth and induction of a leaf protein are decreased in an Arabidopsis thaliana mutant. Proc Natl Acad Sci U S A 89:6837-6840.

Staswick PE, and Tiryaki I (2004) The oxylipin signal jasmonic acid is activated by an enzyme that conjugates it to isoleucine in Arabidopsis. Plant Cell 16:2117-2127.

Staswick PE, Tiryaki I, and Rowe ML (2002) Jasmonate response locus *JAR1* and several related Arabidopsis genes encode enzymes of the firefly luciferase superfamily that show activity on jasmonic, salicylic, and indole-3-acetic acids in an assay for adenylation. Plant Cell 14:1405-1415.

Staswick PE, Yuen GY, and Lehman CC (1998) Jasmonate signaling mutants of Arabidopsis are susceptible to the soil fungus Pythium irregulare. Plant J 15:747-754.

Stelmach BA, Muller A, Hennig P, Gebhardt S, Schubert-Zsilavecz M, and Weiler EW (2001) A novel class of oxylipins, sn1-O-(12-oxophytodienoyl)-sn2-O-(hexadecatrienoyl)-monogalactosyl Diglyceride, from Arabidopsis thaliana. J Biol Chem 276:12832-12838.

Stenzel I, Hause B, Miersch O, Kurz T, Maucher H, Weichert H, Ziegler J, Feussner I, and Wasternack C (2003) Jasmonate biosynthesis and the allene oxide cyclase family of *Arabidopsis thaliana*. Plant Mol Biol 51:895-911.

Stintzi A, and Browse J (2000) The Arabidopsis male-sterile mutant, opr3, lacks the 12-oxophytodienoic acid reductase required for jasmonate synthesis. Proc Natl Acad Sci U S A 97:10625-10630.

Stintzi A, Weber H, Reymond P, Browse J, and Farmer EE (2001) Plant defense in the absence of jasmonic acid: the role of cyclopentenones. Proc Natl Acad Sci U S A 98: 12837-12842.

Strassner J, Schaller F, Frick UB, Howe GA, Weiler EW, Amrhein N, Macheroux P, and Schaller A (2002) Characterization and cDNA-microarray expression analysis of 12-oxophytodienoate reductases reveals differential roles for octadecanoid biosynthesis in the local versus the systemic wound response. Plant J 32:585-601.

Stumpe M, and Feussner I (2006) Formation of oxylipins by CYP74 enzymes. Phytochem Rev 5:347-357.

Suza WP, and Staswick PE (2008) The role of JAR1 in Jasmonoyl-L: -isoleucine production during Arabidopsis wound response. Planta 227:1221-1232.

Tani T, Sobajima H, Okada K, Chujo T, Arimura S, Tsutsumi N, Nishimura M, Seto H, Nojiri H, and Yamane H (2008) Identification of the *OsOPR7* gene encoding 12-oxophytodienoate reductase involved in the biosynthesis of jasmonic acid in rice. Planta 227:517-526.

Thatcher LF, Manners JM, and Kazan K (2009) Fusarium oxysporum hijacks COI1-mediated jasmonate signaling to promote disease development in Arabidopsis. Plant J 58:927-939.

Theodoulou FL, Job K, Slocombe SP, Footitt S, Holdsworth M, Baker A, Larson TR, and Graham IA (2005) Jasmonic acid levels are reduced in COMATOSE ATP-binding cassette transporter mutants. Implications for transport of jasmonate precursors into peroxisomes. Plant Physiol 137:835.

Thines B, Katsir L, Melotto M, Niu Y, Mandaokar A, Liu G, Nomura K, He SY, Howe GA, and Browse J (2007) JAZ repressor proteins are targets of the SCF(COI1) complex during jasmonate signalling. Nature 448:661-665.

Thomma BP, Eggermont K, Penninckx IA, Mauch-Mani B, Vogelsang R, Cammue BP, and Broekaert WF (1998) Separate jasmonate-dependent and salicylate-dependent defense-response pathways in Arabidopsis are essential for resistance to distinct microbial pathogens. Proc Natl Acad Sci U S A 95:15107-15111.

Tilton GB, Shockey JM, and Browse J (2004) Biochemical and molecular characterization of ACH2, an acyl-CoA thioesterase from Arabidopsis thaliana. J Biol Chem 279:7487-7494.

Traw MB, and Bergelson J (2003) Interactive effects of jasmonic acid, salicylic acid, and gibberellin on induction of trichomes in Arabidopsis. Plant Physiol 133:1367-1375.

Turner JG, Ellis C, and Devoto A (2002) The jasmonate signal pathway. Plant Cell 14 Suppl:S153-164.

Ueda J, and Kato J (1980) Isolation and Identification of a Senescence-promoting Substance from Wormwood (Artemisia absinthium L.). Plant Physiol 66:246-249.

Umate P (2011) Genome-wide analysis of lipoxygenase gene family in Arabidopsis and rice. Plant Signal Behav 6:335-338.

Utsunomiya Y, Nakayama T, Oohira H, Hirota R, Mori T, Kawai F, and Ueda T (2000) Purification and inactivation by substrate of an allene oxide synthase (CYP74) from corn (Zea mays L.) seeds. Phytochemistry 53:319-323.

Vanholme B, Grunewald W, Bateman A, Kohchi T, and Gheysen G (2007) The tify family previously known as ZIM. Trends Plant Sci 12:239-244.

Vaz AD, Chakraborty S, and Massey V (1995) Old Yellow enzyme: aromatization of cyclic enones and the mechanism of a novel dismutation reaction. Biochemistry 34:4246-4256.

Vick BA, and Zimmerman DC (1983) The biosynthesis of jasmonic acid: a physiological role for plant lipoxygenase. Biochem Biophys Res Commun 111:470-477.

Vijayan P, Shockey J, Lévesque CA, Cook RJ, and Browse J (1998) A role for jasmonate in pathogen defense of Arabidopsis. Proc Natl Acad Sci U S A 95:7209-7214.

von Malek B, van der Graaff E, Schneitz K, and Keller B (2002) The Arabidopsis male-sterile mutant *dde2-2* is defective in the *ALLENE OXIDE SYNTHASE* gene encoding one of the key enzymes of the jasmonic acid biosynthesis pathway. Planta 216:187-192.

Wasternack C (2007) Jasmonates: an update on biosynthesis, signal transduction and action in plant stress response, growth and development. Ann Bot 100:681-697.

Weber H, Vick BA, and Farmer EE (1997) Dinor-oxo-phytodienoic acid: a new hexadecanoid signal in the jasmonate family. Proc Natl Acad Sci U S A 94:10473-10478.

Xiao S, Dai L, Liu F, Wang Z, Peng W, and Xie D (2004) COS1: an Arabidopsis coronatine insensitive1 suppressor essential for regulation of jasmonate-mediated plant defense and senescence. Plant Cell 16:1132-1142.

Xie DX, Feys BF, James S, Nieto-Rostro M, and Turner JG (1998) COI1: an Arabidopsis gene required for jasmonate-regulated defense and fertility. Science 280:1091-1094.

Xu D, Kohli RM, and Massey V (1999) The role of threonine 37 in flavin reactivity of the old yellow enzyme. Proc Natl Acad Sci U S A 96:3556-3561.

Xu LH, Liu FQ, Lechner E, Genschik P, Crosby WL, Ma H, Peng W, Huang DF, and Xie DX (2002) The SCF^{COI1} ubiquitin-ligase complexes are required for jasmonate response in Arabidopsis. Plant Cell 14:1919-1935.

Xu LH, Liu FQ, Wang ZL, Peng W, Huang RF, Huang DF, and Xie DX (2001) An Arabidopsis mutant *cex1* exhibits constant accumulation of jasmonate-regulated *AtVSP, Thi2.1* and *PDF1.2*. FEBS letters 494:161-164.

Yan J, Zhang C, Gu M, Bai Z, Zhang W, Qi T, Cheng Z, Peng W, Luo H, Nan F, Wang Z, and Xie D (2009) The Arabidopsis CORONATINE INSENSITIVE1 protein is a jasmonate receptor. Plant Cell 21:2220-2236.

Yan Y, Christensen S, Isakeit T, Engelberth J, Meeley R, Hayward A, Emery RJ, and Kolomiets MV (2012) Disruption of *OPR7* and *OPR8* reveals the versatile functions of jasmonic acid in maize development and defense. Plant Cell 24:1420-1436.

Yan Y, Stolz S, Chételat A, Reymond P, Pagni M, Dubugnon L, Farmer EE (2007) A downstream mediator in the growth repression limb of the jasmonate pathway. Plant Cell 19:2470-83.

Yoon JY, Hamayun M, Lee SK, and Lee IJ (2009) Methyl jasmonate alleviated salinity stress in soybean. Journal of Crop Science and Biotechnology 12:63.

Yoshida Y, Sano R, Wada T, Takabayashi J, and Okada K (2009) Jasmonic acid control of GLABRA3 links inducible defense and trichome patterning in Arabidopsis. Development 136:1039-1048.

Zhang J, Simmons C, Yalpani N, Crane V, Wilkinson H, and Kolomiets M (2005) Genomic analysis of the 12-oxo-phytodienoic acid reductase gene family of Zea mays. Plant Mol Biol 59:323-343.

Zhang Y, and Turner JG (2008) Wound-induced endogenous jasmonates stunt plant growth by inhibiting mitosis. Plos One 3:e3699.

Zhou N, Tootle TL, and Glazebrook J (1999) Arabidopsis *PAD3*, a gene required for camalexin biosynthesis, encodes a putative cytochrome P450 monooxygenase. Plant Cell 11:2419-2428.

Zhu Z, An F, Feng Y, Li P, Xue L, A M, Jiang Z, Kim JM, To TK, Li W, Zhang X, Yu Q, Dong Z, Chen WQ, Seki M, Zhou JM, and Guo H (2011) Derepression of ethylene-stabilized transcription factors (EIN3/EIL1) mediates jasmonate and ethylene signaling synergy in Arabidopsis. Proc Natl Acad Sci U S A 108:12539-12544.

Ziegler J, Hamberg M, Miersch O, and Parthier B (1997) Purification and Characterization of Allene Oxide Cyclase from Dry Corn Seeds. Plant Physiol 114:565-573.

Ziegler J, Stenzel I, Hause B, Maucher H, Hamberg M, Grimm R, Ganal M, and Wasternack C (2000) Molecular cloning of allene oxide cyclase. The enzyme establishing the stereochemistry of octadecanoids and jasmonates. J Biol Chem 275:19132-19138.

Ziegler J, Wasternack C, and Hamberg M (1999) On the specificity of allene oxide cyclase. Lipids 34:1005-1015.

Zolman BK, Silva ID, and Bartel B (2001) The Arabidopsis *pxa1* mutant is defective in an ATP-binding cassette transporter-like protein required for peroxisomal fatty acid beta-oxidation. Plant Physiol 127:1266-1278.

Chapter 17

The Effect of Probiotics on Lipid Metabolism

Yong Zhang and Heping Zhang

Additional information is available at the end of the chapter

http://dx.doi.org/10.5772/51938

1. Introduction

Probiotics are defined as viable microorganisms that exhibit beneficial effects on the health of the host [1]. Now, probiotics are known to possess physiological functions such as inhibition to pathogens, assisting digestion, immunoregulatory activity and antitumor activity [2]. Here, we discuss the effects of probiotic on lipid metabolism from seven main aspects including history, antioxidant effect, impact on lipoprotein, microflora view, hormones, receptors and new mechanisms.

1.1. Past and present

As early as in 1974, Mann and Spoerry observed that inhabitants from African Maasai tribes maintained a lower level of blood lipids due to a high fermented milk intake [3]. Further perspective suspected that live Lactobacilli included in fermented milk may contribute to reducing cholesterol [4]. The cholesterol-reducing effect of probiotic has become more apparent with the discovery of bile salt deconjugating and cholesterol assimilating ability of *Lactobacillus* [5] [6]. Thereafter, a set of screening procedures both *in vitro* and *vivo* was established for evaluation of cholesterol-reducing probiotics [7]. Many probiotic strains mostly *L. acidophilus* were screened out with cholesterol-reducing property [8].

A new study by Lye et al showed that there existed five possible probiotic mechanisms including assimilation of cholesterol during growth, binding of cholesterol to cellular surface, disruption of cholesterol micelle, deconjugation of bile salt and bile salt hydrolase (BSH) activity [9]. Now with the development of molecular biology, we can judge cholesterol-lowering effect firstly by detection of BSH gene and its expression in a probiotic genome. A recent study by Sridevi et al showed that *Lactobacillus buchneri* ATCC 4005 exhibited a great cholesterol-lowering property through an optimal condition of bile salt hydrolase production [10]. In conclusion from a meta-analysis, administration of probiotic can exect benefits on total cholesterol and LDL-cholesterol level of human [11].

There are some reports that fermented soy milk by probiotics also showed favorable function of regulating lipids level [12]. The advantages of fermented soy milk are that undesirable soybean oligosaccharides can be hydrolysed which provide nutritional components for probiotic and a large variety of peptides and amino acids are produced as well as active aglycon form of isoflavones [13]. An improved cholesterol profile was observed with daily intake of a probiotic soy product [14]. It seems possible that living probiotics and functional isoflavones cooperated in regulating lipid profile.

2. Antioxidant effect

Probiotic originated from longevity research by the well-known Eli Metchnikoff. As we all known, various published evidence suggested reduction of oxidative stress led to longevity-promoting consistent with Harman's Free Radical Theory of Aging [15]. These two observations inspired the investigation of antioxidant ability of probiotics.

Oxidative stress induced by obesity tend to produce surplus reactive oxygen species (ROS) which may cause further damage by free radical chain reaction mechanism [16]. ROS have some deleterious effects on polyunsaturated lipids in cell membrane leading to damage of cell structure and malondialdehyde (MDA), which was also toxic to DNA and protein and formed as a marker of lipid peroxidation at the same time [17] [18]. As for the oxidative stress, human body has its own antioxidant defense system including superoxide dismutase (SOD), catalase (CAT), glutathione peroxidase (GSH-Px) , glutathione (GSH) and so on [19]. Many *Lactobacillus* strains with antioxidative effects were not only reducing MDA level, but also enhance the antioxidants production (Table1).

Strains	Model	Antioxidant effects	Renferences
Probiotic yoghurt containing *Lactobacillus acidophilus* La5 and *Bifidobacterium lactis* Bb12	Type 2 diabetic patients	Serum MDA concentration significantly decreased	[20]
Probiotic yoghurt containing *Lactobacillus acidophilus* LA-5 and *Bifidobacterium* BB-12	Pregnant Women	Increased erythrocyte glutathione reductase levels, plasma glutathione and 8-oxo-7,8-dihydroguanine levels	[21]
Lactobacillus casei Zhang	High-fat fed rat	A decrease of MDA and increase of SOD and GSH-Px in serum and liver	[22]
Lactobacillus fermentum	pigs	Increased total antioxidant capacity, SOD and GSH-Px activity in serum as well as hepatic CAT and muscle SOD; Decreased MDA level in serum and muscle	[23]

Strains	Model	Antioxidant effects	Renferences
Probiotic yoghurt containing *Lactobacillus acidophilus* LA-5 and *Bifidobacterium* BB-12	human	An increase of SOD and catalase activity	[24]
Bacillus polyfermenticus	Rats with colon carcinoge-nesis	Lower plasma lipid peroxidation levels and higher plasma total antioxidant levels	[25]
Probiotic dahi containing *Lactobacillus acidophilus* and *Lactobacillus casei*	High fructose fed rats	Lower values of TBARS and higher values of glutathione in liver and pancreatic tissues	[26]
Lactobacillus fermentum ME-3	human	Enhanced total antioxidative status	[27]
Bacillus polyfermenticus SCD	High-Fat and cholestero-l fed rat	An increase in total radical trapping antioxidant potential (TRAP) and a decrease in conjugated dienes in plasma	[28]
Streptococcus thermophilus YIT 2001	Iron overloade-d mice	A significant decrease of lipid peroxide in the colonic mucosa	[29]
VSL#3	ob/ob mice	Lower fatty acid beta-oxidation	[30]
L. acidophilus	rats	Higher GSH-Px activity in red blood cells	[31]
L .rhamnosus SBT 2257	rats	Inhibition of hemolysis of red blood cell under the condition of vitamin E dificient	[32]

Table 1. Antioxidative effects of probiotics

3. Impact on lipoprotein

Lipoprotein transport play an important role in accumulation of host lipopolysaccharide level (LPS) [33]. Studies by Cani et al showed that elevated LPS level was considered as a trigger factor involved in the pathogenesis of obesity and metabolic risk via innate immune mechanism [34]. LPS-binding protein (LBP) and lipoproteins exert a synergistic effect on reducing the toxic LPS level[35].

Several fermented milk containing probiotics were demonstrated to reduce low-density lipoprotein cholesterol(LDL-c) level and very-low-density lipoprotein cholesterol (VLDL-c) in animal and human [26] [36] [37].Recently, *L. casei* Shirota had been proved a plasma LBP-lowering effect in obesity mice and *L. reuteri* NCIMB 30242 yoghurt could improve ApoB-100 level in hypercholesterolaemic subjects, suggesting that probiotic possess LPS-reducing function to delay the obesity risk [38] [39].

4. The whole microflora view

Intestinal microbes not only *Lactobacillus* could also exhibit a bile salt deconjugating effect [40], suggesting that other microbes had lipid-reducing potential. Thus, overall intestinal microflora was taken into account for lipid metabolism evaluation. In the past few years, research has focused on new areas of microflora and lipid metabolism with the development of culture-independent methods for understanding the total microbial diversity [41].

The human gut is consisting of a microbial community of 10^{14} bacteria with at least 1000 species and the whole microbiome is more than 100-fold the human genome [42].These researches highlight the significance of the whole gut microbiome contribute to energy harvest and the relationship between obesity and changes of gut microbiome [43]. More detailed, obese is mainly characterized by elevated *Firmicutes/Bacteroidetes* ratio in gut [44]. Probiotics serve as one of effective agents for regulation of gut microflora, they can exext benefits on lipid metabolism through downregulating the ratio of *Firmicutes/Bacteroidetes*. Other bacteria such as *Methanobrevibacter smithii* are also at low level in obese people [45]. Interestingly, atherosclerotic disease, which caused by accumulation of cholesterol and inflammation, was recently found its atherosclerotic plaque microbiota was associated with oral and gut microbiota through high throughput 454 pyrosequencing of 16S rRNA genes [46].

Besides, such a huge microflora provide a large reservoir of LPS molecules to circulation through colonizing of Gram-negative bacteria in the gut [47]. A recent study showed *Bifidobacteria* with genes encoding an ATP-binding-cassette-type carbohydrate transporter could protect against Gram-negative *E. coli* O157:H7 colonization in gut due to acetate production [48]. Thus, probiotic can restrict LPS-related microbial communities in the gut.

The whole gut microflora is also known as a target for drug metabolism because of diverse microbial transformations [49]. Manipulation of commensal microbial composition through antibiotics, probiotics or prebiotics was thought to enhance the metabolic activity and production of effective metabolites [50]. Simvastatin, which is an inhibitor of HMG-CoA and widely used for regulating hepatic cholesterol production, was proposed to possess altered pharmacological properties by microflora degradation via changing its capacity to bind to the corresponding receptors [51]. It is indicated that probiotics have potential to influence the metabolism of lipid-regulating drugs in gut.

5. Regulation of leptin, adiponectin and osteocalcin

Hormones such as leptin, adiponectin and osteocalcin play an important role in lipid metabolism. Obese population was characterized by significant lower levels of osteocalcin and adiponectin as well as high leptin level (leptin-resistant) which have been reported in literature. It is now increasingly accepted that leptin can regulate food intake and energy expenditure through hypothalamus and adiponectin can enhance tissue fat oxidation to downstream fatty acids levels and tissue triglyceride content associated with insulin sensitivity [52]. As for osteocalcin, leptin assumed to modulate osteocalcin bioactivity and osteocalcin could stimulate the adiponectin synthesis [53] [54].

5.1. Leptin

Leptin, an antiobesity hormone produced by adipose tissue, has been reported to regulate body weight by controlling food intake and energy expenditure [55]. However, obesity tend to display markedly higher serum leptin level with a leptin-resistant symptom. Several studies reported a decrease of leptin by probiotic administration. In high-fat fed mice, Lee et al confirmed that *Lactobacillus rhamnosus* PL60 exhibited a reduction in leptin level and anti-obesity effect due to production of conjugated linoleic acid [56]. Moreover, serum leptin concentration was reduced by *Lactobacillus gasseri* SBT205 in lean Zucker rats linked with lowered adipocyte size [57]. Another study also report leptin level was reduced by a combined bifidobacteria (*B. pseudocatenulatum* SPM 1204, *B. longum* SPM 1205, and *B. longum* SPM 1207) in obese rats [58]. Interestingly and controversially, direct injection of *Lactobacillus acidophilus* supernatants (germ free) into the brains of rats lead to weight loss with an increase in leptin expression in neurons and adipose tissue [59].

Leptin-lowering effect of probiotics was also observed in human. Similarly, Naruszewicz et al investigated whether oral administration of *L. plantarum* 299v exert beneficial effect on smokers by detection of cardiovascular risk factors [60]. In this study, smokers showed a great decrease in plasma leptin concentrations and anti-inflammatory properties when supplement of probiotic. Discouragingly, two months of *Lactobacillus acidophilus* and *Bifidobacterium longum* consumption failed to lower plasma leptin levels in male equol excretors [61].

5.2. Adiponectin

As an adipocyte-derived serum protein, adiponectin play an important role in glucose and lipid metabolism since adiponectin deficiency are associated with insulin resistance, inflammation, dyslipidemia and risk of atherogenic vascular disease [62]. In parallel, adiponectin has also been shown to suppress macrophage foam cell formation in atherosclerosis [63]. Several studies showed that probiotic therapy improved adiponectin level or adiponectin gene expression. One comparative research performed in normal microflora (NMF) and germ-free (GF) mice revealed that adiponectin gene expression (Adipoq) was up-regulated in the groups of *Lactobacillus*-treated germ free mice [64]. Moreover, Higurashi et al reported a probiotic cheese could prevent abdominal adipose accumulation and maintained serum adiponectin concentrations in high-calorie fed rats [65]. However, *Lactobacillus plantarum* strain No. 14 exert a white adipose-reducing effect in high-fat fed mice with no change of adiponectin [66].

Kadooka et al used a probiotic *L. gasseri* SBT2055 to regulate abdominal adiposity in obese adults, where the probiotic treatment involved a significant reduction in abdominal visceral and subcutaneous fat areas from baseline and significantly increased high-molecular weight adiponectin in their serum [67]. Furthermore, a recent large scale clinical study conducted by Luoto et al confirmed that pregnant women with a consumption of combined *Lactobacillus rhamnosus* GG and *Bifidobacterium lactis* probiotics possessed higher colostrum adiponectin concentration compared to placebo which was correlated inversely with maternal weight gain during pregnancy [68].

5.3. Osteocalcin

In recent years, osteocalcin secreted by osteoblasts has aroused great interest linked to β cell function, adiponectin production, energy expenditure and adiposity [69]. In humans, fat individuals kept a low level of serum osteocalcin [70]. The only study by Naughton et al showed that osteocalcin levels was slightly increased in middle aged rats by consumption of inulin-rich milk fermented by *Lactobacillus* GG and *Bifidobacterium lactis* [71]. It is interesting that osteocalcin is an vitamin K-dependent protein and two main types including vitamin K1 and vitamin K2 are respectively produced from dietary vegetable and microflora [72]. As an effective way to alter microflora, probiotics have potential to enhance vitamin K2 production and related osteocalcin level through changing the microflora.

6. Interaction with receptors

Various Receptors are involved in regulating important genes in lipid transport and metabolism and selected as potential therapeutic targets for dyslipidemia and atherosclerosis. Recent studies have focused on nuclear receptors (NRs), G protein-coupled receptor (GPRs) and Toll-like receptors (TLRs) as factors regulated by probiotics administration. But the crosstalk among NRs,TLRs and GPRs have not been clearly elucidated. The only investigation about crosstalk of NRs,TLRs and microflora between specific pathogen-free (SPF) mice and germ-free (GF) mice have revealed that LXR alpha, ROR gamma and CAR expression were reduced while TLR-2 and TLR-5 increased in SPF compared with GF mice [73].

6.1. Nuclear receptors

According to the stated above, some probiotics were found to be effective in reducing blood cholesterol level and one possible mechanism is enhanced fecal bile acids level. As one of important lipid mediators, bile acids have been confirmed to influence a series of NRs including farnesoid X receptor (FXR), pregnane-X-receptor (PXR), constitutive androstane receptor (CAR), peroxisome proliferator-activated receptor (PPAR), liver X receptor (LXR), glucocorticoid receptor(GR) and vitamin D receptor(VDR) [74-76].

Recently, *Lactobacillus acidophilus* ATCC 4356 could act as a liver X receptor (LXR) receptor agonist and inhibited the cellular uptake of micellar cholesterol in Caco-2 cells [77]. A similar study conducted with Yoon et al using a combination of *L. rhamnosus* BFE5264 and *L. plantarum* NR74 also showed a up-regulating the expression of LXR and promotion of cholesterol efflux in Caco-2 cells [78]. This is identical to effect of bile acid sequestrants drug which can also induce an increase of LXR activity in liver[79].

As we all known, PPARs play a key role in inflammation and blood glucose metabolism. Some studies have indicated that probiotic regulated the expression of PPARs in experimetal inflammatory model [80]. In fact, PPARs is also a target gene of energy homeostasis and adipogenesis [81]. Linked to ApoE gene transcription, PPAR-γ need LXR pathway for regulating adipocyte triglyceride balance [82]. Avella et al reported that dietary probiotics could modify the expression of PPAR-α, PPAR-β, VDR-α, RAR-γand GR in a marine fish, suggesting extensive crosstalk among NRs activated by probiotic [83]. Concerning about NRs and lipid metabolism linked with probiotic, Aronsson et al observed that *L. paracasei* F19 could reduce the fat storage associated with the drastic changes of PPARs [84]. One most recent study by Zhao et al have also demonstrated probiotic *Pediococcus pentosaceus* LP28 could also acted as a PPAR-γ agonist concomitantly with the great reduction of triglyceride and cholesterol in obese mice [85].

6.2. Toll-like receptors

As important pattern recognition receptors, TLRs participate in distinguishing and recognizing a range of microbial components such as peptidoglycan (TLR2) and LPS (TLR4) to activiate immune responses [86]. Up to date, the relationship between TLRs and lipid metabolism is mainly from two aspects. On one hand,TLRs signaling can directly contact and interfere with cholesterol metabolism in macrophages [87]. On the other hand, TLRs signaling (mainly TLR4) are involved in interaction LPS with fatty acid, lipoprotein and organ injury(especially liver and intestine). There is evidence that low dose of LPS can boost *de novo* fatty acid synthesis and lipolysis and lipoprotein production in liver which leading to hepatic hypertriglyceridemia [88]. In mice, moderately higher LPS level could be increased by a fat-enriched diet and contributed to low grade inflammation [34]. In rabbits, high cholesterol intake plus with low dose LPS accelerated the development of atherosclerosis [89]. These two studies are considered as the result of crosstalk between LPS and TLRs leads to intestinal mucosal injury associated with inflammatory response. Besides, foam cell formation in atherosclerosis has been shown to be mediated by TLR2 and 4 and other TLRs such as TLR3, 7, and 9 may also participate in atherosclerosis [90] [91].

TLR4 appears to be tightly linked to high-fat intake, LPS and inflammation. Probiotics are known to reduced LPS-containing gram-negative organisms (such as *E. coli*) in the gut and influx of LPS into circulation [92] [93]. A great number of probiotics are also able to specifically modulate the NF-κB pathway (one of most important inflammatory pathways)in intestinal epithelial cells and macrophages [94].

Due to TLR4 deficiency with anti-obesigenic effects and susceptible to colitis, little information about influence of probiotic on lipid metabolism is obtained in TLR4 knockout model whereas protective effect of probiotic VSL#3 from inflammation was observed in TLR4 knockout mice [95] [96]. With regard to the role of TLR4 in the development of metabolic disorders, Andreasen et al have considered that *L. acidophilus* NCFM may reduce overflow of LPS from the gut to the circulation and downregulate the TLR4 signalling and pro-inflammatory cytokines in human subjects [97].

Immunity homeostasis also have important effect on lipid metabolism. In general, it is well accepted that probiotic bacteria are able to maintain the Th1 and Th2 banlance of immunity through regulating pro-inflammatory and anti-inflammatory cytokines [98]. In addition, Agrawal et al documented that TLR2-derived signaling mainly enhance Th2-cytokine release, while TLR4 triggered by LPS stimulates Th1-type responses [99]. Interestingly,

Voltan et al found that *L. crispatus* M247 could increase TLR2 mRNA level and reduced TLR4 mRNA and protein levels in the colonic mucosa, suggesting that *L. crispatus* M247 maintain the Th1 / Th2 homeostasis through TLR2 / TLR4 banlance [100].

6.3. G protein-coupled receptors

It has been well-established that probiotic bacteria exert beneficial effects on the intestine especially the antimicrobial property by producing organic acids or regulating the organic acid-producing flora [93]. It has been also reported that GPR41 and GPR43 can be activated by short-chain fatty acids(SCFAs)[101]. Thus, it is possible that probiotic may affect GPRs through production of SCFAs in gut. However, this relationship among these have not yet been well-established. Study performed in Gpr41-deficient mice under germ free or conventional environment revealed that present of microflora was associated with harvest of short-chain fatty acids from the diet which control the degree of adiposity [102].

By our knowledge, only one study has investigated the effect of prebiotic which can specifically increase intestinal probiotic bifidobacteria on GPR43 expression through modified lipid profile [103]. Using a high-fat fed rodent model, the authors studied the effects of prebiotic on changes of microflora, adipose fatty acid profile and receptors expression. High fat diet is able to increase GPR43 and TLR4 expression as well as PPAR-γ expression due to oleic acid and α-linolenic acid production, while prebiotic decreases GPR43 and TLR4 overexpression.

7. New mechanisms exploration

In the past recent years, new mechanisms of probiotics on lipid metabolism were proposed. A research by Khedara et al showed lower nitric oxide level has been responsible for hyperlipidemia since endogenous nitric oxide can reduce fatty acid oxidation [104]. Some probiotics had ability to induce nitric oxide synthesis through activation of inducible nitric oxide synthase [105] [106]. Thus, modified NO availability by probiotics play an important role in lipid metabolism.

Moreover, Tanida et al demonstrated that *Lactobacillus paracasei* ST11 could increase adipose tissue lipolysis through enhancing the autonomic nerve activity [107]. In liver, probiotics also exhibited lipid-reducing effects [108]. Ma et al demostrated that VSL#3 probiotics could increase hepatic NKT cell numbers to attenuate high fat diet-induced steatosis [109]. Huang et al found that *L. acidophilus* 4356 could downregulate the Niemann-Pick C1-Like 1 (NPC1L1) level in the duodenum and jejunum of high-fat fed rats [110]. Another recent study by Aronsson et al revealed a new mechanism of *Lactobacillus paracasei* F19 to reduce fat storage by up-regulating levels of Angiopoietin-Like 4 Protein (ANGPTL4) in mice [84].

Omics technology provide a new insight into the mechanisms of lipid metabolism influenced by probiotics. Lee et al demostrated that gene ccpA (encodes catabolite control protein A) had function in cholesterol reduction in vivo by comparation of cholesterol-reducing strain *L. acidophilus* A4 and the BA9 mutant strain with no lipid-lowering effect

[111]. In addition, six main different expressed proteins involved in these two different strains *in vitro* were identified by proteomic analysis including transcription regulator, FMN-binding protein, major facilitator superfamily permease, glycogen phosphorylase, YknV protein, and fructose/tagatose bisphosphate aldolase.

Microarray analysis of probiotic *L. casei* Zhang effect on liver of high fat diet-fed rats revealed that *L. casei* Zhang administration promote the β-oxidation of fatty acid metabolism through up-regulating five genes expression (Acsl1, Hadh, Acaa2, Acads, and gcdH). Moreover, *L. casei* Zhang could strongly activate expression of glucocorticoid receptor (NR3C1 gene) which might be related to protect against high-fat induced low grade inflammation [112].

Recently, small intestinal proteomes in weanling piglets that respond differently to probiotic (*Lactobacillus fermentum* I5007) and antibiotic (Aureomycin) supplementation in terms of lipid metabolism have shown that probiotic enhanced mucosal SAR1B abundance could prevent weanling piglets from fat malabsorption. More importantly, high mucosal abundance of EIF4A and KRT10 in probiotic-treated piglets may contribute to improve overall gut integrity, suggesting a potential reduction of LPS influx [113].

8. Conclusion

In conclusion, probiotic is a better prevention and treatment strategy for regulating lipid homeostasis with the high prevalence of obesity, burden of amazing overweight and developing chronic diseases in the modern world. Despite the fact that people too pay attention to the thin result to neglect the drug side effect, probiotic can avoid this to achieve a healthy weight. Enhancing bile acids enflux and gut cholesterol assimilation was considered as the classic theory for cholesterol-reducing probiotics. Nevertheless, rencent studies focus on antioxidant activity and interaction with lipoprotein, hormones and the whole microbiota. Besides, crosstalk among NRs, GPRs and TLRs by probiotics is new frontiers for mechanical research. However, further investigations are needed to identify various responses related to lipid metabolism influenced by probiotics.

Author details

Yong Zhang and Heping Zhang
Key Laboratory of Dairy Biotechnology and Engineering, Education Ministry of P. R. China, Department of Food Science and Engineering, Inner Monglia Agricultural University, Hohhot, China

Acknowledgement

We thank professor Heping Zhang for revising this article. We also thank the members of the Laboratory in Department of Biological Science and Engineering directed by Yuzhen Wang at our university for useful advice on molecular biology.

9. References

[1] FAO/WHO. Guidelines for the evaluation of probiotics in food. Food and Agriculture Organization of the United Nations and World Health Organization Working Group Report.2002.http://www.fao.org/es/ESN/food/foodandfood_probio_en.stm (accessed 11 December 2011).

[2] Parvez S, Malik KA, Ah Kang S, Kim HY. Probiotics and their fermented food products are beneficial for health. Journal of Applied Microbiology 2006;100(6)1171-1185.

[3] Mann G V, Spoerry A. Studies of a surfactant and cholesteremia in the Maasai. American Journal of Clinical Nutrition 1974; 27(5) 464–469.

[4] Speck ML. Interactions among lactobacilli and man. Journal of Dairy Science 1976; 59(2)338-343.

[5] Gilliland SE and Speck ML. Deconjugation of bile acids by intestinal lactobacilli. Applied and Environmental Microbiology 1977;33(1)15-18.

[6] Gilliland SE, Nelson CR and Maxwell C. Assimilation of cholesterol by *Lactobacillus acidophilus*. Applied and Environmental Microbiology, 1985;49(2)377–381.

[7] Lin SY, Ayres JW, Winkler W, Sandine WE. *Lactobacillus* effects on cholesterol: in vitro and in vivo results. Journal of Dairy Research 1989;72(11)2885–2899.

[8] Ooi LG and Liong MT. Cholesterol-lowering effects of probiotics and prebiotics: a review of in vivo and in vitro findings. International Journal of Molecular Sciences 2010;11(6) 2499-2522.

[9] Lye HS, Rusul G, Liong MT. Mechanisms of Cholesterol Removal by Lactoballi Under Conditions That Mimic the Human Gastrointestinal Tract. International Dairy Journal 2010; 20(3)169–175.

[10] Sridevi N,Vishwe P, Prabhune A. Hypocholesteremic effect of bile salt hydrolase from *Lactobacillus buchneri* ATCC 4005. Food Research International 2009;42(4) 516-520.

[11] Guo Z, Liu XM, Zhang QX, Shen Z, Tian FW, Zhang H, Sun ZH, Zhang HP, Chen W. Influence of consumption of probiotics on the plasma lipid profile: A meta-analysis of randomised controlled trials. Nutrition, Metabolism & Cardiovascular Diseases 2011; 21(11)844-850.

[12] Izumi T, Piskula MK, Osawa S, Obata A, Tobe K, Saito M, Kataoka S, Kubota Y, Kikuchi M. Soy isoflavone aglycones are absorbed faster and in higher amounts than their glucosides in humans. Journal of Nutrition 2000;130(7)1695–1699.

[13] Buckley ND, Champagne CP, Masotti AI, et al. Green-Johnson Harnessing functional food strategies for the health challenges of space travel—Fermented soy for astronaut nutrition.Acta Astronautica 2011; 68(7–8) 731–738.

[14] Cavallini DC, Suzuki JY, Abdalla DS, Vendramini RC, Pauly-Silveira ND, Roselino MN, Pinto RA, Rossi EA. Influence of a probiotic soy product on fecal microbiota and its association with cardiovascular risk factors in an animal model. Lipids in Health and Disease. 2011 ;10:126.

[15] Andziak B, O'Connor TP, Qi W, DeWaal EM, Pierce A, Chaudhuri AR, Van Remmen H, Buffenstein R. High oxidative damage levels in the longest-living rodent, the naked mole-rat. Aging Cell 2006;5(6)463–471.

[16] Furukawa S, Fujita T, Shimabukuro M, Iwaki M, Yamada Y, Nakajima Y, Nakayama O, Makishima M, Matsuda M, Shimomura I. Increased oxidative stress in obesity and its impact on metabolic syndrome. Journal of Clinical Investigation 2004;114(12)1752-1761.

[17] Girotti A W. Lipid hydroperoxide generation, turnover, and effector action in biological systems. Journal of Lipid Research 1998; 39(8)1529-1542.

[18] Niedernhofer LJ, Daniels SJ, Rouzer CA, Greene RE, Marnett LJ. Malondialdehyde, a Product of Lipid Peroxidation, Is Mutagenic in Human Cells. Journal of Biological Chemistry 2003; 278(33) 31426-31433.

[19] Araujo FB, Barbosa DS, Hsin CY, Maranhão RC, Abdalla DS. Evaluation of oxidative stress in patients with hyperlipidemia. Atherosclerosis 1995; 117(1)61-71.

[20] Ejtahed HS, Mohtadi-Nia J, Homayouni-Rad A, et al. Probiotic yogurt improves antioxidant status in type 2 diabetic patients.Nutrition 2012;28(5) 539–543.

[21] Asemi Z, Jazayeri S, Najafi M, Samimi M, Mofid V, Shidfar F, Shakeri H, Esmaillzadeh A. Effect of daily consumption of probiotic yogurt on oxidative stress in pregnant women: a randomized controlled clinical trial. Annals of Nutrition and Metabolism 2012;60(1):62-68.

[22] Zhang Y, Du R, Wang L, Zhang H. The antioxidative effects of probiotic *Lactobacillus casei* Zhang on the hyperlipidemic rats. European Food Research and Technology 2010; 231(1)151-158.

[23] Wang AN,Yi XW, Yu HF, Dong B, Qiao SY. Free radical scavenging activity of *Lactobacillus fermentum* in vitro and its antioxidative effect on growing-finishing pigs. Journal of Applied Microbiology 2009; 107(4)1140-1148.

[24] Chamari M, Djazayery A, Jalali M. The effect of daily consumption of probiotic and conventional yoghurt on some oxidative stress factors in plasma of young healthy women. ARYA Atherosclerosis Journal 2008; 4(4) 175-179.

[25] Park E, Jeon GI, Park JS, Paik HD. A probiotic strain of *Bacillus polyfermenticus* reduces. DMH induced precancerous lesions in F344 male rat.Biological and Pharmaceutical Bulletin 2007;30(3)569-574.

[26] Yadav H, Jain S, Sinha PR. Antidiabetic effect of probiotic dahi containing *Lactobacillus acidophilus* and *Lactobacillus casei* in high fructose fed rats. Nutrition 2007;23(1):62-68.

[27] Songisepp E, Kals J, Kullisaar T, Mandar R, Hutt P, Zilmer M, Mikelsaar M. Evaluation of the functional efficacy of an antioxidative probiotic in healthy volunteers. Nutrition Journal 2005;4: 22–31.

[28] Paik HD, Park JS, Park E. Effects of *Bacillus polyfermenticus* SCD on lipid and antioxidant metabolisms in rats fed a high-fat and high-cholesterol diet.Biological and Pharmaceutical Bulletin 2005; 28(7) 1270-1274.

[29] Ito M, Ohishi K, Yoshida Y, Yokoi W, Sawada H. Antioxidative effects of lactic acid bacteria on the colonic mucosa of iron-overloaded mice. Journal of Agricultural and Food Chemistry 2003; 51 (15) 4456–4460.

[30] Li Z, Yang S, Lin H, Huang J, Watkins PA, Moser AB, Desimone C, Song XY, Diehl AM. Probiotics and antibodies to TNF inhibit inflammatory activity and improve nonalcoholic fatty liver disease. Hepatology 2003;37(2):343-350.

[31] Zommara M, Tachibana N, Sakono M, Suzuki Y, Oda T, Hashiba H, Imaizumi K. Whey from cultured skim milk decreases serum cholesterol and increases antioxidant enzymes in liver and red blood cells in rats. Nutrition Research 1996;16(2) 293–302.

[32] Kaizu H, Sasaki M, Nakajima H, Suzuki Y. Effect of antioxidative lactic acid bacteria on rats fed a diet deficient in vitamin E. Journal of Dairy Science 1993; 76(9) 2493-2499.

[33] Rauchhaus M, Coats AJ, Anker SD. The endotoxin-lipoprotein hypothesis. Lancet 2000; 356 (9247) 930–933.

[34] Cani PD, Amar J, Iglesias MA, Poggi M, Knauf C, Bastelica D, Neyrinck AM, Fava F, Tuohy KM, Chabo C, Waget A, Delmée E, Cousin B, Sulpice T, Chamontin B, Ferrières J, Tanti JF, Gibson GR, Casteilla L, Delzenne NM, Alessi MC, Burcelin R. Metabolic endotoxemia initiates obesity and insulin resistance.Diabetes 2007;56(7)1761-1772.

[35] Vreugdenhil AC, Snoek AM, van 't Veer C, Greve JW, Buurman WA. LPS-binding protein circulates in association with apoB-containing lipoproteins and enhances endotoxin-LDL/VLDL interaction. Journal of Clinical Investigation 2001;107(2)225–234.

[36] Abd El-Gawad IA, El-Sayed EM, Hafez SA, El-Zeini HM, Saleh FA.The hypocholesterolaemic effect of milkyoghurt and soy-yoghurt containing bifidobacteria in ratsfed on acholesterol-enriched diet. International Dairy Journal 2005; 15(1) 37-44.

[37] Xiao JZ, Kondo S, Takahashi N, Miyaji K, Oshida K, Hiramatsu A, Iwatsuki K, Kokubo S, Hosono A. Effects of milk products fermented by *Bifidobacterium longum* on blood lipids in rats and healthy adult male volunteers. Journal of Dairy Science 2003; 86(7) 2452-2461.

[38] Naito E, Yoshida Y, Makino K, Kounoshi Y, Kunihiro S, Takahashi R, Matsuzaki T, Miyazaki K, Ishikawa F. Beneficial effect of oral administration of *Lactobacillus casei* strain Shirota on insulin resistance in diet-induced obesity mice. Journal of Applied Microbiology 2011; 110(3)650-657.

[39] Jones ML, Martoni CJ, Parent M, Prakash S. Cholesterol-lowering efficacy of a microencapsulated bile salt hydrolase-active *Lactobacillus reuteri* NCIMB 30242 yoghurt formulation in hypercholesterolaemic adults. British Journal of Nutrition 2012;107(10) 1505-1513.

[40] Shimada K, Bricknell KS, Finegold SM. Deconjugation of bile acids by intestinal bacteria: review of literature and additional studies. Journal of Infectious Diseases 1969;119(3)273-281.

[41] Eckburg PB, Bik EM, Bernstein CN, et al. Diversity of the human intestinal microbial flora. Science 2005; 308(5728) 1635–1638.

[42] Qin J, Li R, Raes J, et al. A human gut microbial gene catalogue established by metagenomic sequencing. Nature 2010; 464(7285) 59–65.

[43] Turnbaugh PJ, Ley RE, Mahowald MA, Magrini V, Mardis ER, Gordon JI. An obesity-associated gut microbiome with increased capacity for energy harvest. Nature 2006; 444(7122) 1027–1031.

[44] Tilg H, Moschen AR, Kaser A. Obesity and the microbiota.Gastroenterology 2009;136(5)1476-1483.

[45] Million M, Maraninchi M, Henry M, Armougom F, Richet H, Carrieri P, Valero R, Raccah D, Vialettes B, Raoult D. Obesity-associated gut microbiota is enriched in

Lactobacillus reuteri and depleted in *Bifidobacterium animalis* and *Methanobrevibacter smithii*. International Journal of Obesity. 2011; In Press.

[46] Koren O, Spor A, Felin J, Fåk F, Stombaugh J, Tremaroli V, Behre CJ, Knight R, Fagerberg B, Ley RE, Bäckhed F. Human oral, gut, and plaque microbiota in patients with atherosclerosis. Proceedings of the National Academy of Sciences USA 2011;108(Suppl 1) 4592-4598.

[47] Ghoshal S, Witta J, Zhong J, de Villiers W, Eckhardt E. Chylomicrons promote intestinal absorption of lipopolysaccharides. Journal of Lipid Research 2009;50(1)90–97.

[48] Fukuda S, Toh H, Hase K, Oshima K, Nakanishi Y, Yoshimura K, Tobe T, Clarke JM, Topping DL, Suzuki T, Taylor TD, Itoh K, Kikuchi J, Morita H, Hattori M, Ohno H. *Bifidobacteria* can protect from enteropathogenic infection through production of acetate. Nature 2011;469 (7331) 543-547.

[49] Sousa T, Paterson R, Moore V, Carlsson A, Abrahamson B, Basit AW. The gastrointestinal microbiota as a site for the biotransformation of drugs. International Journal of Pharmaceutics 2008; 363(1-2) 1–25.

[50] Jia W, Li H, Zhao L, Nicholson J K. Gut microbiota: a potential new territory for drug targeting, Nature Reviews Drug Discovery 2008; 7, 123-131.

[51] Aura AM, Mattila I, Hyötyläinen T, Gopalacharyulu P, Bounsaythip C, Orešič M, Oksman-Caldentey KM.Drug metabolome of the Simvastatin formed by human intestinal microbiota in vitro. Molecular BioSystems 2011;7, 437-446

[52] Satoh N, Naruse M, Usui T, Tagami T, Suganami T, Yamada K, Kuzuya H, Shimatsu A, Ogawa Y. Leptin-to-adiponectin ratio as a potential atherogenic index in obese type 2 diabetic patients. Diabetes Care 2004;27(10)2488-2490.

[53] Gravenstein KS, Napora JK, Short RG, Ramachandran R, Carlson OD, Metter EJ, Ferrucci L, Egan JM, Chia CW. Cross-sectional evidence of a signaling pathway from bone homeostasis to glucose metabolism. Journal of Clinical Endocrinology & Metabolism 2011;96 (6)884-890.

[54] Bacchetta J, Boutroy S, Guebre-Egziabher F, Juillard L, Drai J, Pelletier S, Richard M, Charrié A, Carlier MC, Chapurlat R, Laville M, Fouque D. The relationship between adipokines, osteocalcin and bone quality in chronic kidney disease. Nephrology Dialysis Transplantation 2009;24(10)3120-3125.

[55] Friedman JM. The function of leptin in nutrition, weight, and physiology.Nutrition Reviews 2002; 60(10) 1-14.

[56] Lee HY, Park JH, Seok SH, Baek MW, Kim DJ, Lee KE, Paek KS, Lee YH,Park JH. Human originated bacteria, *Lactobacillus rhamnosus* PL60,produce conjugated linoleic acid and show anti-obesity effects in dietinduced obese mice. Biochimica et Biophysica Acta 2006; 1761(7)736-744.

[57] Hamad EM, Sato M, Uzu K, Yoshida T, Higashi S, Kawakami H, Kadooka Y, Matsuyama H, Abd El-Gawad IA, Imaizumi K. Milk fermented by *Lactobacillus gasseri* SBT2055 influences adipocyte size via inhibition of dietary fat absorption in Zucker rats. British Journal of Nutrition 2009;101(5)716-724.

[58] An HM, Park SY, Lee do K, Kim JR, Cha MK, Lee SW, Lim HT, Kim KJ, Ha NJ. Antiobesity and lipid-lowering effects of *Bifidobacterium* spp. in high fat diet-induced obese rats. Lipids in Health and Disease 2011;10:116.

[59] Sousa R, Halper J, Zhang J, Lewis SJ, Li WI. Effect of *Lactobacillus acidophilus* supernatants on body weight and leptin expression in rats. BMC Complementary and Alternative Medicine 2008;8:5.

[60] Naruszewicz M, Johansson ML, Zapolska-Downar D, Bukowska H.Effect of *Lactobacillus plantarum* 299v on cardiovascular disease risk factors in smokers. American Journal of Clinical Nutrition 2002;76(6)1249-1255.

[61] McMullen MH, Hamilton-Reeves JM, Bonorden MJ, Wangen KE, Phipps WR, Feirtag JM, Kurzer MS. Consumption of *Lactobacillus acidophilus* and *Bifidobacterium longum* does not alter phytoestrogen metabolism and plasma hormones in men: a pilot study. Journal of Alternative and Complementary Medicine 2006;12(9)887-894.

[62] Kadowaki T, & Yamauchi T. Adiponectin and adiponectin receptors. Endocrine Reviews,2005; 26(3) 439–451.

[63] Tian L, Luo N, Klein RL, Chung BH, Garvey WT, Fu Y. Adiponectin reduces lipid accumulation in macrophage foam cells.Atherosclerosis 2009;202(1) 152-161.

[64] Nerstedt A, Nilsson EC, Ohlson K, Håkansson J, Thomas Svensson L, Löwenadler B, Svensson UK, Mahlapuu M.Administration of *Lactobacillus* evokes coordinated changes in the intestinal expression profile of genes regulating energy homeostasis and immune phenotype in mice. British Journal of Nutrition 2007; 97(6)1117-1127.

[65] Higurashi S, Kunieda Y, Matsuyama H, Kawakami H. Effect of cheese consumption on the accumulation of abdominal adipose and decrease in serum adiponectin levels in rats fed a calorie dense diet.International Dairy Journal 2007;17(10) 1224–1231.

[66] Takemura N, Okubo T, Sonoyama K. *Lactobacillus plantarum* strain No. 14 reduces adipocyte size in mice fed high-fat diet. Experimental Biology and Medicine 2010;235(7) 849-856

[67] Kadooka Y, Sato M, Imaizumi K, Ogawa A, Ikuyama K, Akai Y, Okano M, Kagoshima M, Tsuchida T.Regulation of abdominal adiposity by probiotics (*Lactobacillus gasseri* SBT2055) in adults with obese tendencies in a randomized controlled trial. European Journal of Clinical Nutrition 2010; 64(6)636-643.

[68] Luoto R, Laitinen K, Nermes M, Isolauri E.Impact of maternal probiotic-supplemented dietary counseling during pregnancy on colostrum adiponectin concentration: A prospective, randomized, placebo-controlled study.Early Human Development 2012;88(6) 339–344.

[69] Fukumoto S, Martin TJ.Bone as an endocrine organ. Trends in Endocrinology & Metabolism. 2009;20(5)230-236.

[70] Holecki M, Zahorska-Markiewicz B, Janowska J, Nieszporek T, Wojaczyńska-Stanek K, Zak-Gołab A, Wiecek A. The influence of weight loss on serum osteoprotegerin concentration in obese perimenopausal women. Obesity 2007; 15 (8)1925–1929.

[71] Naughton V, McSorley E, Naughton PJ.Changes in calcium status in aged rats fed *Lactobacillus* GG and *Bifidobacterium lactis* and oligofructose-enriched inulin. Applied Physiology, Nutrition and Metabolism. 2011;36(1) 161-165.

[72] Merli GJ, Fink J. Vitamin K and thrombosis. Vitamins & Hormones 2008;78:265-279.

[73] Lundin A, Bok CM, Aronsson L, Björkholm B, Gustafsson JA, Pott S, Arulampalam V, Hibberd M, Rafter J, Pettersson S. Gut flora, Toll-like receptors and nuclear receptors: a tripartite communication that tunes innate immunity in large intestine. Cellular Microbiology 2008;10(5) 1093-1103.

[74] Vavassori P, Mencarelli A, Renga B, Distrutti E, Fiorucci S. The bile acid receptor FXR is a modulator of intestinal innate immunity. Journal of Immunology 2009;183(10) 6251-6261.

[75] Fiorucci S, Cipriani S, Baldelli F, Mencarelli A.Bile acid-activated receptors in the treatment of dyslipidemia and related disorders. Progress in Lipid Research 2010;49(2) 171-185.

[76] Rose AJ, Díaz MB, Reimann A, Klement J, Walcher T, Krones-Herzig A, Strobel O, Werner J, Peters A, Kleyman A, Tuckermann JP, Vegiopoulos A, Herzig S. Molecular control of systemic bile acid homeostasis by the liver glucocorticoid receptor. Cell Metabolism 2011; 14(1) 123-130.

[77] Huang Y, Zheng Y.The probiotic *Lactobacillus acidophilus* reduces cholesterol absorption through the down-regulation of Niemann-Pick C1-like 1 in Caco-2 cells. British Journal of Nutrition 2010; 103(4)473-478.

[78] Yoon H, Ju J, Kim H, Lee J, Park H, Ji Y, Shin H, Do MS, Lee J and Holzapfel W. *Lactobacillus rhamnosus* BFE 5264 and *Lactobacillus plantarum* NR74 Promote Cholesterol Excretion Through the Up-Regulation of ABCG5/8 in Caco-2 Cells. Probiotics and Antimicrobial Proteins 2011;3(3-4)194-203.

[79] Brendel C, Schoonjans K, Botrugno OA, Treuter E, Auwerx J. The small heterodimer partner interacts with the liver X receptor alpha and represses its transcriptional activity. Molecular Endocrinology 2002; 16(9) 2065-2076.

[80] Marion-Letellier R, Déchelotte P, Iacucci M, Ghosh S.Dietary modulation of peroxisome proliferator-activated receptor gamma. Gut 2009;58(4) 586-593.

[81] Ahmed W, Ziouzenkova O, Brown J, Devchand P, Francis S, Kadakia M, Kanda T, Orasanu G, Sharlach M, Zandbergen F, Plutzky J. PPARs and their metabolic modulation: new mechanisms for transcriptional regulation? Journal of Internal Medicine 2007;262(2) 184–198.

[82] Yue L, Mazzone T.Peroxisome proliferator-activated receptor-gamma stimulation of adipocyte ApoE gene transcription mediated by the liver receptor X pathway. Journal of Biological Chemistry 2009; 284(16) 10453-10461.

[83] Avella MA, Olivotto I, Silvi S, Place AR, Carnevali O.Effect of dietary probiotics on clownfish: a molecular approach to define how lactic acid bacteria modulate development in a marine fish. American Journal of Physiology-Regulatory, Integrative, and Comparative Physiology 2010;298(2) 359-371.

[84] Aronsson L, Huang Y, Parini P, Korach-André M, Håkansson J, Gustafsson JÅ, Pettersson S, Arulampalam V, Rafter J. Decreased fat storage by *Lactobacillus paracasei* is associated with increased levels of angiopoietin-like 4 protein (ANGPTL4). PLoS One 2010; 5(9): e13087.

[85] Zhao X, Higashikawa F, Noda M, Kawamura Y, Matoba Y, Kumagai T, Sugiyama M(2012) The Obesity and Fatty Liver Are Reduced by Plant-Derived *Pediococcus pentosaceus* LP28 in High Fat Diet-Induced Obese Mice. PLoS One 2012;7:e30696

[86] Takeda K, Kaisho T, Akira S. Toll-like receptors. Annual Review of Immunology. 2003;21:335-376.

[87] Castrillo A, Joseph SB, Vaidya SA, Haberland M, Fogelman AM, Cheng G, Tontonoz P. Crosstalk between LXR and Toll-like receptor signaling mediates bacterial and viral antagonism of cholesterol metabolism. Molecular Cell 2003;12(4)805-816.

[88] Feingold KR, Staprans I, Memon RA, Moser AH, Shigenaga JK, Doerrler W, Dinarello CA, Grunfeld C. Endotoxin rapidly induces changes in lipid metabolism that produce hypertriglyceridemia: low doses stimulate hepatic triglyceride production while high doses inhibit clearance. Journal of Lipid Research 1992;33(12)1765-1776.

[89] Lehr HA, Sagban TA, Ihling C, Zähringer U, Hungerer KD, Blumrich M, Reifenberg K, Bhakdi S. Immunopathogenesis of atherosclerosis: endotoxin accelerates atherosclerosis in rabbits on hypercholesterolemic diet. Circulation 2001;104(8) 914-920.

[90] Michelsen KS, Doherty TM, Shah PK, Arditi M. TLR signaling: an emerging bridge from innate immunity to atherogenesis. Journal of Immunology 2004;173(10) 5901-5907.

[91] Curtiss LK, Tobias PS. Emerging role of Toll-like receptors in atherosclerosis. Journal of Lipid Research 2009;50 Suppl 340-345.

[92] Griffiths EA, Duffy LC, Schanbacher FL, Qiao H, Dryja D, Leavens A, Rossman J, Rich G, Dirienzo D, Ogra PL. In vivo effects of bifidobacteria and lactoferrin on gut endotoxin concentration and mucosal immunity in Balb/c mice. Digestive Diseases and Sciences 2004;49(4)579–589.

[93] Gareau MG, Sherman PM, Walker WA. Probiotics and the gut microbiota in intestinal health and disease. Nature Reviews Gastroenterology & Hepatology 2010;7(9)503-514.

[94] Thomas CM, Versalovic J. Probiotics-host communication: Modulation of signaling pathways in the intestine. Gut Microbes 2010;1(3) 148-163.

[95] Davis JE, Gabler NK, Walker-Daniels J, Spurlock ME.Tlr-4 deficiency selectively protects against obesity induced by diets high in saturated fat. Obesity 2008;16(6)1248-1255.

[96] Lee J, Mo JH, Katakura K, Alkalay I, Rucker AN, Liu YT, Lee HK, Shen C, Cojocaru G, Shenouda S, Kagnoff M, Eckmann L, Ben-Neriah Y, Raz E. Maintenance of colonic homeostasis by distinctive apical TLR9 signalling in intestinal epithelial cells. Nature Cell Biology 2006; 8(12) 1327-1336.

[97] Andreasen AS, Larsen N, Pedersen-Skovsgaard T, Berg RM, Møller K, Svendsen KD, Jakobsen M, Pedersen BK.Effects of *Lactobacillus acidophilus* NCFM on insulin sensitivity and the systemic inflammatory response in human subjects. British Journal of Nutrition. 2010;104(12) 1831-1838.

[98] Delcenserie V, Martel D, Lamoureux M, Amiot J, Boutin Y, Roy D.Immunomodulatory effects of probiotics in the intestinal tract. Current Issues in Molecular Biology 2008;10(1-2) 37-54.

[99] Agrawal S, Agrawal A, Doughty B, Gerwitz A, Blenis J, Van Dyke T, Pulendran B. Cutting edge: different Toll-like receptors agonist instruct dendritic cells to induce

distinct Th responses via different modulation of extracellular signal-regulated kinase-mitogen-activated protein kinase and c-Fos. Journal of Immunology 2003; 171(10)4984–4989.

[100] Voltan S, Castagliuolo I, Elli M, Longo S, Brun P, D'Incà R, Porzionato A, Macchi V, Palù G, Sturniolo GC, Morelli L, Martines D. Aggregating Phenotype in Lactobacillus crispatus Determines Intestinal Colonization and TLR2 and TLR4 Modulation in Murine Colonic Mucosa. Clinical and Vaccine Immunology 2007; 14(9) 1138–1148.

[101] Brown AJ, Goldsworthy SM, Barnes AA, Eilert MM, Tcheang L, Daniels D, Muir AI, Wigglesworth MJ, Kinghorn I, Fraser NJ, Pike NB, Strum JC, Steplewski KM, Murdock PR, Holder JC, Marshall FH, Szekeres PG, Wilson S, Ignar DM, Foord SM, Wise A, Dowell SJ. The Orphan G protein-coupled receptors GPR41 and GPR43 are activated by propionate and other short chain carboxylic acids. Journal of Biological Chemistry 2003;278(13) 11312-11319.

[102] Samuel BS, Shaito A, Motoike T, Rey FE, Backhed F, Manchester JK, Hammer RE, Williams SC, Crowley J, Yanagisawa M, Gordon JI.Effects of the gut microbiota on host adiposity are modulated by the short-chain fatty-acid binding G protein-coupled receptor, Gpr41. Proceedings of the National Academy of Sciences U S A. 2008; 105(43) 16767–16772.

[103] Dewulf EM, Cani PD, Neyrinck AM, Possemiers S, Van Holle A, Muccioli GG, Deldicque L, Bindels LB, Pachikian BD, Sohet FM, Mignolet E, Francaux M, Larondelle Y, Delzenne NM.Inulin-type fructans with prebiotic properties counteract GPR43 overexpression and PPARγ-related adipogenesis in the white adipose tissue of high-fat diet-fed mice. Journal of Nutritional Biochemistry 2011;22(8)712-722.

[104] Khedara A, KawaI Y, Kayashita J, Kato N. Feeding rats the nitric oxide synthase inhibitor, l-nxnitroarginine, elevates serum triglyceride and cholesterol and lowers hepatic fatty acid oxidation. Journal of Nutrition 1996;126(10)2563–2567.

[105] Korhonen R, Korpela R, Saxelin M, Mäki M, Kankaanranta H, Moilanen E. Induction of nitric oxide synthesis by probiotic *Lactobacillus rhamnosus* GG in J774 macrophages and human T84 intestinal epithelial cells. Inflammation 2001;25(4)223-232.

[106] Ulisse S, Gionchetti P, D'Alò S, Russo FP, Pesce I, Ricci G, Rizzello F, Helwig U, Cifone MG, Campieri M, De Simone C. Expression of cytokines, inducible nitric oxide synthase, and matrix metalloproteinases in pouchitis: effects of probiotic treatment. American Journal of Gastroenterology 2001; 96(9)2691-2699.

[107] Tanida M, Shen J, Maeda K, Horii Y, Yamano T, Fukushima Y, Nagai K.High-fat diet-induced obesity is attenuated by probiotic strain *Lactobacillus paracasei* ST11 (NCC2461) in rats. Obesity Research & Clinical Practice 2008; 2(3) 159-169.

[108] Fukushima M,Yamada A, Endo T, Nakano M. Effects of a mixture of organisms, *Lactobacillus acidophilus* or *Streptococcus faecalis* on delta6-desaturase activity in the livers of rats fed a fat- and cholesterol-enriched diet. Nutrients 1999; 15(5)373-378.

[109] Ma X, Hua J, Li Z. Probiotics improve high fat diet-induced hepatic steatosis and insulin resistance by increasing hepatic NKT cells. Journal of Hepatology 2008; 49(5)821-830.

[110] Huang Y, Wang J, Cheng Y, Zheng Y.The hypocholesterolaemic effects of *Lactobacillus acidophilus* American type culture collection 4356 in rats are mediated by the down-regulation of Niemann-Pick C1-like 1. British Journal of Nutrition 2010;104(6)807-812.
[111] Lee J,Kim Y,Yun HS, Kim JG,Oh S, Kim SH. Genetic and proteomic analysis of factors affecting serum cholesterol reduction by *Lactobacillus acidophilus* A4. Applied and Environmental Microbiology 2010; 76(14) 4829-4835.
[112] Zhong Z, Zhang W, Du R, Meng H, Zhang H. Effect of *Lactobacillus casei* Zhang on global gene expression in the liver of hypercholesterolemic rats. European Journal of Lipid Science and Technology 2012; 114(3) 244-252.
[113] Wang X, Yang F, Liu C, Zhou H, Wu G, Qiao S, Li D, Wang J.Dietary supplementation with the probiotic *Lactobacillus fermentum* I5007 and the antibiotic aureomycin differentially affects the small intestinal proteomes of weanling piglets. Journal of Nutrition 2012; 142(1) 7-13.